INTRODUCTION TO BIOMEDICAL EQUIPMENT TECHNOLOGY

INTRODUCTION TO BIOMEDICAL EQUIPMENT TECHNOLOGY

FOURTH EDITION

JOSEPH J. CARR

JOHN M. BROWN

Prentice
Hall

Upper Saddle River, New Jersey
Columbus, Ohio

Library of Congress Cataloging-in-Publication Data
Carr, Joseph J.
  Introduction to biomedical equipment technology / Joseph J. Carr.
John M. Brown.—4th ed.
    p.;   cm.
  Inclues bibliographical references and index.
  ISBN 0-13-010492-2
  1. Medical instruments and apparatus.   I. Brown, John M. (John
Michael), 1944-.   II. Title.
DNLM: 1. Equipment and Supplies. 2. Biomedical Engineering—instrumentation. 3.
Electronics, Medical—instrumentation. WB26C3lli2000
R856.C33 2000
610′.28—dc21

                                                                    00-038505

Vice President and Publisher: Dave Garza
Editor in Chief: Stephen Helba
Assistant Vice President and Publisher: Charles E. Stewart, Jr.
Production Editor: Alexandrina Benedicto Wolf
Production Coordinator: Clarinda Publication Services
Design Coordinator: Robin G. Chukes
Cover Designer: Linda Fares
Cover Image: Index Stock
Production Manager: Matthew Ottenweller
Marketing Manager: Barbara Rose

This book was set in Times Roman by The Clarinda Company. It was printed and bound by R. R. Donnelley & Sons Company. The cover was printed by Phoenix Color Corp.

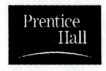

Prentice Hall

PREFACE

This textbook is the fourth edition of a premier book used to educate biomedical and other technical professionals over the last two decades. Since technology advances at an ever-increasing pace, we have included some new and exciting changes, which reflect the modern world of medical instrumentation.

Part of the revision effort was a survey of instructors, successful students, managers, and clinical and biomedical engineers and technicians who ultimately employ the readers of this book. New features were added mostly in response to comments and request of the academic reader.

Since this text is broadly organized, working professionals in biomedical electronics and related fields will find it useful for looking up topics of interest and refreshing selected areas, while bypassing more familiar material. In addition, engineers and technologists, who design biomedical equipment, can easily revisit material covering the broad overview or delve into the critical points of pertinent subjects.

Important chapters added to the third edition and retained in this latest edition include information fundamental to a basic education. Chapter 3 is "Introduction to Biomedical Equipment Instru-

mentation and Measurement." Chapter 4 covers the "Basic Theories of Measurement" technology. Chapter 22 discusses "Computers in Biomedical Equipment," which, among other topics, includes sections on microprocessors and signal acquisition systems, as applied to medical and laboratory instrumentation. This is directed at signal measurement, analog signal processing, analog-to-digital conversion, digital-to-analog conversion, and digital signal processing. These chapters were added to reinforce the concept that many medical instruments are basically electronic measuring devices. The authors believe students need to put into action concepts of accuracy and precision when diagnosing problems and maintaining medical and laboratory equipment. Basic theory of signals and noise provides a necessary background for understanding commonly encountered signals and what to expect from observing them in analog, digital or software form, in addition to windows pull-down menus. In this way, the authors share their savvy with the reader, which has been formulated from theory and years of personal experience. Also, some of the original chapters were enhanced to better cover essential topics, such as the nature and impact of the Internet in medicine and the use of computers in analyzing medical signals, X-ray films, and patient records. In addition, we have extended many block and circuit diagrams with descriptions to improve the reader's working knowledge of biomedical equipment.

In the fourth edition, chapter 24 on "Electromagnetic Interference to Medical Electronic Equipment," including electromagnetic compatibility has been improved, because this is a major issue today, especially with the FDA. In concert, a new chapter 25 is provided on "Quality Assurance and Continuous Quality Improvement" for two reasons: First, most medical equipment manufacturers must meet ISO-9000 quality assurance standards to sell their equipment in Europe and, increasingly, also in the United States and Canada. Adherence to the recommendations of ISO-9000 may also prove beneficial in defending product liability challenges, because it reflects a manufacturer's ability to set up and consistently apply company and production procedures. Second, hospitals are being forced to provide continuous quality improvement by accreditation authorities, such as the FDA, and their ability to meet these requirements facilitates their competitive edge in the medical marketplace. In addition, chapter 16, "Medical Laboratory Instrumentation," now includes a section on hemodialysis machines to treat kidney failure, because of the increasing requirement for this technology from our aging population. Also, a description of the important Y2K problem now appears in chapter 22, "Computers in Biomedical Equipment," as well as a description of new computer devices in medicine, such as the extended interactive computer system and the palmtop or personal digital assistant (PDA).

We appreciate the cooperation of the Burr-Brown Corp. in providing circuit diagrams. Burr-Brown does not authorize or warrant any Burr-Brown prdouct for use in life support devices and/or systems.

Again, we thank our families for their continuing encouragement in the researching and writing of this latest edition.

Joseph J. Carr, MSEE
Falls Church, VA

John M. Brown,
MSEE, DEng
Tucson, AZ

CONTENTS

INTRODUCTION TO BIOMEDICAL EQUIPMENT TECHNOLOGY

CHAPTER 1
The Human Body: An Overview

1-1 Objectives

1. Be able to list the major systems of the body.
2. Know how to describe the principal functions of body systems.
3. Be able to describe how the body controls and regulates itself.
4. Be able to state the relationships among body systems.

1-2 Self-evaluation questions

These questions test your prior knowledge of the material in this chapter. Look for the answers as you read the text. After you have finished studying the chapter, try answering these questions and those at the end of the chapter.

1. Two fluid transport systems in the body are the _____ system and the _____ system.

2. Define *homeostasis* in your own words.

3. List the principal organs in the gastrointestinal (GI) system.

4. Roughly sketch the blood circulatory system.

5. List the principal systems in the body.

1-3 Introduction

The purpose of this chapter is to make you broadly aware of the structure of the human body, but not in such detail as you would find in anatomy and physiology courses. More detailed information on each system is given in later chapters of this book. Students wishing to attempt independent study should consult a college-level textbook on physiology.

In this chapter we discuss the major systems of the body and how they work together to produce an essentially self-regulating machine. The body contains literally hundreds of feedback control systems that attempt to keep the body's internal environment constant. This process is called homeostasis, and it allows the body to respond to changes in the environment and to illness, as well as to accomplish the regulation of levels of sugar, salt, water, acid-base balance, oxygen, carbon dioxide, and the other materials that make up the living organism.

1-4 The cell

All mammals, including humans, are made up of basic building blocks called *cells*. Although many different types of cells are known, they differ according to function, but they are all similar in their basic constituents. The different types of cells perform different jobs and so have different gross structures. Figure 1-1 shows several types of human and mammalian cells.

The size of cells also varies, ranging from 200 nm (1 nm $= 10^{-9}$ m) to several centimeters

in length. Most cells, however, fall within the range of 0.5 to 20 μm (1 μm $= 10^{-6}$ m). An ostrich egg is a single cell that may reach 20 cm in length.

The cell contains material that is used in chemical reactions that keep the cell functioning. The cell is surrounded by a *semipermeable membrane*. This membrane not only contains the substance of the cell but also allows selective passage of materials in and out of the cell. There may also be membrane structures inside the cell that compartmentalize the various chemical reactions taking place.

The structure of most cells includes a *nucleus* inside of the cell, separated from the surrounding *cytoplasm* by its own membrane. The nucleus contains the genetic coding of reproducible cells.

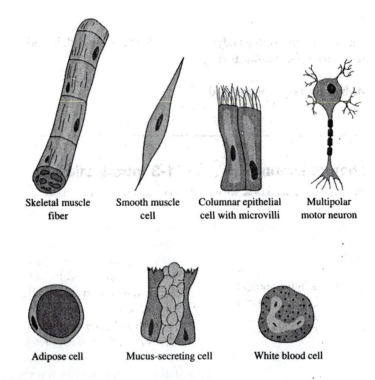

Skeletal muscle fiber   Smooth muscle cell   Columnar epithelial cell with microvilli   Multipolar motor neuron

Adipose cell   Mucus-secreting cell   White blood cell

Figure 1-1
Diverse forms of mammalian cells (not to the same scale). (From *Human Anatomy and Physiology*, 2nd edition, by James E. Crouch, Ph.D. and J. Robert McClintic, Ph.D. John Wiley & Sons, New York, 1976. Used by permission.)

Cells in the human body are quite numerous. It has been estimated that there are approximately 75 trillion cells in the body, of which one-third (25 trillion) are red blood cells. The red blood cells transport oxygen to body tissues.

All cells in a many-celled animal retain certain powers or characteristics, such as organization, irritability (i.e., response to external stimuli), nutrition, metabolism, respiration, and excretion. Some cells also possess the power of *reproduction*. All cells arise from preexisting cells through a process of cell division. In the process called *mitosis*, there is a nonexact quantitative division of cell cytoplasm and an exact qualitative division of the nucleus material.

1-5 Body fluids

The body is almost two-thirds fluid (actually, approximately 56%). Intracellular fluid contains large concentrations of potassium, magnesium, and phosphate ions; extracellular fluid contains significant concentrations of sodium, chloride, bicarbonate ions, oxygen, amino acids, fatty acids, glucose, and carbon dioxide.

1-6 Musculoskeletal system

The muscles and bones of the body provide *locomotion* (i.e., the ability to move around and manipulate our surroundings). If it were not for locomotion, humans would be more dependent on the local environment. Humans would not be able to move to avoid danger, find food and water, or erect shelter from the elements.

Figure 1-2 shows the principal structures of the musculoskeletal system. The skeletal system (Figure 1-2a) consists mostly of *bones* and some *cartilage*. The bones are joined together to form *articulations* and *joints* and so are able to move with respect to each other. In general, muscles (Figure 1-2b) are connected between bones across a joint, so that the bones move with respect to each other when the muscle contracts.

1-7 Respiratory system

The respiratory system takes oxygen into the body and gives off carbon dioxide waste products from the cells. The respiratory system includes the mouth; nose; trachea, or windpipe; bronchii; and lungs. Deoxygenated blood from the right side of the heart passes through the lungs: only 0.4 to 2.0 μm of membrane separates the air-carrying *alveoli* from the pulmonary *capillaries* (i.e., tiny blood vessels). Gaseous oxygen diffuses across this membrane into the blood-stream, while carbon dioxide comes out of the blood, into the alveoli, to be exhaled into the atmosphere.

1-8 Gastrointestinal system

The GI system takes in raw materials in the form of food and liquids and processes them so that they are absorbed into the body. Certain digestive organs are needed to chemically and physically process these raw materials: the liver, gall bladder, salivary glands, pancreas, stomach, and intestinal tract. The system includes the mouth, esophagus, stomach, small intestine, and large intestine.

Digestion of food is the process of breaking down, liquefying, and chemically processing foodstuffs so that they can be used by the body. The process of digestion begins in the mouth, where the teeth and jaw mechanically break down the food material, and the saliva begins the chemical breakdown.

Both mechanical mixing and chemical breakdown occur in the stomach. Gastric juices mix with the food material to form a milky paste called *chyme*. Contractions, called *peristaltic waves*, in the stomach mix the foodstuffs together with the juices. These waves occur approximately every 20 seconds. These waves can reach magnitudes of 50 to 70 cm H_2O. Every contraction will cause a few milliliters of stomach contents to enter the intestine.

Nutrients and fluid are absorbed by the body from the chyme as it moves through the intestine. The chyme is propelled at a rate of approximately 1 cm/min by weak peristaltic waves in the intestine.

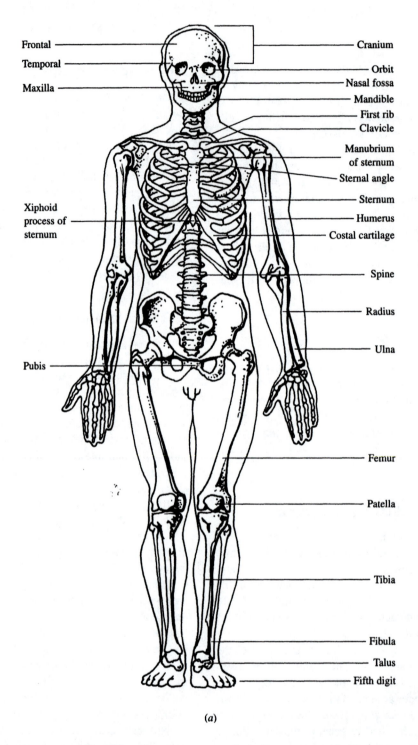

Frontal — Cranium
Temporal — Orbit
Maxilla — Nasal fossa
— Mandible
— First rib
— Clavicle
Manubrium of sternum
Sternal angle
— Sternum
Xiphoid process of sternum — Humerus
Costal cartilage
— Spine
— Radius
— Ulna
Pubis —
— Femur
— Patella
— Tibia
— Fibula
— Talus
— Fifth digit

(*a*)

Figure 1-2a
The human skeleton. (From *Human Anatomy and Physiology*, 2nd edition, by James E. Crouch, Ph.D. and J. Robert McClintic, Ph.D. John Wiley & Sons, New York, 1976. Used by permission.)

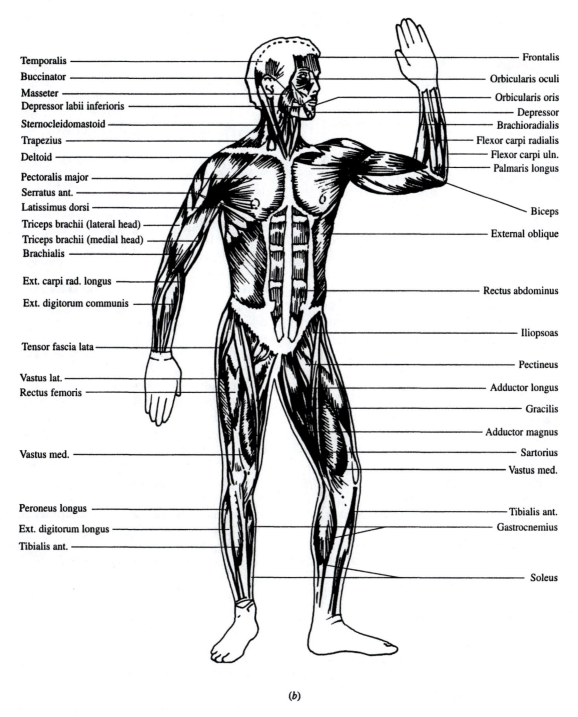

Temporalis

Buccinator

Masseter

Depressor labii inferioris

Sternocleidomastoid

Trapezius

Deltoid

Pectoralis major

Serratus ant.

Latissimus dorsi

Triceps brachii (lateral head)

Triceps brachii (medial head)

Brachialis

Ext. carpi rad. longus

Ext. digitorum communis

Tensor fascia lata

Vastus lat.

Rectus femoris

Vastus med.

Peroneus longus

Ext. digitorum longus

Tibialis ant.

Frontalis

Orbicularis oculi

Orbicularis oris

Depressor

Brachioradialis

Flexor carpi radialis

Flexor carpi uln.

Palmaris longus

Biceps

External oblique

Rectus abdominus

Iliopsoas

Pectineus

Adductor longus

Gracilis

Adductor magnus

Sartorius

Vastus med.

Tibialis ant.

Gastrocnemius

Soleus

(b)

Figure 1-2b
Muscular system. (From *Human Anatomy and Physiology*, 2nd edition, by James E. Crouch,
Ph.D. and J. Robert McClintic, Ph.D. John Wiley & Sons, New York, 1976. Used by permission.)

Waste products and undigested foodstuffs are expelled from the body in the form of fecal material from the anus.

1-9 Nervous system

The nervous system is essential to the functioning of the human organism. It regulates our automatic control systems, integrates and assimilates data from the outside world and our internal organs, and regulates and controls the locomotor system. It has been compared to a computer with an electrical communications system.

The *autonomic nervous system* is responsible for regulating the automatic functions of the body—heartbeat, gland secretions, GI system, and so forth. The autonomic nervous system operates at a subconscious level—you are not generally aware of its functioning.

The *sensory nervous system* receives data from the outside world and certain internal organs through cells that function as sensory receptors (i.e., transducers, in electrical terminology). The eyes and ears are sensory receptors for light and sound, respectively. But there are also other sensory structures that are sensitive to pain, heat, and pressure.

The *central nervous system* (CNS) gathers, assimilates, and integrates data from the outside world, information on the state of internal organs, etc. The brain is the principal organ of the CNS, and, like a computer, it can store, process, and generate information and react to stimuli. The CNS also includes the spinal cord.

1-10 Endocrine system

Whereas the CNS is an electrical communications and control system within the body, the endocrine system is a *chemical* communications/control system and aids in the regulation of internal body states.

Chemicals called *hormones* are secreted by the eight major endocrine glands into the bloodstream, in which they act as control agents to regulate various organic functions.

In general, the endocrine system controls slow-acting phenomena, mainly metabolic functions, while the CNS regulates fast-acting phenomena.

1-11 The circulatory system

The circulatory system transports body fluids around the body from one organ to another. Although the *blood* circulatory system is the most well known, there is also a *lymph* transport system within the body.

Figure 1-3 shows a schematic representation of the blood circulatory system. The transport of blood is caused by a pressure built up when the heart, a pump, contracts. Oxygenated blood from the left ventricle is pumped throughout the body, delivering oxygen to the various organs and tissues. It is claimed that the human blood circulatory system is so extensive that no cell in the body is farther than one cell's diameter (Section 1-4) from a small vessel, or capillary.

The oxygenated blood flows in *arteries* to the organs. The blood flowing into the vessels of the GI tract picks up nutrients and water. The portion of the blood that flows into the kidneys is cleaned of impurities and waste products, which are excreted through the bladder and urethra. The kidneys act as a blood *filter*. The blood gives up much of its oxygen to the tissues, and the deoxygenated blood returns to the heart in the *veins*.

Deoxygenated blood enters the right side of the heart at the right atrium. It is then pumped into the right ventricle and out of the heart to the lungs. In the lungs the blood gives up its carbon dioxide and takes on a fresh supply of oxygen.

1-12 The body as a control system

Many functions of the body (estimates range from hundreds to thousands) are regulated in automatic *negative feedback loops*. Engineering and technology students should be at ease when studying these systems because they behave very much like the control systems we study in engineering and technology schools. Conceptually, then, they are

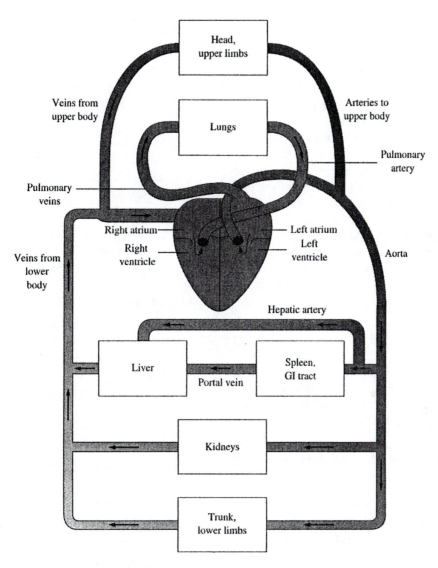

Figure 1-3
Circulatory system. (From *Human Anatomy and Physiology*, 2nd edition, by James E. Crouch,
Ph.D. and J. Robert McClintic, Ph.D. John Wiley & Sons, New York, 1976. Used by permission.)

identical, if functionally different, and obey the same laws. Common electrical control systems include amplifiers, servomechanisms, and the old fashioned home furnace controller, the thermostat.

Any negative feedback control system compares *actual* conditions with *optimal* conditions (those that should exist) and then causes a correction that cancels part of the difference, or *error* (i.e., the difference between the actual and the optimal).

The usual model of a simple control system is the home furnace system, regulated by a simple on-off thermostat. The thermostat measures the temperature in the room and then compares it with the temperature set on the dial. When the room temperature drops below the set point, the thermostat closes a switch that turns on the furnace. The furnace remains on until the error is corrected.

A phenomenon often used as an example of a physiological control system is the automatic regulation of blood pressure. Pressure sensors in the circulatory system, called *baroreceptors,* tell the CNS of the conditions that exist. If the pressure drops below a certain normal point, then the brain issues a command that causes the blood vessels to *constrict,* which brings the pressure up. But if the pressure increases above a normal point, then the brain causes the vessels to *dilate* (i.e., increase their cross-sectional area, thereby reducing the pressure on the system).

1-13 Summary

1. The human body is a homeostatic mechanism; that is, it is self-regulating through a series of negative feedback control systems to maintain a constant internal environment.

2. The cell is the basic building block of the body. Different types of cells perform different functions.

3. Roughly two-thirds of the body is fluid.

4. Major body systems include the nervous, circulatory, musculoskeletal, respiratory, digestive, and endocrine systems.

1-14 Recapitulation

Now return to the objectives and self-evaluation questions at the beginning of the chapter and see how well you can answer them. If you cannot answer certain questions, place a check mark next to each, and reread appropriate parts of the text. Next, try to answer the following questions, using the same procedure.

Questions

1. The ability to maintain a constant internal environment in the body is called _____.

2. _____ are considered to be the basic building blocks of the body.

3. The sizes of various cells in humans range from _____ to _____.

4. One of the largest cells known is the _____ _____, and it may reach 8 in. in length.

5. The cell material is enclosed by a covering called a _____.

6. There are approximately _____ cells in the human body, of which _____ are red blood cells.

7. List six properties common to all cells.

8. The process called _____ is the qualitative reproduction of a cell by division.

9. The body is approximately _____ percent fluid.

10. List the principal ingredients of intracellular fluid.

11. List the principal ingredients of extracellular fluid.

12. The musculoskeletal system provides _____.

13. _____ and _____ are the principal types of tissue forming the skeleton.

14. Define *membrane* in your own words.

15. What is the function of the respiratory system?

16. List the principal components of the respiratory system.

17. What is the function of the GI tract?

18. What is *chyme*?

19. The _____ _____ system integrates and assimilates data.

20. The _____ nervous system provides information on the external and internal environments.

21. The _____ nervous system operates mostly at the subconscious level.

22. The _____ system is a chemical communications and control system within the body.

23. List the components of the circulatory system.

24. The two major fluid transport systems in the body are _____ and _____.

25. _____ is the process by which the body responds to the environment and regulates levels of sugars, salts, water, acid-base balance, oxygen, and carbon dioxide.

26. A _____ membrane selectively permits materials to pass between the inside of a cell and its external environment.

27. The _____ system takes in oxygen and gives off carbon dioxide.

28. The _____ system processes food so that it is absorbed into the body.

29. The _____ system provides locomotion.

30. The musculoskeletal system consists mostly of bones and _____.

31. _____ waves occur in the intestine about every _____ seconds and can reach magnitudes of _____ cm H_2O to _____ cm H_2O.

32. Chemicals called _____ are secreted by eight major glands of the _____ system.

33. The kidneys act to _____ the blood.

34. Much of the body's functions are controlled by internal negative _____ loops that operate much like a _____ control system in engineering.

35. An example of a control system in the body is the control of blood pressure. Sensors called _____ tell the CNS what pressure exists.

36. Blood vessels _____ to reduce pressure and _____ to increase pressure.

Suggested readings

1. Crouch, James E. and J. Robert McClintic, *Human Anatomy and Physiology,* 2nd ed., John Wiley and Sons (New York, 1976).

2. Guyton, Arthur C., *Textbook of Medical Physiology,* W. B. Saunders Company (Philadelphia, 1971).

3. Van DeGraaff, Kent M. and Stuart Ira Fox, *Concepts of Human Anatomy and Physiology,* 3rd ed. Wm. C. Brown Publishers (Dubuque, Ia. 1992).

4. Carola, Robert, John P. Harley, and Charles R. Noback, *Human Anatomy and Physiology,* 2nd ed., McGraw-Hill (New York, 1992).

CHAPTER 2
The Heart and Circulatory System

2-1 Objectives

1. Be able to state the biological principles behind the human cardiovascular system.
2. Be able to describe the anatomy of the heart.
3. Be able to describe the dynamics of blood flow.

4. Know how to explain the generation and propagation of bioelectric potentials in tissue.
5. Be able to describe the general details of the internal electroconduction system of the human heart.

2-2 Self-evaluation questions

These questions test your prior knowledge of the material in this chapter. Look for the answers as you read the text. After you have finished studying the chapter, try answering these questions and those at the end of the chapter.

1. Define *action potential.*

2. Name the four chambers of the heart.

3. Describe the location of the tricuspid valve.

4. What are the *sinoatrial* (SA) and *artioventricular* (AV) nodes?

5. Describe the general path of the blood as it travels through the circulatory system.

6. Define the term *systole.*

7. What is the velocity of propagation of the action potential in the bundle branches following the AV node?

2-3 The circulatory system

The circulatory system carries nourishment and oxygen (O_2) to, and waste and carbon dioxide (CO_2) from, the tissues and organs of the body. The system may be considered as a closed loop hydraulic system, and indeed, you will find that it possesses many of the properties of such a system.

Elementary circulatory system

Figure 2-1 shows the human circulatory system in simplified form. The heart serves as a pump to move blood through vessels called arteries and veins. Blood is carried away from the heart in arteries and is brought back to the heart in veins.

The heart is a dual pump, consisting of a two-chambered pump on both the left and right sides. The upper chambers are inputs to the pumps and are called *atria* (singular, *atrium*). The lower

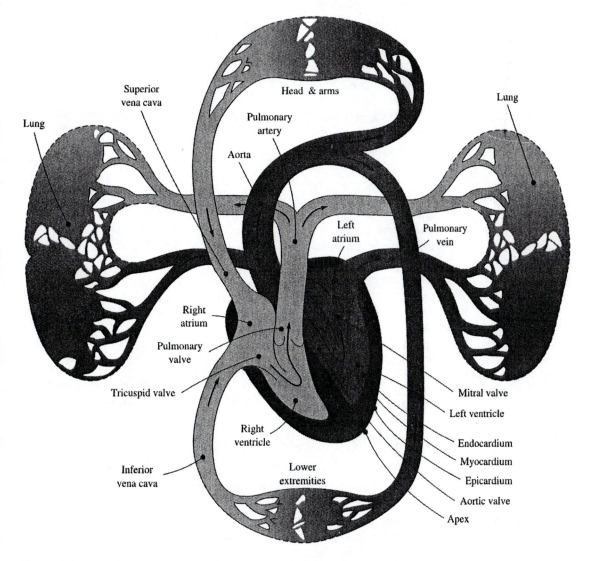

Figure 2-1
The human circulatory system. (Reprinted courtesy of Hewlett-Packard.)

chambers of the heart are called *ventricles* and are the pump outputs.

When blood is circulated through the body, it carries O_2 and nutrients to the organs and tissues and returns carrying CO_2 to be excreted through the lungs and various waste products to be excreted through the kidneys. The deoxygenated blood is returned to the right side of the heart via the venous system. Blood from the head and arms, as well as the rest of the upper portion of the body, returns to the heart through the *superior vena cava;* blood from the lower portion of the body returns through the *inferior vena cava.* Note that the terms *inferior* and *superior* refer not to some qualitative assessment, but to the respective positions of the two vessels. The inferior is generally placed lower in the body than the superior. (Similarly, *great,* as used later in this section, means large.)

Blood leaves the right atrium through the *tricuspid valve* to enter the *right ventricle.* From the right ventricle it passes through the *pulmonary semilunar valve* to the *pulmonary artery.* This vessel carries blood to the lungs, where CO_2 is given up and O_2 is taken on. This gas exchange is studied in greater detail in chapter 6.

Blood returning from the lungs via the pulmonary vein reenters the heart through the *left atrium.* It then passes through the *mitral valve* to the *left ventricle,* and then back into the mainstream of the circulatory system via the *aortic valve.* The great artery attached to the left ventricle is called the *aorta.* Blood then circulates through the body to again return to the right side of the heart via the superior and inferior vena cava.

The blood flowing in the vessels of the body may be viewed as analogous to an electrical circuit. In your elementary electronics courses, you may have learned the old "plumbing analogy" of electricity, in which an electric current is likened to water or fluid in a hydraulic system. Here we use the converse analogy, in which blood flow and pressure are compared to an electrical circuit. We will even introduce an "Ohm's law" relationship for blood flow rate (Equation 2-1).

Blood

Blood has two main components: *cells* and *plasma.* Blood cells make up approximately 40% of the total blood volume, and the remaining 60% is plasma. Since approximately 99% of the cells are red cells, it may be said that 40% of the blood volume consists of red cells. White cells play only a small role in determining the physical properties and composition of blood.

Blood *flow rate* (measured in volume per unit of time) in a blood vessel is described by two factors: the *pressure difference* along the vessel and the *resistance* offered by the vessel (a function of its cross-sectional area). Does this sound familiar? It should, because similar factors in an electrical circuit control the flow of current. In an electrical circuit, we use Ohm's law to describe the relationship between potential difference (analogous to pressure) and current (analogous to blood flow rate). The same sort of relationship describes blood flow:

$$R = \frac{P}{F} \qquad (2\text{-}1)$$

where

   P is the pressure difference in millimeters of mercury (mm Hg)

   F is the flow rate, in milliliters per second (mL/s) or cm^3/s

   R is the resistance of the vessel in *peripheral resistance units* (PRU) (1 PRU is the vessel resistance that allows a flow of 1 mL/s under a pressure of 1 mm Hg).

Example 2-1

Find the resistance of a blood vessel in which the flow rate is 1.7 mL/s at a blood pressure of 6.8 mm Hg.

Solution

$$R = \frac{P}{F}$$

$$R = \frac{6.8 \text{ mm Hg}}{1.7 \text{ mL/s}} = \textbf{4 PRU} \qquad (2\text{-}1)$$

Note that Equation 2-1 shows that a vessel that has a higher resistance (in PRU) would require a higher blood pressure to produce the same flow.

The situation in most cases is a little more complex than that given in Equation 2-1 because the resistance is *not* constant; that is, the vessel walls are *not* rigid (the radius of the vessel varies), and the blood itself is subject to changes in viscosity. The walls of the arteries and the veins are continuously distensible, so the pulsating blood flow will continuously vary some of the parameters. The flow quantity *(F)*, for example, is more precisely described by Poiseuille's law, which gives the factors affecting flow rate or

$$F = \frac{P}{R} = P \times \frac{\pi r^4}{8\eta L} \qquad (2\text{-}2)$$

where

η is the coefficient of blood viscosity in dyne seconds per square centimeter (dyne-s/cm^2)

P is the pressure difference in dyne/cm^2

r is the vessel radius in centimeters

L is the vessel length in centimeters

Example 2-2 _____

A blood vessel has an average radius of 0.5 mm and a length of 20 mm. If the blood pressure is 7.2 mm Hg at an average viscosity of 0.01 dyne-s/cm^2, calculate the blood flow rate in (a) cm^3/s; (b) mL/s. Hint:

$$1 \text{ mm Hg} = 1330 \text{ dyne/cm}^2$$

Solution

a. $F = \dfrac{P}{R} = \dfrac{P\pi r^4}{8\eta L}$

$$= \frac{7.2 \text{ mm} \times 1330 \text{ dyne/cm}^2/\text{mm} \times \pi \times (0.5 \text{ mm} \times 0.1 \text{ cm/mm})^4}{8 \times 0.01 \text{ dyne-s/cm}^2 \times (20 \text{ mm} \times 0.1 \text{ cm/mm})}$$

$$= \mathbf{1.175 \text{ cm}^3/s} \qquad (2\text{-}2)$$

b. $1.175 \text{ cm}^3/\text{s} \times 1 \text{ mL/cm}^3 = \mathbf{1.175 \text{ mL/s}}$

The reader should perform a dimensional analysis to verify the units of flow rate (in cm^3/s) using the values substituted in Example 2-2a in Equation 2-2. When data are given in units other than those specified in Equation 2-2, it is first necessary to convert that data to appropriate units before substituting in Equation 2-2. This is done in Example 2-2a for units of *P, r,* and *L,* respectively, as shown. Note that Example 2-2 shows that a constricted blood vessel impedes the flow rate drastically. If the radius of the vessel is reduced by 50% (or one-half), the flow rate is reduced to one-sixteenth of its original value.

Blood is carried throughout the body in several different types of vessels. Those leading from the heart to tissue and organs are called arteries. Arteries tend to be *elastic,* allowing diameter changes to regulate the blood flow to various parts of the body. The diameter constrictions reflect ordinary changes in demand or emergency situations. Very small arteries are called *arterioles.*

The veins carry blood back to the heart and lungs (where it is reoxygenated). O_2 is transferred to cells of the tissue in *capillary beds* that permeate the entire body. Capillaries are small vessels connecting veins and arteries in a meshlike structure and have a diameter (i.e., $2r$) of only a few micrometers. Capillaries are so numerous and widespread that it is claimed that no cell in the human body is more than its own diameter away from a capillary.

Note that blood flow rate is greatest in the aorta and least in the capillaries (Equation 2-2). The diameter of the capillaries is so small that blood cells must pass through them single file, one by one.

2-4 The heart

The human heart is located in the upper middle portion of the chest *(thorax)*. Although many people believe that the heart is clearly on the left side of the body, it is actually a little more centered, with the lower tip pointed toward the left hip. About one-third of the heart lies to the right of the midline of the body; the rest lies to the left.

The size and weight of the heart vary from one individual to another. In most people, the heart is approximately the size of the person's clenched fist, and the average weight of the heart is about 300 g.

The heart is a muscle that is encased in a sac called the *pericardium.* This double layer of tissue helps the heart stay in position and protects it from harm. The pericardium creates a lubricating fluid on its inside surface so that the friction between it and the heart wall is reduced, allowing the heart to beat freely within the walls of the sac.

A cutaway view of the human heart is shown in Figure 2-2. Besides the two layers of pericardium, there is an *epicardium* and a *myocardium,* the main muscle tissue of the heart. The thick myocardium accounts for approximately 75% of the heart wall thickness.

The heart contains four chambers, which are used to form two separate pumps. Each pump consists of an upper chamber (atrium) and a lower chamber (ventricle). The high pressure *output* side of each pump is the ventricle, so the myocardium thickness in the ventricular region is considerably greater than it is in the atrial region.

There are four *valves* in the human heart. The valve between the right atrium and the right ventricle is known as the tricuspid valve. It gets its name from the fact that it is formed of three cusp-shaped flaps of tissue arranged so that they will shut off and block passage of blood in the reverse direction (from ventricles back to the atrium).

These valves are attached at their bases to a fibrous strand of tissue ringing the opening between upper and lower chambers and at their ends to *chordae tendinae.* These structures are attached to the muscle tissue in the ventricle and keep the tricuspid valve closed as the right ventricular pressure builds up to force blood out of the heart into the pulmonary artery.

The valve between the right ventricle and the pulmonary artery is named for its shape: *semilunar* (half moon) valve. It also consists of three flaps, but it lacks the chordae tendinae of the tricuspid valve. It prevents reverse flow (regurgitation) of blood from the pulmonary artery to the right ventricle.

Blood returning to the heart from the lungs must pass through the left atrium and the mitral valve (also known as a *bicuspid valve* for its shape) to the left ventricle. This valve is formed of two flaps of cusp-shaped pieces of tissue.

The last valve is the *aortic-valve.* Its shape is similar to the pulmonary valve and prevents regurgitation of blood from the aorta back to the left ventricle.

The heart serves as a pump because of its ability to contract under an electrical stimulus. When an electrical triggering signal is received (see section 2-5), the heart will contract, starting in the atria, which undergo a shallow, ripplelike contracting motion. A fraction of a second later, the ventricles also begin to contract, from the bottom up, in a motion that resembles wringing out a dishrag or sponge. The ventricular contraction is known as *systole.* The ventricular relaxation is known as *diastole.*

The heart in a resting adult pumps approximately 3 to 5 liters of blood per minute (3 to 5 L/min). This figure is called *cardiac output* (CO) and is defined as the product of heart rate in beats per minute (beats/min). The volume of blood ejected from the ventricles during systole.

$$CO = heart\ rate\ \text{(beats/min)}$$
$$\times\ stroke\ volume\ \text{(L/beat)} \qquad (2\text{-}3)$$

Example 2-3 _____

Find the CO for:

a. A patient whose heart rate is 60 beats/min if the stroke volume is 50 mL/beat.
b. A heart rate of 90 beats/min and a stroke volume of 80 mL/beat.

Solution

a. $CO = heart\ rate \times stroke\ volume$

$\qquad = 60\ \text{beats/min} \times 50\ \text{mL/beat} \qquad (2\text{-}3)$

$\qquad \times \dfrac{1\,\text{L}}{1000\,\text{mL}}$

$\qquad = \textbf{3 L/min}$

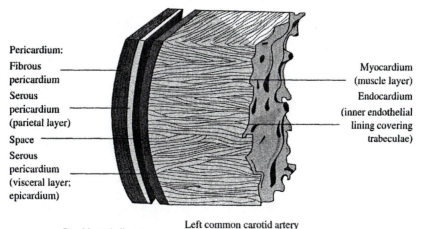

Pericardium:

Fibrous pericardium

Serous pericardium (parietal layer)

Space

Serous pericardium (visceral layer; epicardium)

Myocardium (muscle layer)

Endocardium (inner endothelial lining covering trabeculae)

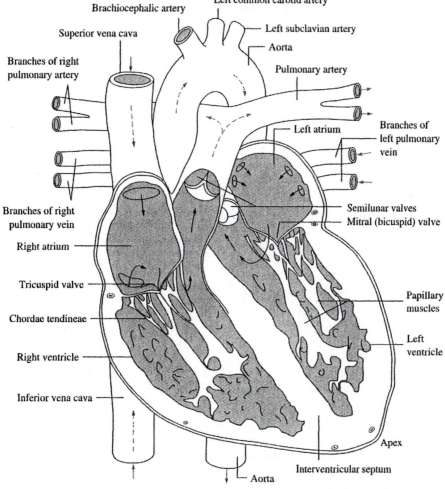

Brachiocephalic artery

Superior vena cava

Branches of right pulmonary artery

Left common carotid artery

Left subclavian artery

Aorta

Pulmonary artery

Left atrium

Branches of left pulmonary vein

Branches of right pulmonary vein

Semilunar valves

Mitral (bicuspid) valve

Right atrium

Tricuspid valve

Chordae tendineae

Right ventricle

Inferior vena cava

Papillary muscles

Left ventricle

Apex

Aorta

Interventricular septum

Figure 2-2
Cross-sectional view of the human heart. (From Human Anatomy and Physiology, 2nd ed., by James E. Crouch, Ph.D. and J. Robert McClintic, Ph.D. John Wiley & Sons, New York, 1976. Used by permission.)

b. CO = 90 beats/min $\times$ 80 mL/beat

$$\times \frac{1\,L}{1000\,mL}$$

$$= 7.2\,L/min$$

Note that the values of CO for the parameters given in the problem are extremes. Most human CO values are in the range of 3 to 5 L/min.

2-5 Bioelectricity

Ionic potentials are formed in certain cells of the body due to differences in the concentrations of certain chemical ions, notably sodium (Na^+), chloride (Cl^-, and potassium (K^+) ions.

The cell wall is a *semipermeable membrane*. Permeability is a measure of the ability of the membrane to pass certain ions. In the case of a semipermeable membrane, a selective process allows some ions to pass while restricting or rejecting others. Such a membrane will not allow the free diffusion of all ions but only a limited few. It is thought that this selective phenomenon is due to ion size differences, their respective electrical charges, and certain other factors. The end result, however, is that cell membranes at rest tend to be more permeable to some ions (e.g., potassium and chloride) than to others (e.g., sodium). As a result, the concentration of positive sodium ions inside a cell (see Figure 2-3a) is *less* than the concentration of sodium ions in the intracellular fluid (outside the cell). A phenomenon known as the *sodium-potassium pump* keeps the sodium largely outside the cell and potassium ions inside.

Potassium is thus pumped into the cell while sodium is pumped out, but the *rate* of sodium pumping is roughly two to five times that of potassium. These rates result in a *difference* of ion *concentraton*, creating an electrical potential, and this causes the cell to be polarized. The inside of the cell is *less positive* than the *outside,* so the cell is said to be *negative* with respect to its outside. Various authorities give slightly different figures for the value of this *resting potential,* but all fall within the 70- to 90-millivolt (mV) range. Guyton

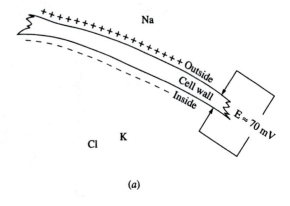

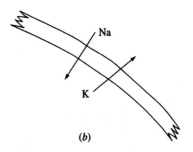

(a)

(b)

Figure 2-3
Cell polarization at rest and during stimulation. (*a*) Resting (diffusion) potential; polarized cell. (*b*) Action potential; depolarized cell.

(1) uses 85 mV, Crouch and McClintic (2) offer 70 mV as the figure, and Strong (3) uses 90 mV. All agree, however, that the cell polarity is negative, so in this text we will use -70 mV as the nominal value of the resting potential. The actual potential is derived from the Nernst equation, which is given in simplified form as

$$E_{(mV)} = \pm\,61\,Log\,\frac{C_o}{C_i} \qquad (2\text{-}4)$$

where

E is the *resting* potential, in millivolts

C_i is the concentration inside the cell in moles/cm^3

C_o is the concentration outside of the cell in moles/cm^3

Log indicates that the logarithm (base ten) of
the concentration ratio is used

Example 2-4 _____

The intracellular K^+ concentration of a group of
cells averages 150×10^{-6} moles/cm^3. The extracellular concentration of K^+ averages 6×10^{-6}
moles/cm^3.
Calculate (a) The concentration ratio.
          (b) Diffusion potential for K^+.

Solution

a. $\dfrac{C_o}{C_i} = \dfrac{6 \times 10^{-6}\,\text{moles/cm}^3}{150 \times 10^{-6}\,\text{moles/cm}^3} = \dfrac{5}{20} = \mathbf{1/4}$

b. $E^{K^+} = 61 \log C_o/C_i = 61 \log 1/25 = \mathbf{-85.3\,mV}$

_____

When the cell is stimulated, the nature of the
cell membrane wall changes abruptly, and it becomes permeable to sodium ions. The sodium ions
rush into the cell (Figure 2-3b) and potassium ions
rush out. The result is an *action potential* (Figure
2-4) that sees the inside of the cell at a potential of
20 to 40 mV more positive than the outside (i.e., a
polarity reversal lasting a few milliseconds).

The cell showing a resting potential is *polarized*
(Figure 2-3a), but when it is generating an action
potential, it is said to be *depolarized.* There is a *refractory period* following depolarization, during
which the cell becomes repolarized (Figure 2-4).
In this period the cell is resistant to another depolarization. To the electronics student this action
might resemble the monostable multivibrator: the
action potential, once triggered, cannot be retrig-
gered until the cell has again become repolarized.

Repolarization occurs when the cell membrane
again changes its properties, forcing sodium out of
the cell and drawing potassium ions to the inside
of the cell wall.

Although ordinary ionic electrical conduction
occurs, action potentials as such tend to be localized phenomena. But conduction does occur because depolarized cells trigger adjacent cells, causing them to produce an action potential. Returning
to our multivibrator analogy from electronics, we
could view this situation as a chain of monostable

multivibrators in cascade so that the output of one
will trigger the next.

2-6 Electroconduction system of the heart

The conduction system of the heart (Figure 2-5)
consists of the *sinoatrial* (SA) *node, bundle of His,
atrioventricular* (AV) *node, the bundle branches,*
and *Purkinje fibers.*

The SA node serves as a *pacemaker* for the
heart, and it provides the trigger signal mentioned
earlier. It is a small bundle of cells (approximately
3×10 mm) located on the rear wall of the right
atrium, just below the point where the superior
vena cava is attached. The SA node fires electrical
impulses through the bioelectric mechanism discussed in the previous section. It is capable of *self-
excitation* (firing on its own) but is under control
of the CNS so that the heart rate can be adjusted
automatically to meet varying requirements.

When the SA node discharges a pulse, then electrical current spreads across the atria (auricles),
causing them to contract. Blood in the atria is forced
by the contraction through the valves to the ventricles. The velocity of propagation for the SA node
action potential is about 30 cm/s in atrial tissue.

There is a band of specialized tissue between
the SA node and the AV node, however, in which
the velocity of propagation is faster than it is in
atrial tissue, on the order of 45 cm/s (Figure 2-5).
This internal conduction pathway carries the signal
to the ventricles.

It would *not* be desirable for the ventricles to
contract in response to an action potential *before*
the atrial are empty of their contents. A *delay* is
needed, therefore, to prevent such an occurrence;
this is the function of the AV node. At 45 cm/s the
action potential will reach the AV node 30 to 50
ms after the SA node discharges, but another 110
ms will pass before the pulse is transmitted from
the AV node. The AV node, then, operates like a
delay line to retard the advance of the action potential along the internal electroconduction system
toward the ventricles.

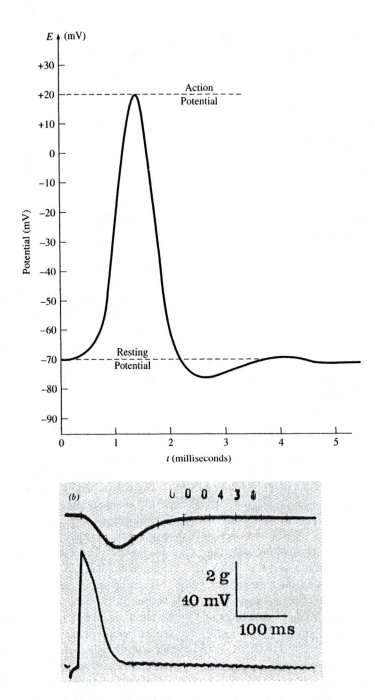

Figure 2-4
Action potential duration with time. (*a*) Typical cell action potential. (*b*) Contraction (upper trace) and action potential (lower trace) from a guinea pig myocardium. (Photo courtesy of Dr. Martin Frank, Dept. of Physiology, The George Washington University Medical School.)

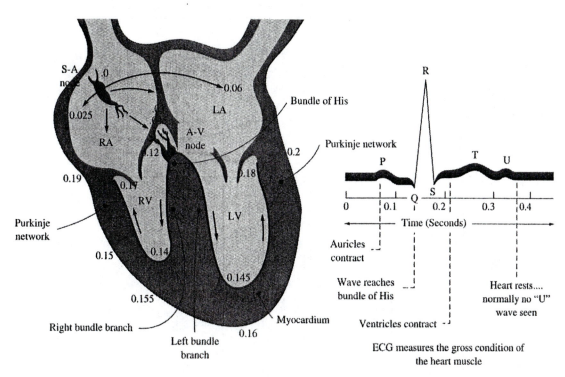

Figure 2-5
Electroconduction system of the heart and resulting ECG waveform. (Reprinted courtesy of Hewlett-Packard.

The muscle cells of the ventricles are actually excited by the Purkinje fibers (Figure 2-5). The action potential travels along these fibers at a much faster rate, on the order of 2 to 4 m/s (i.e., 200 to 400 cm/s). The fibers are arranged in two bundles, one branch to the left and one to the right.

Conduction in the Purkinje fibers is very rapid. (Note that timing is given in Figure 2-5). The action potential traverses the distance between the SA and AV nodes in about 40 ms and is delayed by the AV node for about 110 ms so that the contraction of the lower chambers can be synchronized with the emptying of the upper chambers. Conduction into the bundle branches is rapid, consuming only another 60 ms to reach the furthest Purkinje fibers.

The action potential generated in the SA node stimulates the muscle fibers of the myocardium, causing them to contract. When the muscle is in contraction, it is shorter, and the volume of the ventricular chamber is less, so blood is squeezed out. The contraction of so many muscle cells at one time creates a mass electrical signal that can be detected by electrodes placed on the surface of the patient's chest or the patient's extremities. This electrical discharge can be mechanically plotted as a function of time, and the resultant waveform is called an *electrocardiogram* (ECG). An example of a typical ECG waveform is shown as part of Figure 2-5.

The different parts of the ECG waveform are designated by letters. The P-wave indicates *atrial* contraction; ventricular systole occurs immediately following the QRS complex, and a refractory period *(resting* for *repolarization)* is indicated by the T-wave.

Oddly enough, the duration of the ECG features is relatively constant over a wide range of heart rates. The *QRS* complex (see waveform in Figure 2-5), for example, requires approximately 90 ms, the PR interval roughly 150 to 200 ms, and

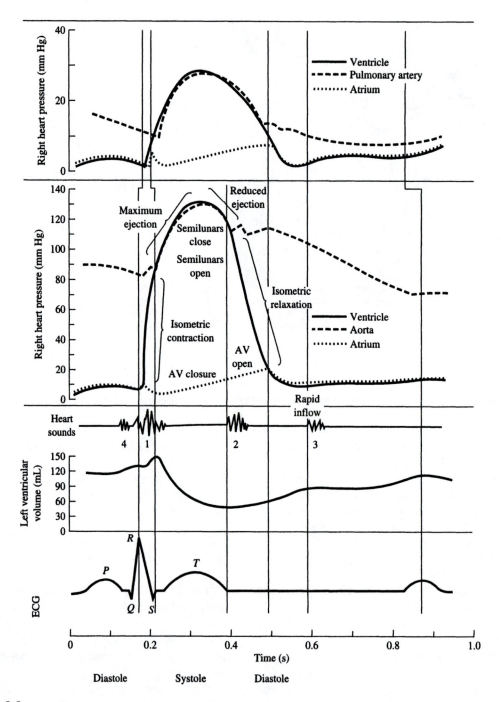

Figure 2-6
Pressures, ECG tracings, and heart sounds over time.

the ST segment about 50 to 150 ms. Right atrial pressure changes from a diastolic value of approximately 3 mm Hg to a systolic value of approximately 8 mm Hg.

By now you should be ready to correlate the ECG features, contraction of the heart, and pulsatile flow of blood from the heart. Figure 2-6 shows the ECG and its relationship to the various pressures existing in the left and right sides of the heart. Notice that the ventricular pressure begins rising sharply as the heart begins to contract. This occurs in the period immediately following the R wave of the ECG. It reaches a peak and then subsides, returning to its resting value. The peak pressure is known as the *systolic pressure,* because it occurs during systole. The resting pressure is known as the *diastolic pressure,* and it occurs during the period called *diastole.* The period of systole lasts about 350 ms, while diastole is a little longer, about 550 ms.

Also shown in Figure 2-6 are certain heart sounds labeled 1, 2, 3, and 4. These sounds are attributed to the mechanical action of the four valves.

Contraction of the atria is triggered by the SA node and begins immediately after the P wave on the ECG. The pressure in the right and left atria will begin to rise as the contraction commences. Right atrial pressure changes from a 2 to 3 mm Hg diastolic value to a systolic value of 7 to 8 mm Hg. The pressure in the left atrium rises from about 3 mm Hg in diastole to about 10 mm Hg in systole.

The pressure in the atria does not actually cause the transfer of blood from the atria to ventricles. Valve openings, which allow blood transfer, are due mostly to changes in differential pressure. During diastole the pressure in the ventricles drops to less than the atrial pressure. This causes the valves (tricuspid on the right and mitral on the left) to open, allowing blood to be drawn into the ventricles under the influence of the pressure difference.

The ventricular contraction commences immediately after the R wave on the ECG. The ventricular pressure increases to a level greater than atrial pressure, forcing shut the tricuspid and mitral valves. These valve closures give rise to the first

heart sound. The pressure in the right ventricle will rise from a pressure slightly less than atrial pressure during diastole to 28 to 30 mm Hg during systole. A pressure of 18 to 20 mm Hg is sufficient to overcome the reverse pressure in the pulmonary artery and open the pulmonary valve. The left ventricle, however, faces a higher pressure situation and so must attain a pressure of 75 to 80 mm Hg to open the aortic valve and reaches a peak pressure of 120 to 130 mm Hg.

The ventricles will begin to relax following the peak of systole, and the ventricular pressure will begin to drop. When the ventricular pressure is less than the pressure in the arteries, the respective valves will close. During this period of pressure reversal, blood attempts to flow back into the ventricles. The valve closure and blood flow dynamics at this time give rise to the second heart sound. Also noted is a *dicrotic notch,* occurring just past 0.4 s in Figure 2-6, in the aortic pressure waveform. Following valve closure is a period of relaxation during which the ventricles will again fill with blood.

Note that in all phases of the heart cycle, it is pressure changes that actuate valve opening and closing. There is no fancy control system in operation here, just the results of ordinary pressure differences, such as you may have studied in an introductory physics course.

2-7 Heart problems

The physician uses the ECG and other tests to determine the gross condition of the heart. Although a complete discussion of heart problems is beyond the scope of this book, we can discuss some of the more common problems in generalized terms.

The heart is a muscle and, as such, must be *perfused* with blood to keep it healthy. Blood is supplied to the heart through the coronary arteries that branch off from the aorta just before it joins the heart.

If an artery bringing blood to the heart becomes partially or totally occluded (i.e., blocked off), the area of the heart served by that vessel will suffer damage from the loss of the blood flow. That area of the heart is said to be *infarcted* and is dysfunctional. This type of damage is referred to as a *myocardial infarction* (MI), another term for heart attack.

Another class of heart problem is cardiac *arrhythmias.* These are abnormal heartbeat rhythms and may be seen as ECG changes. Conditions under this classification include extremes in heart rate, premature contractions, heart block, and fibrillation.

The human heart rate varies normally over a range of 60 to 110 beats/min. Rates faster than this are called *tachycardia.* Various authorities list slightly different figures as the threshold for defined tachycardia, but most list 120 beats/min, with the range being 110 to 130 beats/min.

The opposite condition, too slow a heart rate, is called *bradycardia,* and again different sources list slightly different thresholds, but all are within the 40- to 60-beats/min range.

Premature contractions occur when an area of the heart becomes irritable enough to produce a *spurious* action potential at a time *between* normal beats. The action potential spreads across the myocardium in much the same manner as the regular discharge. Beats occurring at improper times are called *ectopic beats.* If they result in atrial contraction, then it is a *premature atrial contraction* (PCA), and if in the ventricle, a *premature ventricular contraction* (PVC).

Heart block occurs when the internal electroconduction system of the heart is interrupted or significantly impeded. Among the more common forms is the atrioventricular block occurring at the junction of the atria and ventricles. More on this subject is covered later when we discuss pacemakers.

Fibrillation is a condition in which the muscle cells discharge asynchronously in a random manner. In *ventricular fibrillation* the major features of the ECG disappear and the waveform takes on a low-amplitude, "jittery" appearance, indicating that the ventricles are not contracting but only quivering. Ventricular fibrillation is a fatal arrhythmia that will kill the patient in a few minutes if not corrected.

Atrial fibrillation is an arrhythmia in which the atria quiver rather than beat. The cause is believed to be the existence of numerous pacemaker sites in addition to the SA node. It is characterized on the ECG tracing by the disappearance of the P wave. This arrhythmia is less serious than ventricular tachycardia or ventricular fibrillation because the ventricles beat, as indicated by a normal QRS complex in the ECG. Symptoms of atrial fibrillation include shortness of breath, profound fatigue, and an irregular heartbeat that might reach well over 120 beats/min while resting. If blood clots form in the atria, they can cause infarction or death. Patients are usually put on a regime of daily aspirn or warfarin to prevent clotting.

Wolf-Parkinson-White (WPW) syndrome (or preexcitation syndrome) and reentry node problems are associated with sudden death in young athletes. The reentry node defect is related to the AV node in the electroconduction system. The AV node has two pathways, one fast and one slow. The signal propagates through one of the paths, and then feeds back into the other pathway. Often the first symptom is a heart rate in excess of 200 beats/min, which in all but the young and fit may cause blackouts.

Both WPW syndrome and reentry node defects are often treated using an RF ablation technique, in which a radio frequency current is introduced to destroy the extra pathways. The procedure is done in conjunction with a cardiac catheterization, in which a catheter is inserted into the heart so that an electrophysiology study can be conducted by a specially trained cardiologist called an *electrophysiologist.*

2-8 Summary

1. The heart is a dual two-chambered pump that supplies pressure to circulate the blood throughout the body.

2. Blood is carried from the heart in arteries and returns to the heart in veins.

3. Blood returns to the heart on the right side and is pumped from the heart on the left side.

4. An internal pacemaker (SA node) generates an electrical signal to initiate contraction of the heart. This signal is an action potential and is propagated by the electroconduction system to the ventricles.

5. Contracting heart muscle cells generate a mass action potential that may be picked up by electrodes on the surface of the body. The tracing of this potential is called an electrocardiogram (ECG).

2-9 Recapitulation

Now return to the objectives and self-evaluation questions at the beginning of the chapter and see how well you can answer them. If you cannot answer certain questions, place a check mark next to each and review appropriate parts of the text. Next, try to answer the following questions using the same procedure. When you have answered all of the questions, solve the problems.

Questions

1. The upper chambers of the heart are called _____.

2. The lower chambers of the heart are called _____.

3. The superior and inferior _____ return blood to the _____ atrium.

4. The _____ valve is located between the right atrium and the right ventricle.

5. Blood leaves the right ventricle via the _____ artery.

6. The _____ valve is located between the left atrium and the left ventricle.

7. The great artery leaving the left side of the heart is called the _____.

8. State Ohm's law for blood flow.

9. Blood is about _____% red cells by volume.

10. Very small vessels called _____ have diameters in the micrometer range.

11. Blood velocity in the capillaries is (faster) (slower) than its velocity in the aorta.

12. The average human heart weighs about _____ g.

13. The sac surrounding the heart is the _____.

14. Heart muscle is called _____.

15. The _____ are the heart chambers that are subject to the highest pressures.

16. Name four valves in the heart.

17. The _____ is the heart's pacemaker.

18. The period of contraction is called _____.

19. An electrical potential is generated across a cell wall because of a difference in _____ concentration.

20. The potential across a cell wall is called a _____ potential.

21. The cell wall is a _____ membrane.

22. A phenomenon known as the _____ pump keeps _____ ions predominantly outside of the cell wall.

23. Action potentials have an amplitude of about _____ mV.

24. Write the simplified Nernst equation.

25. Resting potentials are about _____ mV.

26. The delay line in the heart's electroconduction system is called the _____.

27. The five principal structures of the heart's electroconduction system are _____, _____, _____, _____, and _____.

28. Action potentials travel down the conduction system at rates of _____ cm/s between SA and AV nodes, and at _____ cm/s after the SA node.

29. The AV delay is about _____ ms.

30. The _____ is a recording of the heart's electrical activity.

31. A pressure of about _____ mm Hg is required to open the aortic valve.

32. The _____ notch in the aortic pressure waveform indicates the onset of diastole.

33. A heart rate that is too slow is called _____.

34. A heart rate that is too fast is called _____.

35. _____ _____ is an arrhythmia in which the upper chambers of the heart quiver rather than beat.

36. Which arrhythmia is characterized by the disappearance of the P wave on the ECG, even though the QRS complex is still present?

37. List several symptoms of atrial fibrillation.

38. List two cardiac arrhythmias that are associated with sudden, unexpected death in young athletes.

39. _____ _____ is a treatment for WPW syndrome in which extra pathway tissue is burned away during a cardiac catheterization procedure.

Problems

1. Find the resistance of a blood vessel that has a flow rate of 1.8 mL/s and a pressure of 7.6 mm Hg.

2. Find the resistance of a blood vessel that has a flow rate of 2 mL/s and a pressure of 7.3 mm Hg.

3. Find the flow rate if the resistance is 6 PRU and the pressure difference is 8.5 mm Hg.

4. Find the flow rate if the resistance is 5.2 PRU and ΔP is 7.9 mm Hg.

5. Find the resistance of a blood vessel that has a pressure of 4 mm Hg and a flow rate of 0.5 mL/s.

6. Find the resistance of a blood vessel that has a pressure of 4.5 mm Hg and a flow rate of 0.75 mL/s.

7. Calculate the flow rate in a blood vessel with an average diameter of 12 mm if the pressure drop over a length of 25 mm is 8.4 mm Hg and the blood viscosity is 0.015 dyne-s/cm^2.

8. Calculate the flow rate in a blood vessel with an average diameter of 9 mm if the pressure drop over a 22 mm length is 9.8 mm Hg and the blood viscosity is 0.015 dyne-s/cm^2.

9. Find the resistance in PRU of the vessels in problems 7 and 8 above.

10. Find the flow rate of the vessel in problem 7 if the diameter (a) increases to 18 mm and (b) decreases to 6 mm.

11. Find the flow rate of the vessel in problem 7 if the diameter decreases to 6 mm.

12. Calculate the CO for a heart rate of 70 beats/min and a stroke volume of 60 mL.

13. Calculate the CO for a heart rate of 130 beats/min and a stroke volume of 55 mL.

14. Find the diffusion potential across a membrane if the K^+ concentration is 4×10^{-6} moles/cm^3 on one side and 9×10^{-6} moles/cm^3 on the other side.

15. Find the diffusion potential across a membrane if the K^+ concentration is 5×10^{-6} moles/cm^3 on one side and 9.6×10^{-6} moles/cm^3 on the other side.

16. The K^+ concentration is 6×10^{-6} moles/cm^3 in the intracellular fluid and 1.2×10^{-5} moles/cm^3 inside of a cell. Find the diffusion potential.

17. The K^+ concentration is 5.8×10^{-6} moles/cm^3 in the intracellular fluid and 2×10^{-5} moles/cm^3 inside of a cell. Find the diffusion potential.

References

1. Guyton, Arthur C., *Basic Human Physiology: Normal Function and the Mechanisms of Disease,* W. B. Saunders Company (Philadelphia, 1977).

2. Crouch, James E. and J. Robert McClintic, *Human Anatomy and Physiology,* 2nd ed. John Wiley and Sons (New York, 1976).

3. Strong, Peter, *Biophysical Measurements,* Tektronix, Inc. Measurement Concept Series (Beaverton, Ore., 1976).

4. Van De Graaff, Kent M. and Stuart I. Fox, *Concepts of Human Anatomy and Physiology,* 3rd ed. Wm. C. Brown Publishers (Dubuque, IA, 1992).

CHAPTER 3
Introduction to Biomedical Instrumentation and Measurement

3-1 Objectives

1. Be able to understand *variation* and its effect on measurements.
2. Be able to recognize and correctly use *significant figures,* especially in the context of measurement.
3. Be able to understand and use *decibel* notation in systems and signals calculations.
4. Be able to use scientific notation.
5. Be able to explain the differences among *mean, median, mode, harmonic average, root mean square,* and *root of the sum of squares* averages of a data set.
6. Know the meaning of *standard deviation* and *variance* in measurement data.

3-2 Self-evaluation questions

These questions test your prior knowledge of the material in this chapter. Look for the answers as you read the text. After you have finished studying the chapter, try answering these questions and those at the end of the chapter.

1. _____ _____ is the square root of the variance of a data set.

2. The number of significant figures in a measurement can be increased by multiplying the result by another measured value (true or false).

3. Express 0.0000000826 A in scientific notation.

4. Name four different measures of the *average* of a data set.

3-3 Introduction

The British physicist and mathematician William Thompson, Lord Kelvin (1824-1907), reportedly once said something to the effect that one cannot really claim to know much about a thing until one can measure it. Much of the history of science and engineering in general and electronics and biomedical instrumentation in particular has been based on measuring things. Whether a measurement is made to troubleshoot an existing circuit, characterize and define a new circuit, or find the value of some nonelectronic physical variable (e.g., pressure or temperature), the common thread is the need for using some instrument (usually an electronic device) to make a measurement.

In this book you will learn about biomedical instrumentation devices. Although the entire universe of possible electronic measurement devices could never be included in a single text, or indeed a shelf full of texts, we will discuss the generic types used in a wide variety of biomedical applications.

You will also learn about the theory of measurement. In the naive sense it is possible to measure a voltage and use the information gained for some particular purpose without knowing much about measurement theory. However, there comes a point when it becomes necessary to understand a little of what you are doing in order to gain the maximum utility from your practical measurements.

Before beginning our discussions, some readers may wish to undertake a quick review of some arithmetic basics; these are found in the remainder of this chapter. For some students this material is simple, while for others it is new; for still others it is a necessary refresher. If you feel no need for the material in the following sections, then please feel free to skip ahead to the next chapter. Although not strictly needed, an understanding of the basic concepts of calculus would be helpful, at least in a descriptive sense. For those readers who have not had an introductory course in calculus, a quick overview of the basic principles is provided in appendix A. You need not be highly trained in mathematics to understand the basics presented in this text.

3-4 Significant figures

Much of our everyday experience deals with exact numbers of things: six stamps, $7.50, and seven people. These items can be counted and an exact numerical representation provided; all figures are significant in such cases. But in other situations you may take measurements that are subject to errors. For example, you might measure the height of a person as 67, 68, or 69 in., depending on how straight the person stands. Or what about the answer you give when asked a person's weight? The scale may register 162 lb, but one of the balance weights may not be perfect, or perhaps the scale dial at rest sticks a little off zero. How many people do you know who own a perfectly accurate watch that never needs to be reset? None, of course. These flaws are implicitly resolved when we apply the concept of *significant figures* to the measurements. This concept demands that we *impute no more precision or accuracy to a measurement or calculation than the natural physical reality of the situation permits.*

The counting numbers (1, 2, 3, 4, 5, 6, 7, 8, and 9) are always significant. Zero (0) is significant only if it is used to indicate exactly zero, or a truly null case. Zero is not significant if it is used merely as a place holder to make the numbers more easily read on the printed page. For example, if the number is properly written, then "0.60" means *exactly* six-tenths and not approximately 0.6; the zero used here is significant. If the number is written "0.6," then we may assume that it means six-tenths plus or minus some amount of either error or uncertainty.

When we use numbers to indicate a quantity, then the concept of significant figures becomes important. For example, "16 gallons" has two significant figures but can reasonably be taken to mean that the quantity of liquid is somewhere between 15 and 17 gallons. But if our device for measuring liquids is better, then we might write "16.0" gallons to indicate precisely 16 gallons plus or minus a very small error; i.e., perhaps the real value is between 15.9 and 16.1 gallons. Consider a pressure gauge that is guaranteed to an accuracy of ±5%. A reading of 100 torr has three figures, meaning that the actual pressure is between (100 − 5%) and (100 + 5%), or 95 to 105 torr (two significant figures).

Consider a practical measurement situation. A digital voltmeter is used to measure an electrical potential difference of exactly 15 volts (V). The instrument reads from 00.00 to 19.99 V, with an accuracy of ±1%. In addition, digital voltmeters typically have a ±1 digit error in the least significant position because of their design; this problem is called *last digit bobble*. For the digital voltmeter in question:

$$19.99$$

Most significant digit $\uparrow$ $\uparrow$ least significant digit

The last digit bobble problem means that a reading of 15.00 V could represent any value between (15.00 − 00.01), or 14.99 V, and (15.00 + 00.01), or 15.01 V. In addition, the error of 1% means that the actual voltage could be ±(15 × 0.01), or ±0.15 V. Thus, the actual voltage could be (15.00 − 0.15) V to (15.00 + 0.15) V, or a range of +14.84 to +15.16 V.

If both errors are minus:

Reading: 15.00 V
            −0.01 V
            −0.15 V
            14.84 V (worst case)

or, if both errors are positive:

Reading: 15.00 V
            +0.15 V
            +0.01 V
            15.16 V (worst case)

Significant figure errors are propagated in calculations. A rule to remember is that *the number of significant figures is not improved by combining the numbers with other numbers.* For example, multiplying a significant digit by a nonsignificant digit yields a result that has at least one nonsignificant digit. Often, the number of significant figures decreases in calculation, but it does not increase. Suppose we measure a voltage as 15.65 V and a current (I) in the same electrical circuit as 0.025 amperes (A). The power (P) is the product VI. Let's find that product, placing a little hat (^) over

each digit that is not significant, and then carry that notation down wherever a nonsignificant digit is a factor with another digit.

$$
\begin{array}{r}
15.6\hat{5} \\
\times\ 0.02\hat{5} \\
\hline
78\hat{2}\hat{5} \\
313\hat{0} \\
000\hat{0} \\
\underline{000\hat{0}} \\
00.39\hat{1}\hat{2}\hat{5}
\end{array}
$$

As can be seen, only the 3 and one of the leading zeros are significant. Thus, we claim more precision than is truly available if we list the power as 0.39 watts (W) when the 9 is not significant. We might better list this value as 0.4 W.

The reason scientists and engineers are so particular about significant figures is that it is bad form, and potentially dangerous under some circumstances, to claim more precision or accuracy than is truly the case. For this reason, we typically limit the figures to the number of decimal places for which a reasonable expectation of physical reality obtains.

Significant figure rules were perhaps a little easier to understand and use in the days when scientists and engineers calculated on slide rules. Those tools were limited to two or three digits, so one was less tempted to write down a very long number. But in this age of inexpensive 10-digit scientific pocket calculators, and the nearly universal distribution of personal computers, the distinction often gets lost. Consider a simple electrical problem as an example. One expression of Ohm's law states that the current (I) flowing in a circuit is the quotient of the voltage (V) and the resistance (R). Suppose 10 V is applied to a resistance of 3 ohms (Ω). According to a pocket scientific calculator, the current is 10 V/3 Ω = 3.333333333 A. Does anyone really think that an ordinary laboratory ammeter can measure to within 10^{-9} A (i.e., 3.33 *nanoamperes*)? In most cases, we could not claim more than 3.33 or 3.333 A (at most) with very high-quality meters that have been recently calibrated. Indeed, on most lower quality instruments 3 or 3.3 would be a more reasonable statement of the current reading.

Being mindful of significant figures is a key factor in making good measurements and maintaining the integrity and credibility of the measurement system.

3-5 Scientific notation

Scientific notation is a simple arithmetic shorthand that allows one to deal with very large or very small numbers using only a few digits between 1 and 10, and *power-of-ten exponents*. The form of a number in scientific notation is:

$$n.ij \times 10^x$$

Numbers — base-10, exponent

For example, if the age of a college professor is 47 years, then it could be written:

$$\text{Age} = 4.7 \times 10^1 \text{ years} \qquad (3\text{-}1)$$

(Note the unit *years* in the equation. The *specification of a value is never complete if the units are not included*; $47 \times 4.7 \times 10^1$ is *not* the same as 47 *years* or 4.7×10^1 *years*. The only exception is when the quantity is inherently nondimensional.)

When the exponent is negative, it is the same as saying $1/10^x$. In other words:

$$10^{-x} = \frac{1}{10^x} \qquad (3\text{-}2)$$

Some of the standard values in power-of-ten notation, along with their respective prefixes for use with units, are:

1/1,000,000,000	=	0.000000001 = 10^{-9}	nano
1/1,000,000	=	0.000001 = 10^{-6}	micro
1/100,000	=	0.00001 = 10^{-5}	
1/10,000	=	0.0001 = 10^{-4}	
1/1,000	=	0.001 = 10^{-3}	milli
1/100	=	0.01 = 10^{-2}	centi

1/10	=	0.10 = 10^{-1}	deci
1.0	=	10^0	
10	=	10^1	deka
100	=	10^2	hecto
1,000	=	10^3	kilo
10,000	=	10^4	
100,000	=	10^5	
1,000,000	=	10^6	mega
1,000,000,000	=	10^9	giga[1]

Scientific notation is especially appealing when dealing with numbers for which there are only a few significant figures. If we measure a human brain wave scalp surface potential (electroencephalogram, or EEG) as 143.6 microvolts (μV), then we may reasonably prefer to represent it as 1.44×10^{-4} V.

The prefixes listed above are used to subdivide units. For example, *milli* means 1/1000 (or 0.001), so a millimeter is 0.001 m, and a milliampere is 0.001 A. Similarly, *kilo* means 1,000, so a kilometer is 1,000 m, and a kilohertz is 1,000 Hz.

3-6 Units and physical constants

In accordance with standard medical, engineering, and scientific practice, all units in this text will be in either the centimeter-gram-second (CGS) or the meter-kilogram-second (MKS) system, unless otherwise specified. These units are taken from the Système International (SI), otherwise known as the *metric system*. Because the SI depends on using multiplying prefixes in the basic units, we include a table of common metric prefixes (Table 3-1). Table 3-2 gives the standard physical units; Table 3-3 shows physical constants of interest, including those used in problems in this and other chapters; and Table 3-4 lists some common conversion factors.

---

[1]Note: 1,000,000,000 (10^9) is called 1 *billion* in the United States but 1000 *million* in England and most of the rest of the world. The term *milliard* was once applied to 10^9. To be 1 billion outside of the United States the number would have to be 1,000,000,000,000 (10^{12}).

TABLE 3-1   METRIC PREFIXES

Metric prefix	Multiplying factor	Symbol
tera	10^{12}	T
giga	10^{9}	G
mega	10^{6}	M
kilo	10^{3}	k
hecto	10^{2}	h
deka	10^{1}	da
deci	10^{-1}	d
centi	10^{-2}	c
milli	10^{-3}	m
micro	10^{-6}	μ
nano	10^{-9}	n
pico	10^{-12}	p
femto	10^{-15}	f
atto	10^{-18}	a

TABLE 3-2   STANDARD PHYSICAL UNITS

Quantity	Unit	Symbol
Capacitance	farad	F
Electric charge	coulomb	C
Conductance	siemens	S
Conductivity	siemens/meter	S/m
Current	ampere	A
Energy	joule (watt-second)	J
Field	volts/meter	E
Flux linkage	weber(volt-second)	
Frequency	hertz	Hz
Inductance	henry	H
Length	meter	m
Mass	gram	g
Power	watt	W
Resistance	ohm	Ω
Time	second	s
Velocity	meter/second	m/s
Electric potential	volt	V

TABLE 3-3   PHYSICAL CONSTANTS

Constant	Value	Symbol
Boltzmann's constant	1.38×10^{-23} J/K	K
Electric charge (e^{-})	1.6×10^{-19} C	q
Electron (volt)	1.6×10^{-19} J	eV
Electron (mass)	9.12×10^{-31} kg	m
Permeability of free space	$4\pi \times 10^{-7}$ H/m	U_o
Permittivity of free space	8.85×10^{-12} F/m	ϵ_o
Planck's constant	6.626×10^{-34} J-s	h
Velocity of electromagnetic waves	3×10^{8} m/s	c
Pi	3.141592654	π

TABLE 3-4   CONVERSION FACTORS

1 in.	=	2.54 cm
1 in.	=	25.4 mm
1 ft	=	0.305 m
1 mile	=	1.61 km
1 nautical mile	=	6,080 ft
1 statute mile	=	5,280 ft
1 mil	=	2.54×10^{-5} m
1 kg	=	2.2 lb
1 kg	=	1,000 g
1 g	=	1,000 mg
1 neper	=	8.686 dB
1 gaus	=	10,000 teslas
1 torr	=	1 mm Hg

3-7 What is average?

What is *average?* That's a common question, and the answer is not always as obvious as it might seem to be. There are several different kinds of average, and all of them are valid in the right situa-tions. Various areas of biomedical equipment technology use different types of averages in different cases.

The word *average* refers to the *most typical value,* or *most expected value,* in a collection of numerical data. When you collect data, the results can vary from one observation to another in a number of ways (even when conditions are supposed to be the same).

First, of course, there is old-fashioned measurement and observational error. Not all rulers are truly the same, and not all applications of the same ruler to the same object turn out the same. Nor is it probable that even the same pair of perfect eyes will correctly read the scale every time a measurement is taken. In short, there will always be some *variability* in the measurements from one trial to another.

Next, there will be some actual variability in the events being recorded. Natural phenomena do, in fact, vary for one reason or another; blood pressure and heart rate may change slightly from heartbeat to heartbeat quite apart from any external factor. One way to handle these variations is to find the most typical value for the lot. Consider the case in which a student observed a red berry bush over a period of time. At one point, the observer counted 28 bunches of berries and found one to eight berries in the different bunches. What does average mean in this case? There are actually several different kinds of average, but the most commonly encountered are the *arithmetic mean* (usually called simply the *mean*), the *median,* and the *mode*. These are each different from the others, and all of them are correct averages when used in the right context. Let's look at the data a little more closely (Table 3-5).

The arithmetic mean is the type of average that most people use everyday. The mean is the sum of all values divided by the number (n) of different values. Or, to put it in proper form:

$$\overline{X} = \frac{X_1 + X_2 + X_3 + \cdots + X_n}{n} \qquad (3\text{-}3)$$

The sum of all 28 values in Table 3-5 is 125, so what is the average?

$$\overline{X} = \frac{125}{28} = 4.46 \qquad (3\text{-}4)$$

The mean average is 4.46, but don't expect to actually find a 0.46 berry. This average is the arithmetic mean.

TABLE 3-5 DATA VALUES

4 6 5 5 3 6 4 33 4 5 3 1 6 5 2 5 2 3 4 4 5 7
7 8 4 6 5

The *median* is another type of average: it is the *middle value in the data set;* that is, the value at the point where exactly *half of the values are above it and half are below it.* In our berry example there are 28 values, an even number, so the median will be midway between two of them (with 14 above and 14 below). Figure 3-1 shows the data distribution in a crude kind of bar graph. Count the X's in each category from one end to the middle, and then the other end. Note that there are 14 values between 0 and 4 and 14 values from 5 to 9. That means the median value will be half-way between 4 and 5, or 4.5. If there were an odd number of data points, then the middle point—the median—would be the data point that has an equal number of points above it and below it.

The *mode* is also an average of sorts and is defined as the *most frequently occurring value* in the data set. In the data in Table 3-5, the mode is easily seen in the X-chart (Figure 3-1). There were

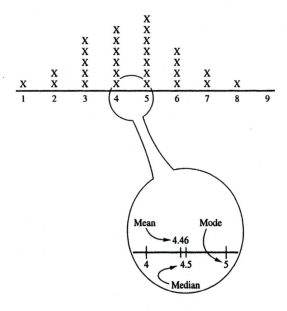

Figure 3-1
Data distribution (X chart) for 28 data values.
Source: Carr, J. J., *Elements of Electronic Instrumentation and Measurement,* (EEIM), Prentice Hall (Englewood Cliffs, N.J., 1996). Subsequent source notes will specify EEIM only.

more bunches with five berries than any other number, so 5 is the mode. So now we have an arithmetic mean of 4.46, a median of 4.5, and a mode of 5, and all are the average of the same data set depending on the definition of *average.*

Different averages are used for different situations. If the data is *perfectly symmetrical,* then the mean, median, and mode are the same number. In fact, that's nearly the case in the data above. If the mean, median, and mode are not the same, then the data is not symmetrical around the mean, and the difference is a test of that symmetry. In the berry bush data, the distribution is nearly symmetrical, so the mean could be used. But in other situations the mean is not terribly useful, especially if one or two data points have very large or very small values compared with the rest of the data.

The mean is best used when the measurement data is symmetrical, the median is often used when the data is highly asymmetrical due to outliers, and the mode is used to answer questions, such as: What is the most common cause of death? Or what is the most popular TV show on Friday night?

Other averages include the *geometric mean* and the *harmonic mean* (H.M.). The geometric mean is often used when the data is not symmetrical, especially in biological studies. For example, suppose you have $48 to spend, and you spend half of your available money each day for 5 days. The data would tabulate as shown in Table 3-6. The arithmetic mean of the five values is:

$$\frac{48 + 24 + 12 + 6 + 3}{5} = \frac{93}{5} = 18.6$$

TABLE 3-6   TABULATION OF GEOMETRIC MEAN (EXAMPLE)

Day	Amount ($)	Amt spent	Amt remaining
1	48	24	24
2	24	12	12
3	12	6	6
4	6	3	3
5	3	1.50	1.50

If we graph these values (Figure 3-2a), we note that the line connecting the tops of the bar graphs is not straight. To find the geometric mean, we need to find the *logarithm* of each value, add the logarithms up, and then take the *logarithmic mean.* Then we take the *antilog* of the log-mean. The log-mean is:

$$\frac{\text{Log}48 + \text{Log}24 + \text{Log}12 + \text{Log}6 + \text{Log}3}{5}$$

$$= \frac{1.68 + 1.38 + 1.08 + 0.778 + 0.477}{5}$$

$$= \frac{5.395}{5}$$

$$= 1.079$$

Now take the antilog of the answer:

$$\text{Log}^{-1}(1.079) = 11.99$$

The logarithmic chart (Figure 3-2a) is not a straight line. If we want to straighten that line, we use *semilog paper* (Figure 3-2b) or make the translation with a computer graphing program.

The H.M. is a bit more complicated and is used when data are expressed in *ratios,* such as miles per hour or dollars per dozen. The expression for H.M. reflects the fact that it is the *reciprocal of the mean of the reciprocals of the data:*

$$\text{H.M.} = \frac{1}{\left(\dfrac{\dfrac{1}{X_1} + \dfrac{1}{X_2} + \dfrac{1}{X_3} + \cdots + \dfrac{1}{X_n}}{n}\right)} \quad (3\text{-}5)$$

Suppose we compare the price of eggs in the local store over 1 month (Table 3-7):

The arithmetic mean is:

$$\frac{\$2.29 + \$1.98 + \$1.56 + \$2.04}{4}$$

$$= \frac{7.87}{4} = \$1.9675 \approx \$1.97$$

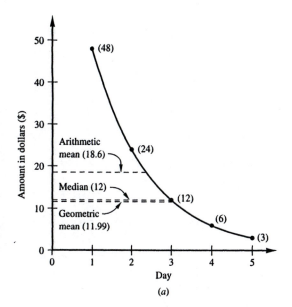

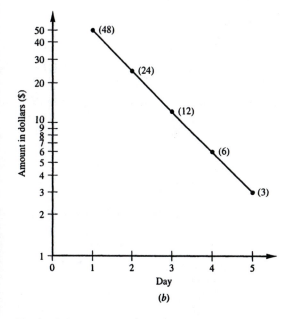

Figure 3-2
(*a*) Linear graph of data, (*b*) semilogarithmic graph of same data. Source: EEIM.

TABLE 3-7   TABULATION OF HARMONIC MEAN (EXAMPLE)

Week	Price ($/doz)
1	2.29
2	1.98
3	1.56
4	2.04

but the harmonic mean is:

$$\text{H.M.} = \cfrac{1}{\left(\cfrac{\cfrac{1}{\$2.29} + \cfrac{1}{\$1.98} + \cfrac{1}{\$1.56} + \cfrac{1}{\$2.04}}{4}\right)}$$

$$\text{H.M.} = \cfrac{1}{\left(\cfrac{0.437 + 0.505 + 0.641 + 0.490}{4}\right)}$$

$$\text{H.M.} = \frac{\$2.073}{4} = \frac{\$1}{0.518} = \$1.929 \approx \$1.93$$

Root-mean-square and root-sum-squares average

Other averages are sometimes seen in biomedical science, engineering, and technology: *integrated average*, *root-mean-square* (rms) and *root-sum-squares* (rss). The integrated average is the *area under the curve of the function* (Figure 3-3) divided by the segment of the range over which the average is taken:

$$\overline{X} = \frac{1}{T}\int_{t1}^{t2} X\,dt \qquad (3\text{-}6)$$

The integrated average is often found in electronic circuits in which either a resistor-capacitor (RC) low-pass filter or an RC operational amplifier circuit, called a Miller integrator, is used. This circuit has an RC product much greater than the period of the applied input waveform. The output of

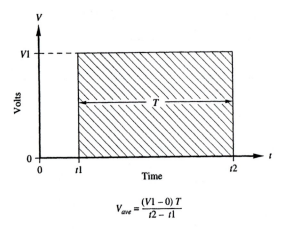

$$V_{ave} = \frac{(V1 - 0)\, T}{t2 - t1}$$

Figure 3-3
Integrated average. Source: EEIM.

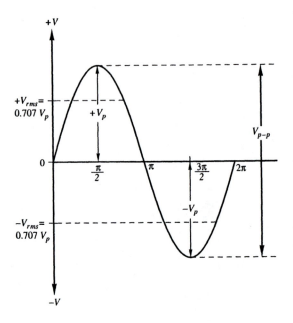

Figure 3-4
Peak value of a sine wave voltage. Source: EEIM.

the circuit is proportional to the time average of the input signal. In computer-based instruments the integrated average is found either by using a numerical integration algorithm or by adding up a large number of sequential samples, spaced equally in time, and then dividing by the total time period.

The rms value is used extensively in electrical circuits and certain other technologies. For example, a sinewave alternating current (AC) wave may be compared with the direct current (DC) voltage level that will produce the same amount of heating in an electrical resistance. The value of the AC wave that is the DC heating equivalent is the rms value. The definition of rms is:

$$V_{rms} = \sqrt{\frac{1}{T} \int_{t1}^{t2} (V(t))^2 \, dt} \qquad (3\text{-}7)$$

where

V_{rms} is the rms value

T is the time interval t1 to t2

$V(t)$ is a time-varying voltage function

For the special case of the sinewave, the rms value of voltage is $V_p/\sqrt{2}$, or 0.707 V_p, where V_p is the peak voltage (Figure 3-4). For waveshapes other than sinusoidal, however, Equation 3-7 will evaluate differently.

The rss average is used when pieces of different data are combined to form a single number, even though they are in no way correlated with each other. For example, noise signals in electronic circuits are errors and may come from several different *independent* sources. Suppose we have n independent noise voltage sources (Vn_1, Vn_1, $\cdots$ Vn_n). Where these sources are truly independent of each other, they are *decorrelated* and therefore cannot be simply combined in a linear additive manner but rather must be combined using the rss method:

$$V_{rss} = \sqrt{\sum_{i=1}^{n} (Vn_i)^2} \qquad (3\text{-}8)$$

$$V_{rss} = \sqrt{(Vn1)^2 + (Vn2)^2 + (Vn3)^2 + \cdots + (Vn_n)^2} \qquad (3\text{-}9)$$

The rss method is used sometimes to define a single valued error term from a number of uncorrelated error terms or, alternatively, to find a single standard error of a number of measurements of the same value.

Example 3-1

An electronic amplifier circuit contains five independent noise sources that produce the following decorrelated noise signal voltage levels: $Vn1 = 25$ nanovolts (nV); $Vn2 = 56$ nV; $Vn3 = -33$ nV; $Vn4 = -10$ nV; and $Vn5 = 62$ nV. What is the rss value of a composite noise signal?

Solution:

$$V_{rss} = \sqrt{(Vn1)^2 + (Vn2)^2 + (Vn3)^2 + (Vn4)^2 + (Vn5)^2}\, nV$$

$$= \sqrt{(25)^2 + (56)^2 + (-33)^2 + (-10)^2 + (62)^2}\, nV$$

$$= \sqrt{625 + 3136 + 1089 + 100 + 3844}\, nV$$

$$= \sqrt{8794} = 93.8\, nV$$

Note that the rss value in the example above is not the same as the summation of the components.

Although it is common practice in biomedical measurements, and in science experiments in general, to quote the average value of the data acquired, one must be cautious in using the correct average (or the most reasonable average) and to correctly interpret what *average* means in context.

3-8 Logarithmic representation of signal levels: decibel notation

The subject of decibels (dB) frequently confuses the newcomer to electronics, and even many an old-timer seems to have occasional memory lapses regarding the subject. For the benefit of both, and because the subject is so vitally important to understanding instrumentation and measurement systems, we will review the decibel.

The decibel measurement originated in the telephone industry and was named after telephone inventor Alexander Graham Bell. The original unit was the *bel*. The prefix *deci* means one-tenth, so the decibel is one-tenth of a bel. The bel is too large for most common applications, so it is rarely, if ever, used. Thus, we will concentrate only on the more familiar decibel.

The decibel is nothing more than a means of logarithmically expressing the ratio between two signal levels; for example, the output-over-input signal ratio (gain) of an amplifier. Because the decibel is a ratio, it is also dimensionless, despite the fact that dB looks like a dimension to some people.

Consider the voltage amplifier as an example of dimensionless gain; its gain is expressed as the output voltage over the input voltage (V_o/V_{in}). It is dimensionless because the units are volts/volts, which *cancel out*.

Example 3-2

A voltage amplifier outputs 6 V when the input signal has a potential of 0.5 V. Find the voltage gain (A_v).

$$A_v = \frac{V_o}{V_{in}}$$

$$A_v = \frac{6\ V}{0.5\ V} = 12$$

Note above that volts (V) units appeared in both numerator and denominator and thus cancelled out, leaving only a dimensionless 12 behind (*Cancel out* is a short way to express the situation in which units in the numerator and denominator are the same and thus evaluate to 1).

To analyze system gains and losses using simple addition and subtraction rather than multiplication and division, we use a little "math trick" on the ratio. We take the base-10 logarithm of the ratio and multiply it by a scaling factor (either 10 or 20). For voltage systems such as our voltage amplifier, the expression becomes:

$$dB = 20\, LOG \left(\frac{V_o}{V_{in}} \right) \quad (3\text{-}10)$$

In the earlier example, we had a voltage amplifier with a gain of 12 because 0.5 V input produced a 6-V output. How is this same gain (i.e., V_o/V_{in} ratio) expressed in decibels?

$$dB = 20\ LOG\ (V_o/V_{in})$$
$$dB = 20\ LOG\ (6/0.5)$$
$$dB = 20\ LOG\ (12) = \mathbf{21.6}$$

Despite the fact that we have changed the ratio by converting it to a logarithm, *the decibel is nonetheless nothing more than a means for expressing a ratio*. Thus, a voltage gain of 12 can also be expressed as a gain of 21.6 dB.

A similar expression can be used for current amplifiers, where the gain ratio is I_o/I_{in}:

$$dB = 20\ LOG\ \left(\frac{I_o}{I_{in}}\right) \qquad (3\text{-}11)$$

For power measurements we need a modified expression to account for the fact that power is proportional to the square of the voltage or current:

$$dB = 10\ LOG\ \left(\frac{P_o}{P_{in}}\right) \qquad (3\text{-}12)$$

We now have three basic equations for calculating decibels, which are summarized in Figure 3-5.

Adding it all up

So why bother converting seemingly easy-to-handle, dimensionless numbers like voltage or power gains to a logarithmic number like decibels? Because it makes calculating signal strengths in a system easier. To see this effect, let's consider the multistage system in Figure 3-6. Here we

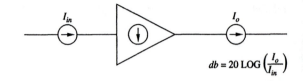

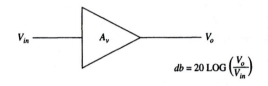

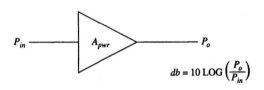

Figure 3-5
Three basic equations for calculating decibels.
Source: EEIM.

have a hypothetical electronic circuit that has three amplifier stages and an attenuator pad. The stage gains are as follows:

$$A1 = V_1/V_{in} = 0.2/0.010 = 20$$
$$Atten = V_2/V1 = 0.1/0.2 = 0.5$$
$$A2 = V_3/V_2 = 1.5/0.1 = 15$$
$$A3 = V_o/V_3 = 6/1.5 = 4$$

The overall gain is the product of the stage gains in the system:

$$A_v = A1 \times Atten \times A2 \times A3$$
$$A_v = (20)(0.5)(15)(4) = \mathbf{600}$$

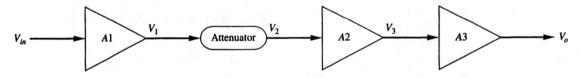

Figure 3-6
Three-stage amplifier with attenuator pad. Source: EEIM.

When converted to decibels, the gains are expressed as:

$$A1 = 26.02$$
$$\text{Atten} = -6.02$$
$$A2 = 23.52$$
$$A3 = 12.04$$

The overall gain of the system (in decibels) is the sum of these numbers:

$$A_{v(dB)} = A1 + \text{Attn} + A2 + A3$$
$$A_{v(dB)} = (26.02) + (-6.02) + (23.52) + (12.04)$$
$$A_{v(dB)} = 55.56 \text{ dB}$$

The system gain calculated earlier was 600, and this number should be the same as above:

$$A_{dB} = 20 \text{ LOG } (600)$$
$$A_{dB} = \textbf{55.56 dB}$$

They're the same.

One convenience of the decibel scheme is that gains are expressed as positive numbers and losses as negative numbers. Conceptually, it seems easier to understand a loss of −6.02 dB than a loss represented as a gain of +0.50.

Converting between decibel and gain notation

We sometimes face situations in which gain is expressed in decibels, and we want to calculate the gain in terms of the output-input ratio. Common values of gain and loss expressed in decibels are shown in Table 3-8. Suppose we have an amplifier of +20 dB with an input signal of 1 mV (1 mV = 0.001 V), as shown in Figure 3-7. What is the expected output voltage? It is 20 dB higher than 0.001 V. However, your meter or oscilloscope is probably not calibrated in decibels but rather in volts. (Note: Some instruments are indeed calibrated in logarithmic units or decibels, e.g., audio voltmeters are often calibrated in both volts and decibels or volume units). By using a little algebra, we can rearrange the expression (dB = 20 LOG

TABLE 3-8 COMMON GAINS AND LOSSES EXPRESSED IN DECIBELS

Ratio (out/in)	Voltage gain (dB)	Power gain (dB)
1/1000	−60	−30
1/100	−40	−20
1/10	−20	−10
1/2	−6.02	−3.01
1	0	0
2	+6.02	+3.01
5	+14	+7
10	+20	+10
100	+40	+20
1,000	+60	+30
10,000	+80	+40
100,000	+100	+50
1,000,000	+120	+60

$[V_o/V_{in}]$) to solve for output voltage, V_o. The new expression is:

$$V_o = V_{in} \, 10^{dB/20} \qquad (3\text{-}13)$$

which is also sometimes written in the alternative form:

$$V_o = V_{in} \, EXP \, (dB/20) \qquad (3\text{-}14)$$

In the example above we want to calculate V_o if the gain in dB and the input signal voltage are known. We can calculate it from the equations above. Using the values given above (20 dB and 1 mV):

$$V_o = V_{in} \, EXP \, (dB/20)$$
$$V_o = (0.001) \, EXP \, (20/20)$$
$$V_o = (0.001) \, EXP \, (1)$$
$$V_o = (0.001)(100) = \textbf{0.01 V}$$

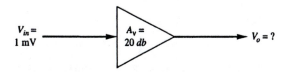

Figure 3-7
20-dB amplifier with 1-mV input signal.
Source: EEIM.

For those who don't want to make the calculation, Table 3-8 shows common voltage and power
gains and losses expressed both ways.

Again, we see the convenience of decibel scales
over gain ratios. If we want to calculate the system
gain of a circuit that has a gain of 10,000 and an
attenuation of 1/1000 in series, then we can do it
either way:

$$A_v = (10,000)(0.001) = 10$$

or

$$A_v = (+80 \text{ dB}) + (-60 \text{ dB}) = +20 \text{ dB}$$

Special decibel scales

Various user groups have defined special decibel-
based scales that meet their own needs. They make
a special scale by defining a certain reference signal level as 0 dB and comparing all other signal
levels to that defined point. In the dimensionless
dB scale, 0 dB corresponds to a gain of unity
(Table 3-8). But if we define 0 dB as a particular
signal level, then we obtain one of the special
scales. Below are listed several such scales commonly used in electronics.

dBm Used in reference frequency (RF) measurements, 0 dBm is defined as 1 mW of RF
signal dissipated in a 50-Ω resistive load.

VU (volume units) The VU scale is used in
audio work and defines 0 VU as 1 mW of
1,000 Hz audio signal dissipated in a 600-Ω
resistive load.

dB (telephone) The dB scale, now obsolete,
defined 0 dB as 6 mW of a 1,000 Hz audio
signal dissipated in a 500-Ω load (once used in
telephone work). (Note: One source listed 400
Hz as the reference frequency.)

dBmV Used in television antenna coaxial cable systems with a 75-Ω resistive impedance,
the dBmV system uses 1,000 μV (1 mV)
across a 75-Ω resistive load as the 0 dBmv
reference point.

Consider the case of the RF signal generator. In
RF systems using standard 50-Ω input-and-output
impedances, all power levels are referenced to 0
dBm being 1 mW (0.001 W). To write signal levels
in dBm, we use the modified power dB expression:

$$dBm = 10 \ LOG \left(\frac{P}{1 \ mW} \right) \qquad (3\text{-}15)$$

Example 3-3 _____

What is the signal level 9 mW as expressed in
dBm?

$$dBm = 10 \ LOG \ (P/1 \ mW)$$
$$dBm = 10 \ LOG \ (9/1)$$
$$dBm = \textbf{9.54 dBm}$$

Thus, when we refer to a signal level of 9.54
dBm, we mean an RF power of 9 mW dissipated
in a 50Ω load.

_____

Signal levels less than 1 mW show up as negative dBm. For example, 0.02 mW is also written as
−17 dBm.

Converting dBm to voltage

Signal generator output controls and level meters
are frequently calibrated in microvolts or millivolts
(although some are also calibrated in dBm). How
do we convert dBm to volts or volts to dBm?
Microvolts to dBm Use the expression $P = V^2/R$
$= V^2/50$ to find milliwatts, and then use the dBm
expression given above.

Example 3-4 _____

Express a signal level of 800 μV (i.e., 0.8 mV)
rms in dBm.

$$P = V^2/50$$
$$P = (0.8m)^2/50$$
$$P = 0.64\mu/50 = 0.0128 \ \mu W$$
$$dBm = 10 \ LOG \ (P/1 \ mW)$$
$$dBm = 10 \ LOG \ (0.0128 \ \mu W/1 \ mW)$$
$$dBm = -48.9$$

Converting dBm to microvolts or millivolts Find the power level represented by the dBm level, and then calculate the voltage using 50 Ω as the load.

Example 3-5

What voltage exists across a 50-Ω resistive load when -6 dBm is dissipated in the load?

$$P = (1 \text{ mW})(10^{\text{dBm}/10})$$
$$P = (1 \text{ mW})(10^{-6 \text{ dBm}/10})$$
$$P = (1 \text{ mW})(10^{-0.6})$$
$$P = (1 \text{ mW})(0.25) = \textbf{0.25 mW}$$

If $P = V^2/50$, then $V = (50P)^{1/2} = 7.07(P^{1/2})$, so:

$$V = (7.07)(P^{1/2})$$
$$V = (7.07)(0.25^{1/2}) = \textbf{3.54 mV}$$

Note: Because power is expressed in milliwatts, the resulting answer is in millivolts. To convert to microvolts, multiply the result by 1,000.

3-9 The basics of measurement theory

Measurements are ". . . the assignment of numerals to represent [physical] properties." Measurements are made to fulfill one or more of several different goals: obtain information about a physical phenomenon, assign a value to some fundamental constant, record trends, control some process, correlate behavior with other parameters to obtain insight into their relationships, or determine how much to pay for a beef cow. A measurement is an act that is designed to ". . . derive quantitative information about. . . [some physical phenomenon] . . . by comparison to a reference . . ." (Herceg 1972) or a standard (1). The physical quantity being measured is called the *measurand,* or *factor.*

Data classes

The data that result from measurements can be divided into two major classes, which are each divided into two subclasses. The major divisions include *qualitative* data and *quantitative* data.

Qualitative data Qualitative data is nonnumerical, or categorical. It includes information, such as the presence or nonpresence of some factor, good or bad, defective or not defective, gender, and race.

Qualitative data does not inherently result in numbers, and thus is sometimes held in less esteem than quantitative data. This attitude is misguided unless there is an inherent need for numbers in a particular case.

Qualitative data can be further broken into two subgroups: *nominal* data and *ordinal* data.

Nominal data is qualitative data that has no inherent order or rank. Examples include lists of names, labels, and groupings.

Ordinal data allows ranking, but differences between data points are either nonexistent or meaningless.

Qualitative data can sometimes be given a numerical flavor by correct collection techniques. For example, because many of these data are binary (i.e., has only two possible results), one can assign the digits 0 and 1 (e.g., 1 for yes and 0 for no). Another popular method is to assign some arbitrary but consistent scale indicating depth of feeling, preferences, and so forth. For example, a five-point scale (Figure 3-8) is often used to assign numerals to questions that are largely value judgments.

Quantitative data Quantitative data are those which naturally result in some number to represent a factor. Examples include amount of money, length, temperature, number of defects per unit, number of defective units, voltage, pressure, and weight.

Quantitative data can be further divided into two subclasses: *interval* data and *ratio* data.

Interval data allow for a meaningful comparison of differences but not the relative values of

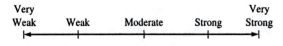

Association of Two Factors

| Very Weak | Weak | Moderate | Strong | Very Strong |

Figure 3-8
Five-point scale for use with qualitative data.

two or more factors. Such measurements are made relative to an arbitrarily selected standard zero point. For example, Western cultures assign calendar dates according to the supposed birth date of Christ. In other cultures, the zero point is some other fixed historical event.

Other examples of interval measures include the Celsius (centigrade) and Fahrenheit temperature scales (°C and °F, respectively). The Celsius scale sets the zero degree point at the freezing point of water. Another arbitrary (but convenient) reference point on the Celsius scale is 100°C, which is the boiling point of water. These points are used because they are easy to replicate whenever one wants to calibrate a Celsius thermometer. The Celsius scale is also called *centigrade* because there are 100 *(centi)* equal divisions between the arbitrarily set 0°C and 100°C points. The zero point on the Fahrenheit scale is equally arbitrary, but its selection seems to us a bit irrational (water freezes at 32°F).

The 0°C and 100°C points on the Celsius scale are arbitrary because there is no particular reason to select these points except for calibration convenience. After all, there are temperatures colder than 0°C and hotter than 100°C.

The selection of zero points on the temperature scale illustrates the properties of interval data: We can make meaningful statements about differences of temperature, but differences cannot be scaled up (i.e., 40°C is *not* twice the temperature of 20°C).

Ratio data is based on some fixed or natural zero point, such as weights, pressures, and temperatures (e.g., the Kelvin scale). Retaining our temperature scale example, the Kelvin scale uses degrees the same size as those used in the Celsius scale (a change of 1°C is the same as a change of 1°K), but the zero reference point is what physicists call *absolute zero,* i.e., the temperature at which all molecular motion ceases (0°K is about −273.16°C). Thus, 0°K represents a natural zero point.

A consequence of having a natural zero reference point is that ratios as well as differences are meaningful. Raising a temperature from 100°K to 200°K is an increase of twice the temperature.

Measurement standards

Metrology, the science of measurement, requires a *rule* to which things are compared; that rule is called a *standard.* Not all standards are equal, so there is a hierarchy of standards (Figure 3-9): *international reference standards, primary standards, transfer standards, working standards,* and *shop-level standards, secondary standards,* and *gauges* and *instruments.*

International reference standards These standards are agreed on by the International Standards Institute (ISI). For years the reference standard for the meter was a platinum bar 1.000 m long, which was stored in a vault in Paris and maintained by the ISI. Other international standards are kept by various authorities around the world.

Primary standards These are the principal standards maintained at a national level in the various countries. In the United States these standards are maintained by the National Institutes of Standards and Technology (NIST), formerly the National Bureau of Standards. Some primary standards are periodically taken to Paris, where they are compared with an international reference standard maintained by the ISI.

Transfer standards These standards are second level and are periodically compared with the primary standard. They are used to calibrate lower-order standards used in the country so that wear and tear on the primary standard is reduced.

Working standards Working standards are compared with transfer standards in a nationally certified laboratory or at the NIST. Such standards are said to be *NIST-traceable.*

Secondary standards These standards are used locally (e.g., in the plant) to calibrate instruments and gauges (see p. 41).

Gauges and instruments The lowest order of standards, these are the devices actually used to make measurements and collect data on the ob-

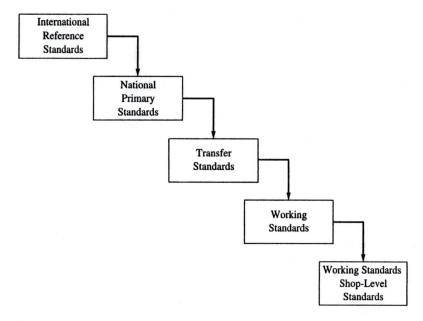

Figure 3-9
Hierarchy of standards.

jects being measured. Gauges and instruments are compared with either working standards or secondary standards.

Examples of these standards can be seen in the hierarchical chain leading from the local grocery checkout counter weighing scale all the way back to the NIST. The scale used to weigh the product sold by the pound is a gauge or an instrument standard (shop-level). In most states, a local (county or city) weights-and-measures inspector visits the stores and checks the calibration of the produce scales at each checkout counter to make sure that consumers get what they pay for. The inspector is equipped with a set of standard weights that can be placed on the scale. These are secondary standards. Once every 6 months, the inspector must take the secondary standards to a laboratory at the state level and compare the secondary standard weight set to a master set kept at the lab (the working standard). Once a year, the lab weight set is taken to either the NIST or a designated metrology

laboratory for comparison to a transfer standard. That transfer standard is, in turn, compared with the primary standard periodically.

Variation and error

All measurements are subject to a certain amount of *variation* caused by small *errors* in the measurement process, and by actual variation in the measured parameter. In this context, the idea of error does not mean mistake, but rather a normal random variation resulting from inherent limitations of the system. There are many different causes of random variation. Some errors are dependent on the particular type of measurement being made (and are a function of the type of meter being used), while other errors are caused by inherent variation in the process being measured.

Consider an ordinary meter stick as an analogy. It is divided into 100 large divisions of 1 cm each and 1000 small divisions of 1 mm each. Or is it? In truth, the distance from 0 to 100 cm is not *exactly* 100.0000 cm, but rather 100 ± ε cm, where ε is some small error. In addition, the spaces between divisions (either 1 mm or 1 cm) are not exactly the same size but vary somewhat from mark to mark. As a result, when you measure the size of, say, a printed circuit board, there will be some error.

Random variation causes the data obtained when making measurements to *disperse.* Consider a practical situation. Suppose we want to measure the mass of an electronic component, say a capacitor. The design specification weight is supposed to be 1.45 g, but when a sample of 30 identical capacitors are weighed on a very good scale, the results shown in Figure 3-10 and Table 3-9 were obtained. Even though the capacitors were all identical, there was a dispersion of the data points. Not one capacitor in the sample lot actually met the 1.45-g specification exactly, but rather were dispersed around 1.45 g.

If you examine a large number of capacitors and plot their weights on a histogram as in Figure 3-10a, you will find that a pattern emerges. As long as certain conditions are met, then the various weights will form into the familiar *bell-shaped curve* (Figure 3-10b), which is called (depending on country and context) the *normal distribution curve,* the *Gaussian curve,* and the *Laplacean.* Regardless of what it is called, the normal distribution pattern shown in Figure 3-10b is extremely common in science and technology.

The normal distribution curve plots frequency of occurrence against some other parameter. Note in Figure 3-10a that even with only a few data points, some values begin to stack up more than others. When thousands of capacitor weights are measured, it is likely that the resultant histogram will very nearly resemble the bell-shaped curve. The *mean* is usually designated by the Greek letter mu (μ) when the entire population of values is plotted or by an x-bar $(\overline{X})$ when only a sample of the population is taken.

One of the uses of the normal distribution curve is that it offers us a measure of the dispersion of

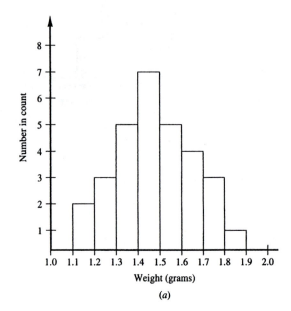

(a)

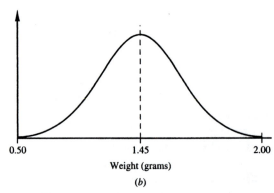

(b)

Figure 3-10
Weights of 30 capacitors plotted (*a*) in bar graph and (*b*) in line graph (normal distribution curve).
Source: EEIM.

TABLE 3-9   SORTED DATA POINTS (LOW-TO-HIGH)

1.16 1.18 1.2 1.26 1.26 1.3 1.3 1.3 1.33 1.35 1.4 1.4 1.4 1.4 1.4 1.43 1.48 1.5 1.5 1.5 1.5 1.53 1.6 1.6 1.62 1.65 1.7 1.7 1.7 1.81

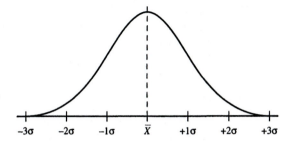

Figure 3-11
Standard deviation. Source: EEIM.

the data. This property of the data can be summed up as the *variance* and *standard deviation* of the data. For the entire population, standard deviation is denoted by Greek letter sigma (σ) and variance by σ^2. Variance is defined by:

$$\sigma^2 = \frac{\sum_{i=1}^{N}(X_i - \overline{X})^2}{N} \qquad (3\text{-}16)$$

Standard deviation, which is the square root of variance, is defined by:

$$\sigma = \sqrt{\frac{\sum_{i=1}^{N}(X_i - \overline{X})^2}{N}} \qquad (3\text{-}17)$$

Equations 3-16 and 3-17 define the variance and standard deviation for the entire population of data. If a small sample is taken, then replace σ^2 with s^2, σ with s, and N in the denominators with $N - 1$, as shown below:

$$\sigma^2 = \frac{\sum_{i=1}^{N}(X_i - \overline{X})^2}{N-1} \qquad (3\text{-}18)$$

and

$$\sigma = \sqrt{\frac{\sum_{i=1}^{N}(X_i - \overline{X})^2}{N-1}} \qquad (3\text{-}19)$$

If the process is truly random, then the value that one would report in making the measurement is the mean value, μ. But it is also necessary to specify either the variance or the standard deviation. We know that any particular measurement may or may not be μ. We also know that 68.27% of all values lie between $\pm 1\sigma$ (Figure 3-11), 98.45% between $\pm 2\sigma$, and 99.73% between $\pm 3\sigma$.

3-10 Summary

1. We recognize and use only the significant figures so that we impute no more precision or accuracy to a measurement than is justified by the situation.

2. The number of significant figures in a measurement is not improved by mathematically combining them with other numbers.

3. Scientific notation is an arithmetic shorthand that represents very large and very small quantities using power-of-ten exponents.

4. In the metric system, a base unit (e.g., the *meter* as the unit of length) is combined with a prefix that either multiplies or divides the units for larger or smaller quantities (e.g., *kilo*meters and *milli*meters).

5. The *average* of a number set is considered the most typical, or most expected, value. Three types of averages are commonly used (mean, median, and mode); other types are less commonly used (geometric, harmonic, and logarithmic mean; rms and rss).

6. Signal levels are often represented on a logarithmic scale called the *decibel scale*. Gains and losses expressed in decibels can be directly added or subtracted in making circuit and systems calculations. The decibel is an expression of the ratio of two signals. Standardized decibel notations are often used by setting one signal level to a standard value.

7. When measurements are made, the quantity being measured is called the *measurand.*

3-11 Recapitulation

Now return to the objectives and self-evaluation questions at the beginning of the chapter and see how well you can answer them. If you cannot answer certain questions, place a check mark next to each and review appropriate parts of the text. Next, try to answer the following questions and problems using the same procedure.

Questions

1. State the number of significant figures used in each of the following: (a) 1, (b) 22, (c) 5, (d) 245.

2. State the number of significant figures in each of the following: (a) 2.4, (b) 4.32, (c) 256.322, (d) 32.

3. Zero is always a significant figure. True or false?

4. Identify the least significant digit and the most significant figure in each of the following: (a) 12.25, (b) 9.99, (c) 2.56, (d) 234.0.

5. A digital instrument display bounces between two readings: 14.56 and 14.57 V. This phenomenon is called _____ _____ _____.

6. Give the power-of-ten equivalent for the following metric prefixes: (a) pico, (b) milli, (c) micro, (d) deci, (e) kilo, (f) mega, (g) giga.

7. Which of the following represents a 6-dB loss? (a) 6 dB, (b) −6 dB.

8. Errors in measurement are the same as operator mistakes. True or false?

9. Random variation causes data obtained when measuring a fixed value _____ _____ around a mean value.

10. The dispersion of a data set is measured by the _____ and the _____ _____.

11. Factors such as good/bad, defective/not defective, gender, race, and presence/nonpresence are examples of _____ data.

12. _____ data has no inherent order or rank.

13. _____ data allows ranking, but the differences between data are meaningless.

14. _____ data allows comparison of differences but is based on an arbitrary zero point.

15. _____ data allows comparison of differences but is based on a natural or inherent zero point.

16. The Fahrenheit and Celsius temperature scales represent _____ data, while the Kelvin scale represents _____ data.

17. List four levels of standards and describe their use.

Problems

1. A digital voltmeter reads 18.85 V. If the accuracy is 1%, and considering the phenomenon in question 5, in which range is the actual voltage likely to be?

2. Multiply 2.345 and 2.22. (a) What is the product? (b) How many significant figures are there in the answer?

3. A digital voltmeter of 0 to 1999 mV is used to measure two voltages. One is 1230 mV and the other is 758 mV. A calculator shows that the quotient of these voltages is 1.622691293. If the voltmeter has an accuracy limit of 1%, what is a more reasonable expression of this ratio?

4. Express the following as scientific notation: (a) 1.00, (b) 125, (c) 0.0000127, (d) 1,500,000, (e) 10,000, (f) 56,000.

5. Express the following in regular notation: (a) 2×10^{-2}, (b) 3.4×10^{5}, (c) 10^{-4}.

6. Convert the following to meters: (a) 25.4 mm, (b) 2.54 cm, (c) 0.100 km, (d) 123 cm.

7. A human ECG produces a peak signal of 1.6 mV riding on a 1.45-V DC pedestal. Com-

bine these two voltages and express them in: (a) volts, (b) millivolts.

8. The most expected value of a single data set is called the _____.

9. Find the *arithmetic mean* of the following data: 12.2, 5, 8.5, 14.32, 7.5, 6.5, 6.5, 5.5.

10. Find the *median* of the following data: 5, 6, 4, 3, 2, 9, 7.

11. Find the *mode* of the following data: 5, 6, 4, 3, 4, 2, 4, 7, 2, 9, 4.

12. You have $480 to spend. You spend half of your money each day. Tabulate the amount spent and then calculate the logarithmic mean.

13. The following prices are found for a certain brand of canned peas over a period of 6 weeks. Calculate both the arithmetic mean and the H.M. of the following data: $1.96, $2.05, $1.75, $1.94, $2.25, and $2.10.

14. Find the rms value of a sinewave AC signal that has a peak voltage of 45.3 V.

15. Find the rss value of the following signal levels: 25.6 μV, 22 μV, 56.5 μV, 33 μV.

16. An amplifier has an output signal of 3.6 V rms when a sinewave input signal of 0.1 V rms is present. State its gain in decibels.

17. An amplifier has a gain of 20 dB. This represents an output-to-input ratio of _____.

18. An amplifier has three amplification stages and a 1-dB attenuator in cascade. Assuming that all impedances are properly matched, what is the overall gain if the amplification factors are 5, 10, and 6 dB? Express your answer in decibels and in nondecibel form.

19. A double-balanced modulator is rated to accept signals up to +7 dBm. What is this signal level expressed in: (a) watts, (b) volts rms? Assume that all impedances are 50 Ω and are matched.

20. A signal level of 145 μV is found across a 50-Ω load. What is this signal level expressed in dBm?

21. The data below were collected by measurement with a voltmeter. Calculate: (a) mean voltage, (b) variance, (c) standard deviation.

4.35 6.21 5.02 3.99 3.02 6.0 4.77 3.3
4.05 5.43 3.45 1.99 6.15 5.75 2.98 5.43
2.22 3.49 4.0 4.4 5.2 5.7 7.01 8.1 4.33
4.0 5.2 4.65 4.34 3.9 5.45 6.9

Reference

1. Herceg, E.E., *Handbook of Measurement and Control,* Schaevitz Engineering (Pennsauken, N.J., 1972).

Suggested readings

1. Campbell, N.R., *Foundations of Science,* Dover (New York, 1957). Cited in John Mandel, *The Statistical Analysis of Experimental Data,* John Wiley & Sons (New York, 1964, Dover paperback edition 1984).

2. Carr, J.J., *The Art of Science,* HighText Publications (Solana Beach, Calif., 1992).

3. Carr, J.J., *A CrashCourse in Statistics.* HighText Publications (Book and CD-ROM) (Solana Beach, Calif., 1994).

CHAPTER 4
Basic Theories of Measurement

4-1 Objectives

1. Be able to list the basic categories of measurements.
2. Know the meanings of the terms *accuracy, precision, resolution, reliability,* and *validity* of measurements.
3. Be able to understand and evaluate the role and nature of measurement *error.*
4. Know how to minimize error in measurements.

4-2 Self-evaluation questions

These questions test your prior knowledge of the material in this chapter. Look for the answers as you read the text. After you have finished studying the chapter, try answering these questions and those at the end of the chapter.

1. Measurement errors usually result from human error. True or false?

2. Blood pressure measurement by use of an external cuff is an example of a _____ measurement.

3. If a voltage changes when a voltmeter is connected into the circuit, the resultant error is an example of _____ _____ error.

4. A defined procedure that yields consistent results from one measurement to the next is an example of a(n) _____ definition.

4-3 Introduction

In this chapter you will learn the fundamentals of measurement, electronic or otherwise. This material is critical to making measurements in bio medical and scientific instruments, as well as in most other fields. The material starts out with a discussion of the various categories of measurement (e.g., direct, indirect, null). Also discussed are issues such as *precision* and *accuracy* (often confused), *resolution, validity,* and *reliability* of a measurement. We also explain *measurement error* and how to avoid some of the most serious and most common errors.

4-4 Categories of measurement

There are three general categories of measurement: *direct, indirect,* and *null.* Electronic instruments are available based on all three categories.

Direct measurement

Direct measurements are made by holding the measurand up to some calibrated standard and comparing the two. A good example is the meter stick ruler used to cut a piece of coaxial cable to the correct length. You know that the cable must be cut to a length of 24 cm, so you hold a meter stick (the standard or reference) up to the piece of cable (Figure 4-1), set the 0-cm point at one end, make a mark on the cable adjacent to the 24 mark on the meter stick, and make your cut at the appropriate point.

Indirect measurement

Indirect measurements are made by measuring something other than the actual measurand. Although frequently considered second best from the perspective of measurement accuracy, indirect methods are often used when direct measurements are either difficult or dangerous. For example, one might measure the temperature of a point on the wall of a furnace that is melting metal (Figure 4-2*a*), knowing that it is related to the interior temperature by a certain factor (Figure 4-2*b*).

There was a minicomputer manufacturer who used an indirect temperature measurement to ease the job of the service technicians. The equipment was one of the first commercial (i.e., nonresearch) computer-based systems for monitoring coronary care unit (CCU) patients' analog ECG and pressure waveforms. The manufacturer created a small hole at the top of the rack-mounted cabinet where the temperature would be less than 39°C when the temperature on the electronic circuit boards deep inside the cabinet was within specification. Although they were interested in the temperature at the board level, they made a measurement that correlated to the desired measurement.

The system manufacturer specified this method for two reasons: (1) The measurement point was easily available (while the boards were not) and thus did not require any disassembly, and (2) the service technician could use an ordinary medical fever thermometer (30°C to 42°C) as the measurement instrument, which was easily available wherever the computer was installed. No special laboratory thermometers were needed.

Perhaps the most common example of an indirect measurement is the way human blood pressure is measured: the pressure in an occluding cuff placed around the arm is measured, a process called *sphygmomanometry* (Figure 4-3; see chapter 9). Research around 1905 showed that the cuff pressures at two easily heard events (onset and cessation of Korotkoff's sounds) are correlated with the systolic (P_s) and diastolic (P_d) arterial blood pressures. Direct blood pressure measurement may be more accurate, but is dangerous

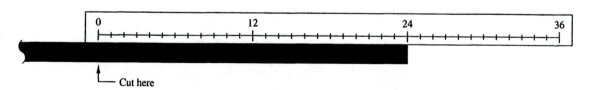

Figure 4-1
Measuring cable with a meter stick. Source: EEIM.

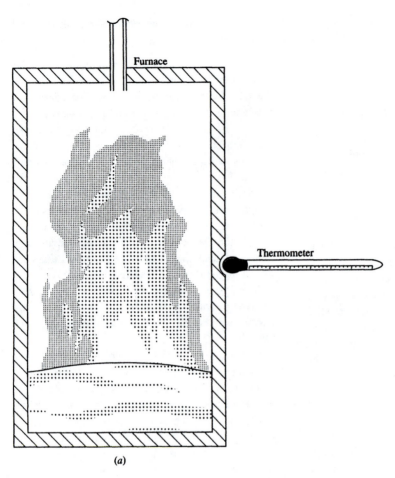

Furnace

Thermometer

(a)

Figure 4-2
(a) Measuring point on furnace wall, (b) graph of measured vs. interior temperature.
Source: EEIM.

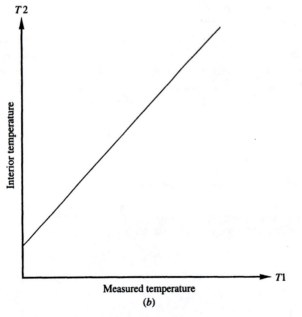

$T2$

Interior temperature

Measured temperature

$T1$

(b)

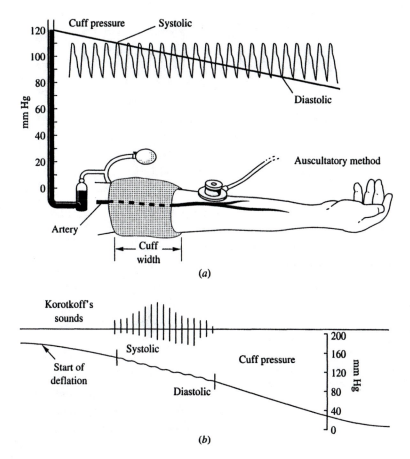

Figure 4-3
Indirect measurement of blood pressure. Source: EEIM.

because it is an invasive surgical procedure. This method does not actually measure the blood pressure, but rather measures cuff pressure. By correlating cuff pressure with the onset and cessation of Korotkoff's sounds, it is possible to measure blood pressure.

Null measurements

Null measurements are made by comparing a calibrated source to an unknown measurand and then adjusting either one or the other until the difference between them is zero. An *electrical poten-tiometer* is such an instrument; it is an adjustable calibrated voltage source and a comparison meter (zero-center galvanometer). The reference voltage from the potentiometer is applied (Figure 4-4) to one side of the zero-center galvanometer (or one input of a difference-measuring voltmeter), and the unknown is applied to the other side of the galvanometer (or remaining input of the differential voltmeter). The output of the potentiometer is adjusted until the meter reads zero difference. The setting of the potentiometer under the nulled condition is the same as the unknown measurand voltage.

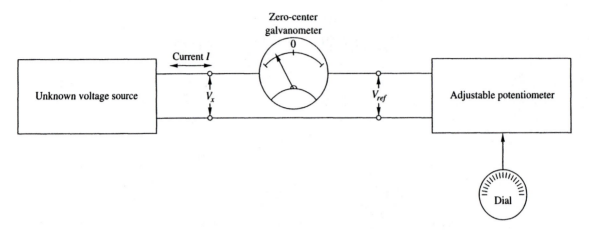

Figure 4-4
Example of null measurement. Source: EEIM.

4-5 Factors in making measurements

The goodness of measurements involves several concepts that must be understood. Some of the more significant of these are: *error, validity, reliability* and *repeatability, accuracy* and *precision,* and *resolution.*

Error

In all measurements a certain degree of error is present. The word *error* in this context refers to normal random variation and in no way means mistakes. In short order, we will discuss error in greater depth.

If measurements are made repeatedly on the same parameter (which is truly unchanging), or if different instruments or instrument operators are used to make successive measurements, the measurements will tend to cluster around a central value (X_o in Figure 4-5). In most cases, it is assumed that X_o is the true value, but if there is substantial inherent error in the measurement process, then it may deviate from the true value (X_i) by a certain amount (ΔX), which is the error term. The assumption that the central value of a series of

measurements is the true value is only valid when the error term is small. As $\Delta X \rightarrow 0$, $X_o \rightarrow X_i$.

Validity

The *validity* of a measurement is a statement of how well the instrument actually measures what it purports to measure. An electronic blood pressure sensor may actually be measuring the deflection of a thin metallic diaphragm of known area, which is in turn measured by the strain applied to a strain gauge element cemented to the diaphragm. What

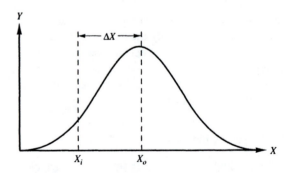

Figure 4-5
The accuracy of a measurement is indicated by the size of ΔX.

determines the validity of a sensor measurement is the extent to which the measurement of the deflection of that diaphragm relates to applied pressure, and over what range or under what conditions. In many measurement devices, the output readings are only meaningful under certain specified conditions or over a specified range.

Reliability and repeatability

The *reliability* of the measurement is a statement of its *consistency* when discerning the values of the measurand on different trials, when the measurand may take on very different values. In the case of the pressure sensor discussed above, a deformation of a diaphragm may change its characteristics sufficiently to alter future measurements of the same pressure value.

Related to reliability is the idea of *repeatability,* which refers to the ability of the instrument to return the same value when repeatedly exposed to the exact same stimulant. Neither reliability nor repeatability is the same as accuracy, for a measurement may be both reliable and repeatable while being quite wrong.

Accuracy and precision

The *accuracy* of a measurement refers to the freedom from error, or the degree of conformity between the measurand and the standard. *Precision,* on the other hand, refers to the exactness of successive measurements, also sometimes considered the degree of refinement of the measurement. Accuracy and precision are often confused with one another, and these words are often erroneously used interchangeably. One way of stating the situation is to note that *a precise measurement has a small standard deviation and variance under repeated trials, but in an accurate measurement, the mean value of the normal distribution curve is close to the true value.*

The relationship between precision and accuracy can be seen in the target-shooting example in Figure 4-6. In all of these cases, the data form a normal distribution curve over a large number of iterations of the measurement. Four targets are shown in a precision-versus-accuracy matrix. The target in Figure 4-6a has *good accuracy* because the shots are clustered on the bullseye. It also has *good precision,* as seen by the fact that the cluster has a small dispersion; i.e., it is a *tight group,* as target shooters say. The target in Figure 4-6b has good precision (small dispersion, good clustering), but bad accuracy (the cluster is off center, high, and to the left). The target in Figure 4-6c has good accuracy because the cluster is centered, but the bullet holes are all over the paper. The clustering is poor, which indicates a lack of precision. The target in Figure 4-6d lacks both accuracy and precision.

Target shooting is a good analogy for measurement processes and how to solve problems with them. Shooting instructors know that it's better to work on precision first, i.e., getting the cluster smaller (called *grouping* in shooting). That's analogous to reducing the random or inherent variation in a measurement process (it also works for other work processes, see chapter 27). Some of the clustering is the result of the mechanics of the gun, but most of it is caused by the shooter. Once the shooter (or worker) is consistently shooting tight clusters, then it's time to worry about moving the impact point (i.e., the average). How is this done? Not by adjusting the worker (i.e.,shooter), but adjusting the process (i.e., the gun). The gun that shot the target in Figure 4-6b can be brought into working order by adjusting the movable sights about two clicks to the right and two clicks down.

A mistake often made by novice shooters and poor managers is to adjust the sights with too few shots on the paper. Enough shots (data points) must be collected to truly see the clustering before any meaningful change can be made. One author (J.J.C.) has observed shooters fire two shots and then adjust the sights; fire two more shots and adjust; fire two more shots and adjust; fire. . . . They wonder why the gun never seems to come into regulation. They blame the gun, the ammuni-

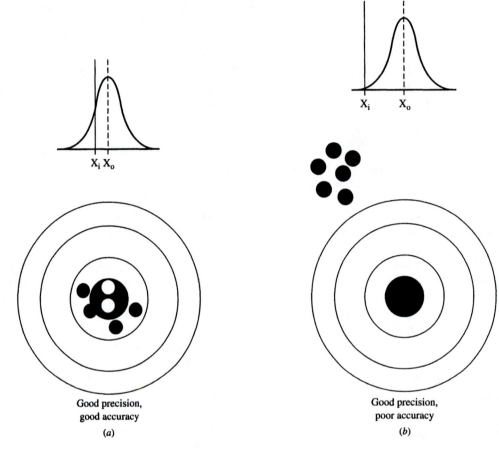

Figure 4-6
(a) Good accuracy, good precision, (b) poor accuracy, good precision.

tion, and the lighting on the range, but never their methods.

The standard deviation (which is the square root of variance) of the measurement is a good indication of its precision, which also means the inherent error in the measurement.

Several tactics help reduce the effects of error on practical measurements:

1. Make the measurement many times and then average the results.

2. Make the measurement several times using different instruments, if feasible.

3. When using instruments, such as rulers or analog meters, try making the successive measurements on different parts of the scale. For example, on rulers and analog meter dials the distance between tick marks is not really constant because of manufacturing error. The same is also true of electrical meter scales. Measure lengths using different points on the scale as the zero reference point (e.g., on a meter stick use 2, 12, 20, and 30 cm as the zero point), and then average the results. By taking the measurements from different sections of the scale, individual errors and

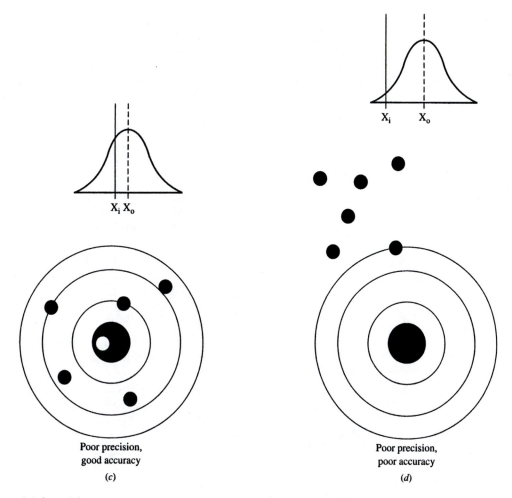

Poor precision,
good accuracy
(c)

Poor precision,
poor accuracy
(d)

Figure 4-6 (cont'd)
(c) Good accuracy, poor precision, (d) poor precision, poor accuracy.

biases that accumulate will be averaged to a lower overall error.

Resolution

Resolution refers to the degree to which the measurand can be broken into identifiable adjacent parts. An example can be seen on the standard television test pattern broadcast by some stations in the early morning hours between broadcast days. Various features on the test pattern will in-

clude parallel vertical or horizontal lines of different densities. One patch may be 100 lines per inch, another 200 lines per inch, and so forth up the scale. The resolution of the video system is the maximum density *at which it is still possible to see adjacent lines with space between them.* For any system, there is a limit above which the lines are blurred into a single entity.

In a digital electronic measuring instrument, the resolution is set by the number of bits used in the data word. Digital instruments use the binary (base-2) number system in which the only two permissible digits are 0 and 1. The binary *word* is a binary number representing a quantity. For example, binary 0001 represents decimal 1, while binary 1001 represents decimal 5. An 8-bit data word, the standard for many small embedded computers, can take on values from 00000000_2 to 11111111_2, so it can break the range into 2^8 (256) distinct values, or 2^8-1 (255) different segments. The resolution of that system depends on the value of the measured parameter change that must occur to change the least significant bit in the data word. For example, if 8 bits are used to represent a voltage range of 0 to 10 V, then the resolution is $(10 - 0)/255$, or 0.039 V (39 mV) per bit. This resolution is often specified as the 1-LSB (least significant bit) resolution.

4-6 Measurement errors

No measurement is perfect, and measurement apparatus is never ideal, so there will always be some *error* (not mistakes) in all forms of measurement. An error is a deviation between the actual value of a measurand and the indicated value produced by the sensor or instrument used to measure the value. To reiterate: *Error is inherent, and is NOT the fault of the person making the measurement.* Error is not the same as mistake, and understanding error can greatly improve our effectiveness in making measurements.

Error can be expressed in *absolute* terms or by using a relative scale. An absolute error would be expressed in terms of X $\pm$ x cm, or some other such unit, while a relative error expression would be X cm $\pm$ 1%. In an electrical circuit, a voltage might be stated as 4.5 V $\pm$ 1%. Which expression to use may be a matter of custom, convention, personal choice, or utility, depending on the situation.

4-7 Categories of error

There are four general categories of error: *theoretical, static, dynamic,* and *instrument insertion.*

Theoretical error

All measurements are based on some measurement theory that predicts how a value will behave when a certain measurement procedure is applied. The measurement theory is usually based on some theoretical model of the phenomenon being measured, i.e., an intellectual construct that tells us something of how that phenomenon works. It is often the case that the theoretical model is valid only over a specified range of the phenomenon. For example, nonlinear phenomena that have a quadratic, cubic, or exponential function can be treated as a straight line linear function over small, carefully selected sections of the range. Electronic sensor outputs often fall into this class.

Alternatively, the actual phenomenon may be terribly complex, or even chaotic, under the right conditions, so the model is therefore simplified for many practical measurements. An equation that is used as the basis for a measurement theory may be only a first-order approximation of the actual situation. For example, consider the *mean arterial pressure* (MAP) that is often measured in clinical medicine and medical research situations. The MAP approximation equation used by clinicians is:

$$\overline{P} = Diastolic + \frac{Systolic - Diastolic}{3}$$

$$(4\text{-}1)$$

This equation is really only an approximation (and holds true mostly for well people, but not for some sick people to whom it is applied) of the equation that expresses the mathematical integral of the blood pressure over a cardiac cycle, i.e., the time average of the arterial pressure. The actual expression is written in calculus notation, which is beyond the math abilities of many of the people who use the clinical version above:

$$\overline{P} = \frac{1}{T}\int_{t_1}^{t_2} P(t)\, dt \qquad (4\text{-}2)$$

The approximation (Equation 4-1) works well but is subject to greater error than Equation 4-2 because of the theoretical simplification of the first equation.

Static error

Static errors include a number of subclasses that are all related because they are always present, even in unchanging systems (and thus are not dynamic errors). These errors are not functions of the time or frequency variation.

Reading static errors These errors result from misreading the display output of the sensor system. An analog meter uses a pointer to indicate the measured value. If the pointer is read at an angle other than straight on, then a *parallax reading error* occurs. Another reading error is the *interpolation error,* i.e., an error made in judging or estimating the correct value between two calibrated marks on the meter scale (Figure 4-7). Still another reading error occurs if the pointer on a meter scale is too broad and covers several marks at once.

A related error seen in digital readouts is the *last digit bobble error.* On digital displays, the least significant digit on the display often will flip back and forth between two values. For example, a digital voltmeter might read 12.24 and 12.25 alternately, depending on when you looked at it, despite the fact that absolutely no change occurred in the voltage being measured. This phenomenon occurs when the actual voltage is midway between the two indicated voltages. Error, noise, and uncertainty in the system will make a voltage close to 12.245 V bobble back and forth between the two permissible output states (12.24 V and 12.25 V) on the meter. An example in which *bobble* is of significant concern is when some action is taken when a value changes above or below a certain quantity, and the digital display bobbles above and below the critical threshold.

Environmental static errors All sensors and instruments operate in an environment that can affect the output states. Factors such as temperature (perhaps the most common error-producing agent), pressure, electromagnetic fields, and radiation must be considered in some electronic sensor systems.

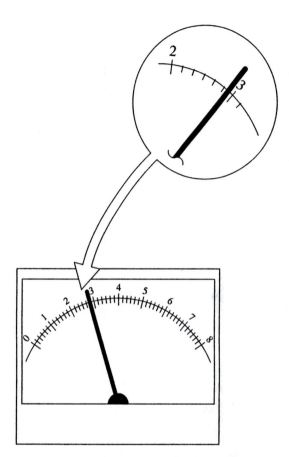

Figure 4-7
Interpolation error. Source: EEIM.

Characteristic static errors These static errors are still left after reading errors and environmental errors are accounted for. When the environment is well within the allowable limits and is unchanging, when there is no reading error, a residual error will remain that is a function of the measurement instrument or process itself. Errors found under this category include zero offset error, gain error, processing error, linearity error, hysteresis error, repeatability error, and resolution error.

Also included in the characteristic error are any design or manufacturing deficiencies that lead to error. Not all of the ticks on the ruler are truly 1.0000 mm apart at all points along the ruler.

While it is hoped that the errors are random, so that the overall error is small, there is always the possibility of a distinct bias or error trend in any measurement device.

For digital systems, *a quantization error* must be added to the resolution error. Quantization error emerges from the fact that the output data can only take on certain discrete values. For example, an 8-bit analog-to-digital converter allows 256 different states, so a 0-V to 10-V range is broken into 256 discrete values in 39.06-mV steps. A potential that is between two of these steps is assigned to one or the other according to the rounding protocol used in the measurement process. An example is the weight sensor that outputs 8.540 V, on a 10-V scale, to represent a certain weight. The actual 8-bit digitized value may represent 8.502, 8.541, or 8.580 V because of the ± 0.039-V quantization error.

Dynamic error

Dynamic errors arise when the measurand is changing or in motion during the measurement process. Examples of dynamic errors include the inertia of mechanical indicating devices (such as analog meters) during measurement of rapidly changing parameters. A number of limitations in electronic instrumentation fall into this category, especially when a frequency, phase, or slew rate limitation is present.

Instrument insertion error

A fundamental rule of making measurements is that *the measurement process should not significantly alter the phenomenon being measured.* Otherwise, the measurand is actually the altered situation, not the original situation that is of true interest. Examples of this error are found in many places. One is that pressure sensors tend to add volume to the system being measured and thus slightly reduce the pressure indicated below the actual pressure. Similarly, a flowmeter might add length, a different pipe diameter, or turbulence to a system being measured. A voltmeter with a low

impedance of its own could alter resistance ratios in an electrical circuit and produce a false reading (Figure 4-8). This problem is especially seen when using cheap analog volt-ohm-milliammeters, which have a low sensitivity and hence a low impedance (R_m in Figure 4-8), to measure a voltage in a circuit. The meter resistance R_m is effectively shunted across the circuit resistance across which the voltage appears.

Instrument insertion errors can usually be minimized by good instrument design and good practices. No measurement device has zero effect on

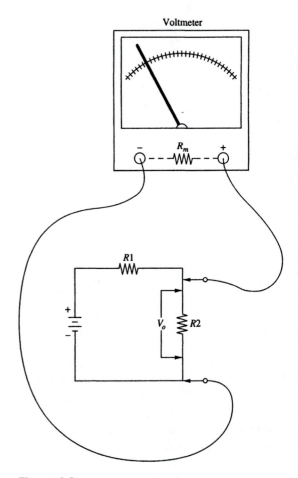

Figure 4-8
False reading caused by instrument insertion error.
Source: EEIM.

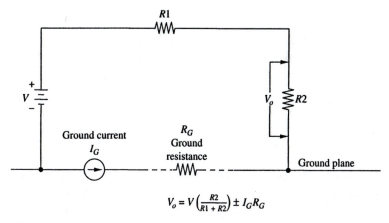

$$V_o = V\left(\frac{R2}{R1 + R2}\right) \pm I_G R_G$$

Figure 4-9
Ground loop voltage drop and ground plane noise. Source: EEIM.

the system being measured, but one can reduce the error to a very small value by appropriate selection of methods and devices.

4-8 Dealing with measurement errors

Measurement errors can be minimized through several methods, some of which are combined under the rubric *procedure,* and others under the legend *statistics.*

Under procedure one can find methods that will reduce, or even minimize, error contributions to the final result. For example, in an electrical circuit, a voltmeter that has an extremely high input impedance compared with circuit resistances should be used. The idea is to use an instrument (whether a voltmeter, a pressure meter, or whatever) that least disturbs the thing being measured.

A significant source of measurement error in some electronic circuits is ground loop voltage drops and ground plane noise. Figure 4-9 shows how this problem occurs. The circuit seen by the user of the instrument is a *dc* voltage source driving a resistor voltage divider. An unseen ground current (I_G) flows through the resistance of the

ground plane (R_G) to produce a voltage drop $I_G R_G$. This voltage may add or subtract from the reading of output voltage V_o, depending on its phase and polarity.

A way to reduce total error is to use several different instruments to measure the same parameter. In Figure 4-10 we see an example in which the current flow in a circuit is being measured by three different ammeters: M_1, M_2, and M_3. Each of these instruments will produce a result that contains an error term that is decorrelated from the er-

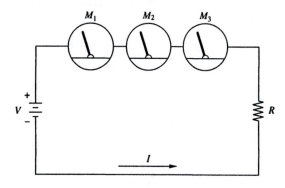

Figure 4-10
Current measured by three ammeters to reduce measurement error.

ror of the others and is not biased (unless, by selecting three identical-model meters we inherit the characteristic error of that type of instrument). We can estimate the correct value of the current flow rate by taking the average of the three:

$$M_o = \frac{M_1 + M_2 + M_3}{3} \qquad (4\text{-}3)$$

One must either be careful to randomize the system in cases in which the sensor or instruments used tend to have large error terms biased in one direction or calibrate the average error so that it may be subtracted out of the final result.

4-9 Error contributions analysis

An *error analysis* can be performed to identify and quantify all contributing sources of error in the system. A determination is then made regarding the randomness of those errors, and a *worst case analysis* is made. Under the worst case, one assumes that all of the component errors are biased in a single direction and are maximized. We then attempt to determine the consequences (to our purpose for making the measurement) if these errors line up in that manner, even if such an alignment is improbable. The worst-case analysis should be done on both the positive and negative side of the nominal value. An *error budget* is then created to allocate an allowable error to each individual component of the measurement system to ensure that the overall error is not too high for the intended use of the system.

If errors are independent of each other and are random rather than biased in one direction, and if they are of the same order of magnitude, then one can find the *root of the sum of the squares, or root-sum-square, (rss)* value of the errors and use it as a composite error term in planning a measurement system. The rss error is:

$$\epsilon_{rss} = \sqrt{\sum \epsilon_i^2} \qquad (4\text{-}4)$$

The rss error term is a reasonable estimate or approximation of the combined effects of the individual error components.

A collection of repetitive measurements of a phenomenon can be considered a *sampled population* and treated as such. If we take N measurements (M_1 through M_n) of the same parameter and then average them, we get:

$$\overline{M} = \frac{M_1 + M_2 + M_3 + \cdots + M_n}{N}$$
$$(4\text{-}5)$$

The average value obtained in Equation 4-5 is the *mean arithmetic average*. This value is usually reported as the correct value for the measurement, but when taken alone does not address the issue of error. For this purpose we add a correction factor by quoting the *standard error of the mean,* or

$$\sigma_{\overline{m}} = \frac{\sigma_m}{\sqrt{N}} \qquad (4\text{-}6)$$

Which is reported in the result as:

$$M = \overline{M} \pm \sigma_{\overline{m}} \qquad (4\text{-}7)$$

Any measurement contains error, and this procedure allows us to estimate that error and thereby understand the limitations of that particular measurement.

4-10 Operational definitions in measurement

Some measurement procedures suggest themselves immediately from the nature of the phenomenon being measured. In other cases, however, there is a degree of ambiguity in the process, and it must be overcome. Sometimes the ambiguity results from the fact that there are many different ways to define the phenomenon, or perhaps no single way is well established. In cases such as these, one might wish to resort to an *operational definition,* i.e., a procedure that will produce consistent results from measurement to measurement or when measurements are taken by different people.

An operational definition, therefore, is a defined, standardized procedure that must be followed, and it specifies as many factors as necessary to control the measurement, so that changes can be properly attributed only to the unknown variable. The need for operational (as opposed to absolute) definitions arises from the fact that things are only rarely so neat, clean, and crisp as to suggest their own natural definition. By its very nature, the operational definition does not ask true-or-false questions; rather, it asks what happens under given sets of assumptions or conditions. What an operational definition can do for you, however, is standardize a measurement in a clear and precise way so that it remains consistent across numerous trials. Operational definitions are used extensively in science and technology. When widely accepted, or promulgated by a recognized authority, they are called *standards*.

An operational definition should embrace what is measurable quantitatively, or at least in nonsubjective terms. For example, in measuring the *saltiness* of a saline solution (salt water), one might taste it and render a subjective judgment, such as *weak* or *strong*. Alternatively, one can establish an operational definition that calls for measuring the electrical resistance of the saline under certain specified conditions:

1. Immerse two 1-cm diameter circular nickel electrodes, spaced 5 cm apart and facing each other, to a depth of 3 cm into a 500-mL beaker of the test solution.

2. Bring the solution to a temperature of 4°C.

3. Measure the electrical resistance (R) between the electrodes using a Snotz model 1120 digital ohmmeter.

4. Find the conductance (G) by taking the reciprocal of resistance (G = 1/R).

You can probably come up with a better definition of the conductance of saline solution that works for some peculiar situation. The procedure above was once used as the basis for conductivity meters used to test dialysate mix used in kidney dialysis. Keep in mind that only rarely does a preferred definition suggest itself naturally, so one must be defined through consensus of the users.

The use of operational definitions results in both strengths and weaknesses. One weakness is that the definition might not be honed finely enough for the purpose at hand. Sociologists and psychologists often face this problem because of difficulties in dealing with nonlinearities, such as human emotions. But such problems also point to a strength. We must recognize that scientific truth is always tentative, so we must deal with uncertainties in experimentation. Sometimes the band of uncertainty around a point of truth can be reduced by the use of several operational definitions in different tests of the same phenomenon. By taking different looks from different angles, we may get a more refined idea of what is actually happening.

When an operational definition becomes widely accepted and is used throughout an industry, it may become part of a formal standard or test procedure. You may, for example, see a procedure listed as "performed in accordance with NIST[1] XXXX.XXX," "ANSI Standard XXX," or "AAMI Standard XYZ." These notations mean that whoever made the measurement followed some published standard.

4-11 Summary

1. There are three basic categories of measurement: *direct, indirect*, and *null*.

2. Factors involved in measurement include *error, validity, reliability, repeatability, accuracy, precision*, and *resolution*.

3. Error is inherent in measurements and in no way indicates that mistakes were made.

4. Validity of a measurement is a statement of how well the measurement measures what it purports to measure.

5. Reliability of a measurement is a statement of its consistency.

---

[1]*National Institute for Standards and Technology*, formerly called *National Bureau of Standards*.

6. Accuracy refers to the measurement's freedom from error.

7. Precision refers to the exactness of successive measures of the same unchanging quantity.

8. Resolution refers to the degree to which the measurand can be broken into identifiable adjacent parts.

9. The basic categories of error are: *theoretical, static, dynamic,* and *instrument insertion.*

10. Measurements that are difficult, complex, or ambiguous are often accomplished with an operational definition, i.e., a standard procedure for making the measurement. If all users consistently apply the standard method, then the results are comparable.

4-12 Recapitulation

Now return to the objectives and self-evaluation questions at the beginning of the chapter and see how well you can answer them. If you cannot answer certain questions, place a check mark next to each and review appropriate parts of the text. Next, try to answer the following questions and problems using the same procedure.

Questions and problems

1. List the three categories of measurements: _____, _____, and _____.

2. A meter stick is an example of a _____ measurement.

3. Measuring human blood pressure by sphygmomanometry is an example of an _____ measurement.

4. A potentiometer and a zero-center galvanometer are used to measure an unknown potential. This is a _____ measurement.

5. List seven factors in making a good measurement: _____, _____, _____, _____, _____, _____, and _____.

6. Random variation in the value reported by successive measurements of the same unchanging quantity is called _____.

7. The statement of how well a measurement method actually measures the quantity it purports to measure is its _____.

8. The _____ of a measurement is a statement of the amount by which a measurement departs from the actual value of the measurand.

9. The _____ of a measurement is a statement of the dispersion of the values of an unchanging measurand in a large number of successive trials.

10. The standard deviation of a set of measurements made on an unchanging measurand is a good indication of its _____.

11. On a TV test pattern, a series of lines radiating out from a central point is used to measure the _____ of the TV set.

12. _____ is found in all forms of measurement, no matter how accurate or how well the procedure is carried out.

13. List four general categories of measurement error: _____, _____, _____, and _____.

14. Which of the types of measurement error in question 13 are normally the fault of the instrument user?

15. The _____ category of error results from the theory of measurement used in the particular case, e.g., in measuring mean arterial blood pressure by calculation from the minimum (diastolic) and maximum (systolic) values over one heart beat cycle.

16. Parallax error is an example of a _____ error in reading an analog meter scale.

17. _____ _____ _____ is an example of a static error in reading a digital voltmeter.

18. List several types of characteristic static errors.

19. For digital systems, overall error must include the _____ error caused by the digital nature of the circuits.

20. A reading of the value of a rapidly changing near-*dc* voltage lags because of inertia in the meter movement. This is an example of _____ error.

21. A voltage measurement error is caused by the integration time window of a digital voltmeter. This is a _____ error.

22. If a low-impedance voltmeter is inserted into a high-resistance *dc* circuit, a _____ _____ error is created.

23. Three voltmeters are connected in parallel across the output of a voltage source: No. 1 reads 12.23 V, No. 2 reads 12.1 V, and No. 3 reads 12.2 V. What is the probable voltage indicated by this set of readings?

24. If a set of n measurements are made of an alternating current measurand, and the errors are independent of each other, an appropriate measurement calculation method is the _____ _____ square.

25. Find the mean and the standard deviation of the set of weight measurements given below:

1.6 1.8 1.2 1.26 1.26 1.3 1.3 1.3 1.33
1.35 1.4 1.4
1.4 1.4 1.4 1.43 1.48 1.53 1.5 1.5 1.5
1.53 1.6 1.6
1.62 1.65 1.74 1.79 1.7 1.81

26 Calculate the standard error of the mean for the sample above and report it in the standard manner.

CHAPTER 5
Signals and Noise

5-1 Objectives

1. Be able to understand the different classes of signals.
2. Be able to describe waveforms in terms of a Fourier series.

3. Be able to understand noise and signals and their relationship.
4. Be able to describe noise factor, noise figure, and noise temperature.

5-2 Self-evaluation questions

These questions test your prior knowledge of the material in this chapter. Look for the answers as you read the text. After you have finished studying the chapter, try answering these questions and those at the end of the chapter.[1]

1. Write the equation for the Fourier series.

2. Describe the harmonic content of a squarewave.

3 Describe the differences between analog and sampled analog signals.

4. A noise figure of 5.8 dB corresponds to a noise factor of _____.

5-3 Types of signals

Signals are the grist for the instrumentation designer's mill, and it is to the processing of signals that we will soon direct our attention. But the nature of signals, and their relationship to noise and interfering signals, determines appropriate design all the way from the system level down to the component selection level. In this chapter, we will take a look at signals and noise and how each affects the design of instrumentation circuits.

---

[1]Some of the material in this chapter uses the notation of calculus. You do not need a course in calculus to understand this material, as it is explained in the text, but you might wish to read Appendix A ("Some Math Notes") before you proceed further.

Signals can be categorized in several ways, but one of the most fundamental is according to time domain behavior (the other major category is frequency domain). We will therefore consider signals of the form $v = f(t)$ or $i = f(t)$. The time domain classes of signals include *static* and *quasistatic, periodic, repetitive, transient,* and *random*. There is also a *chaotic* class of signals. Each of these categories has certain properties that can profoundly influence appropriate design decisions.

Static and quasistatic signals

A *static* signal (Figure 5-1a) is, by definition, unchanging over a very long period of time (T_{long} in Figure 5-1a). Such a signal is essentially a dc level, so must be processed in low-drift dc amplifier circuits. The term *quasistatic* means nearly unchanging, so a quasistatic signal (Figure 5-1b) refers to a signal that changes so slowly over a long time that it possesses characteristics more like those of static signals than dynamic (rapidly changing) signals.

Periodic signals

A *periodic* signal (Figure 5-1c) is one that repeats itself on a regular basis. Examples of periodic signals include sine waves, square waves, sawtooth waves, and triangle waves. The nature of the periodic waveform is such that each waveform is identical to others at like points along the time line. In other words, if you advance along the time line by exactly one period (T), then the voltage, polarity, and direction of change of the waveform will be repeated. That is, for a voltage waveform, $V(t) = V(t + T)$.

Repetitive signals

A *repetitive* signal (Figure 5-1d) is quasiperiodic and thus bears some similarity to the periodic waveform. The principal difference between repetitive and periodic signals is seen by comparing the signal at f(t) and f(t + T), where T is the period of the signal. These points might not be identical in repetitive signals but are identical in periodic signals. The repetitive signal might contain either transient or stable features that vary from period to period. An example is the human arterial blood pressure waveform, or the voltage representation of it obtained from a blood pressure transducer (Figure 5-1d). While the waveform tends to vary from a minima (diastolic) to a maxima (systolic) in a quasiperiodic manner, there are both normal and pathological anomalies from one cycle to another. For example, the amplitudes of the maxima and minima, and the repetition rate (heart rate) tend to vary quite normally in healthy humans. In addition, events such as *premature ventricular contractions* (PVCs) are anomalies that may be pathological. (PVCs tend to be purely transient events superimposed on the repetitive signal.) Thus, the repetitive signal may bear characteristics of both transient and periodic signals.

Transient signals

A *transient* signal (Figure 5-1e) is either a one-time event or a periodic event in which the event duration is very short compared with the period of the waveform. In terms of Figure 5-1f, the latter definition means that $t_1 < < < t_2$. These signals can be treated as if they are transients.

5-4 Fourier series

All continuous periodic signals can be represented by a fundamental frequency sine wave and a collection of harmonics of that fundamental sine wave that are summed together linearly. These frequencies make up the *Fourier series* of the waveform. The elementary sine wave (Figure 5-2) is described by:

$$v = V_M \sin (2\omega t) \qquad (5\text{-}1)$$

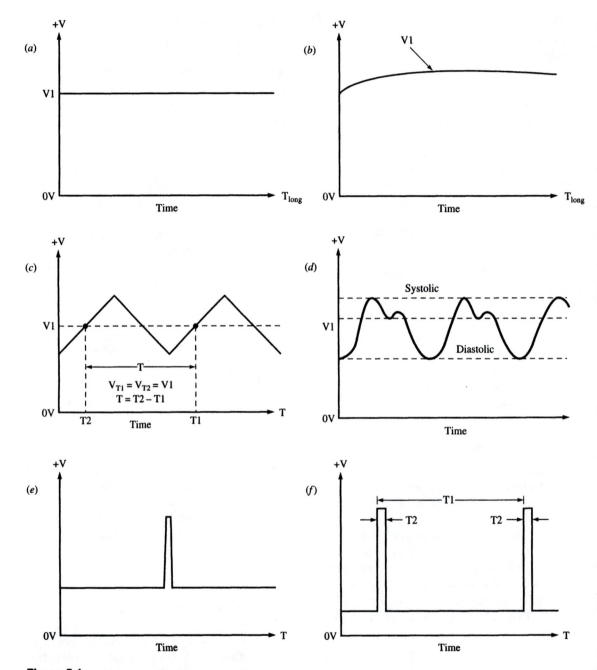

Figure 5-1
Signal types. (*a*) Static signal. (*b*) Quasistatic signal. (*c*) Periodic signal. (*d*) Repetitive signal.
(*e*) Single-event transient signal. (*f*) Repetitive-transient or quasi-transient signal.

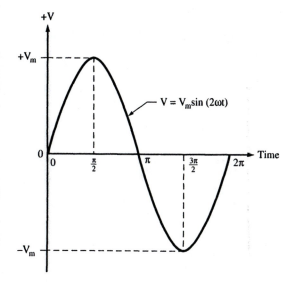

Figure 5-2
Sinusoidal waveform.

where

v   is the instantaneous amplitude of the sine
     wave

V_M is the peak amplitude of the sine wave

ω   is the angular frequency $(2\pi F)$ of the sine
     wave

t   is the time in seconds

The *period* of the sine wave is the time between recurrence of identical events, or $T = 2\pi/\omega = 1/F$ (where F is the frequency in cycles per second).

The Fourier series that makes up a waveform can be found if a given waveform is decomposed into its constituent frequencies by either a bank of frequency-selective filters or a digital signal processing algorithm called the *fast Fourier transform* (FFT). The Fourier series can also be used to construct a waveform from the ground up. Figure 5-3 shows square wave (Figure 5-3*a*), sawtooth wave (Figure 5-3*b*), and peaked wave (Figure 5-3*c*) signals constructed from fundamental sine waves and their harmonic sine and cosine functions.

The Fourier series for any waveform can be expressed in the form:

$$f(t) = \frac{a_o}{2} \int_{n=1}^{\infty} [a_n\cos(n\omega t) + b_n\sin(n\omega t)] \quad (5\text{-}2)$$

where

a_n and b_n represent the amplitudes of the
harmonics (see later)

n is an integer
(Other terms are as previously defined)

The amplitude coefficients (a_n and b_n) are expressed by:

$$a_n = \frac{2}{T}\int_0^T f(t)\cos(n\omega t)\, dt \quad (5\text{-}3)$$

and

$$b_n = \frac{2}{T}\int_0^T f(t)\sin(n\omega t)\, dt \quad (5\text{-}4)$$

The amplitude terms are nonzero at the specific frequencies determined by the Fourier series. Because only certain frequencies, determined by integer *n*, are allowable, the spectrum of the periodic signal is said to be *discrete*.

The term $a_o/2$ in the Fourier series expression (Equation 5-2) is the average value of $f(t)$ over one complete cycle (one period) of the waveform. In practical terms, it is also the *dc component* of the waveform. When the waveform possesses *half-wave symmetry* (i.e., the peak amplitude above zero is equal to the peak amplitude below zero at every point in *t*, or $+V_m = |-V_m|$), there is no dc component, so $a_o = 0$.

An alternative Fourier series expression replaces the $a_n\cos(n\omega t) + b_n\sin(n\omega t)$ with an equivalent expression of another form:

$$f(t) = \frac{2}{T}\sum_{n=1}^{\infty} C_a(n\omega t - \phi) \quad (5\text{-}5)$$

where

$C_n = [(a_n)^2 + (b_n)^2]^{1/2}$

$\phi_n = \arctan(a_n/b_n)$
(Other terms as previously defined)

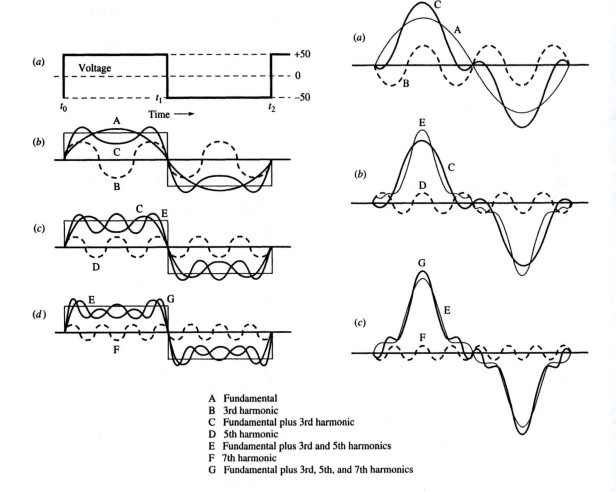

A Fundamental
B 3rd harmonic
C Fundamental plus 3rd harmonic
D 5th harmonic
E Fundamental plus 3rd and 5th harmonics
F 7th harmonic
G Fundamental plus 3rd, 5th, and 7th harmonics

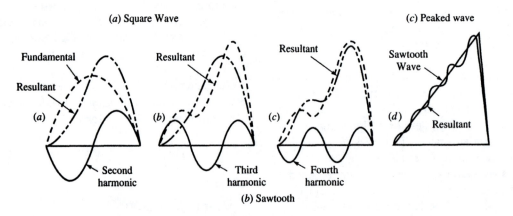

(a) Square Wave

(c) Peaked wave

Fundamental

Resultant

Resultant

Resultant

Sawtooth
Wave

Resultant

(a)

(b)

(c)

(d)

Second
harmonic

Third
harmonic

Fourth
harmonic

(b) Sawtooth

Figure 5-3
The Fourier series makes up waveforms. (a) Square wave. (b) Sawtooth wave. (c) Peaked wave.

One can infer certain things about the harmonic content of a waveform by examination of its symmetries. One would conclude from the above equations that the harmonics extend to infinity on all waveforms. Clearly, in practical systems a much less than infinite bandwidth is found, so some of those harmonics will be removed by the normal action of the electronic circuits. Also, it is sometimes found that higher harmonics might not be truly significant, and so can be ignored. As n becomes larger, the amplitude coefficients a_n and b_n tend to become smaller. At some point, the amplitude coefficients are reduced sufficiently that their contribution to the shape of the wave is either negligible for the practical purpose at hand or totally unobservable in practical terms. The value of n at which this occurs depends partially on the *rise time* of the waveform. Rise time is usually defined as the time required for the waveform to rise from 10% to 90% of its final amplitude. Let's consider a practical example from biomedical instrumentation.

Figure 5-4 shows the human arterial pressure waveform superimposed on the same time line as the ECG waveform. These waveforms are time-correlated because they both represent different views of the same physical event, i.e., the beating of the human heart. Suppose that the heart rate is 72 beats/min, or 1.2 Hz. The pressure waveform has a slower rise time than the ECG waveform, and so contains a smaller number of harmonics. The pressure waveform can be accurately reproduced with about 25 harmonics (e.g., an approximately 30 Hz bandwidth), while the ECG waveform requires 70 to 80 harmonics for faithful reproduction (e.g., approximately a 100 Hz bandwidth). To adequately process these two waveforms, the instrument must have upper −3 dB frequency responses of 30 and 100 Hz for the pressure and ECG channels, respectively. Because both pressure and ECG waveforms have significantly rounded features, the lower −3 dB frequency response (a function of subharmonic content) must be 0.05 Hz.

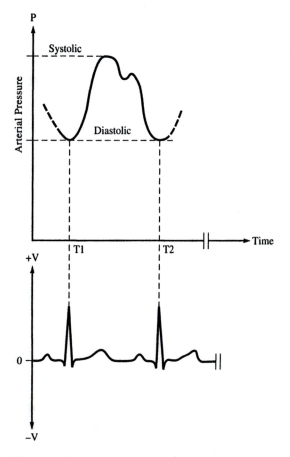

Figure 5-4
Human arterial pressure wave.

The square wave represents another case altogether because it has a very fast rise time. Theoretically, the square wave contains an infinite number of harmonics, but not all of the possible harmonics are present. For example, in the square wave, only the odd harmonics are typically found (e.g., third, fifth, seventh). According to some standards, accurately reproducing the square wave requires 100 harmonics, while others claim that 1000 harmonics are needed. Which standard to use may depend on the specifics of the application.

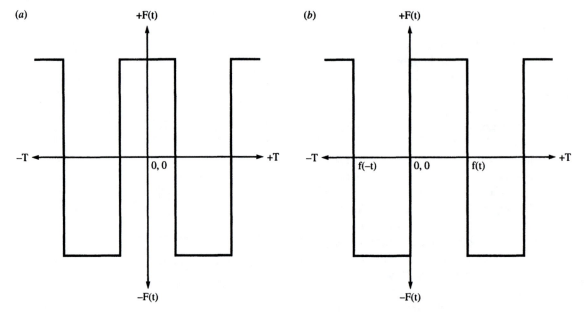

Figure 5-5
Odd and even Fourier series waveforms. (a) Odd-function square wave. (b) Even-function square wave.

Another factor that determines the profile of the Fourier series of a specific waveform is whether the function is *odd* or *even*. Figure 5-5a shows an odd-function square wave, and Figure 5-5b shows an even-function square wave. Even function is one in which $f(t) = f(-t)$, while for odd function, $-f(t) = f(-t)$. In even function, only cosine harmonics are present, so the sine amplitude coefficient b_n is zero. Similarly, in odd function only sine harmonics are present, so the cosine amplitude coefficient a_n is zero.

5-5 Waveform symmetry

Both *symmetry* and *asymmetry* can occur in several ways in a waveform (Figure 5-6), and those factors can affect the nature of the Fourier series of the waveform. Figure 5-6a shows a waveform with a dc component. Or, in terms of the Fourier series equation, the term a_o is nonzero. The dc compo-

nent represents a case of asymmetry in a signal. This offset can seriously affect instrumentation electronic circuits that are dc-coupled and thereby can result in serious artifact.

Two different forms of symmetry are shown in Figure 5-6b. *Zero-axis symmetry* occurs when, on a point-for-point basis, the wave shape and amplitude above the zero baseline are equal to the amplitude below the baseline (or $|+V_m| = |-V_m|$). When a waveform possesses zero-axis symmetry, it will usually not contain even harmonics; only odd harmonics are present. This situation is found in square waves, for example (Figure 5-7a). Zero-axis symmetry is not found only in sine and square waves, however, as the sawtooth waveform in Figure 5-6c demonstrates.

An exception to the *no even harmonics* general rule is that even harmonics will be present in the zero-axis symmetrical waveform (Fig. 5-7B) if the *even harmonics are in phase with the fundamental*

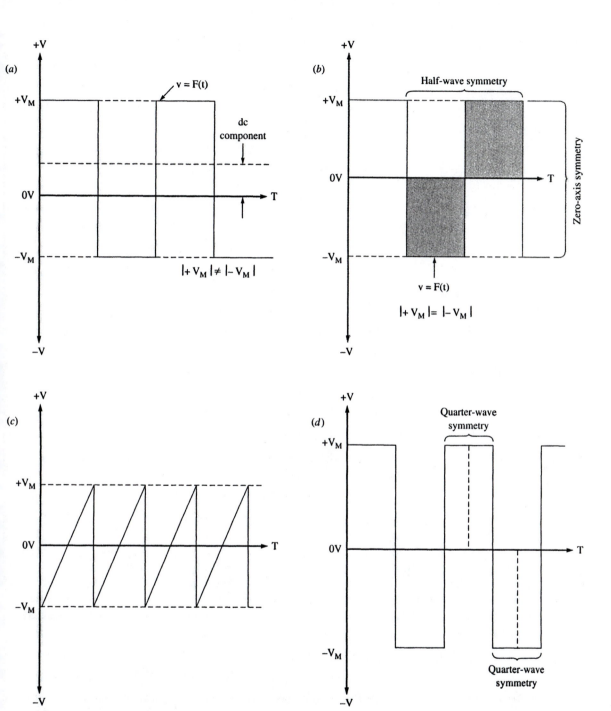

Figure 5-6
Waveform symmetry. (*a*) Square wave with DC component that causes asymmetry.
(*b*) Symmetrical square wave. (*c*) Sawtooth waveform forms mirror image across zero
baseline. (*d*) Quarter-wave symmetry.

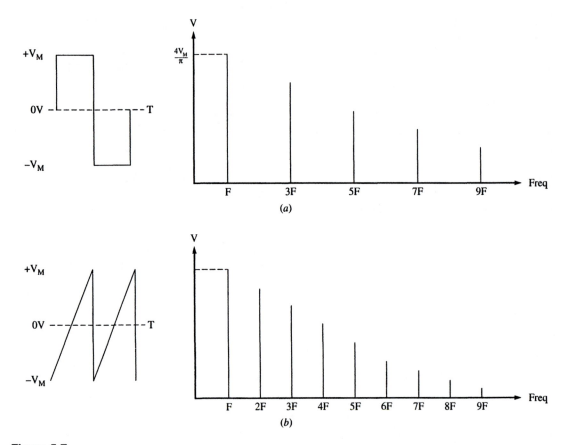

Figure 5-7
Fourier series for two waveforms: (*a*) Square wave. (*b*) Sawtooth wave.

sine wave. This condition will neither produce a dc component or disturb the zero-axis symmetry.

Also shown in Figure 5-6*b* is *half-wave symmetry*. In this type of symmetry the *shape* of the wave above the zero baseline is a mirror image of the shape of the waveform below the baseline (shaded region in Figure 5-6*b*). Half-wave symmetry also implies a lack of even harmonics.

Quarter-wave symmetry (Figure 5-6*d*) exists when the left and right sides of the waveforms are mirror images of each other on the same side of the zero-axis. Note that in Figure 5-6*d*, above the zero-axis the waveform is like a square wave, and indeed the left and right sides are mirror images of each other. Similarly, below the zero-axis the

rounded waveform has a mirror-image relationship between the left and right sides. In this case, there is a full set of even harmonics, and any odd harmonics that are present are in phase with the fundamental sine wave.

5-6 Transient signals

A transient signal is an event that occurs once only, occurs randomly over a long period of time, or is periodic but has a very short duration compared with its period (i.e., it is a very short duty cycle event). Many pulse signals fit the latter criterion, even though mathematically they are periodic.

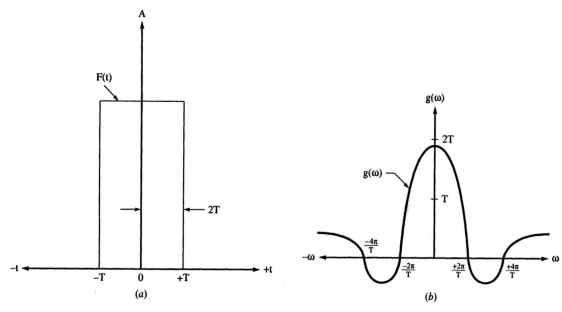

Figure 5-8
Transient signal has continuous spectrum. (*a*) Transient signal of duration 2T. (*b*) Spectral density region.

Transient signals are not represented properly by the Fourier series but can nonetheless be represented by sine waves in a spectrum. The difference is that the spectrum of the transient signal is *continuous* rather than discrete (as in a periodic signal). Consider a transient signal of period 2T, as in Figure 5-8*a*. The *spectral density*, g(ω), is:

$$g(\omega) = \int_{-\infty}^{+\infty} f(t) e^{-j\omega t}\, dt \qquad (5\text{-}6)$$

Equation 5-6 represents the spectral density g(ω). Given a spectral density, however, the original waveform can be reconstructed from:

$$f(t) = \frac{1}{2\pi} \int_{-\infty}^{+\infty} g(\omega)\, e^{j\omega t}\, d\omega \qquad (5\text{-}7)$$

The shape of the spectral density region is shown in Figure 5-8*b*. Note that the negative frequencies are a product of the mathematics and do not have physical reality. The shape of Figure 5-8*b* is expressed by:

$$g(\omega) = \frac{\sin \omega t}{\omega t} \qquad (5\text{-}8)$$

The general form *SIN x/x* is used also for repetitive pulse signals as well as the transient form shown in Figure 5-8*b*.

5-7 Sampled signals

The digital computer is incapable of accepting analog input signals, but rather requires a digitized representation of that signal. The *analog-to-digital (A/D) converter* will convert an input voltage (or current) to a representative binary word. If the A/D converter is either clocked or allowed to run asynchronously according to its own clock, then it will take a continuous string of samples of the signal as a function of time. When combined, these signals represent the original analog signal in binary form.

But the sampled signal is not exactly the same as the original signal, and some effort must be expended to ensure that the representation is as accurate as possible. Consider Figure 5-9. The

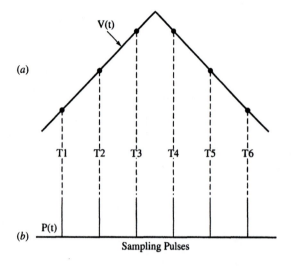

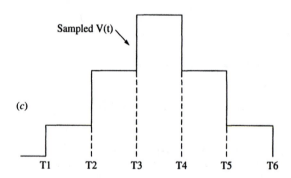

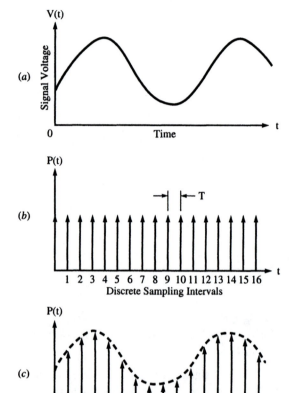

Figure 5-9
Sampled signal. (*a*) Continuous waveform.
(*b*) Sampled version of continuous waveform.
(*c*) Reconstructed waveform.

Figure 5-10
Sampled signal. (*a*) Sine wave. (*b*) Sampling of sine wave. (*c*) Sampled sine wave.

waveform in Figure 5-9*a* is a continuous voltage function of time, V(t); in this case a triangle waveform is seen. If the signal is sampled by another signal, P(t), with frequency F_s and sampling period $T = 1/F_s$, as shown in Figure 5-9*b,* and then later reconstructed, the waveform may look something like Figure 5-9*c*. While this may be sufficiently representative of the waveform for many purposes, it would be reconstructed with greater fidelity if the sampling frequency (F_s) were increased. Figure 5-10 shows another case in which a sine wave, V(t) in Figure 5-10*a*, is sampled by a pulse signal, P(t) in Figure 5-10*b*. The sampling signal, P(t), consists of a train of equally spaced

narrow pulses spaced in time by T. The sampling frequency $F_s = 1/T$. The result is shown in Figure 5-10*c* and is another pulsed signal in which the amplitudes of the pulses represent a sampled version of the original sine wave signal.

The sampling rate, F_s, must by *Nyquist's theorem* be twice the maximum frequency (F_m) in the Fourier spectrum of the applied analog signal, V(t). To reconstruct the original signal after sampling, it is necessary to pass the sampled waveform through a low-pass filter that limits the bandpass to F_s.

The sampling process is analogous to a form of *amplitude modulation* (AM), in which V(t) is the

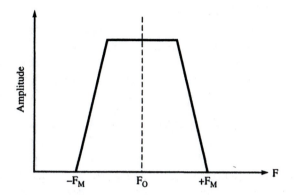

Figure 5-11
Spectrum of sampled signal.

modulating signal, with spectrum from dc to F_m, and P(t) is the carrier frequency. The resultant spectrum is shown partially in Figure 5-11, and resembles the double sideband with carrier AM spectrum. The spectrum of the modulating signal appears as sidebands around the carrier frequency, shown here as F_o. The actual spectrum is a bit more complex, as shown in Figure 5-12. Like an unfiltered AM radio transmitter, the same spectral information appears not only around the fundamental frequency (F_s) of the carrier (shown at zero in Figure 5-12), but also at the harmonics and subharmonics spaced at intervals of F_s up and down the spectrum.

Provided that the sampling frequency $F_s \geq 2F_m$, the original signal is recoverable from the sampled version by passing it through a low-pass filter with a cutoff frequency F_c, set to pass only the spectrum of the analog signal but not the sampling frequency. This phenomenon is shown with the dotted line in Figure 5-12.

A problem occurs when the sampling frequency F_s is less than $2F_m$, (Figure 5-13). The spectrum of the sampled signal looks as it did before, but the regions around each harmonic overlap so that the value of $-F_m$ for one spectral region is less than $+F_m$ for the next lower frequency region. This overlap results in a phenomenon called *aliasing*. That is, when the sampled signal is recovered by low-pass filtering, it will produce not the original sine wave frequency F_o but a lower frequency equal to ($F_s - F_o$), and the information carried in the waveform is thus lost or distorted.

The solution, for high-fidelity sampling of the analog waveform for input to a computer, is as follows:

1. Bandwidth-limit the signal at the input of the sampler or A/D converter with a low-pass filter that has a cutoff frequency F_c that is selected to pass only the maximum frequency in the waveform (F_m) and not the sampling frequency (F_s).

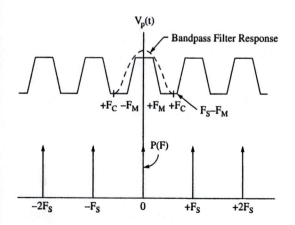

Figure 5-12
Wider view of sampled signal spectrum.

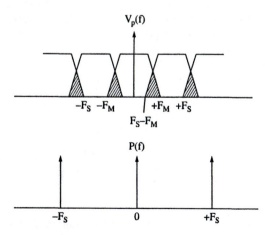

Figure 5-13
Aliasing occurs when $F_s < 2F_M$.

2. Set the sampling frequency F_s at a minimum of twice the maximum frequency in the applied waveform's Fourier spectrum, i.e., $F_s \geq 2F_m$.

Note: Experience has shown that some users will not accept a reconstructed sampled waveform if the sample rate is $2F_m$; for example, medical ECG waveforms—in which $F_m = 100$ Hz—tend to look "blocky" when sampled at 200 Hz and then reconstructed. User acceptance is much better when the waveform is sampled at 500 Hz, or $5F_m$. While that rate once was expensive to accommodate in an eight-bit A/D converter, it is now very inexpensive and should be used—Nyquist's theorem notwithstanding.

5-8 Noise

An ideal electronic circuit produces no noise of its own, so the output signal from the ideal circuit contains only the noise that was in the original signal. But real electronic circuits and components do produce a certain level of inherent noise of their own. Even the simple fixed-value resistor is noisy. Figure 5-14a shows the equivalent circuit for an ideal, noise-free resistor. The inherent noise is represented in Figure 5-14b by a noise voltage source, V_n, in series with the ideal, noise-free resistance, R_i. At any temperature above *absolute zero* (0°K, or about −273°C), electrons in any material are in constant random motion. Because of the inherent randomness of that motion, however, there is no detectable current in any one direction. In other words, electron drift in any single direction is cancelled over short time periods by equal drift in the opposite direction. Electron motions are therefore statistically decorrelated. There is, however, a continuous series of random current pulses generated in the material, and those pulses are seen by the outside world as a noise signal. This signal is called by several names: *Johnson noise, thermal agitation noise,* or *thermal noise.*

This noise is called *white noise* because it has a very broadband (nearly Gaussian) spectral density. The thermal noise spectrum is dominated by mid-frequencies (10^4 to 10^5 Hz) and is essentially flat. The term *white noise* is a metaphor similar to the term *white light,* which is composed of all visible color frequencies. The expression for Johnson noise is:

$$(V_n)^2 = 4KTRB \; V^2/\text{Hz} \qquad (5\text{-}9)$$

where

V_n is the noise voltage (V)

K is Boltzmann's constant (1.38×10^{23} J/°K)

T is the temperature in degrees kelvin (°K)

R is the resistance in ohms (Ω)

B is the bandwidth in hertz (Hz)

With the constants collected, and the expression normalized to 1 kΩ, Equation 5-9 reduces to:

$$V_n = 4\sqrt{\frac{R}{1 \text{ k}\Omega}} \; \frac{nV}{\sqrt{\text{Hz}}} \qquad (5\text{-}10)$$

The evaluated solution of Equation 5-10 is normally read *nanovolts per square root hertz.* In this equation, a 1-MΩ resistor will have a thermal noise of 126 nV/$\sqrt{\text{Hz}}$.

Several other forms of noise are present in linear integrated circuits (ICs) and other semiconductor amplifiers to some extent. For example, because current flow at the quantum level is not smooth and predictable, an intermittent burst phenomenon sometimes occurs. This noise, called *popcorn noise,* consists of pulses of many mil-

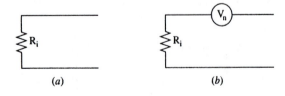

(a)   (b)

Figure 5-14
Resistor noise. (a) Ideal, noise-free resistor. (b) Practical resistor has internal thermal noise source.

liseconds' duration. Another form of noise is *shot noise* (also called *Schottky noise*). The term *shot* is derived from the fact that the noise sounds like a handful of BB shot thrown against a metal surface. Shot noise is a consequence of dc current flowing in any conductor and is found from:

$$(I_n)^2 = 2qIB \ A^2/Hz \qquad (5\text{-}11)$$

where

I_n is the noise current in amperes (A)

q is the elementary electric charge
   $(1.6 \times 10^{-19}$ coulombs)

I is the current in amperes (A)

B is the bandwidth in hertz (Hz)

Finally, there is *flicker noise* also called *pink noise* or *l/f noise*. The latter name applies because flicker noise is predominantly a low-frequency ($<$ 1000 Hz) phenomenon. This type of noise is found in all conductors and becomes important in IC devices because of manufacturing defects.

The noise spectrum in any given instrumentation system will contain elements of several kinds of noise, although in some systems one form may dominate the others. It is common to characterize noise from a single source using the *root mean square* (rms) value of the voltage amplitudes:

$$V_{n(rms)} = \sqrt{\frac{1}{T} \int_0^T [F(t)]^2 \, dt} \qquad (5\text{-}12)$$

Figure 5-15 shows the noise spectrum profile for a typical system that contains l/f noise, thermal or white noise, and some high frequency noise.

5-9 Signal-to-noise ratio

Amplifiers can be evaluated on the basis of *signal-to-noise ratio* (SNR), denoted S_n. The goal of the circuit or instrument designer is to enhance the SNR as much as possible. Ultimately, the minimum signal level detectable at the output of an amplifier is the level that appears above the noise

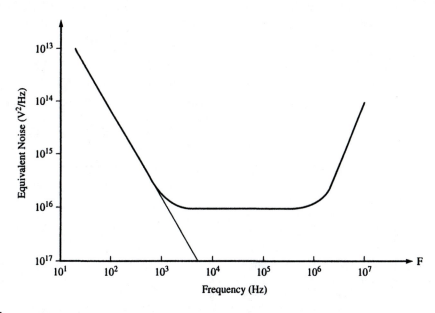

Figure 5-15
Noise spectrum profile when l/f noise, thermal ("white") noise, and high frequency noise are present.

floor level. Therefore, the lower the system noise floor, the smaller the *minimum allowable signal.* Although often thought of as a radio receiver parameter, SNR is applicable in other amplifiers in which signal levels are low and gains are high. This situation occurs in scientific, medical, and engineering instrumentation as well as in other applications.

Noise resulting from thermal agitation of electrons is measured in terms of *noise power* (P_n) and carries the units of power (watts). Noise power is found from:

$$P_n = KTB \qquad (5\text{-}13)$$

where

P_n is the noise power in watts (W)

K is Boltzmann's constant $(1.38 \times 10^{-23} \text{ J/}°\text{K})$

B is the bandwidth in hertz (Hz)

T is the temperature in Kelvins

Notice in Equation 5-13 that there is no center frequency term, only the bandwidth (B). True thermal noise is Gaussian (or near-Gaussian), so frequency content, phase, and amplitudes are equally distributed across the entire spectrum. Thus, in bandwidth-limited systems, such as a practical amplifier or network, the total noise power is related to temperature and bandwidth. We can conclude that a 200-Hz bandwidth centered on 1 kHz produces the same thermal noise level as a 200-Hz bandwidth centered on 600 Hz or any other frequency.

Noise sources can be categorized as either *internal* or *external*. Internal noise sources are caused by thermal currents in the semiconductor material resistances. Internal noise is the noise component contributed by the amplifier under consideration. When noise, or SNR, is measured at both input and output of an amplifier, the output noise is greater. The internal noise of the device is the difference between output noise level and input noise level.

External noise is the noise produced by the signal source, so it is often called *source noise*. This noise signal is caused by thermal agitation cur-

rents in the signal source, and even a simple zero-signal input termination resistance has some amount of thermal agitation noise. In fact, the simple terminated noise level might be higher than V_n because of component construction. For example, the noise signal produced by a carbon composition resistor has an additional noise source modeled as V_{na} in Figure 5-16. This noise generator is a function of resistor construction and manufacturing defects.

Figure 5-17a shows a circuit model showing that several voltage and current noise sources exist in an operational amplifier (op-amp). The relative strengths of these noise sources, hence their overall contribution, varies with op-amp type. In a field effect transitor (FET)–input op-amp, for example, the current noise sources are tiny, but voltage noise sources are very large. On bipolar op-amps the exact opposite situation obtains.

All of the noise sources in Figure 5-17a are uncorrelated with respect to each other, so one cannot simply add noise voltages; only noise power can be added. To characterize noise voltages and currents they must be added in the rss manner.

Models, such as the one shown in Figure 5-17a, are too complex for most situations, so it is standard practice to combine all of the voltage noise sources into one source and all of the current noise sources into another source. The composite sources have a value equal to the rss voltage (or current) of the individual sources. Figure 5-17b is such a model, in which only a single current source and a single voltage source are used. The *equivalent ac noise* in Figure 5-17b is the overall

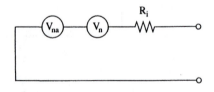

Figure 5-16
Noise source Vna is due to resistor construction and manufacturing defects.

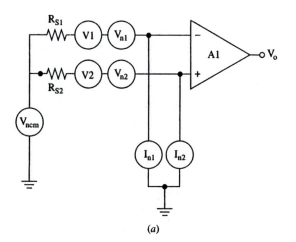

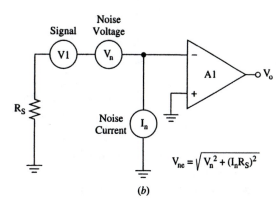

$$V_{ne} = \sqrt{V_n^2 + (I_n R_S)^2}$$

(a) (b)

Figure 5-17
Voltage and current noise sources. (a) Multiple uncorrelated noise sources. (b) Equivalent
noise source makes calculations easier.

noise, given a specified value of source resistance, R_s, and is found from the rss value of V_n and I_n:

$$V_{nT} = \sqrt{V_n^2 + (I_n R_s)^2} \qquad (5\text{-}14)$$

5-10 Noise factor, figure, and temperature

The noise of a system or network can be defined in three different but related ways: *noise factor* (F_n), *noise figure* (NF) and *equivalent noise temperature* (T_e); these properties are definable as a simple ratio, decibel ratio, or temperature, respectively.

Noise factor

For components such as resistors, the noise factor is the ratio of the noise produced by a real resistor to the simple thermal noise of an ideal resistor. The noise factor of a system is the ratio of output noise power (P_{no}) to input noise power (P_{ni}).

$$F_n = \frac{P_{no}}{P_{ni}}\Big|_{T = 290°K} \qquad (5\text{-}15)$$

To make comparisons easier, the noise factor is always measured at the standard temperature (T_o) of 290°K which is (standardized room temperature).

The input noise power, P_{ni}, is defined as the product of the source noise at standard temperature (T_o) and the amplifier gain (G):

$$P_{ni} = GKBT_o \qquad (5\text{-}16)$$

It is also possible to define noise factor F_n in terms of output and input SNR:

$$F_n = \frac{S_{ni}}{S_{no}} \qquad (5\text{-}17)$$

which is also:

$$F_n = \frac{P_{no}}{KT_o BG} \qquad (5\text{-}18)$$

where

S_{ni} is the input signal-to-noise ratio

S_{no} is the output signal-to-noise ratio

P_{no} is the output noise power

K is Boltzmann's constant (1.38×10^{-23} J/°K)

T_o is 290°K

B is the network bandwidth in hertz (Hz)

G is the amplifier gain

The noise factor can be evaluated in a model that considers the amplifier ideal and therefore amplifies only through gain G the noise produced by the input noise source:

$$F_n = \frac{KT_oBG + \Delta N}{KT_oBG} \qquad (5\text{-}19)$$

or

$$F_n = \frac{\Delta N}{KT_oBG} \qquad (5\text{-}20)$$

where

ΔN is the noise added by the network or amplifier
(Other terms as previously defined)

Noise figure

The noise figure is a frequently used measure of an amplifier's *goodness,* or its departure from the ideal. Thus it is a *figure of merit.* The noise figure is the noise factor converted to decibel notation:

$$NF = 10 \, LOG \, F_n \qquad (5\text{-}21)$$

where

NF   is the noise figure in decibels (dB)

F_n is the noise factor

LOG refers to the system of base-10 logarithms

Noise temperature

The noise temperature is a means for specifying noise in terms of an equivalent temperature. Evaluating Equation 2-16 shows that the noise power is directly proportional to temperature in degrees kelvin and that noise power collapses to zero at absolute zero ($0°K$).

Note that the equivalent noise temperature T_e is not the physical temperature of the amplifier, but rather a theoretical construct that is an *equivalent* temperature that produces that amount of noise power. The noise temperature is related to the noise factor by:

$$T_e = (F_n - 1) \, T_o \qquad (5\text{-}22)$$

and to noise figure by:

$$T_e = \left[antilog\left(\frac{NF}{10}\right) - 1 \right] K T_o \qquad (5\text{-}23)$$

Now that we have noise temperature T_e, we can also define noise factor and noise figure in terms of noise temperature:

$$F_n = \frac{T_e}{T_o} + 1 \qquad (5\text{-}24)$$

and

$$NF = 10 \, LOG\left(\frac{T_e}{T_o} + 1\right) \qquad (5\text{-}25)$$

The total noise in any amplifier or network is the sum of internally and externally generated noise. In terms of noise temperature:

$$P_{n(total)} = GKB(T_o + T_e) \qquad (5\text{-}26)$$

where

$P_{n(total)}$ is the total noise power
(Other terms as previously defined)

5-11 Noise in cascade amplifiers

A noise signal is seen by a following amplifier as a valid input signal. Thus, in a cascade amplifier, the final stage sees an input signal that consists of the original signal and noise amplified by each successive stage. Each stage in the cascade chain amplifies signals and noise from previous stages and contributes some noise of its own. The overall noise factor for a cascade amplifier can be calculated from the *Friis noise equation:*

$$F_N = F_1 + \frac{F_2 - 1}{G1} + \frac{F_3 - 1}{G1G2}$$
$$+ \cdots + \frac{F_n - 1}{G1G2\cdots G_n} \qquad (5\text{-}27)$$

where

F_N is the overall noise factor of N stages in cascade

F_1 is the noise factor of stage 1

F_2 is the noise factor of stage 2

F_n is the noise factor of the nth stage

G1   is the gain of stage 1

G2   is the gain of stage 2

G_{n-1} is the gain of stage $(n - 1)$

As you can see from Equation 5-27, the noise factor of the entire cascade chain is dominated by the noise contribution of the first stage or two. High-gain, low-noise amplifiers (such as electroencephalogram [EEG] preamplifiers) typically use a low-noise amplifier circuit for only the first stage or two in the cascade chain.

5-12 Noise reduction strategies

Although noise is a serious problem for the designer, especially when low signal levels are present, a number of commonsense approaches can be used to minimize the effects of noise on a system. In this section we will examine several of these methods. For example:

1. Keep the source resistance and the amplifier input resistance as low as possible. Using high value resistances will increase thermal noise proportionally.

2. Total thermal noise is also a function of the bandwidth of the circuit. Therefore, reducing

the bandwidth of the circuit to a minimum will also minimize noise. But this job must be done mindfully, because signals have a Fourier spectrum that must be preserved for faithful reproduction or accurate measurement. The solution is to match the bandwidth to the frequency response required for the input signal.

3. Prevent external noise from affecting the performance of the system by appropriate use of grounding, shielding, and filtering.

4. Use a low-noise amplifier in the input stage of the system.

5. For some semiconductor circuits, use the lowest dc power supply potentials that will do the job.

Using feedback to reduce noise

Negative feedback is well known for reducing amplitude and phase errors, thereby reducing the distortion of an amplifier. Judicious use of feedback can also reduce the output noise of a signal conditioning amplifier.

Consider Figure 5-18. This circuit model shows gain distributed into two blocks, G1 and G2. The total gain of the circuit (G) is the product G1G2. A noise source produces a noise signal, V_n, and injects it into a summation junction between G1 and

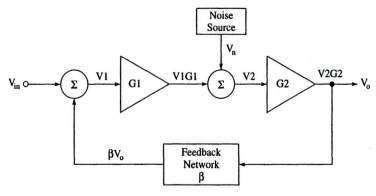

Figure 5-18
Cascade two-stage amplifier block diagram.

G2. A feedback network with a transfer function β produces a signal βV_o that is summed with input signal V_{in}. By inspection of Figure 5-18 we know:

$$V1 = V_{in} + \beta V_o \qquad (5\text{-}28)$$

$$V2 = V1G1 + V_n \qquad (5\text{-}29)$$

$$V2 = (V_{in} + \beta V_o)G1 + V_n \qquad (5\text{-}30)$$

and

$$V_o = V2G2 \qquad (5\text{-}31)$$

Substituting Equation 5-30 into Equation 5-31:

$$V_o = [((V_{in} + \beta V_o)G1 + V_n)G2] \qquad (5\text{-}32)$$

$$V_o = G1G2V_{in} + \beta V_o G1G2 + V_n G2 \qquad (5\text{-}33)$$

which, when rearranged, leads to:

$$V_o = \frac{G1G2V_{in} + NG2}{1 - \beta G1G2} \qquad (5\text{-}34)$$

and finally:

$$V_o = \frac{G1G2}{1 - \beta G1G2}\left[V_{in} + \frac{N}{G1}\right] \qquad (5\text{-}35)$$

The result shown in Equation 5-35 is consistent with *Black's equation* for feedback amplifiers $[G_o = G/(1 - \beta G)]$, and demonstrates that the noise is reduced by the gain factor (G1). This result is also consistent with the design philosophy inherent in the Friis equation.

Noise reduction by signal averaging

If a signal is either periodic or repetitive, or can be made so, then it is possible to enhance signal-to-noise ratio (SNR, or S_n) by signal averaging. The basis for this simple signal-processing technique is the assumption that noise meets the definition of either random or chaotic processes. If so, then noise tends to integrate to zero or near zero over time. If time-averaging integration is performed in a coherent manner, then a repetitive signal tends to build in value, while noise levels (being decorrelated) decrease. If we assume that the SNR is:

$$S_n = 20\ LOG\left(\frac{V_{in}}{V_n}\right) \qquad (5\text{-}36)$$

Then, for systems in which $V_i < V_n$, the noise reduction by time averaging is:

$$\bar{S} = 20\ LOG\left(\frac{V_{in}}{V_n/\sqrt{N}}\right) \qquad (5\text{-}37)$$

where

$\bar{S}$ is the time-averaged SNR

S_n is the unprocessed SNR

N is the number of repetitions of the signal

Example

An EEG system processes a 5-μV signal in the presence of a 100-μV random noise level. Calculate the unprocessed SNR, the processed SNR for 1000 repetitions of the signal, and the processing gain.

Solution

a. *Unprocessed SNR:*

$$S_n = 20\ LOG(V_{in}/V_n)$$
$$= 20\ LOG(5\ \mu V/100\ \mu V) = -26\ \textbf{dB}$$

b. *Processed SNR:*

$$\bar{S}_n = 20\ LOG[V_{in}/(V_n/\sqrt{N})]$$
$$= 20\ LOG[5\mu V/(100\mu V/\sqrt{1000})]$$
$$= +4\ \text{dB}$$

c. *Processing Gain:*

$$G_p = \bar{S}_n - S_n$$
$$= (+4\ \text{dB}) - (-26\ \text{dB}) = +\textbf{22 dB}$$

The effect of time averaging is to increase the time required to collect data, so (by F = 1/T), time averaging is effectively a means of decreasing the bandwidth of the system.

Coherency is maintained in a system by ensuring that repetitive data points are processed in a consistent time relationship with respect to each other. The averager will be triggered by a repetitive event, and that action starts the process. Data points are always matched to other data points taken at the same elapsed time after the trigger for previous iterations. For example, the *ith* data point following a current sweep is paired with all other *ith* points from previous sweeps, and none other.

An example of signal averaging used to extract weak signals from larger noise signals is found in *evoked potential* studies of EEG waveforms (chapter 13).

5-13 Summary

1. There are several classes of signals: *static* and *quasistatic, periodic, repetitive, transient,* and *random.* These signals differ in how they behave in time (e.g., repetitive, periodic, or unchanging) and in the frequency domain.

2. All waveforms can be represented by a mathematical statement called a *Fourier series,* i.e., a collection of sine and cosine harmonics of the fundamental frequency. The Fourier series is represented graphically by a series of bars that each represent a different harmonic, and the length of each represents the strength of that component. The Fourier series of the signal is important to understanding signal processing and circuit requirements. The ECG waveform, for example, has a fundamental repetition rate of around 70 beats/min (at rest) and Fourier components up to about 100 Hz.

3. Waveform symmetry can be used to guess the Fourier content of the waveform.

4. *Sampled signals* are obtained by repetitively measuring the amplitude of an analog signal.

5. Electrical noise signals caused by thermal agitation are present even when there are no active devices (e.g., transistors, ICs) in the circuit, at all temperatures above absolute zero (0°K or about -273.2°C). Additional forms of noise are contributed by active circuits.

6. A critical requirement for signals to be useful is the signal-to-noise ratio (SNR, or S_n). The noise performance of circuits can be represented by the noise factor, noise figure, or noise temperature of the circuit.

7. The Friis equation represents the noise performance of a chain of cascade amplifiers. The equation demonstrates that the noise performance of the cascade chain is set mostly by the noise performance of the first stage.

8. Several strategies are available for reducing noise, among which are signal averaging, filtering, and integration.

5-14 Recapitulation

Now return to the objectives and self-evaluation questions at the beginning of the chapter and see how well you can answer them. If you cannot answer certain questions, place a check mark next to each and review appropriate parts of the text. Next, try to answer the following questions using the same procedure. When you have answered all of the questions, solve the problems.

Questions

1. List five different time domain classes of signals: _____, _____, _____, _____, and _____.

2. Sketch the time-series waveforms of the signals in question 1.

3. A _____ signal is unchanging over time.

4. A _____ signal is nearly unchanging, or changes very slowly, over time.

5. A _____ signal repeats itself exactly over time such that $V(t) = V(t + T)$.

6. A _____ signal is basically repetitive, but there may be wave shape or duration differences from repetition to repetition, as well as occasional anomalous events that are different from the rest of the waveform.

7. The human _____ _____ _____ waveform is an example of the signal in question 6.

8. A _____ signal is a one-time event, or occurs periodically, but with a duration that is very short relative to its period.

9. A _____ _____ is the mathematical expression of a series of discrete harmonic components and a fundamental frequency that make up a continuous waveform.

10. The _____ of a repeating waveform is the time between recurrence of identical events.

11. Write the relationship between frequency and the period of a sine wave.

12. The harmonic content of a waveform can be found using a computer algorithm called the _____ _____ transform.

13. A waveform with half-wave symmetry can have a dc component. True or false?

14. The number of harmonics present in a waveform depends in part on the _____ time of the waveform.

15. In _____-_____ symmetry waveforms, usually no even-order harmonics are present.

16. State an exception to the rule in question 15.

17. The frequency spectrum of a _____ signal is discrete, while that of a _____ signal is continuous.

18. The _____ density pertains to which type of signal in question 17?

19. A _____ signal is made by repetitively measuring the amplitude of a waveform over time.

20. An _____-to-_____ converter can be used to create the signal in question 19.

21. According to Nyquist's theorem, the minimum sampling frequency for reconstructing or representing a signal is _____ the maximum frequency component in the waveform's spectrum.

22. _____ is a phenomenon that occurs when the sampling frequency is too low.

23. All conductors generate random electrical noise at all temperatures above _____ _____ (use either the name or numerical representation of that temperature).

24. What are three names used to describe thermal noise?

25. _____ noise has an intermittent burst characteristic.

26. _____-noise, also called _____ noise or _____ noise, is primarily a low-frequency component.

27. The _____ _____ _____ average is used to characterize the noise sources in a circuit.

28. Why is the SNR important in signals acquisition?

29. List three different ways that the noise performance of an amplifier or circuit can be expressed.

30. The noise performance of a cascade chain of amplifiers is dominated by the (first/last) stage, which can be seen by evaluating the _____ noise equation.

31. Write the equation in question 30.

32. List three noise-reduction methods. Describe each using a few sentences (in your own words).

33. Sketch periodic waveforms that exhibit: (a) quarter-wave symmetry, (b) half-wave symmetry.

34. Sketch a squarewave with a dc component that is one-third the peak amplitude (not peak to peak) of the waveform.

Problems

1. What is the period, in seconds, of a 100-Hz sine wave?

2. The amplitude of a 100-Hz sine wave at time t_1 is 0.55 V. What is the amplitude at time $t_1 + T$?

3. A sine wave has a peak amplitude of 2 V and a frequency of 1000 Hz. Calculate the instantaneous voltage at a time of 250 μs after the waveform passes through the 0-V baseline in a positive direction.

4. Calculate the noise voltage between dc and 1000 Hz due to thermal agitation in a circuit containing only a 75-Ω resistor.

5. What is the noise level of a 4.7 kΩ ideal resistor, expressed in $nV/\sqrt{Hz}$?

6. What is the shot-noise level over the bandwidth dc to 20 kHz in a conductor in which 100 mA flows?

7. Two noise sources are present in a circuit: a voltage source that produces 50 μV (rms), and a current source in which a 120-nA current flows in a 100-Ω resistance. What is the average noise voltage of this circuit?

8. A circuit has a noise figure of 4.7 dB. Calculate the noise factor.

9. Calculate the noise temperature of the circuit in problem 8.

10. Three amplifiers in cascade have the following characteristics:

Amplifier	Gain	Noise Figure (dB)
A1	100	2.1 d
A2	10	10.8 d
A3	5	5.4 d

Calculate the noise factor for the entire chain.

11. Reverse the order of the amplifiers in problem 10 (i.e., exchange A1 and A3), and recalculate the noise factor. Compare the results.

12. An operational amplifier has an open-loop gain of 1,000,000. Calculate the closed loop gain when $\beta = 0.10$.

13. An EEG signal processes a 10-μV signal in the presence of 125 μV of random noise. Calculate the processing gain and processed SNR if signal averaging of 256 repetitions of the waveform is performed.

CHAPTER 6
Electrodes, Sensors, and Transducers

6-1 Objectives

1. Be able to list the problems associated with the acquisition of biopotentials.
2. Be able to list the different types of electrodes used to acquire biopotentials.

3. Be able to list and describe the types of transducers used to measure physiological parameters.

6-2 Self-evaluation questions

These questions test your prior knowledge of the material in this chapter. Look for the answers as you read the text. After you have finished studying the chapter, try answering these questions and those at the end of the chapter.

1. Define the terms *half-cell* and *electrode offset potentials.*

2. Describe the *column electrode.* What is the principal advantage of the column electrode?

3. Describe the operation of a *Wheatstone bridge.* What factors determine the output voltage? What is the *null condition?*

4. What are the differences between *bonded* and *unbonded* strain gauges?

5. List three types of temperature transducers.

6-3 Signal acquisition

Most medical instruments are *electronic* devices and so *must* have an electrical signal for an input. When a biopotential must be acquired, some form of *electrode* is used between the patient and the instrument. In other cases, a *transducer* is used to convert some nonelectrical physical parameter or stimulus, such as force, pressure, or temperature, to an analogous electrical signal proportional to the value of the original stimulus parameter.

Definition: A *transducer,* in this context, is a device that will *convert* some form of *energy* produced by a physical stimulus to an *electrical analog* of the stimulus.

6-4 Transduction

It is necessary to understand the linked concepts of *transduction* and *transducible property.* A transducible property is a characteristic of the physical event that is singularly able to represent that parameter and be transformed into an electrical signal by some device or process. For example, carbon dioxide (CO_2) absorbs electromagnetic wavelengths of 2.7, 4.3, and 14.7 μm. Although water also absorbs 2.7-μm radiation to a small degree, it is possible to make an infrared (IR) sensor that will respond to either 4.3 or 14.7 μm or all three wavelengths to measure CO_2 content of a gas, such as air. End-tidal CO_2 monitors, used in respiratory therapy, intensive care, and anesthesia, use infrared sensors. Transduction is the process of converting the transducible property into an electrical signal that can be input to an instrument.

6-5 Active versus passive sensors

Another ambiguity found in discussions of biomedical sensors is the distinction between *active* and *passive sensors.* Unfortunately, competing texts use opposite definitions of these terms. This text adopts the form that is used by most people in the medical instruments field, which is also consistent with usage in other areas of electronics.

An *active sensor* requires an external ac or dc electrical source to power the device. An example is the resistive strain gauge blood pressure sensor that requires a $+7.5$-V dc-regulated power supply to operate. Without that external excitation potential, there is no output from the sensor.

A *passive sensor,* on the other hand, either provides its own energy or derives its energy from the phenomenon being measured. An example is the thermocouple, which is often used to measure temperature in research settings.

It is unfortunate that some textbook authors invert these definitions, but if the above definitions are accepted, you will be consistent with the most common usage.

6-6 Sensor error sources

Sensors, like all other devices, sustain certain errors. To maintain consistency, error is defined as the *difference between the measured value and the true value.* While the full range of possible errors is beyond the scope of this book, it is possible to break them into five basic categories: *insertion, application, characteristic, dynamic,* and *environmental errors.*

Insertion errors

This class of error occurs during the act of inserting the sensor into the system being measured. This is a general problem with electronic measurements, indeed, with all measurements. For example, when measuring the voltage in a circuit, one must be certain that the inherent impedance of the voltmeter is much larger than the circuit impedance; otherwise circuit loading will occur, and the reading will be in significant error. Possible sources of this form of error include using a transducer that is too large for the system (e.g., pressures), one that is too sluggish for the dynamics of the system, or one that self-heats to the extent that excessive thermal energy is added to the system. Nineteenth-century British physicist Lord Kelvin formulated a *first rule of instrumentation,* to the effect that *the measuring instrument must not alter the event being measured.*

Application errors

These errors are caused by the operator, such as the proverbial *cockpit trouble* referred to by airplane mechanics. Again, far too many of these errors are possible, so we must settle on a couple of illustrative examples. One error seen in temperature measurements is either incorrect placement of the probe or erroneous insulation of the probe from the measurement site. This problem often occurs in clinical medicine when the sanitary cover over the probe of a digital thermometer is not properly seated. Examples seen in blood pressure sensor applications include failure to purge the system of air and other gases (bubbles in the line), and incorrect physical placement of the transducer (above or below the heart line) so that a positive or negative pressure head is erroneously added to the correct reading.

Characteristic errors

This category is most often meant when discussing errors without otherwise qualifying the term. These are errors inherent in the device itself, i.e., the difference between the ideal published characteristic transfer function of the device and the actual characteristic. This form of error may include a dc offset value (a false pressure head), an incorrect slope, or a slope that is not perfectly linear.

Dynamic errors

Many sensors are characterized and calibrated in a static condition, i.e., with an input parameter that is either static or quasistatic. Many sensors are heavily damped, so that they will not respond to rapid changes in the input parameter. For example, thermistors tend to require many seconds to respond to a step-function change in temperature. That is, a thermistor in equilibrium will not jump immediately to the new resistance on an abrupt change in temperature; rather, the device will change slowly toward the new value. Thus, if an attempt is made to follow a rapidly changing temperature with a sluggish sensor, the output waveform will be distorted and therefore contain error. The issues to confront with respect to dynamic errors include response time, amplitude distortion, and phase distortion.

Environmental errors

These errors are derived from the environment in which the sensor is used. They most often include

temperature but may also include vibration, shock, altitude, chemical exposure, or other factors. These factors most often affect the characteristic errors of the sensor, so are often combined with that category in practical application.

6-7 Sensor terminology

Sensors, like other areas of technology, have a specific terminology that must be understood before they can be properly applied. Some of the most common terms are discussed below.

Sensitivity

The sensitivity of the sensor is defined as the slope of the output characteristic curve ($\Delta Y/\Delta X$ in Figure 6-1) or, more generally, the *minimum input of physical parameter that will create a detectable output change.* In some sensors, the sensitivity is defined as the input parameter change required to produce a standardized output change. In others, it is defined as an output voltage change for a given change in input parameter. For example, a typical blood pressure transducer may have a sensitivity rating of 10μV/V/mm Hg; that is, there will be a 10-μV output voltage for each volt of excitation potential and each millimeter of mercury of applied pressure.

Sensitivity error

The sensitivity error (shown as a dotted curve in Figure 6-1) is a departure from the ideal slope of the characteristic curve. For example, the pressure transducer discussed above may have an actual sensitivity of 7.8 μV/V/mm Hg instead of 10 μV/V/mm Hg.

Range

The range of the sensor is the maximum and minimum values of applied parameter that can be measured. For example, a given pressure sensor may have a range of −400 to +400 mm Hg. Alternatively, the positive and negative ranges often

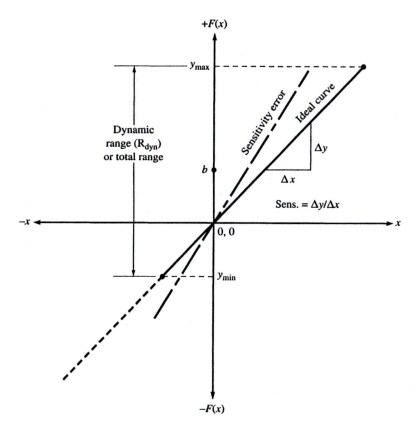

Figure 6-1
Ideal curve and sensitivity error. Source: J.J. Carr, *Sensors and Circuits*, Prentice Hall.

are unequal. For example, a certain medical blood pressure transducer is specified to have a minimum (vacuum) limit of −50 mm Hg (Y_{min} in Figure 6-1) and a maximum (pressure) limit of +450 mm Hg (Y_{max} in Figure 6-1). This specification is common, incidentally, and is one reason doctors and nurses sometimes destroy blood pressure sensors when attempting to draw blood through an arterial line without being mindful of the position of the fluid stopcocks in the system. A small syringe can exert a tremendous vacuum on a closed system.

Dynamic range

The dynamic range is the total range of the sensor from minimum to maximum. That is, in terms of Figure 6-1, $R_{dyn} = Y_{max} - |-Y_{min}|$.

Precision

The concept of precision refers to the degree of *reproducibility* of a measurement. In other words, if exactly the same value were measured a number of times, an ideal sensor would output exactly the same value every time. But real sensors output a range of values distributed in some manner relative to the actual correct value. For example, suppose a pressure of exactly 150 mm Hg is applied to a sensor. Even if the applied pressure never changes, the output values from the sensor will vary considerably. Some subtle problems arise in the matter of precision when the true value and the sensor's mean value are not within a certain distance of each other (e.g., the 1-σ range of the normal distribution curve).

Resolution

This specification is the smallest detectable incremental change of input parameter that can be detected in the output signal. Resolution can be expressed either as a proportion of the reading (or the full-scale reading) or in absolute terms.

Accuracy

The accuracy of the sensor is the maximum difference that will exist between the actual value (which must be measured by a primary or good secondary standard) and the indicated value at the output of the sensor. Again, the accuracy can be

expressed either as a percentage of full scale or in absolute terms.

Offset

The offset error of a transducer is defined as the output that will exist when it should be zero or, alternatively, the difference between the actual output value and the specified output value under some particular set of conditions. An example of the first situation in terms of Figure 6-1 would exist if the characteristic curve had the same sensitivity slope as the ideal but crossed the Y-axis (output) at *b* instead of zero. An example of the other form of offset is seen in the characteristic curve of a pH electrode shown in Figure 6-2. The ideal

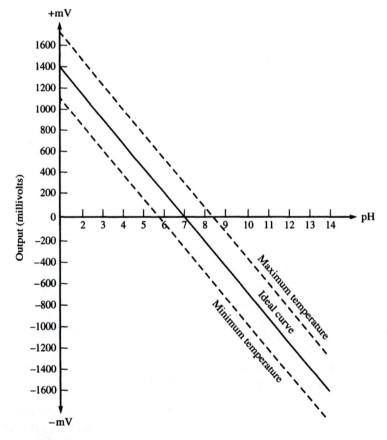

Figure 6-2
Typical pH electrode curve showing temperature sensitivity. Source: J.J. Carr, *Sensors and Circuits*, Prentice Hall.

curve will exist only at one temperature (usually 25°C), while the actual curve will be between the minimum temperature and maximum temperature limits, depending on the temperature of the sample and electrode.

Linearity

The linearity of the transducer is an expression of the extent to which the actual measured curve of a sensor departs from the ideal curve. Figure 6-3 shows a somewhat exaggerated relationship between the ideal, or least-squares-fit, line and the actual measured, or *calibration,* line (Note: in most cases, the static curve is used to determine linearity, and this may deviate somewhat from a dynamic linearity). Linearity is often specified in terms of *percentage of nonlinearity,* which is defined as:

$$Nonlinearity\,(\%) = \frac{D_{in(max)}}{IN_{f.s.}} \times 100 \qquad (6\text{-}1)$$

where

Nonlinearity (%) is the percentage of nonlinearity

$D_{in(max)}$ is the maximum input deviation

$IN_{f.s.}$ is the maximum, full-scale input

The static nonlinearity defined by Equation 6-1 is often subject to environmental factors, including temperature, vibration, acoustic noise level, and humidity. It is important to know under what conditions the specification is valid, and departures from those conditions may not yield linear changes.

Hysteresis

A transducer should be capable of following the changes of the input parameter regardless of in which direction the change is made; hysteresis is the measure of this property. Figure 6-4 shows a

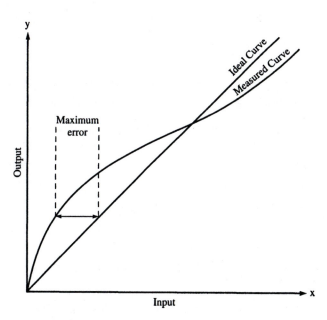

Figure 6-3
Ideal versus measured curve showing linearity error. Source: J.J. Carr, *Sensors and Circuits,* Prentice Hall.

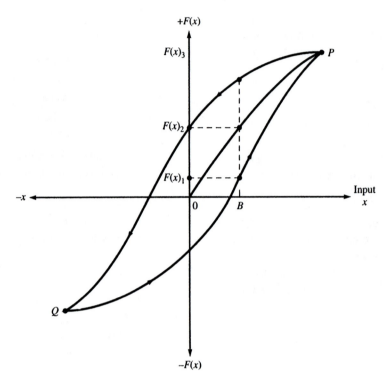

Figure 6-4
Hysteresis curve. Source: J.J. Carr, *Sensors and Circuits*, Prentice Hall.

typical hysteresis curve. Note that it matters from which *direction* the change is made. Approaching a fixed input value (point *B* in Figure 6-4) from a higher value (point *P*) will result in a different indication than approaching the same value from a lesser value (point *Q* or zero). Note that input value *B* can be represented by $F(x)_1$, $F(x)_2$, or $F(x)_3$ depending on the immediate previous value—clearly an error due to hysteresis.

Response time

Sensors do not change output state immediately when an input parameter change occurs. Rather, it will change to the new state over a period of time, called the response time (T_r in Figure 6-5). The response time can be defined as the *time required for a sensor output to change from its previous state to a final settled value within a tolerance band of the correct new value*. This concept is somewhat differ-

ent from the notion of the *time constant* (T) of the system. This term can be defined in a manner similar to that for a capacitor charging through a resistance and is usually less than the response time.

The curves in Figure 6-5 show two types of response time. In Figure 6-5a the curve represents the response time following an abrupt positive step-function change of the input parameter. The form shown in Figure 6-5b is a decay time (T_d to distinguish from T_r, for they are not always the same) in response to a negative step-function change of the input parameter.

Dynamic linearity

The dynamic linearity of the sensor is a measure of its ability to follow rapid changes in the input parameter. Amplitude distortion characteristics, phase distortion characteristics, and response time are important in determining dynamic linearity.

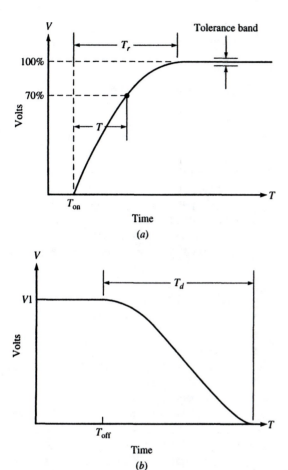

Figure 6-5
(*a*) Rise-time definition; (*b*) fall-time definition.
Source: J.J. Carr, *Sensors and Circuits*, Prentice Hall.

Given a system of low hysteresis (always desirable), the amplitude response is represented by:

$$F(x) = ax + bx^2 + cx^3 + dx^4 + \cdots + K \qquad (6\text{-}2)$$

In Equation 6-2, the term $f(x)$ is the output signal, while the x terms represent the input parameter and its harmonics, and K is an offset constant (if any). The harmonics become especially important when the error harmonics generated by the sensor action fall into the same frequency bands as the natural harmonics produced by the dynamic action of the input parameter. All continuous waveforms are represented by a Fourier series of a fundamental sine

wave and its harmonics. In any nonsinusoidal waveform (including time-varying changes of a physical parameter), the harmonics present will be those that can be affected by the action of the sensor.

The nature of the nonlinearity of the calibration curve (Figure 6-6) tells something about which

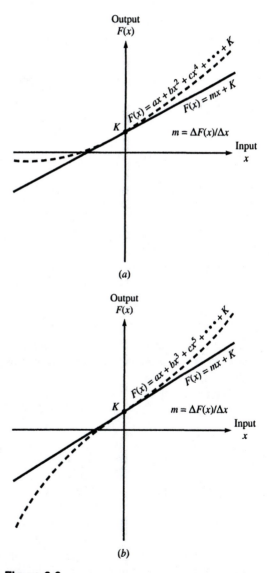

Figure 6-6
Output versus input signal curves showing (*a*) quadratic error; (*b*) cubic error. Source: J.J. Carr, *Sensors and Circuits*, Prentice Hall.

harmonics are present. In Figure 6-6a, the calibration curve (shown as a dotted line) is *asymmetrical*, so only *odd* harmonic terms exist. Assuming a form for the ideal curve of $F(x) = mx + K$, Equation 6-2 becomes, for the symmetrical case:

$$F(x) = ax + bx^2 + cx^4 + \cdots + K \qquad (6\text{-}3)$$

In the other type of calibration curve (Figure 6-6b), the indicated values are *symmetrical* about the ideal $mx + K$ curve. In this case, $F(x) = -F(-x)$, and the form of Equation 6-2 is:

$$F(x) = ax + bx^3 + cx^5 + \cdots + K \qquad (6\text{-}4)$$

Now we will take a look at some of the tactics and signals processing criteria that can be adapted to biomedical applications to improve the nature of the data collected from the sensor.

6-8 Tactics and signals processing for improved sensing

The selection of sensors and the circuits that are connected to them can go a long way toward ensuring that the data acquired will accurately represent the physical phenomenon or event being detected.

For proper operation in a dynamic input environment, the sensor selected should have a flat response curve, i.e., free of amplitude distortion, phase distortion (which almost invariably causes amplitude distortion), ringing, and resonances.

An implication of these problems concerns the *frequency response* of the sensor and its signals processing system. Figure 6-7a shows a perfectly linear system in which the gain is constant over the entire spectrum of frequencies, i.e., in an ideal theoretical system from "dc to daylight" and beyond. But real systems do not have such characteristics. Figure 6-7b shows the type of frequency response that might be found on real systems. In this example, the gain is flat between two frequencies, and over this region the performance is similar to the ideal case. But beyond these points, the gain falls off at a given slope. The breakpoint that defines the flat region is, by convention, taken to be the

frequencies (F_L and F_H) at which the gain falls off to 70.7% of its gain in the flat region. These points are known as the -6 dB points in voltage systems and the -3 dB points in power systems.

When the frequency response is not entirely flat, one can expect to find phase distortion. Figure 6-7c shows the situations in which the phase shift of the system is a linear function of frequency (solid line) and those in which it is a nonlinear function of frequency (dotted line).

We can see the effects of phase distortion in a somewhat simplistic sense in Figure 6-8. Figure 6-8a is the applied signal, e.g., the output of an ideal sensor in response to step-function changes of the measured input parameter. If the signals processing electronics and the sensor mechanism itself are perfectly ideal, then the only effect of the change will be displacement in time (T), as shown in Figure 6-8b. There will be no distortion of the shape of the wave. But in the presence of phase distortion, the wave will be not only time displaced but also distorted. Figures 6-8c and 6-8d show two forms of distortion that can occur with phase nonlinearity.

A slightly different view of the same phenomenon is shown in Figures 6-9 and 6-10. Consider a system in which the bandwidth can be varied across several limits, represented by curves *a*, *b*, and *c* in Figure 6-9. Curve *c* represents the most restrictive because it sharply limits both low and high frequency response, while curve *a* is the least restrictive. Note in Figure 6-10 the various responses to the three bandwidths represented in Figure 6-9.

These curves can be simulated by evaluating the response to squarewaves in resistor-capacitor (RC) filter networks. In fact, one of the problems when using electronic filters is the effects of the -6 dB points on the applied waveform.

One might erroneously assume from the discussion above that the instrument designer should select amplifiers with as wide a band as possible. That is not the case, however, because bandwidth can cause other problems at least as severe as those that are solved. Noise, for example, is proportional to

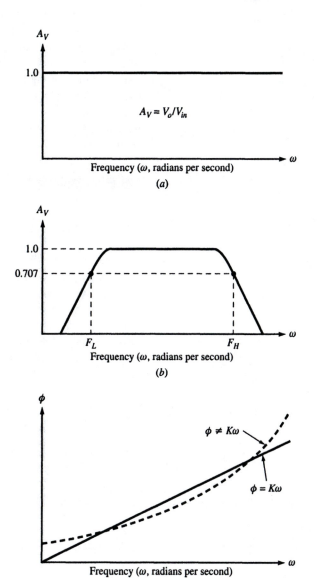

Figure 6-7
Frequency-response characteristics: (*a*) wideband; (*b*) band-pass; (*c*) typical for a sensor.
Source: J.J. Carr, *Sensors and Circuits*, Prentice Hall.

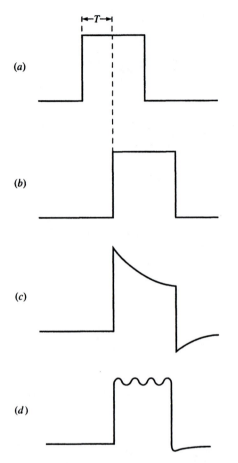

Figure 6-8
(*a*) Square wave; (*b*) propagation delay; (*c*) low-frequency rolloff; (*d*) ringing. Source: J.J. Carr, *Sensors and Circuits*, Prentice Hall.

bandwidth. It is possible to eliminate the problems of noise, plus certain input signal problems, such as ringing or resonances, by proper selection of the frequency-response cutoff points. Thus, the selection of amplifier bandwidth and phase distortion characteristics is a trade-off between the need to make a high-fidelity recording of the input event and the other problems that can occur in the system.

6-9 Electrodes for biophysical sensing

Bioelectricity is a naturally occurring phenomenon that arises from the fact that living organisms are composed of ions in various different quantities. *Ionic conduction* is different from *electronic conduction,* which is perhaps more familiar in the ordinary experience of engineers and technologists. Ionic conduction involves the migration of ions—positively and negatively charged molecules—throughout a region, whereas electronic conduction involves the flow of electrons under the influence of an electrical field. In an *electrolytic solution,* ions are easily available. Potential differences occur when the concentration of ions is different between two points.

When dealing with ionic conduction in depth, you will soon find that it is a very complex, nonlinear phenomenon. But for small signal applications, where there is only a very small—indeed, minuscule—current flowing, modeling it as a flow

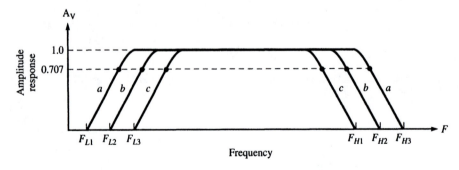

Figure 6-9
Band-pass frequency-response characteristics. Source: J.J. Carr, *Sensors and Circuits*, Prentice Hall.

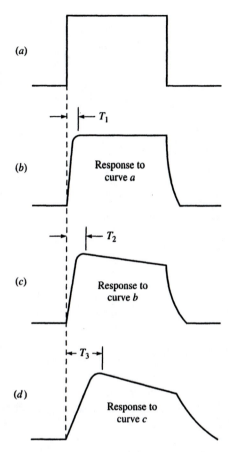

(a)

(b)   Response to
      curve *a*

T_1

(c)   Response to
      curve *b*

T_2

(d)   Response to
      curve *c*

T_3

Figure 6-10
Response of curves to a square wave (*a*). Source:
J.J. Carr, *Sensors and Circuits*, Prentice Hall.

quire medically significant bioelectrical signals, such as *electrocardiographic* (ECG), *electroencephalographic* (EEG), and *electromyographic* (EMG). Both clinical and research examples are easily found, although in many cases the two are the same. Most such bioelectrical signals are acquired from one of three forms of electrode: *surface macroelectrodes, indwelling macroelectrodes,* and *microelectrodes.* Of these, the first two are generally used in vivo, while the latter are used in vitro.

Here we will discuss the acquisition of biopotentials by dealing with the types of electrodes commonly used in biomedical instrumentation. Again, it should be recognized that this discussion is generic and representative, not exhaustive, for the subject is quite complex (indeed, books have been written on bioelectrodes).

Electrode potentials

The skin and other tissues of higher-order organisms, such as humans, are electrolytic and so can be modeled as electrolytic solutions. In some models, the solution is shown as saline, reflecting the fact that we humans are very similar to salt water in our composition. Imagine a metallic electrode immersed in an electrolytic solution (Figure 6-11). Almost immediately after immersion, the electrode

of electrical current between points of potential difference is a fair first-order approximation. Chemists would find this model wanting, except in the most elementary classes, but their needs for understanding are greater than those of the instrumentation specialist. Keep in mind, however, that situations in which a more substantial current flows change the situation entirely, and a higher-order model is needed.

Bioelectrodes are a class of sensors that transduce ionic conduction to electronic conduction so that the signal can be processed in electronic circuits. The usual purpose of bioelectrodes is to ac-

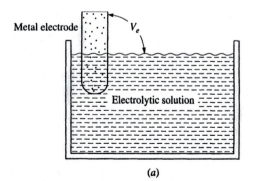

Metal electrode — V_e

Electrolytic solution

(a)

Figure 6-11
Metallic electrode immersed in an electrolytic solution.

will begin to discharge some metallic ions into the solution, while some of the ions in the solution start combining with the metallic electrodes. This is, incidentally, the chemical phenomenon on which the electroplating and anodizing processes are based.

After a short while, a *charge gradient* builds up, creating a potential difference, or *electrode potential* (V_e in Figure 6-11), or *half-cell potential*. Keep in mind that this potential difference can be caused by differences in concentration of a single ion type. For example, if you have two positive ions (++) in one location (call it *A*), and three positive ions (+++) in another location (call it *B*), then there will be a net difference of 3 − 2, or 1, with point *B* being more positive than point *A*. Two basic reactions can take place at the electrode/electrolyte interface. An *oxidizing reaction* involves metal → electrons + metal ions; a *reduction reaction* involves electrons + metal ions → metal.

A complex phenomenon is seen at the interface between the metallic electrode and the electrolyte. Ions migrate toward one side of the region or another, forming two parallel layers of ions of opposite charge. This region is called the *electrode double layer*, and its ionic differences are the source of the electrode or half-cell potential (V_e). Different materials exhibit different half-cell potentials, as shown in Table 6-1.

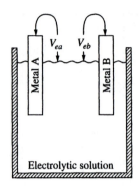

Figure 6-12
Dissimilar metals immersed in a common electrolytic solution produce differential potentials.

TABLE 6-1   HALF-CELL POTENTIALS OF COMMON ELEMENTS

Material	Half-cell potential (V)
Aluminum (Al^{+++})	−1.66
Zinc (ZN^{++})	−0.76
Iron (Fe^{++})	−0.44
Lead (Pb^{++})	−0.12
Hydrogen (H^+)	0
Copper (Cu^{++})	+0.34
Silver (Ag^+)	+0.80
Platinum (Pt^+)	+0.86
Gold (Au^+)	+1.50

By international scientific agreement, the zero reference point when making half-cell potential measurements is the *hydrogen-hydrogen* (H-H) *electrode,* which is assigned a half-cell potential of zero volts by convention. All other electrode half-cell potentials are measured against the H-H zero reference. The half-cell potentials cited for any given electrode are the differential potential between the actual electrode and the H-H reference electrode.

Now, consider what happens when two electrodes (call them *A* and *B*), made of *dissimilar metals,* are immersed in the same electrolytic solution (Figure 6-12). Each electrode will exhibit its own half-cell potential (V_{ea} and V_{eb}), and if the two metals are truly dissimilar the two potentials will be different ($V_{ea} \neq V_{eb}$). Because the two half-cell potentials are different, there is a net potential difference (V_{ed}) between them, which causes an electronic current (I_e) to flow through an external circuit. The differential potential, sometimes called an *electrode offset potential,* is only a first-order approximation for the small signal case and is defined as

$$V_{ed} = V_{ea} - V_{eb} \qquad (6\text{-}5)$$

For example, consider the case in which a gold (Au^+) electrode is immersed in the same electrolyte as a silver (Ag^+) electrode. In that situation

$$V_{ed} = V_{e(Au)} - V_{e(Ag)} \quad (6\text{-}6)$$

$$V_{ed} = (+1.50\text{ V}) - (+0.80\text{ V})$$
$$= +0.70\text{ V} \quad (6\text{-}7)$$

or, in the frequently seen case of copper (Cu^{++}) and silver (Ag^+), which can exist erroneously in electronic circuits that use copper connecting wires,

$$V_{ed} = V_{e(Ag)} - V_{e(Cu)}$$
$$V_{ed} = (+0.80\text{ V}) - (+0.34\text{ V}) \quad (6\text{-}8)$$
$$= 0.46\text{ V}$$

The electrode offset potential will be zero when the two electrodes are made of identical materials, which is the usual case in bioelectric sensing.

Care must be given to the selection of materials when designing electrodes for bioelectric sensing. The choice of materials, as noted earlier, will affect the half-cell and offset potentials. Besides its initial materials dependency, the actual half-cell potential exhibited by any given electrode may change slowly with time. Some candidate materials look good initially but undergo such a large change with time and chemical environment that they are rendered almost useless in practical applications.

There are two general categories of material combinations. A *perfectly polarized* or *perfectly nonreversible* electrode is one in which there is no net transfer of charge across the metal/electrolyte interface; in these electrodes, only one of the two types of chemical reactions can occur. A *perfectly nonpolarizable* or *perfectly reversible* electrode is one in which there is an unhindered transfer of charge between the metal of the electrode and the electrode. Although these idealized situations are obtained in reality, care must be given to selecting the right electrode. In general, we must select a reversible electrode, such as silver-silver chloride (Ag-AgCl).

Body fluids are terribly corrosive to metals, so not all materials are acceptable for bioelectric sensing. In addition, some materials that form reversible electrodes (e.g., zinc-zinc sulphate) are

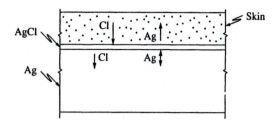

Figure 6-13
Silver-silver chloride biomedical electrode.

toxic to living tissue and so are inherently unsuitable. For these reasons, materials such as the noble metals (e.g., gold and platinum), some tungsten alloys, silver-silver chloride, and a material called platinum-platinum black are used to make practical biopotentials electrodes. In general medical use for simple surface recording of bipotentials, the silver-silver chloride electrode is used most often. Unless otherwise specified, you can generally assume that this material is used in clinical electrodes.

Figure 6-13 shows why the silver-silver chloride electrode is so popular with medical instrument designers. These electrodes consist of a body of silver onto which a thin layer of silver chloride is deposited. The silver chloride provides a free two-way exchange of Ag^+ and Cl^- ions, so that no double layer forms. When manufacturing silver-silver chloride electrodes, it is necessary to use spectroscopically pure silver for the process. Such silver is 0.99999 fine (i.e., 99.999% pure), compared with ordinary jeweler's and silversmith's silver, which is 0.999 fine (i.e., 99.9% pure). Note: Sterling silver is 92.5% 0.999 fine silver and 7.5% copper.

Electrode model circuit

Figure 6-14*a* shows a circuit model of a biomedical surface electrode. This model more or less matches the equivalent circuit of ECG and EEG electrodes. In this circuit a differential amplifier is used for signals processing and so will cancel the effects of electrode half-cell potentials V_{ea} and V_{eb}.

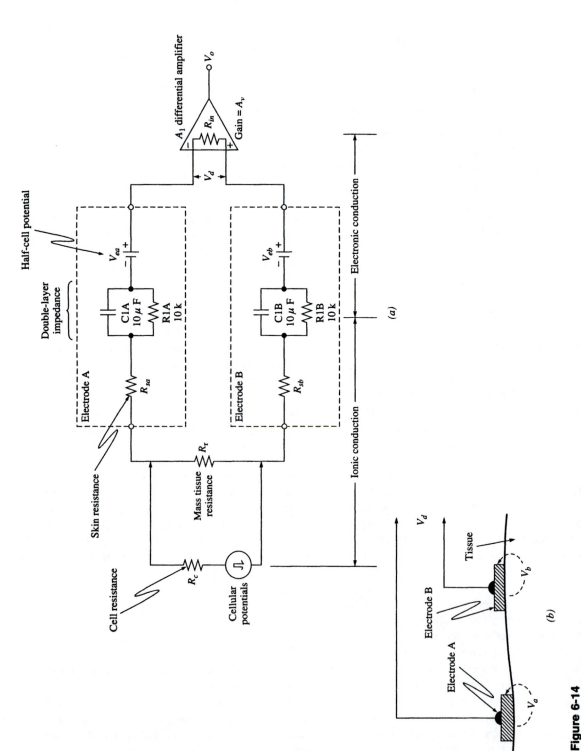

Figure 6-14
Biomedical electrodes. (a) Circuit model for biomedical electrode; (b) two biomedical electrodes produce a differential voltage.

Resistance R_τ represents the internal resistances of the body, which are typically quite low. The biopotentials signal is represented as a differential voltage, V_d. The other resistances in the circuit represent the resistances at the electrode-skin contact interface. The surprising aspect of Figure 6-14a is the usual values associated with capacitors C1A and C1B. While some capacitance is normally expected, it usually surprises people to learn that these contact capacitances can attain values of several microfarads (the value 10 μF is often cited).

When two or more electrodes are used together, as is almost always the case in physiological recording, the differential voltage between them is the algebraic sum of the two. In Figure 6-14b there are two electrodes, A and B, producing voltages V_a and V_b. The differential voltage V_d is $V_a \pm V_b$.

Electrode potentials cause recording problems

The electrode half-cell potential becomes a serious problem in bioelectric signals acquisition because of the tremendous difference between these dc potentials and the biopotentials. A typical half-cell potential for a biomedical electrode is .1.5 V, while biopotentials are more than 1000 times less than the half-cell potential. The surface manifestation of the ECG signal is 1 to 2 mV, while EEG scalp potentials are on the order of 50 μV. Thus, the half-cell electrode voltage is 1500 times greater than the peak ECG potential and 30,000 times greater than the EEG signal.

The instrument designer must provide a strategy for overcoming the effects of the massive half-cell potential offset. Because the half-cell potential forms a large dc component for the minute signal voltage, it is necessary to find an appropriate strategy that uses a combination of the following approaches:

1. We could use a differential dc amplifier to acquire the signal. If the electrodes are identical, then the half-cell potentials should be the same. Theoretically, at least, the equal potentials would be seen as a single common-mode potential and thus would cancel in the output. A limitation on this approach is that the gains required to process low-level signals also act on tiny differences between the two half-cell potentials. A difference of 1 mV between two half-cell potentials—only 0.1% of the total—looks like any other 1-mV dc signal in the gain-of-1000 ECG amplifier.

2. The signals acquisition circuit must be designed to provide a counter-offset voltage to cancel the half-cell potential of the electrode. While this approach has certain appeal, it is limited by the fact that the half-cell potential changes with time and the relative motion between skin and electrode. Electrode motion can cause a wildly varying baseline.

3. We can ac-couple the input amplifier. This approach permits removal of the signal component from the dc offset. This option is, perhaps, the most appealing—especially when variations of the dc offset are of substantially lower frequency than the signal frequency components. In that case, the normal −3 dB frequency response limit can be of use to tailor the attenuation of variations in the dc offset.

In some biomedical applications, however, signal components are near-dc. For example, the frequency content of the ECG signal is 0.05 to 100 Hz. In medical ECG equipment, therefore, one can expect the baseline to shift every time the patient moves around in bed.

In most cases, the first and third options are selected for biopotentials amplifiers. The user will require an ac-coupled, differential input amplifier for signals acquisition.

6-10 Medical surface electrodes

Surface electrodes are those that are placed in contact with the skin of the subject. Also in this category are certain needle electrodes of a size that prevents their being inserted inside a single cell (which a microelectrode is). There is some basis for including needle electrodes under the rubric *indwelling electrodes,* but that is not generally the practice in biomedical engineering.

Surface electrodes (other than needle electrodes) vary in diameter from 0.3 to 5 cm, with most being in the 1-cm range. Human skin tends to have a very high impedance compared with other voltage sources. Typically, normal skin impedance, as seen by the electrode, varies from 0.5 kΩ for sweaty skin surfaces to more than 20 kΩ for dry skin surfaces. Problem skin, especially dry, scaly, or diseased skin, may reach impedances in the 500-kΩ range. In any event, one must treat surface electrodes as a very high impedance voltage source—a fact that seriously influences the design of biopotentials amplifier input circuitry. In most cases, the rule of thumb for a voltage amplifier is to make the input impedance of the amplifier at least 10 times the source impedance. For biopotentials amplifiers this requirement means 5 MΩ or more input impedance—a value easily achieved using either premium bipolar, (BiFET), or (Bi-MOS) operational amplifiers.

Typical medical surface electrodes

A variety of electrodes have been designed for surface acquisition of biomedical signals. Perhaps the oldest form of ECG electrode in clinical use is the strap-on variety (Figure 6-15a). These electrodes are 1- to 2-sq in. brass plates that are held in place by rubber straps. A conductive gel or paste is used to reduce the impedance between the electrode and skin.

A related form of ECG electrode is the suction-cup electrode shown in Figure 6-15b. This device is used as a chest electrode in short-term ECG recording. For longer-term recording or monitoring, such as continuous monitoring of a hospitalized patient in a coronary or intensive care unit, the paste-on column electrode is used instead.

A typical column electrode is shown schematically in Figure 6-16a; photographic examples are shown in Figure 6-16b. The electrode consists of a

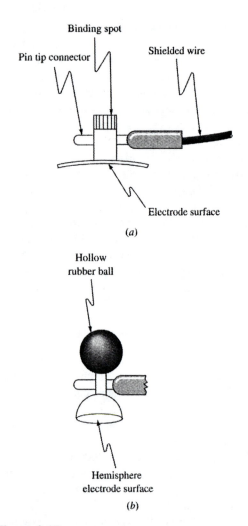

(a)

(b)

Figure 6-15
Typical ECG electrodes. (*a*) Strap-on electrode. (*b*) Suction-cup electrode.

silver-silver chloride metal contact button at the top of a hollow column that is filled with a conductive gel or paste. This assembly is held in place by an adhesive-coated foam rubber disk.

The use of a gel-filled or paste-filled column that holds the actual metallic electrode off the surface reduces movement artifact. For this reason (among several others), the electrodes shown in Figure 6-16 are preferred for monitoring hospitalized patients.

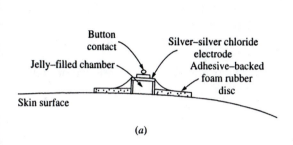

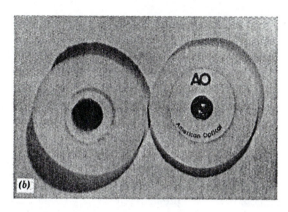

Figure 6-16
Column electrodes. (*a*) Cut-away side view. (*b*) A popular type of foam-backed column electrode.

A convenient form of column electrode often used in monitoring situations is the three-electrode pad. These adhesive pads have a surface area of 20 to 30 sq in. and contain three ECG electrodes (two differential signal pick-up electrodes and a reference electrode) in a single package. They provide a convenient electrode for monitoring, although for diagnostic use, the more traditional electrodes are preferred. The three-electrode pad is a temporary disposable unit that is discarded after use.

Problems with surface electrodes

Several problems are associated with surface electrodes of all types. One of the problems with column electrodes is that the adhesive will not stick for long on sweaty or clammy skin surfaces. The user also must avoid placing the electrode over bony prominences. Usually, the fleshy portions of the chest and abdomen are selected as electrode sites. Various hospitals have different protocols for changing the electrodes, but in general, the electrode is changed at least every 24 hours (it is often changed more frequently because few last as long as 24 hours). In some hospitals, the electrode sites are moved—and electrodes changed—once every 8-hour nursing shift to avoid ischemia of the skin at the site.

Although nearly all forms of electrodes can be used in short-term recording situations, long-term monitoring is a little more difficult. One of the most significant problems is *movement artifact* (spurious signal component), which is generated by patient movements and consists of a small electrical component from the bioelectric signals in the patient's skeletal muscles and a large component from the change in interface between electrode and skin. Movement artifact becomes worse as time goes on and the paste or gel dries out.

For short-term recordings, movement artifact is of little practical importance because most patients can lie still long enough for the recording to be made. But in the intensive and coronary care units it is necessary to do long-term monitoring and recording of ECG signals, so the problem becomes more acute.

The most common mechanism that creates artifact signals is *electrode slippage*. If the electrode position slips, then the thickness of the layer of jelly or paste changes abruptly, and this change is reflected as changes in both the electrode impedance and the electrode offset potential. The outward effect produces an artifact in the recorded signal that could possibly obscure the real signal or be interpreted as a bioelectric event in its own right. In the former case, medical people will probably recognize the artifact; they are generally quite good at differentiating gross artifacts from similar-appearing genuine physiologically based anomalies. In the latter case, however, an artifact could lead to a misinterpretation of the waveform's informational content.

Several attempts have been made to solve the movement artifact problem by securing the electrodes more tightly to the patient's skin. Sometimes adhesive tape is used to hold the electrode in place, and while this approach will work for a while, the electrodes inevitably become loose. In an hour or two the problem returns.

Another popular solution involves the use of a rough (prickly) surface electrode that digs in below the scaly outer layer of skin. But these electrodes are often uncomfortable for the patient, and they fail to solve the problem completely.

Movement artifacts are particularly severe in ECG stress-testing laboratories. The patient walks on a treadmill while the monitoring system records the ECG waveform. The column electrode does fairly well in overcoming the motion artifact, but even so it is often necessary for the medical staff conducting the test to clean and gently abrade the skin at the site where the electrode is attached.

Needle electrodes

The surface electrodes discussed thus far are non-invasive. That is, they adhere to the skin without puncturing it. Figure 6-17 depicts the needle electrode. This type of ECG electrode is inserted into the tissue immediately beneath the skin by puncturing the skin at a large oblique angle (i.e., close to horizontal with respect to the skin surface). The needle electrode is only used for exceptionally poor skin, especially on anesthetized patients, and in veterinary situations. Of course, infection is an issue in these cases, so needle electrodes are either disposable (one-time use) or are resterilized in ethylene oxide gas.

Indwelling electrodes

Indwelling electrodes are intended to be inserted into the body. These are not to be confused with needle electrodes, which are intended for insertion into the layers beneath the skin. The indwelling electrode is typically a tiny, exposed metallic contact at the end of a long, insulated catheter (Figure 6-18). In one application, the electrode is threaded through the patient's veins (usually in the right arm) to the right side of the heart to measure the intracardiac ECG waveform. Certain low-amplitude, high-frequency features (such as the signal from bundle of His) become visible only when an indwelling electrode is used.

EEG electrodes

The brain produces bioelectric signals that can be picked up through surface electrodes attached to the scalp. These electrodes will be connected to an EEG amplifier that drives either an oscilloscope or strip chart recorder.

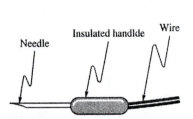

Figure 6-17
Needle ECG electrode.

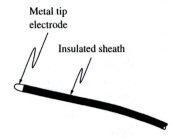

Figure 6-18
Indwelling electrodes.

The typical EEG electrode may be a needle, as in Figure 6-17, but in most cases it is a 1-cm diameter concave disc made either of gold or silver. The disc electrode is held in place by a thick paste that is highly conductive, or by a headband in certain monitoring applications.

6-11 Microelectrodes

The *microelectrode* is an ultrafine device that is used to measure biopotentials at the cellular level (Figure 6-19). In practice, the microelectrode penetrates a cell that is immersed in an infinite fluid (such as physiological saline), which is in turn connected to a reference electrode. Although several types of microelectrodes exist, most of them are of one of two basic forms: metallic-contact or fluid-filled. In both cases, an exposed contact surface of about 1 to 2 μm (1 μm = 10^{-6} m) is in contact with the cell. As might be expected, this fact makes microelectrodes very high impedance devices.

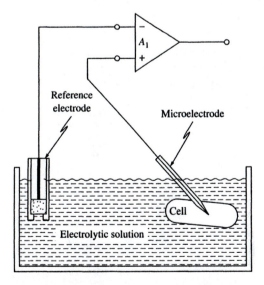

Figure 6-19
ECG microelectrode used to measure cellular potentials.

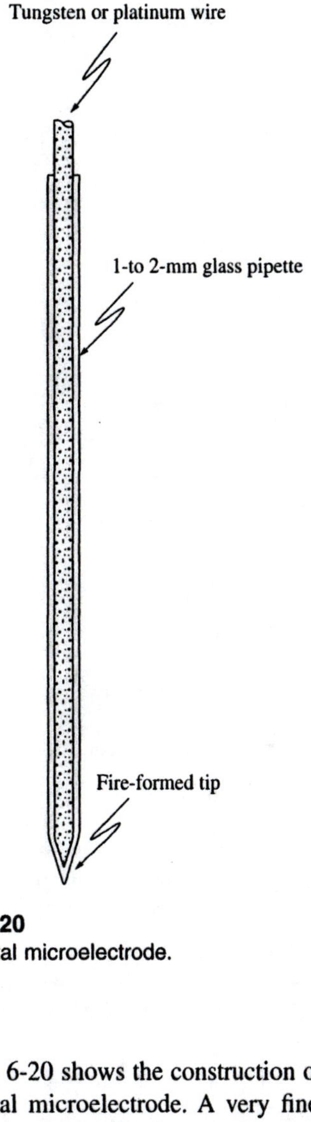

Tungsten or platinum wire

1-to 2-mm glass pipette

Fire-formed tip

Figure 6-20
Glass-metal microelectrode.

Figure 6-20 shows the construction of a typical glass-metal microelectrode. A very fine platinum or tungsten wire is slip-fit through a 1.5- to 2-mm glass pipette. The tip is etched and then fire-formed into the shallow angle taper shown. The electrode can then be connected to one input of the signals amplifier.

There are two subcategories of this type of electrode. In one type, the metallic tip is flush with the end of the pipette taper, while in the other, a thin layer of glass covers the metal point. This glass layer is so thin that it requires measurement

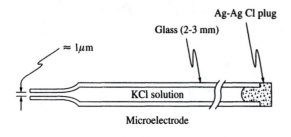

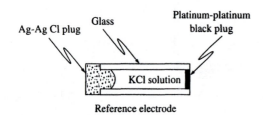

Figure 6-21
Fluid-filled microelectrode.

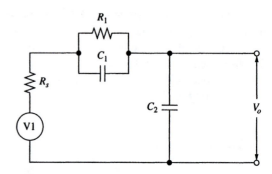

Figure 6-22
Microelectrode equivalent circuit.

in angstroms and drastically increases the impedance of the device.

The fluid-filled microelectrode is shown in Figure 6-21. In this type, the glass pipette is filled with a 3M solution of potassium chloride (KCl), and the large end is capped with an silver-silver chloride plug. The small end need not be capped because the 1-μm opening is small enough to contain the fluid.

The reference electrode is likewise filled with 3M KCl but is much larger than the microelectrode. A platinum plug contains fluid on the interface end, while an silver-silver chloride plug caps the other end.

Figure 6-22 shows a simplified equivalent circuit for the microelectrode (disregarding the contribution of the reference electrode). Analysis of this circuit reveals the signals acquisition problem caused by the RC components. Resistor R_1 and capacitor C_1 are the result of the effects at the electrode/cell interface and are (surprisingly) frequency-dependent. These values fall off to a negligible point at a rate of $1/(2\pi F)^2$ and are generally considerably lower than R_s and C_2.

Resistance R_s in Figure 6-22 is the spreading resistance of the electrode and is a function of the tip diameter. The value of R_s in metallic microelectrodes without the glass coating is approximated by

$$R_s = \frac{P}{4\pi r} \tag{6-9}$$

where

R_s is the resistance in ohms (Ω)

P is the resistivity of the infinite solution outside of the electrode (e.g., 70 Ω-cm for physiological saline)

r is the tip radius (typically 0.5 μm for a 1-μm electrode)

Assuming the aforementioned typical values, calculate the tip-spreading resistance of a 1-μm microelectrode.

$$R_x = \frac{P}{4\pi r} \tag{6-10}$$

$$R_x = \frac{70 \ \Omega\text{-cm}}{(4\pi)\left(0.5 \ \mu\text{m} \times \left(\frac{10^{-4} \text{ cm}}{1 \ \mu\text{m}}\right)\right)} \tag{6-11}$$

$R_s = 111.4 \ \text{k}\Omega$

The impedance of glass-coated metallic microelectrodes is at least one or two orders of magnitude higher than this figure.

For fluid-filled potassium chloride microelectrodes with small taper angles ($\pi/180$ radians), the series resistance is approximated by

$$R_s = \frac{2P}{\pi r \alpha} \qquad (6\text{-}12)$$

where

R_s is the resistance in ohms (Ω)

P is the resistivity (typically 3.7 Ω-cm for 3M KCl)

r is the tip radius (typically 0.1 μm)

α is the taper angle (typically $\pi/180$)

Example 6-1

Find the series impedance of a potassium chloride microelectrode using the aforementioned values.

Solution

$$R_s = \frac{2P}{\pi r \alpha}$$

$$R_s = \frac{(2)(3.7\ \Omega\text{-cm})}{(3.14)\left(0.1\mu\text{m} \times \left(\dfrac{10^{-4}\ \text{cm}}{1\ \mu\text{m}}\right)\right)\left(\dfrac{3.14}{180}\right)}$$

$$R_s = 13.5\ \text{M}\Omega$$

The capacitance of the microelectrode is given by

$$C_2 = \frac{0.55e}{\ln\left(\dfrac{R}{r}\right)}\ \frac{\text{pF}}{\text{cm}} \qquad (6\text{-}13)$$

where

e is the dielectric constant of glass (typically 4)

R is the outside tip radius

r is the inside tip radius (r and R in the same units)

Example 6-2

Find the capacitance of a microelectrode if the pipette radius is 0.2 μm and the inside tip radius is 0.15 μm.

Solution

$$C_2 = \frac{0.55e}{\ln\left(\dfrac{R}{r}\right)}\ \frac{\text{pF}}{\text{cm}}$$

$$C_2 = \frac{(0.55)(4)}{\ln\left(\dfrac{0.2\ \mu\text{m}}{0.15\ \mu\text{m}}\right)}\ \frac{\text{pF}}{\text{cm}}$$

$$C_2 = 7.7\ \frac{\text{pF}}{\text{cm}}$$

How do these values affect performance of the microelectrode? Resistance R_s and capacitor C_2 operate together as an RC low-pass filter. For example, a potassium chloride microelectrode immersed in 3 cm of physiological saline has a capacitance of approximately 23 pF. Suppose it is connected to the amplifier input (15 pF) through 3 ft of small-diameter coaxial cable (27 pF/ft, or 81 pF). The total capacitance is $(23 + 15 + 81)$ pF = 119 pF. Given a 13.5 MΩ-resistance, the frequency response (at the -3 dB point) is

$$F = \frac{1}{2\pi RC} \qquad (6\text{-}14)$$

where

F is the -3 dB point in hertz (Hz)

R is the resistance in ohms (Ω)

C is the capacitance in farads (f)

Example 6-3

For $C = 119$ pF (1.19×10^{-10} farads) and $R = 1.35 \times 10^7\ \Omega$, find the frequency response upper -3 dB point.

Solution

$$F = \frac{1}{(2)(3.14)(1.35) \times 10^7\ \Omega)(1.19 \times 10^{-10}\ \text{f})}$$

$$F = 99\ \text{Hz} \approx \textbf{100 Hz}$$

Clearly, a 100-Hz frequency response, with a -6 dB per octave characteristic above 100 Hz, results

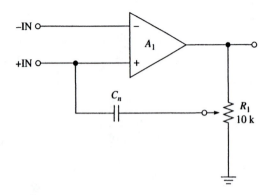

Figure 6-23
Capacitance nulling circuit.

Solution

$$C_n = \frac{C}{A - 1}$$

$$C_n = \frac{100 \text{ pF}}{10 - 1}$$

$$C_n = \frac{100 \text{ pF}}{9} = \textbf{11 pF}$$

in severe rounding of the fast rise-time action potentials. A strategy must be devised in the instrument design to overcome the effects of capacitance in high-impedance electrodes.

Neutralizing microelectrode capacitance

Figure 6-23 shows the standard method for neutralizing the capacitance of the microelectrode and associated circuitry. A neutralization capacitance, C_n, is in the positive feedback path along with a potentiometer voltage divider. The value of this capacitance is

$$C_n = \frac{C}{A - 1} \tag{6-15}$$

where

C_n is the neutralization capacitance

C is the total input capacitance

A is the gain of the amplifier

Example 6-4 _____

A microelectrode and its cabling exhibit a total capacitance of 100 pF. Find the value of neutralization capacitance (Figure 6-23) required for a gain-of-10 amplifier.

6-12 Transducers and other sensors

Transducers are part of an overall class of devices called *sensors,* which also include biophysical electrodes. A general problem with the word *transducer* is that it also refers to devices such as loudspeakers and ultrasonic sender units. To understand this distinction, let us reiterate in different words the definition given in section 6-3: A transducer is a device that converts energy from some other form into electrical energy for the purposes of measurement or control.

Transducers differ from electrodes in that they use some intervening transducible element to make the measurement, while electrodes directly acquire the signal. For example, a pressure transducer may use the change of resistance of a tautwire element when it is flexed as a measure of pressure. Similarly, a thermistor relies on the change of electrical resistance of some materials undergoing temperature changes to measure temperature. Because many transducers use *piezoresistive* elements connected in a Wheatstone bridge, we will begin our study with these highly valuable circuits.

The Wheatstone bridge

Many biomedical transducers are used in a circuit configuration called a *Wheatstone bridge* (see Figure 6-24). Many transducers, not bridges in their own right, are often connected with other

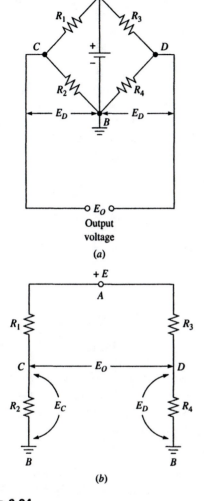

Figure 6-24
The Wheatstone bridge circuit. (a) Original circuit.
(b) Original circuit redrawn.

components to form a Wheatstone bridge. Any discussion of biomedical transducers, therefore, must begin with an introduction to the bridge circuit.

The basic Wheatstone bridge of Figure 6-24a uses one resistor in each of four arms. A battery (E) *excites* the bridge connected across two oppos-

ing resistor junctions (A and B). The bridge output voltage E_o appears across the remaining pair of resistor junctions (C and D).

The original circuit of Figure 6-24a is redrawn in Figure 6-16b, which simplifies analysis.

We may analyze the Wheatstone bridge circuit by initially breaking it into circuits across E: $R_1 - R_2$ and $R_3 - R_4$. Both of these networks are resistor voltage dividers. In fact, the Wheatstone bridge may be viewed as two resistor voltage dividers *in parallel* across the supply E. The output voltage (E_o) is the *difference* between the two ground-referenced potentials E_C and E_D produced by the divider networks. In equation form, this relation is

$$E_o = E_C - E_D \qquad (6\text{-}16)$$

But E_C and E_D may be expressed in terms of the excitation potential E, using the simple voltage divider theorem

$$E_C = E \times \frac{R_2}{R_1 + R_2} \qquad (6\text{-}17)$$

and

$$E_D = E \times \frac{R_4}{R_3 + R_4} \qquad (6\text{-}18)$$

Substituting Equations 6-17 and 6-18 into Equation 6-16, we obtain the output voltage E_o as

$$E_o \frac{ER_2}{R_1 + R_2} - \frac{ER_4}{R_3 + R_4} \qquad (6\text{-}19)$$

$$E_o = E\left(\frac{R_2}{R_1 + R_2} - \frac{R_4}{R_3 + R_4}\right) \qquad (6\text{-}20)$$

Example 6-5

A Wheatstone bridge (Figure 6-24) is excited by a 12-V dc source and contains the following resistances: $R_1 = 1.2$ kΩ, $R_2 = 3$ kΩ, $R_3 = 2.2$ kΩ, and $R_4 = 5$ kΩ. Find the output voltage E_o.

Solution

$$E_o = E\left(\frac{R_2}{R_1 + R_2} - \frac{R_4}{R_3 + R_4}\right)$$

$$E_o = 12\left(\frac{3}{1.2 + 3} - \frac{5}{2.2 + 5}\right)$$

$$E_o = 12\left(\frac{3}{4.2} - \frac{5}{7.2}\right)$$

$$E_o = 12(0.714 - 0.694) = \mathbf{0.24\ V}$$

Note from Example 6-5 and Equation 6-20 that the Wheatstone bridge voltage output is dependent on the resistances in the arms. Changing one or more of these resistances will change the output voltage. This phenomenon is the basis for many biomedical transducers.

The *null condition* in a Wheatstone bridge circuit exists when the output voltage E_o is zero. But from Equation 6-17, if E_o is zero, then either the excitation potential E must be zero (not true) or the expression inside the brackets must be equal to zero (true). The null condition occurs when

$$E_C = E_D \tag{6-21}$$

$$E_{CB} = E_{DB} \tag{6-22}$$

and

$$E_{AC} = E_{AD} \tag{6-23}$$

So equals divided by equals are equal, and

$$\frac{E_{CB}}{E_{AC}} = \frac{E_{DB}}{E_{AD}} \tag{6-24}$$

Since no current flows from C to D at the null and $E_C = E_D$, then from Figure 6-24b,

$$\frac{I_{ACB}R_1}{I_{ACB}R_2} = \frac{I_{ADB}R_3}{I_{ADB}R_4} \tag{6-25}$$

so

$$\frac{R_1}{R_2} = \frac{R_3}{R_4} \tag{6-26}$$

Equation 6-26 gives us the sole necessary condition for the null condition in an excited Wheatstone bridge. Note that it is not necessary

for the resistances to be equal, only that the *ratios* (of the two *half-bridge* voltage dividers) be equal.

Example 6-6

Show that the null condition exists in a Wheatstone bridge consisting of the following resistances: $R_1 = 2$ kΩ, $R_2 = 1$ kΩ, $R_3 = 10$ kΩ, and $R_4 = 5$ kΩ. (*Hint:* Equation 6-26 describes the sole condition necessary for null.)

Solution

$$\frac{R_2}{R_1} = \frac{R_4}{R_3}$$

$$\frac{1}{2} = \frac{5}{10}$$

$$\mathbf{0.5 = 0.5}$$

Since both sides of the equation evaluate to the same quantity, we may conclude that the bridge is in the null condition. A bridge in the null condition is said to be *balanced*.

In many biomedical transducers using the Wheatstone bridge, all four resistances are equal in the null condition. This is not a strict physical requirement, but it is the way many manufacturers choose to build their products. Values for R in the 150- to 800-Ω range are typical.

In most designs, the null condition exists when the parameter stimulating the transducer is at either zero or some predetermined value (e.g., atmospheric pressure) that is taken to be a *zero baseline*. The stimulus (parameter being measured) will cause any or all of the bridge resistance elements to change resistance by some small amount h. (Note that h is sometimes written ΔR, meaning a *small* change in the parameter R.) When the applied stimulus is zero, then all four resistors have a resistance of R, and the output voltage is zero. The bridge is in the null condition.

When the stimulus is *not* zero, each arm takes on a resistance of $R \pm h$, and this unbalances the circuit to produce an output voltage that is proportional to the value of the applied stimulus.

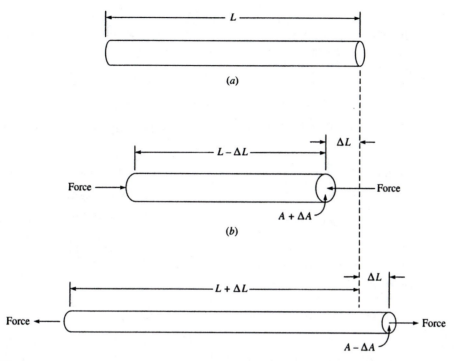

Figure 6-25
Mechanism for piezoresistivity. (*a*) Bar at rest (no force applied). (*b*) Bar under a compression force. (*c*) Bar under a tension force.

6-13 Strain gauges

A *strain gauge* is a resistive element that produces a *change* in its resistance proportional to an applied mechanical *strain*. A strain is a *force* applied in either *compression* (a push along the axis *toward* the center) or *tension* (a pull along the axis *away* from the center).

Figure 6-25*a* shows a small metallic bar with no force applied. It will have a length L and a cross-sectional area A. Changes in length are given by ΔL and changes in area by ΔA.

In Figure 6-25*b* we see the result of applying a *compression* force to the ends of the bar. The length *reduces* to $L - \Delta L$, and the cross-sectional area *increases* to $A + \Delta A$.

Similarly, when a *tension* force of the same magnitude is applied to the bar, the length *increases* to $L + \Delta L$ and the cross-sectional area reduces to $A - \Delta A$.

The resistance of a metallic bar is given in terms of the length and cross-sectional area in the expression

$$R = \rho\left(\frac{L}{A}\right) \qquad (6\text{-}27)$$

where [1]

ρ is the resistivity constant unique to the type of material used in the bar in ohm-meters (Ω-m)

L is the length in meters (m)

A is the cross-sectional area in square meters (m^2)

---

[1] In the British engineering system commonly used in the United States, the units of resistivity are ohms per circular mil foot. A *circular mil* is the area of a circle that has a diameter of 1 mil or $\frac{1}{1000}$ in.

Example 6-7

Find the resistance of a copper bar that has a cross-sectional area of 0.5 mm^2 and a length of 250 mm. (*Hint:* The resistivity of copper is 1.7×10^{-8} Ω-m.)

Solution

$$R = \rho\left(\frac{L}{A}\right)$$

$$R = (1.7 \times 10^{-8}\ \Omega\text{-M}) \times$$

$$\frac{[250\ \text{mm} \times (1\ \text{m}/1000\ \text{mm})]}{0.5\ \text{mm}^2 \times (1\ \text{m}/1000\ \text{mm})^2}$$

$$R = \frac{1.7 \times 10^{-8}\ \Omega \times 0.25}{5 \times 10^{-7}} = \mathbf{0.0085\ \Omega}$$

Equation 6-27 tells us that the resistance varies directly as the length and inversely as the square of the cross-sectional area. Both of these phenomena are crucial to the operation of the resistive strain gauge transducers.

Example 6-7 illustrates the change of resistance with changes in size and shape. This phenomenon is sometimes called *piezoresistivity*. The resistance of the bar will become $R + h$ in tension and $R - h$ in compression. If you examine Equation 6-27 carefully, you will note that changes in both length and cross-sectional area tend to *increase* the resistance in *tension* and *decrease* the resistance in *compression*. The resistances after force is applied are *in tension:*

$$(R + h) = \frac{L + \Delta L}{A - \Delta A} \qquad (6\text{-}28)$$

and in a compression:

$$(R - h) = \frac{L - \Delta L}{A + \Delta A} \qquad (6\text{-}29)$$

Example 6-8

A thin constantan wire stretched taut has a length of 30 mm and a cross-sectional area of 0.01 mm^2. The resistance is 1.5 Ω. The force applied to the wire is increased so that the length increases by 10 mm and the cross-sectional area decreases by 0.0027 mm^2. Find the change in resistance h. (*Hint:* The resistivity of constantan is approximately 5×10^{-7} Ω-m.)

Solution

$$(R + h) = \rho\frac{L + \Delta L}{A - \Delta A}$$

$$(R + h) = (5 \times 10^{-7}\ \Omega\text{-M}) \times$$

$$\frac{[(30 + 10)\text{mm} \times (1\ \text{m}/1000\ \text{mm})]}{(0.01 - 0.0027)\ \text{mm}^2 \times [(1\ \text{m}/1000\ \text{mm})]^2}$$

$$1.5 + h = \frac{(5 \times 10^{-7}\ \Omega)(40)(10^3)}{0.0073}$$

then $1.5 + h = 2.74\ \Omega$

so $h = 2.74 - 1.5 = \mathbf{1.24\ \Omega}$

The change in resistance will be approximately linear for small changes in dimensions provided that ΔL is much less than L. Of course, if too great a force is applied, modulus of elasticity is exceeded and the wire becomes permanently deformed. It is then useless as a transducer.

Gauge factor

The gauge factor (GF) for a strain gauge transducer is a means of comparing it with other similar transducers. The definition of gauge factor is

$$\text{GF} = \frac{\Delta R/R}{\Delta L/L} \qquad (6\text{-}30)$$

where

GF is the gauge factor (dimensionless)

ΔR is the change in resistance in ohms (Ω)

R is the unstrained resistance in ohms

ΔL is the change in length in meters (m)

L is the length in meters

Example 6-9

A 20-mm length of wire used as a strain gauge exhibits a resistance of 150 Ω. When a force is applied in tension, the resistance changes by 2 Ω and the length changes by 0.07 mm. Find the gauge factor GF.

Solution

$$GF = \frac{\Delta R/R}{\Delta L/L}$$

$$GF = \frac{2/150}{0.07/20}$$

$$GF = \frac{0.013}{0.0035} = \textbf{3.71}$$

The gauge factor gives us a means for evaluating the relative *sensitivity* of a strain gauge element. The greater the change in resistance per unit change in length, the greater the *sensitivity* of the element and the greater the gauge factor.

Equation 6-30 is sometimes given in the alternate form

$$GF = \frac{\Delta R/R}{\mathscr{E}} \qquad (6\text{-}31)$$

in which $\mathscr{E}$ (strain) is the factor $\Delta L/L$.

Types of strain gauges

There are two basic forms of piezoresistive strain gauge: *bonded* and *unbonded*. Figure 6-26a shows a crude example of the *unbonded* strain gauge. The resistance element is a *thin* wire of a special alloy that is stretched *taut* between two flexible supports, which are in turn mounted on a thin metal diaphragm. When a force such as F_1 is applied, the diaphragm will flex in a manner that spreads the supports further apart, causing an increased tension in the resistance wire. This *tension* tends to *increase* the resistance of the wire in an amount proportional to the applied force.

Similarly, if a force such as F_2 is applied to the diaphragm, the ends of the supports move *closer* together, *reducing* the tension in the taut wire. This action is the same as applying a compression force to the wire. The electrical resistance in this case will *reduce* in an amount proportional to the applied force.

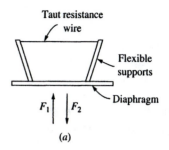

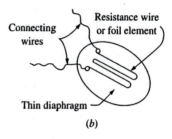

Figure 6-26
Piezoresistive strain gauge. (*a*) The unbonded strain gauge. (*b*) The bonded strain gauge.

A *bonded* strain gauge is made by cementing a thin wire or foil element to a diaphragm, as shown in Figure 6-26b. Flexing the diaphragm *deforms* the element, causing a change in electrical resistance exactly as in the unbonded strain gauge.

Unbonded strain gauges can be constructed so that they are linear over a wide range of applied force but are very delicate. The bonded strain gauge, on the other hand, is generally more rugged but is linear over a smaller range of forces. Note well, however, that *no* piezoresistive strain gauges will take a large amount of abuse, and they should always be treated as *delicate instruments*.

Many biomedical strain gauge transducers are of bonded construction because the linear range is adequate and the extra ruggedness is a desirable feature in medical environments, where people cannot take the kind of precautions that would be required if a more delicate type were used. Note, however, that the Statham P-23 series are of the unbonded type but are made in a very rugged housing. These are among the most common cardiovascular pressure transducers used in medicine.

Very few physiological strain gauge transducers use a single element; most use four strain gauge elements connected in a Wheatstone bridge circuit. In the unbonded types, there will be four supports, one for each bridge junction. Two of the resistance elements will be connected to each support. In the bonded variety there will be foil or wire elements arranged in a bridge configuration.

Both types of transducers are found with an element geometry that places *two* elements in *tension* and *two* elements in *compression* for any applied force. Such a configuration increases the output of the bridge for any applied force and so increases the *sensitivity* of the transducer.

Figure 6-27*a* shows a Wheatstone bridge with strain gage elements for each of the four bridge arms. We may find that R_1 and R_4 are aligned parallel to each other along one axis of the diaphragm, while resistors R_2 and R_3 are parallel to each other and *perpendicular* to R_1/R_4.

Consider a force applied to the diaphragm of a transducer such as Figure 6-27*b*. Resistors R_1 and R_4 will be in compression, while R_2 and R_3 are in tension.

Assume that all resistors are equal ($R_1 = R_2 = R_3 = R_4 = R$) when no force is applied to the diaphragm, and let $\Delta R = h$. When a force is applied, the resistance of R_1 and R_4 will be $R + h$, the resistance of R_2 and R_3 will be $R - h$. From a rewritten version of Equation 6-20, we know that the output voltage is

$$E_o = E \times \left[\frac{(R - h)}{(R + h) + (R - h)} \right.$$
$$\left. - \frac{(R + h)}{(R - h) + (R + h)} \right] \quad (6\text{-}32)$$

$$E_o = E \times \left[\frac{(R - h)}{2R} - \frac{(R + h)}{2R} \right] \quad (6\text{-}33)$$

$$E_o = E\left(\frac{h}{R}\right) = -E\left(\frac{\Delta R}{R}\right) \quad (6\text{-}34)$$

$$E_o = -E\left(\frac{\Delta R}{R}\right) \quad (6\text{-}35)$$

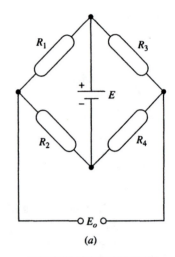

(a)

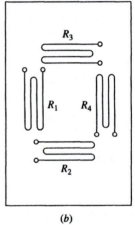

(b)

Figure 6-27
Wheatstone bridge strain gauge. (*a*) Strain gauge elements in a bridge circuit. (*b*) Mechanical configuration using a common diaphragm.

Example 6-10 _____

A strain gauge transducer is constructed to match the one shown in Figure 6-27*b*. In the null condition, each element has a resistance of 200 Ω. When a force is applied, each resistance changes by 10 Ω. Find the output voltage if a 10-V excitation potential is applied to the bridge.

Solution

$$E_o = -E \times \frac{\Delta R}{R}$$
$$E_o = -10 \text{ V} \times 10/200$$
$$E_o = -10 \text{ V} \times 0.05 = -\textbf{0.50 V}$$

Transducer sensitivity (φ)

The *sensitivity* (φ) of a transducer is the rating that allows us to *predict* the output voltage from knowledge of the excitation voltage and the value of the applied stimulus. The units for φ are microvolts per volt of excitation per unit of applied stimulus (μV/V/U).

Let us consider a force transducer. A certain biomedical force transducer is usually calibrated in *grams*. Before you object that this must be wrong (grams are units of *mass*), let us hasten to point out that the force in this case would be the earth's *gravitational attraction* on a mass of 1 g. This convention allows calibration of force transducers using a simple metric weight set from a platform balance, as opposed to conventional force in dynes (1 g-force = 980 dynes).

If the sensitivity factor φ is known for a transducer, then the output voltage may be calculated from

$$E_o = \phi \times E \times F \qquad (6\text{-}36)$$

where

E_o is the output potential in volts (V)

E is the excitation potential in volts

F is the applied force in grams (g)

φ is the sensitivity in μV/V/g

Example 6-11 _____

A transducer has a sensitivity of 10 μV/V/g. Predict the output voltage for an applied force of 15 g if the excitation potential is 5 V dc.

Solution

$$E_o = \phi \times E \times F$$
$$E_o = \frac{10 \text{ μV}}{\text{V-}g} \times 5 \text{ V} \times 15 \text{ g}$$
$$E_o = 750 \text{ μV} = \textbf{0.00075 V}$$

Note that the sensitivity is important in both the design and the repair of medical instruments because it allows us to predict the output voltage for a given stimulus level, and therefore the gain of the amplifier required for processing the signal.

Solid-state piezoresistive strain gauges

In the past, most strain gauge transducers were made using wire elements or vacuum-deposited metallic elements. Today, however, many strain gauge devices are based on solid-state silicon technology, in which all four elements of the Wheatstone bridge are formed of piezoresistive semiconductor material. Some are made similar to bonded strain gauges (i.e., the material is deposited or diffused onto a diaphragm). Others use a cantilever design in which the semiconductor piezoresistive elements are supported between fixed supports.

6-14 Inductive transducers

Almost any electrical property that can be made to vary in a predictable manner under the influence of a physical stimulus may be used for transduction of that stimulus. Inductance, for example, can be varied easily by physical movement of a permeable core within an inductor. Inductors, therefore, can be used to make transducers. There are, in fact, three basic forms of inductive transducer: *single coil, reactive Wheatstone bridge,* and *linear voltage differential transformer* (LVDT).

The first type, single coil devices, are rarely used in modern equipment. They are constructed much like the dynamic microphone, in which a diaphragm affects either the position of an iron or ferrite core

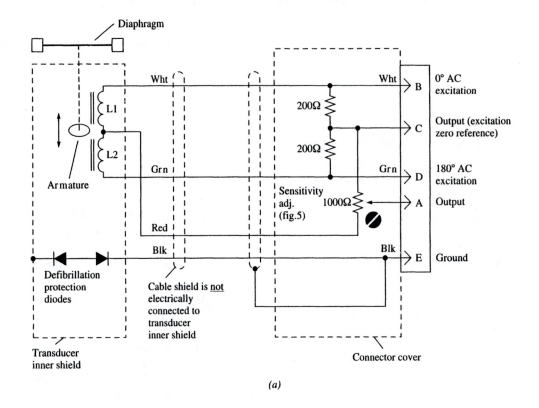

Diaphragm

Wht

L1

L2

Armature

200Ω

200Ω

Wht — B   0° AC excitation

— C   Output (excitation zero reference)

Grn

Grn — D   180° AC excitation

Sensitivity adj. (fig.5)   1000Ω   — A   Output

Red

Blk

Blk — E   Ground

Defibrillation protection diodes

Cable shield is not electrically connected to transducer inner shield

Transducer inner shield

Connector cover

(a)

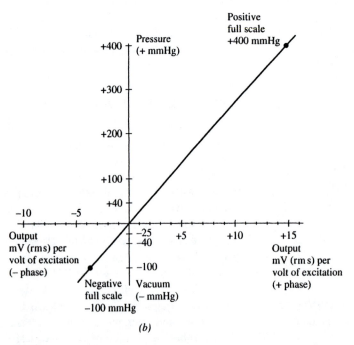

Positive full scale +400 mmHg

Pressure (+ mmHg)

+400

+300

+200

+100

+40

−10   −5

Output mV (rms) per volt of excitation (− phase)

−25
−40   +5   +10   +15

Output mV (rms) per volt of excitation (+ phase)

−100

Negative full scale −100 mmHg

Vacuum (− mmHg)

(b)

Figure 6-28
Inductive Wheatstone bridge strain gauge. (*a*) Circuit for H-P Model 1280. (Reprinted courtesy of Hewlett-Packard) (*b*) Output function. (Reprinted courtesy of Hewlett-Packard)

inside of the coil or the field of a core formed from a permanent magnet. A force applied to the diaphragm creates a current in the winding of the latter and changes the inductance in the former.

An example of an inductive bridge transducer is shown in Figure 6-28a. The output function for this transducer is shown in Figure 6-28b. The Wheatstone bridge circuit consists of the inductive reactances of coils L_1 and L_2, plus the 200-Ω resistors.

Note that alternating current (ac) excitation is required because the reactance of a coil is zero when dc is applied. Hewlett-Packard typically uses an excitation signal of 2400 Hz at 5 V (rms). Other manufacturers use as much as 10 V (rms) at frequencies between 400 and 5000 Hz.

The Hewlett-Packard model 1280 transducer shown in Figure 6-28a is used for measurement of arterial and venous blood pressure in mm Hg. (Note that the accepted units of pressure are torr (1 torr = 1 mm Hg). In medicine, however, the term mm Hg is still used most of the time.)

The transduction occurs because of a change of *position* of the inductor's core. But this yields only position data unless the applied force operates against some other force, such as a *spring*. The force required to compress or stretch a spring is given by Hooke's law: $F = -kX$, in which the term X is a displacement (change of position).

At zero gauge pressure (transducer's diaphragm open to atmosphere) the diaphragm is not distended in either direction, so the armature core is displaced equally in both L_1 and L_2 are equal, so the bridge is *balanced*. There will be no output voltage.

When a pressure *above* or *below* atmospheric pressure is applied, the diaphragm becomes distended in one direction, and this forces the armature further into one coil than the other. The respective inductive reactances of L_1 and L_2 are no longer equal, so the bridge is *unbalanced* and an output voltage develops. The amplitude of the ac-output signal is proportional to the *magnitude* of the applied pressure, while its *phase* indicates whether the pressure is *positive* (a compression) or *negative* (a vacuum) (Figure 6-28b). The sensitivity of the transducer in this case is about 40 μV/V/mm Hg.

Note in Figure 6-28a that the output voltage at pin A of the connector is taken from the wiper of a potentiometer. This sensitivity control is used to trim out *normal* differences between transducers, so that pressure-monitoring instruments can be easily calibrated by less-skilled operators.

An example of an LVDT transducer is shown in Figure 6-29. It is a transformer with a primary (L_1) and *two* secondaries (L_2 and L_3). The secondaries are connected in *opposite sense* so that their respective currents tend to cancel each other. When the stimulus is zero, the core affects L_2 and L_3 *equally* so the current cancellation is *total* and the output voltage is therefore *zero*.

An ac excitation signal is applied to the primary. When the stimulus is applied to the diaphragm, it displaces the core. The inductive reactances of L_2 and L_3 are no longer equal, so their respective currents are no longer equal, so their respective currents are no longer equal. Secondary current cancellation is less than total, so a current flows in the external load, creating an output voltage signal. This output voltage has a magnitude proportional to the applied stimulus and a phase indicating the direction the core was moved. In the case of a pressure transducer, this tells us whether the pressure is positive or negative.

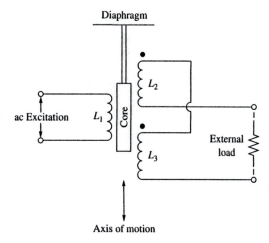

Figure 6-29
Linear voltage differential transformer.

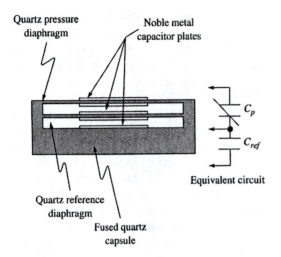

Figure 6-30
Homogeneous fused quartz pressure transducer.

6-15 Quartz pressure sensors

Another modern form of sensor, especially in medical pressure measurements, is the *quartz* transducer. These devices are basically capacitively based (see section 6-16) but are made differently than are other capacitive transducers. The pressure sensor capsule of these devices is made of homogeneous fused quartz (Figure 6-30). There are two capacitors in the capsule: a *pressure* capacitor (C_p) and a reference capacitor (C_{ref}). The capacitor plates are made of noble metals which have been vacuum-deposited onto their respective surfaces of the quartz capsule.

These capacitors are connected in a ratiometric series arrangement (Figure 6-30) so that differences in dialectric properties of the quartz material are compensated. The capacitors can be connected in a capacitive bridge circuit, a mixed RC bridge circuit (both similar to Wheatstone bridges), or in oscillator circuits (Figure 6-31). Several of these circuits are discussed in section 6-16.

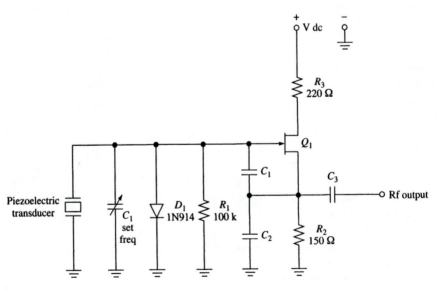

Figure 6-31
Oscillator circuit.

Advantages of the quartz transducer include very low levels of (some sources claim zero) hysteresis, very low levels of slippage of the metals and alloys with respect to the crystal, very low levels of temperature sensitivity, highly elastic properties, and ruggedness.

6-16 Capacitive transducers

Another capacitive transducer that is seen occasionally is the metallic plate *capacitive transducer*. These cause the capacitance of the transducer to vary with the stimulus. Since capacitance is used, ac excitation is necessary.

In almost all varieties, the capacitive transducer uses a stationary plate or plates attached to the housing and a movable plate that changes position under the influence of the stimulus. Recall that the capacitance of a parallel plate capacitor varies *directly* with the *plate area* and *inversely* with the *separation* between the plates. *Either* or *both* may be varied in any given transducer.

One form of capacitive transducer consists of a solid metal disc parallel to a flexible metal diaphragm; the two elements are separated by an air or vacuum dielectric (Figure 6-32). This construc-

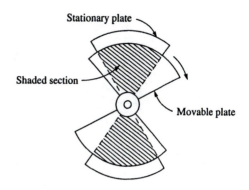

Figure 6-33
Butterfly plate transducer.

tion is very similar to that of the *capacitor microphone*, which is in fact a transducer for *sound waves*. When a force is applied to the diaphragm, it will move either closer to or further from the stationary disc. This increases or decreases the capacitance, respectively.

Another popular form (Figure 6-33) uses a stationary metal plate (i.e., *stator*) and a rotating movable plate. The movable plate usually has a butterfly shape. The capacitance varies because the position of the rotor determines how much of the stator plate is shaded by the rotor. At only one position will the shading be greatest, so the capacitance will also be greatest. At 90° of rotation from that position, the shading is least, so the capacitance is also least.

Figure 6-34 shows still another form of capacitance transducer. In this type of transducer, a movable metal plate (P_3) is placed between two stationary plates (P_1 and P_2). This forms a differential capacitor consisting of two sections (Figure 6-34*b*). Capacitor C_1 is the capacitance between plates P_1 and P_3, while capacitance C_2 is the capacitance between plates P_2 and P_3. When a force is applied to the diaphragm plate, P_3 will move closer to one end plate than the other. If the force is in the direction shown by the arrow, then P_3 is closer to P_2 than P_1, so capacitance C_2 is greater than C_1. In the opposite situation, the movable

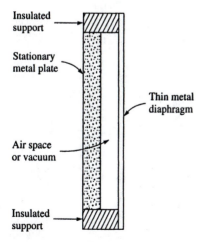

Figure 6-32
Simple capacitance transducer.

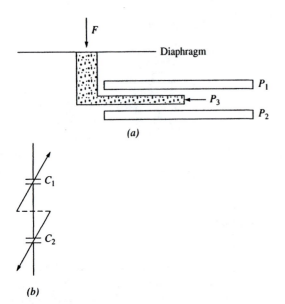

(a)

(b)

Figure 6-34
Differential capacitance transducer. (a) Mechanical structure. (b) Schematic symbol.

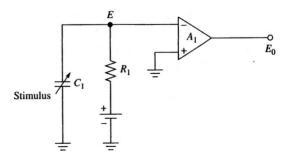

Figure 6-35
Electrometer transducer.

resistances, while two arms are capacitive reactances. Capacitor C_1 represents the capacitance of the transducer, while C_2 is the capacitance of a variable trimmer capacitor used to balance the bridge under zero stimulus conditions.

In some cases resistor R_2 will be the second section of a differential capacitor. Under zero stimulus conditions the capacitance of C_2 and the capacitance that replaces R_2 in Figure 6-36 will be

plate is closer to P_1 than P_2, so capacitance C_1 is greater than C_2.

There are several ways to use capacitance transducers in instrumentation circuits. One method, although rarely used in biomedical applications, is to have the transducer be part of an L-C resonant circuit controlling the frequency of an oscillator. Varying the capacitance under influence of a stimulus will vary the oscillator frequency (i.e., will modulate frequency) an amount proportional to the stimulus.

Another way, shown in Figure 6-35, is called the electrometer technique. In this circuit, the capacitance of the transducer is charged through a constant current source (R_1 and E). The voltage across the capacitance (the voltage applied to the input of the amplifier) depends on the capacitance, which is proportional to an applied stimulus.

One of the most common methods is to use the capacitor transducer in one arm of a Wheatstone bridge (Figure 6-36). Two arms of the bridge are

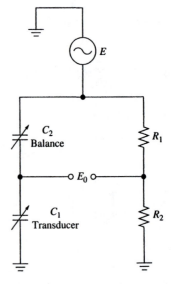

Figure 6-36
Capacitive Wheatstone bridge.

equal, but under the influence of a stimulus, the re-lation changes and balance is upset.

6-17 Temperature transducers

There are three types of common temperature transducers: *thermocouples, thermistors,* and *solid-state PN junctions.* Of these, the latter two find the greatest use in clinical applications, while all three are used in biomedical and biophysical research applications.

A thermocouple (Figure 6-37*a*) consists of two *dissimilar* conductors or semiconductors joined together at one end. Because the *work functions* of the two materials are different, a potential will be generated when this junction is heated. The potential is roughly linear with changes of temperature over a relatively wide range, although at the extreme limits of temperature for any given pair of materials, nonlinearity increases markedly.

Transistors (*thermal resistors*) are resistors that are designed to change value in a predictable manner with changes in temperature (Figure 6-37*b*). A positive temperature coefficient (PTC) device *increases* resistance with increases in temperature, while a negative temperature coefficient (NTC) device *decreases* resistance with increases in temperature.

Most thermistors have a nonlinear curve when the curve is plotted over a wide temperature range, but when limited to a narrow temperature range (such as human body temperatures), the linearity is better. When thermistors are used, it is necessary to ensure that the temperature is not allowed to go into the ranges where the calibration is unknown or extremely nonlinear. Most medical temperature transducers are thermistors.

The last class of thermal transducer is the solid-state PN junction diode (Figure 6-37*c*). If you take an ordinary solid-state rectifier diode and connect it across an ohmmeter, you may observe this phenomenon. Note the forward biased resistance at room temperature, and then heat the diode temporarily with a lamp or soldering iron. The diode resistance drops as temperature increases.

Most temperature transducers, however, use a diode-connected bipolar transistor such as the one in Figure 6-37*c*. We know that the base-emitter voltage of a transistor is proportional to temperature. For the differential pair in Figure 6-37*c* the transducer output voltage is

$$\Delta V_{be} = \frac{KT \ln(I_{c1}/I_{c2})}{q} \qquad (6\text{-}37)$$

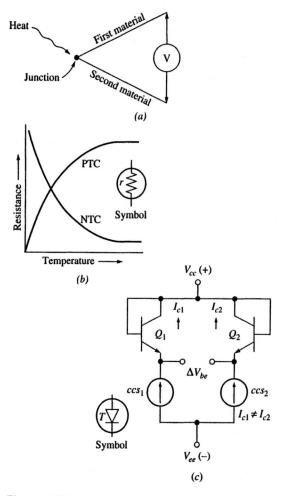

(a)

(b)

(c)

Figure 6-37
Three types of temperature transducers. (*a*) Thermocouple. (*b*) Thermistor. (*c*) PN junction.

where

   K is Boltzmann's constant $(1.38 \times 10^{-23}$ J/°K)

   T is the temperature in degrees kelvin
(*Note:* 0°C = 273°K)

   q is the electronic charge, 1.6×10^{-19}
coulombs per electron

   I_{c1} and I_{c2} are the collector currents of Q_1 and
Q_2, respectively

The quantity K/q is a ratio of constants and is constant under *all* circumstances. The current ratio I_{c1}/I_{c2} is held constant by using constant current sources in the emitter circuits of Q_1 and Q_2. Of course, the *logarithm* of a constant is also a constant. So the only variable in Equation 6-37 is the temperature.

Example 6-12

Find the output voltage of a temperature transducer constructed as Figure 6-37c if I_{c1} is 2 mA

and I_{c2} is 1 mA and the temperature is 37°C. (*Hint:* 37°C is $(37 + 273)$°K, or 310°K.)

Solution

$$\Delta V_{be} = (KT \ln(I_{c1}/I_{c2})/q$$

$$\Delta V_{be} = \frac{(1.38 \times 10^{-23} \text{J/°K})(310 \text{ K°})}{[\ln (2 \text{ mA}/1 \text{ mA})]}{1.6 \times 10^{-19} \text{ °C}}$$

$$\Delta V_{be} = 1.85 \times 10^{-2} \text{ J/°C} = \mathbf{0.0185 \text{ V}}$$

Equation 6-37 yields a value of approximately 59.8 μV/°K. The student should verify that the result in this example is actually *volts*, since 1 V = 1 J/°C.

The circuit in Figure 6-37c has one distinct advantage over others: It is widely linear over most temperatures (up to the point where the thermistors are damaged), so the output voltage ΔV_{be} may be processed in a simple amplifier and requires no special circuitry to linearize the result. If an ampli-

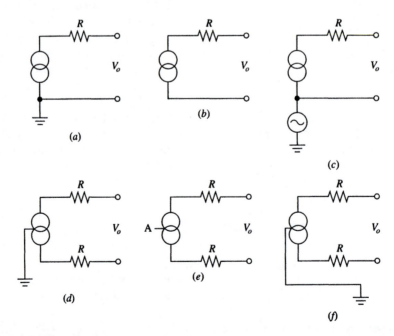

Figure 6-38
Input signal source configurations. Source: J.J. Carr, *Sensors and Circuits*, Prentice Hall.

fier of suitable gain is chosen and provided, then the temperature and the amplifier output voltage can be made numerically equal, allowing a simple voltmeter readout device. Most such instrumental systems are scaled to produce an amplifier output voltage of 10 mV/°K.

6-18 Matching sensors to circuits

Figure 6-38 shows an array of several different forms of model sensor circuits. In each circuit, a current source, source resistance R is shown, and (in some circuits) a voltage source is shown. Figure 6-38a shows the standard single-ended grounded sensor. The term *single-ended* means that one side of the sensor circuit is grounded. If neither side is grounded, then the sensor is said to be a single-ended *floating* sensor (Figure 6-38b). In the single-ended sensor, the output signal is referenced either to ground or to a single common nongrounded point. This form is sometimes subject to serious interference from external fields,

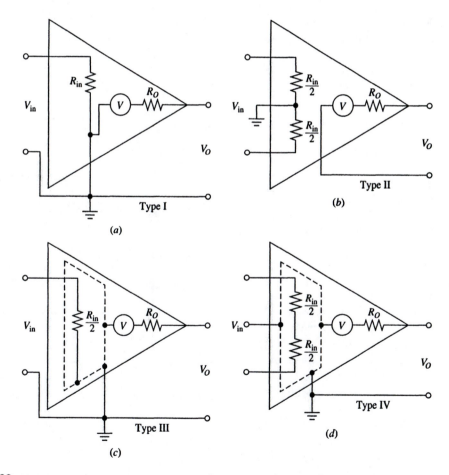

Figure 6-39
(a) Single-ended input equivalent circuit; (b) differential input; (c) single-ended amplifier equivalent circuit; (d) differential amplifier equivalent circuit. Source: J.J. Carr, *Sensors and Circuits*, Prentice Hall.

especially in the presence of strong audio frequency, radio frequency, or 60-Hz ac power-line fields. A variant on the single-ended floating sensor is the single-ended floating driven off-ground sensor shown in Figure 6-38c.

If a sensor drives the output through equal resistances, it is said to be *balanced*. Figure 6-38d shows an example of a balanced grounded sensor. In this form of output circuit, the sensor is referenced to ground through two equal resistances (both designated R). The version shown in Figure 6-38e is an example of a balanced floating sensor. That is, the sensor is connected to a nongrounded common point A and outputs through two equal resistances R. The important point to remember about the balanced floating sensor is that it is both balanced and ungrounded. Finally, in Figure 6-38f we see the balanced driven off-ground sensor circuit.

Amplifier input circuits

The output circuit of the sensor is usually connected to a signal processing circuit, most frequently an amplifier of some sort (although certain other circuits are also used occasionally). Unfortunately, there are several different types of amplifier input circuits, and not all sensors can be easily interfaced with all of them. Figure 6-39 shows four basic types of input circuit. Figure 6-39a depicts the type I circuit, a single-ended amplifier. The input circuit is modeled as a resistance to ground. Figure 6-39b shows the type II circuit, which is modeled as a pair of differential inputs that see equal resistances to ground. In both, the output circuit is a voltage source in series with an output resistance. Figure 6-39c shows the type III input circuit, which is single-ended, floating, and shielded. The input resembles the regular single-ended input shown in Figure 6-39a, but the input is grounded and protected from interference by a shield. In Figure 6-39d we see the type IV input circuit. This circuit resembles type II, except that the input circuit is protected by a shield, is floating, and is guarded.

Matching sensors and amplifiers

One cannot simply connect the various forms of sensors to the various forms of amplifier inputs without careful consideration. Figure 6-40 shows a general table relating the sensor and amplifier circuits. "Yes" in a block means that the combination (row versus column) is recommended. "No" means there are problems with that particular combination, so it is not recommended.

There are two combinations that may or may not work, depending on the circumstances, so some degree of caution is required. For example, mixing a type I input circuit with a form A sensor output circuit requires consideration of signal levels. This combination should not be used when the output of the sensor is in the microvolt or millivolt range. Also, it is not a good idea to mix two grounds, that is, one each on the amplifier and sensor. Either one ground should be eliminated or they should be joined together in a single-point (also called *star*) ground. A similar problem occurs when a form A sensor and a type II amplifier input are interfaced. Some differential amplifiers can be converted into a single-ended amplifier, but one must be certain in each case.

Input circuit type	Sensor Signal Source Form					
	A	B	C	D	E	F
I	See text	Yes	No	No	Yes	No
II	See text	Yes	No	Yes	Yes	No
III	Yes	Yes	Yes	No	Yes	No
IV	Yes	Yes	Yes	Yes	Yes	Yes

Figure 6-40
Chart crossing input amplifier types and signal sources. Sources: J.J. Carr, *Sensors and Circuits*, Prentice Hall.

6-19 Summary

1. When *metallic electrodes* are connected to skin, a *half-cell potential* is formed. The combined half-cell potentials of two or more electrodes form an *electrode offset potential. Polarization* occurs when dc flows through the electrode/skin interface.

2. *Plate* and *suction cup electrodes* are used for making short-term recordings of bioelectric potentials, but for longer recordings, a *column electrode* is used. In all cases, however, an *electrolytic paste* or gel is used between the electrode surface and the skin.

3. Many biomedical transducers are based on the Wheatstone bridge principle.

4. Bonded and unbonded strain gauges use the principle of *piezoresistivity* to make pressure and force transducers.

5. Three basic types of temperature measurement transducers are the *thermocouple, thermistor,* and *solid-state PN junction.*

6. *Transducers or sensors must have some transducible property* to be useful.

7. Transducers can be divided into *active* and *passive* types.

8. Transducer or sensor errors can be classified into five basic categories: *insertion, application, characteristic, dynamic,* and *environmental.*

6-20 Recapitulation

Now return to the objectives and self-evaluation questions at the beginning of the chapter and see how well you can answer them. If you cannot answer certain questions, place a check mark next to each and review appropriate parts of the text. Next, try to answer the following questions using the same procedure. When you have answered all of the questions, solve the problems.

Questions

1. Define *half-cell potential.* Describe the factors that give rise to the half-cell potential.

2. Describe the differences between *electronic conduction* and *ionic conduction.*

3. Define *oxydizing reactions* and *reduction reactions.*

4. What is the *electrode double layer?* Define it in your own words.

5. Define *electrode offset potential.*

6. Two general categories of electrode material combinations are: _____ _____ and _____ _____.

7. List three techniques that might be used to overcome the effects of electrode offset potentials.

8. What is the approximate range of half-cell potentials in the materials normally considered for use in biomedical electrodes?

9. What material is normally employed in biomedical electrodes?

10. Draw the equivalent circuit for a pair of electrodes applied to the skin. Show the amplifier input resistance.

11. Sketch a diagram showing the electrode double-layer phenomenon for: (a) ordinary conductors, (b) silver-silver chloride materials.

12. What is the range of impedance normally found in medical electrodes?

13. Sketch a microelectrode based on platinum wire.

14. Sketch the circuit diagram of an amplifier that can compensate for microelectrode capacitance.

15. Name two forms of electrodes normally used for short-term ECG recording.

16. Describe or draw the diagram for a *column electrode.*

17. Long-term (more than a few minutes) ECG monitoring is usually done with ———— electrodes.

18. Why does the column electrode reduce movement artifacts?

19. State the most common cause of movement artifact in ECG recording.

20. Describe the typical ECG monitoring electrode.

21. EEG electrodes are used to record bioelectric potentials arising in the ————.

22. Draw the circuit of a *Wheatstone bridge*.

23. Define *piezoresistivity*.

24. What are the differences between *bonded strain gauges, unbonded strain gauges,* and *solid-state semiconductor strain gauges?*

25. What are the differences between quartz and moving plate capacitive transducers?

26. A(n) ———— sensor requires an external *ac* or *dc* electrical excitation source.

27. A(n) ———— sensor requires no external electrical source but generates its own electrical energy.

28. List five different forms of sensor error: ————, ————, ————, ———— and ————.

29. Write Kelvin's *first rule of instrumentation*.

30. Bubbles in a blood pressure transducer line and improper placement of the transducer result in what are called ———— errors.

31. Departure of a transducer characteristic from the ideal characteristic is the ———— error.

32. In your own words, describe the difference between *precision* and *accuracy*.

33. The ———— of a sensor describes the smallest incremental change of an input parameter that can be detected in the output signal.

Problems

1. A copper wire, 45 cm long, has a cross-sectional area of 0.05 cm^2. Calculate its resistance. (*Hint:* The resistivity of copper is 17×10^{-8} Ω.)

2. A copper bar is 4.5 in. long and has a cross-sectional area of 100 circular mils. What is its resistance? (*Hint:* The resistivity of any material can be converted to the British engineering units by dividing the meter-kilogram-second units by 6×10^8).

3. In the Wheatstone bridge shown in Figure 6-24, assume that $R_1 = 1.5$ kΩ, $R_2 = 780$ Ω, $R_3 = 990$ Ω, and $R_4 = 1.2$ kΩ. Find the output voltage when an excitation voltage of +5 V *dc* is applied.

4. A blood pressure transducer is based on the Wheatstone bridge. The sensitivity is nominally rated at 50 μV/V/mm Hg. Find the output voltage if an excitation potential of +7.5 V and a pressure of 100 torr is applied.

5. A 40-mm length of wire has a resistance of 100 Ω. When a tension force is applied, the resistance changes to 80 Ω and the length becomes 40.04 mm. Calculate the *gauge factor.*

6. A transducer with a sensitivity of 50 μV/V/g is used to measure a 120-g-force. Find the output voltage if the excitation potential is +7.5 V.

7. A dual transistor is connected as shown in Figure 6-37c to form a temperature transducer. Calculate the output voltage if $I_{C1} = 4$ mA, $I_{C2} = 1.75$ mA, and the applied temperature is 37°C.

8. Show that the following is true:

$$\Delta V_{be} = \frac{KT \ln \left(\dfrac{I_{C1}}{I_{C2}} \right)}{q}$$

Hint: For each transistor in Figure 6-25*c:*
$V_{be} = [KT(\ln(I_c/I_s))]/q$, where I_s is the *reverse saturation current,* which is a constant in matched transistors.

9. Find the capacitance of a microelectrode if the pipette radius is 0.15 μm and the inside tip radius is 0.1 μm. Assume platinum wire is used inside a glass pipette.

10. For electrode capacitance of $C = 122$ pF and an impedance of 25 MΩ, find the frequency response upper -3 dB point.

11. A microelectrode and its cabling exhibit a total capacitance of 44 pF. Find the value of neutralization capacitor required for a gain-of-30 amplifier.

Suggested readings

1. Bryzek, Janusz, "Silicon Low Pressure Sensors Address HVAC Applications," *Sensors,* March 1990, pp. 9ff.

2. Carr, Joseph J., *Elements of Electronic Instrumentation and Measurement,* 3rd ed., Prentice-Hall (Toms River, N.J., 1995).

3. Carr, Joseph J., *A CrashCourse™ in Statistics,* HighText Publications (Solana Beach, Calif., 1994). A combination book and CD-ROM interactive multimedia tutorial software for *Windows®* computers.

4. Carr, Joseph J., *The Art of Science,* HighText Publications (San Diego, 1992).

5. Carr, Joseph J., *Sensors and Circuits: Sensors, Transducers, and Supporting Circuits for Electronic Instrumentation, Measurement, and Control,* Prentice-Hall (Englewood Cliffs, N.J., 1992).

6. Carr, Joseph J., *Designer's Handbook of Instrumentation and Control Circuits,* Academic Press (San Diego, 1991).

7. Carr, Joseph J., *Microcomputer Interfacing: A Practical Guide for Technicians, Engineers and Scientists,* Prentice-Hall (Englewood Cliffs, N.J., 1991).

8. Carr, Joseph J., *Designing Microprocessor-Based Instrumentation,* Reston Publishing Co./Division of Prentice-Hall (Englewood Cliffs, NJ, 1982).

9. Cobbold, Richard S.C., *Transducers for Biomedical Measurements,* Wiley (New York, 1974).

10. Fitzsimmons, J., "New Pressure Sensor Technology," *Sensors,* March 1986, pp. 44ff.

11. Frank, Oliver, *Practical Instrumentation Transducer.* Hayden Books (New York, 1971).

12. Geddes, L.A. and L.E. Baker, *Principles of Applied Biomedical Instrumentation,* Wiley (New York, 1968).

13. Mulkins, Donald F., "The Quartz Capacitive Pressure Sensor," *Sensors,* July 1989, pp. 9ff.

14. Simmons, J. and D. Soderquist, "Temperature Measurement Method Based on Matched Transistor Pair Requires No Reference." (Precision Monolithics, Inc., Applications Note AN-12, Santa Clara, CA 1976).

15. "Low-Cost Catheter Tip Sensor Measures Blood Pressure During Surgery," product feature column, *Sensors,* July 1989, pp. 30ff.

CHAPTER 7

Bioelectric Amplifiers

7-1 Objectives

1. Be able to state the requirements for a *bioelectric amplifier*.
2. Be able to describe the basic principles of *operational amplifiers*.
3. Be able to draw several different bioelectric amplifier configurations.

4. Be able to state the principles of operation of isolation amplifiers.
5. Be able to describe the problems associated with the acquisition of bioelectric phenomena.
6. Be able to draw the elements of a medical data acquisition system.

7-2 Self-evaluation questions

These questions test your prior knowledge of the material in this chapter. Look for the answers as you read the text. After you have finished studying the chapter, try answering these questions and those at the end of the chapter.

1. List the features required in a bioelectric amplifier.

2. List the basic properties of the operational amplifier.

3. Draw the circuit for an operational amplifier integrator, and describe its operation.

4. Find the voltage gain of an inverting follower that has a 100-kΩ feedback resistor and a 5-kΩ input resistor.

5. Describe an isolation amplifier. Why is it used as a bioelectric amplifier?

6. State the mathematical expression that gives the gain of an noninverting follower.

7-3 Bioelectric amplifiers

Amplifiers used to process biopotentials are called *bioelectric amplifiers,* but this designation applies to a large number of different types of amplifiers. The gain of a bioelectric amplifier, for example, may be low, medium, or high (i.e., ×10, ×100, ×1000, ×10,000). Similarly, some bioelectric amplifiers are ac-coupled, while others are dc-coupled. The frequency response of typical bioelectric amplifiers may be from dc (or near-dc, i.e., 0.05 Hz) up to 100 kHz.

Dc-coupling is required where the input signals are clearly dc or change *very slowly* (some in vivo O_2 levels change in *mm Hg per minute* or *per hour*). But even at frequencies as low as 0.05 Hz, ac-coupling may be used instead of dc. The reason for this is to overcome electrode offset potentials. In the ECG amplifier, for example, frequency components as low as 0.05 Hz might be processed. But the electrode-skin connection produces an electrode offset (dc) potential that will interfere with the ECG signal. The amplifier, therefore, must be ac-coupled to block the dc offset in the input signal, yet have a frequency response down to 0.05 Hz to faithfully reproduce the patient's ECG waveform.

The *high-frequency response* is the frequency at which the gain drops 3 dB below its midfrequency value. In some cases the −3 dB high-frequency point will be a frequency as low as 30 Hz, but in most cases it is 10 kHz. Specialized models used to process specific waveforms may have a particular response. ECG amplifiers, for example, usually have a frequency response of 0.05 to 100 Hz.

A few general-purpose amplifiers have *adjustable* frequency response and are thus usable for a wide range of applications. In general, it is wise to use only the minimum frequency response needed to ensure good reproduction of the input waveform. This practice permits rejection of high-frequency noise.

Low-gain amplifiers are those with gain factors between ×1 and ×10. The unity-gain (×1) amplifier is used mostly for isolation, buffering, and possibly impedance transformation between signal source and readout device. Low-gain amplifiers are often used for the measurement of action potentials and other relatively high-amplitude bioelectric events.

Medium-gain amplifiers are those that provide gain factors between ×10 and ×1000 and are used for the recording of ECG waveforms, muscle potentials, and so forth.

High-gain, or *low-level,* signal amplifiers have gain factors over ×1000, with some having factors as high as ×1,000,000. This type of amplifier is used in very sensitive measurements, such as the recording of brain potentials (EEG).

Two important parameters in bioelectric amplifiers, especially those in the high- and medium-gain classes, are *noise* and *drift*. *Drift* is the (spurious) change in output signal voltage caused by changes in operating temperature (rather than input signal changes). *Noise*, in this case, normally is the thermal noise generated in resistances and semiconductor devices. Good design and prudent component selection reduce these problems to the negligible level in modern equipment.

All three classes of bioelectric amplifiers must have a very high *input impedance*. This requirement is the one commonality among *all* bioelectric amplifiers, because almost all bioelectric signal sources exhibit a high *source impedance*. Most bioelectric sources have an impedance between 10^3 and 10^7 Ω, and ordinary engineering design practices dictate an amplifier input impedance that is at least an order of magnitude higher than the source impedance. Modern metal oxide semiconductor field effect transistor (MOSFET) and junction field effect transistor (JFET) amplifier (operational amplifier) devices have input impedances on the order of 1 *teraohm* (10^{12} Ω).

The properties of the integrated circuit (IC) operational amplifier make it especially well suited as a bioelectric amplifier. A discussion of operational amplifier theory follows. A greater understanding will be achieved as we discuss basic principles and then practical circuits made from commercially available components. These parts help make biomedical instrumentation what it is today. In addition, circuit applications are shown to demonstrate the versatility of operational amplifiers and to stress their importance in biomedical instrument circuits.

7-4 Operational amplifiers

The *operational amplifier* (op-amp) is a device that behaves in a unique manner: The properties of the circuit containing an operational amplifier are determined by the properties of the *negative feedback loop*. For the elementary voltage amplifier circuit configurations, we require only the basic properties of the device, Ohm's law, and Kirchhoff's law to derive the transfer equations. The author of one book on op-amp circuit design* was reportedly tempted to title his book *Ohm's Law With Applications.* There are more elegant, more mathematical methods for analyzing the behavior of the voltage amplifier configurations, but none shows circuit action quite as vividly as the simple method presented here, as follows.

The op-amp gets its name from the fact that it was originally conceived to solve mathematical operations in analog computers. Although analog computers are no longer in widespread use, many electronic instruments use operational amplifiers and are, in effect, scaled-down, dedicated, or single-purpose analog computers.

Commercial operational amplifiers have been available since the early 1950s, and integrated circuit op-amps since the mid-60s. Prices of modern IC operational amplifier devices range from less than a dollar for low-quality units to dozens of dollars for high-grade specialized units. Many premium grade op-amps are priced in the less-than-$10 range, and some are in the $2 range.

The circuit symbol for an op-amp is shown in Figure 7-1a. The amplifier must operate in all four quadrants, so the output terminal must be able to swing either to the positive or to the negative. The power supply (Figure 7-1b), therefore, must be *bipolar;* that is, it must consist of two supplies, one positive to ground and a second negative to ground.

---

*John I. Smith, *Modern Operational Circuit Design,* Wiley-Interscience (New York, 1971).

The power supply shown in Figure 7-1b has two batteries, but an ac-mains-operated bipolar supply will also work. Battery E_1 forms the V_{cc} supply and is *positive* with respect to ground. Battery E_2 forms the V_{ee} supply and is connected so that it is *negative* with respect to ground.

Note on the op-amp symbol shown in Figure 7-1a that there is no *ground* terminal on the op-amp. The only ground connection in this operational amplifier is formed at the junction of the two power supplies.

The op-amp has two inputs: the *inverting* input and the *noninverting* input. These are indicated by $(-)$ and $(+)$ signs, respectively.

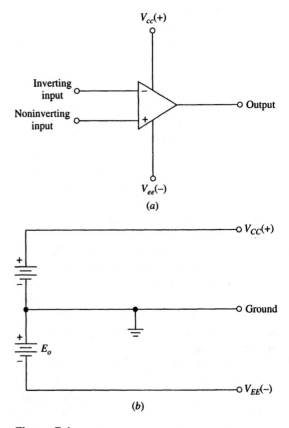

Figure 7-1
The operational amplifier. (*a*) Circuit symbol. (*b*) Power supply configuration.

The inverting input produces an output signal that is 180 degrees out of phase with the input signal. This is called *inversion* of the signal.

The noninverting input produces an output signal that is *in phase* with the input signal. There is *no* phase inversion of the signal between input and output.

Both inverting and noninverting inputs offer the same gain, so we may conclude that these respective inputs have *equal* but *opposite* phase effect at the output.

The various signal voltages that can affect the op-amp output terminal are shown in Figure 7-2. E_1 is applied to the inverting input, while E_2 is applied to the noninverting input. As long as E_1 and E_2 are *not equal* and of the same polarity, the operational amplifier will see a *differential* input voltage consisting of $E_2 - E_1$. The output voltage will be proportional to the gain of the stage and the *difference* between E_1 and E_2.

Common-mode signal voltages are those that are *common* to *both* inputs, such as E_3, or where E_1 and E_2 are of equal magnitude and have the same polarity. In common-mode situations, the differential voltage between the inputs is *zero,* so the output is zero.

The *common-mode rejection ratio* (CMRR) of an op-amp is an expression of how nearly any given device approximates the ideal situation, in which a common-mode signal has *no* effect on the output terminal voltage.

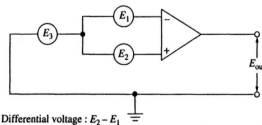

Differential voltage : $E_2 - E_1$
Common voltage : E_3, $E_1 = E_2$

Figure 7-2
Signal voltage sources.

7-4-1 The properties of ideal op-amps

We can analyze the op-amp by considering the following ideal properties:

1. Infinite open-loop (i.e., no feedback) *voltage gain* ($A_{vol} = \infty$).

2. *Zero* output impedance ($Z_o = 0$).

3. *Infinite* input impedance ($Z_i = \infty$).

4. *Infinite* frequency response.

5. *Zero* noise contribution.

6. Both inputs *follow* each other in feedback circuits. That is, in a circuit with negative feedback, a voltage applied to one input allows us to treat the *other* input as if it were at the *same* potential.

These six properties will be cited frequently throughout this chapter.

Before continuing our analysis of the feedback voltage amplifier configurations, let us consider first some implications of these properties.

Infinite open-loop voltage gain. The open-loop voltage gain (A_{vol}) of any amplifier circuit is the gain *without* any feedback. In the *ideal* op-amp, this gain is defined as infinite. An implication of this property is that the closed-loop characteristics of the circuit are determined entirely by the properties of the feedback loop network and are independent of the amplifying device.

Zero output impedance, $Z_o = 0$, implies that the output is an ideal voltage source.

Infinite input impedance, $Z_i = \infty$, tells us that the input terminals neither *sink or source any current,* nor do they load any circuit to which they are connected.

Property 6 is crucial to our circuit analysis: *The inputs tend to follow each other.* This means that we treat both inputs as if they were at the same potential. If a given voltage is applied to, say, the noninverting input, then we must treat the inverting input as if it were at the *same* potential. In fact, if a voltage is applied to one input, a voltmeter would *measure* the *same* voltage at the other input.

In this text, we consider the operational amplifier as a special black box that has the previously cited six properties.†

7-5 Basic amplifier configurations

There are many circuit configurations using op-amps as the active device, but only three basic classes of voltage amplifiers exist: *inverting follower, noninverting follower with gain,* and *unity gain noninverting follower.* The following sections discuss simple circuits and applications of bioelectric amplifiers made from commercially available components.

7-5-1 Inverting followers

Figure 7-3 shows the basic inverting circuit. It consists of an *op-amp,* an *input resistor* (R_1), and a *feedback resistor* (R_2).

The *noninverting* input is *grounded* in this circuit, so by property 6, we treat the *inverting* as if it were also grounded. This idea is sometimes called a *virtual ground,* for want of a better phrase. Point A, the junction of the two resistors and the operational amplifier's inverting input, is properly called the *summing junction,* or *summation node.*

When an input voltage E_{in} is applied, it sees the point A end of R_1 as being at ground potential, so current I_1 flows and is equal to E_{in}/R_1.

By Kirchhoff's law we know that the sum of all currents entering and leaving the summing junction is zero. Property 3 tells us that no current flows in to or out of the inverting input, so we may deduce that only input current I_1 and feedback current I_2 affect the junction. By Kirchhoff's current law, then, current I_2 must have a magnitude and polarity that exactly *cancels* I_1. We may view the

---

†For those desiring a deeper and more mathematical treatment, see the suggested readings at the end of the chapter.

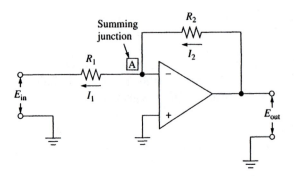

Figure 7-3
Inverting follower.

operational amplifier as a servo system that generates an output voltage that permits I_2 to cancel I_1.

We can derive the *transfer function* of the inverting follower by the following procedure.

(a) By Kirchhoff's current law

$$-I_1 = I_2 \qquad (7\text{-}1)$$

(b) By Ohm's law

$$I_1 = \frac{E_{in}}{R_1} \qquad (7\text{-}2)$$

$$I_2 = \frac{E_{out}}{R_2} \qquad (7\text{-}3)$$

Substituting Equations 7-2 and 7-3 into Equation 7-1 gives us

$$\frac{-E_{in}}{R_1} = \frac{E_{out}}{R_2} \qquad (7\text{-}4)$$

Solving Equation 7-4 for the transfer function E_{out}/E_{in} gives us the voltage gain of the inverting follower configuration.

$$\frac{E_{out}}{E_{in}} = \frac{-R_2}{R_1} = -A_v \qquad (7\text{-}5)$$

The quantity R_2/R_1 gives us the magnitude of the voltage gain for this amplifier configuration, and the minus sign tells us that a 180-degree phase inversion takes place. The voltage amplification or gain expression is often represented by the symbol A_v.

Equation 7-5 is also frequently seen in two alternative but equivalent forms

$$E_{out} = -E_{in}\left(\frac{R_2}{R_1}\right) \qquad (7\text{-}6)$$

and

$$E_{out} = -A_v E_{in} \qquad (7\text{-}7)$$

Example 7-1

Calculate the gain of an inverting follower if the feedback resistor (i,e., R_2) is 120 kΩ, and the input resistor (R_1) is 5.6 kΩ.

Solution

$$A_v = \frac{-R_2}{R_1} \qquad (7\text{-}5)$$

$$A_v = -(120 \text{ k}\Omega)/(5.6 \text{ k}\Omega) = 21$$

Figure 7-4 shows inverting operational amplifier circuit detail. Along with external circuit components, some internal "guts" of the op-amp are revealed. All op-amps have plus and minus bias current (I_{b+} and I_{b-}) and output load current (I_o). Also, all op-amps have three types of internal resistance and capacitance: (1) common-mode R_{cm} and C_{cm} (referenced to ground), (2) differential

R_{diff} and C_{diff} (between op-amp terminals), and (3) output R_o. Notice there is no ground on the op-amp itself. The ground reference is actually the point between the power supplies, where the minus of the $+V_{cc}$ power supply and the plus of the $-V_{cc}$ (sometimes called V_{ee}) come together.

Examining Figure 7-4 reveals that the external components interact with each other and with the op-amp to cause errors. One is a 0.5% gain error from the ideal of -1 V/V. It is caused by the external 50-Ω source resistance, R_s, and the input resistance, R_1. Essentially, R_s becomes part of a voltage divider with R_1 at the input, and some of E_{in} is undesirably dropped across R_s. This may not seem like much gain error, but over a number of op-amp stages, the error could easily accumulate to several percent. Another error occurs at the output where R_o/A_{vol} acts as another voltage divider with the load resistance, R_L. Fortunately, R_o/A_{vol} equals about 1000/100,000 Ω, which is only 0.001 Ω, or 1 mΩ. The quantity 0.001 Ω is so small compared to R_L or 10,000 Ω that the gain error is negligible.

How does internal op-amp resistance cause errors? R_{cm} on the minus op-amp terminal is in parallel with the input resistance, but R_{cm}, usually > 1000 MΩ, causes only a very small error on R_1

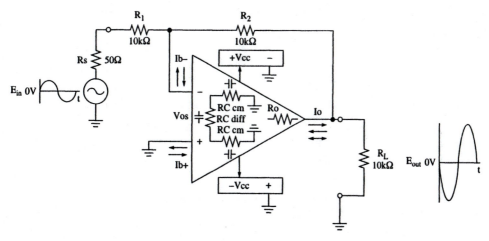

Figure 7-4
Inverting operational amplifier circuit detail.

= 10 kΩ. However, C_{cm}, usually < 5 pico-farad (pF), can cause a gain error at higher frequencies. For example, at a frequency of 1 MHz, the reactance of C_{cm} is 32 kΩ, and this shunts the external resistance, increasing the gain error at 1 MHz. The differential resistance, R_{diff}, also enters the picture, but we will not calculate the error here. The intention of this discussion is to show "real-world" op-amp circuits.

One other error is bias current circulating through the feedback resistance, R_2. If I_{b-} = 10 nA, then 0.1 mV dc will be dropped across R_2, which shows up at the op-amp output as 0.1 mV. Assuming E_{out} = 10 V, a dc error of 0.001% (0.1 mV/10 V × 100) shows up, but it is actually rather small.

Examining op-amp circuit details shows that, although circuit gain is mostly dependent on external resistance such as R_1 and R_2, certain dc and ac errors are always present. Armed with this information, it is easier to understand and use op-amp circuits more fully.

Next is a special inverting op-amp circuit encountered frequently in biomedical instrumentation. It is the transimpedance amplifier or current-to-voltage converter shown in Figure 7-5. This circuit takes an input current I_s, from a current source, and converts it into a voltage, E_o, at the op-amp's output. Notice that a positive input current pulse flowing into the op-amp's summing junction or negative input produces a negative output voltage pulse. The current flowing in the feedback loop is I_f, which is almost equal to I_{in}. The op-amp's bias current will either add to or subtract from I_{in} to produce I_f. If I_b is small, say 1/1000 of I_{in}, then the error is small. Ignoring op-amp error, a 10-nA input gives a 0.1 V output, which can easily be further amplified.

The most common bioelectric (the words *bio-electronic* and *bioelectic* are used interchangeably) transimpedance amplifier circuit is the photodiode amplifier. Figure 7-6 shows a commercially available op-amp, in a real "light-to-voltage" circuit. Notice it is an inverting op-amp configuration.

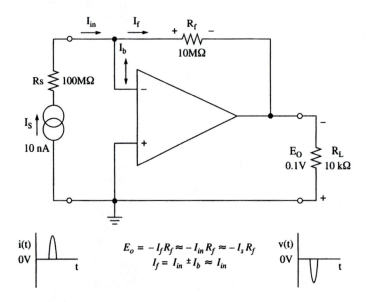

$$E_o = -I_f R_f \approx -I_{in} R_f \approx -I_s R_f$$
$$I_f = I_{in} \pm I_b \approx I_{in}$$

Figure 7-5
Basic transimpedance amplifier (current-to-voltage converter).

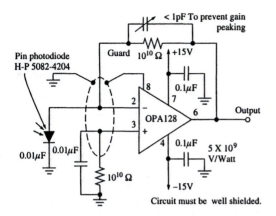

Figure 7-6
Sensitive photodiode amplifier. (Courtesy of Burr-Brown under copyright 1995 Burr-Brown Corporation)

Light shining on the photodiode produces a current that flows into the summing junction of the op-amp and then through the feedback resistance (10,000 MΩ in this highly sensitive photodetector circuit). Remember, ignoring op-amp errors, the voltage across the feedback resistor equals the op-amp output voltage. An input light signal of 0.002 μW will give an output of 10 V, because the overall gain is 5 × 1,000 MV/W. The op-amp's analog output voltage can then be digitized through an analog-to-digital converter and used to record the exact light intensity. Notice that 10,000 MΩ is also placed from the positive input to ground. This tends to cancel the offset error caused by op-amp bias current, since + and − bias currents are nearly equal. Another major error is gain peaking, which is caused by diode capacitance. To minimize this, a 1-pF capacitor is placed in the feedback loop.

Noise or random voltage fluctuation that appears in the output signal is the last error we discuss here. This error is caused by resistor noise, op-amp voltage and current noise, and noise pickup. To keep noise low, the circuit should use the smallest feedback resistor practical, a low-noise op-amp, and shielded op-amp input pins. After that, low-pass filtering must be provided.

Such photodetector circuits are used in optical pulse oximeters to measure human blood oxygen saturation, optical glucose meters to measure human blood sugar levels, and medical lab spectrophotometers to measure blood plasma elements. This circuit shows up often.

7-5-2 Noninverting followers with gain

An example of the *noninverting follower gain* amplifier is shown in Figure 7-7a. In this circuit the input voltage is applied directly to the *noninverting* input terminal of the operational amplifier. Feedback resistor R_2 and input resistor R_1 are the same as in the inverting follower, except that the other end of R_1 is grounded.

By property 6 we know that point A must be treated as if it were at a potential equal to E_{in}. We may derive the transfer equation for this circuit using the same technique that was used in the previous case.

By Kirchhoff's current law

$$I_1 = I_2 \qquad (7\text{-}8)$$

By Ohm's law

$$I_1 = \frac{E_{in}}{R_1} \qquad (7\text{-}9)$$

$$I_2 = \frac{E_{out} - E_{in}}{R_2} \qquad (7\text{-}10)$$

Substituting Equations 7-9 and 7-10 into Equation 7-8 results in

$$\frac{E_{in}}{R_1} = \frac{E_{out} - E_{in}}{R_2} \qquad (7\text{-}10A)$$

$$\frac{E_{in}}{R_1} = \frac{E_{out}}{R_2} - \frac{E_{in}}{R_2} \qquad (7\text{-}10B)$$

$$\frac{E_{in}}{R_1} + \frac{E_{in}}{R_2} = \frac{E_{out}}{R_2} \qquad (7\text{-}10C)$$

$$\frac{E_{in}R_2}{R_1} + \frac{E_{in}R_2}{R_2} = E_{out} \qquad (7\text{-}10D)$$

$$\frac{R_2}{R_1} + 1 = \frac{E_{out}}{E_{in}} = A_v \qquad (7\text{-}11)$$

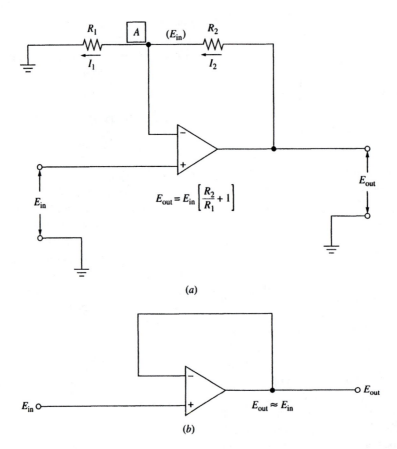

$$E_{out} = E_{in}\left[\frac{R_2}{R_1} + 1\right]$$

(a)

$$E_{out} \approx E_{in}$$

(b)

Figure 7-7
Noninverting followers. (a) With gain. (b) Unity gain.

Example 7-2

Calculate the voltage gain of a noninverting follower if $R_2 = 10$ kΩ and $R_1 = 2.2$ kΩ.

Solution

$$A_v = \frac{R_2}{R_1} + 1 \qquad (7\text{-}11)$$

$$A_v = 10\,k\Omega/2.2\,k\Omega + 1$$

$$A_v = 4.6 + 1 = \mathbf{5.6}$$

At high gains (i.e., circuits with high R_2/R_1 ratios), the gains of the inverting and noninverting followers are very nearly equal but, at low gains, a difference is noted.

7-5-3 Unity gain noninverting followers

A special case of the noninverting follower is the *unity gain noninverting follower* of Figure 7-7b. The resistor network is not used in this circuit, and the output is connected directly to the inverting input, resulting in 100% negative feedback. By Equation 7-11 this yields a gain in Equation 7-11 of $(0 + 1)$, or simply $+1$, *unity.*

The unity gain noninverting follower is used in applications such as output buffering and impedance matching between a high source impedance and a low-impedance input circuit.

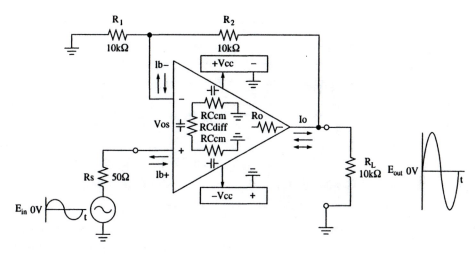

Figure 7-8
Noninverting operational amplifier circuit detail.

A more complete understanding of the noninverting op-amp circuit is gained from the detail in Figure 7-8. Just as in the inverting case, the op-amp possesses internal resistance and capacitance. However, since the input signal is driving a very high impedance (op-amp common-mode and differential R and C), very little gain error occurs. The 50-Ω source resistance is much smaller than the noninverting op-amp input resistance of around 1000 MΩ. Again, as in the inverting case, the R_o/A_{vol} and R_{load} divider cause a small output gain error. Small op-amp bias currents also flow in the source and feedback resistances to cause small offset errors. Thus the circuit gain is 2, with small offset and gain errors created by the op-amp interacting with its surrounding circuit elements.

A main characteristic of op-amp circuits is that the negative terminal is a reflection of its positive terminal. That is, when dc or ac voltages are applied to the positive input, that same dc and/or ac voltage also appears on the negative input. For example, if a 1-V_{p-p} sine wave riding around 0 V dc drives the plus input, then a 1-V_{p-p} sine wave riding around 0 V dc will also be present on the negative input.

A common bioelectronic noninverting amplifier circuit is the pH probe amplifier. Figure 7-9 shows

a commercially available op-amp connected in a gain of 20. The 50-mV probe output is amplified to produce 1 V at the op-amp's output. The 100-kΩ offset trim potentiometer will zero out the op-amp's offset voltage (say 250 μV) and the error caused by the noninverting terminal bias current times the large source resistance (say, 0.5 pA times 500 MΩ = 250 μV). Gain errors are caused mostly by inexact feedback resistances.

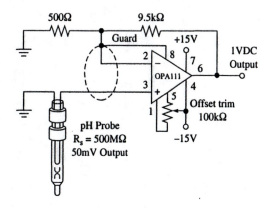

Figure 7-9
High-impedance (10^{14} Ω) pH probe amplifier. (Courtesy of Burr-Brown under copyright 1995 Burr-Brown Corporation)

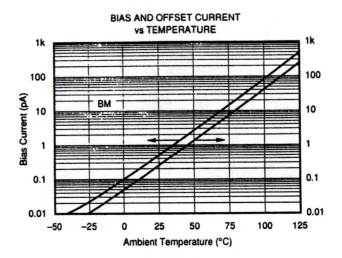

Figure 7-10
Important consideration: temperature effect on bias and offset current from OPA111 FET input op-amp. (Courtesy of Burr-Brown under copyright 1995 Burr-Brown Corporation)

In discussing a "real op-amp circuit," three important considerations show up again and again: bias current, voltage noise, and noise pickup. First, in Figure 7-10, we see from a typical product data sheet curve that bias current increases with temperature. At room temperature of 25°C, the bias is 0.5 pA, but at 75°C it is 10 pA, which is 20 times bigger. This makes the upper temperature offset error (10 pA $\times$ 500 MΩ = 5 mV) much higher than the room temperature error (0.5 pA $\times$ 500 MΩ = 0.25 mV).

The second important consideration is high noise caused by very high source resistance. In Figure 7-11, it is clear that at a source resistance

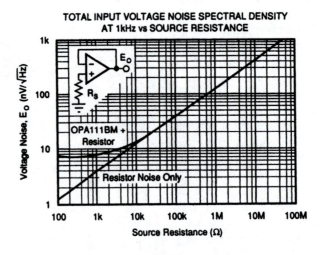

Figure 7-11
Important consideration: source resistance effect on total noise from the OPA111 FET input op-amp. (Courtesy of Burr-Brown under copyright 1995 Burr-Brown Corporation)

of, say, 100 MΩ, the total circuit noise can be big. This noise has three parts: (1) op-amp voltage noise, (2) op-amp current noise times source resistance, and (3) resistor noise (resistors have noise all by themselves just sitting on the table). Sometimes noise is referred to as Johnson, or thermal, noise, because it is the result of agitation of charges in materials. Noise on the typical product data sheet curve is 1000 nV/√Hz. The purpose for showing this graph is to emphasize that unfiltered wideband white noise can be rather high in pH probe circuits. Seeing noise will come as no surprise when it is understood where it comes from.

The third important consideration is the noise pickup. The guard shown in Figure 7-9 is further explained in Figure 7-12. To keep noise low in this noninverting op-amp circuit, the input pins 2 and 3 must be guarded or shielded. The way to do this is to lay out the printed circuit board as shown. Notice that pins 2 and 3 are completely surrounded by metal traces and then connected to pin 8 (the op-amp metal case) of this commercially available op-amp. It works this way: When, say, that 60 Hz

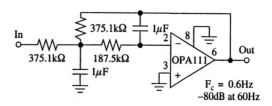

Figure 7-13
0.6-Hz two-pole (second-order) low-pass filter. (Courtesy of Burr-Brown under copyright 1995 Burr-Brown Corporation)

electromagnetic interference (EMI) noise cuts across the metal case, it tends to cause noise currents to flow in the input pins 2 and 3. However, since pins 2 and 3 are connected to the case through pin 8, they are at the same potential as the case (0 V between case and pins). Hence, noise current cannot flow into the input, because the voltage is zero. We say that the input pins are guarded against leakage or stray resistance and capacitance.

Understanding dc and noise errors in pH probe circuits helps technicians appreciate and work more effectively with bioelectric amplifiers.

Inverting and noninverting op-amp circuits are also used to form filters that are commonly found in biomedical equipment. Figure 7-13 shows a 0.6-Hz inverting, low-pass filter using a commercially available op-amp. The circuit has two poles (also called *second order*) because there are two capacitors. One is in parallel with the signal path, and the other is in the feedback loop of the op-amp. This type of filter is often used to reduce wideband or white noise from op-amps and EMI noise from 60-Hz power lines. In fact, any 60-Hz noise present in the input signal will be attenuated by80 dB. This means that the 60-Hz noise at the output will be 10,000 times smaller than at the input. Getting rid of 60-Hz noise is important to many biomedical measurements, such as pH level.

Multipole filters can be made from separate op-amps or from one chip, as shown in Figure 7-14. This circuit is a noninverting, two-pole, 10-kHz low-pass filter. The cut-off frequency of 10 kHz is used in ECG circuits to filter out electrosurgery

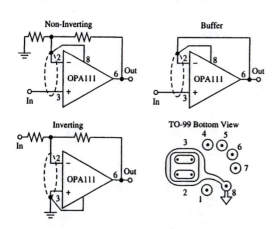

Board layout for input guarding: guard top and bottom of board. Alternate: use Teflon® standoff for sensitive input pins.

Teflon® E.I. Du Pont de Nemours & Co.

Figure 7-12
Important consideration: PC board layout and connection of input guard. (Courtesy of Burr-Brown under copyright 1995 Burr-Brown Corporation)

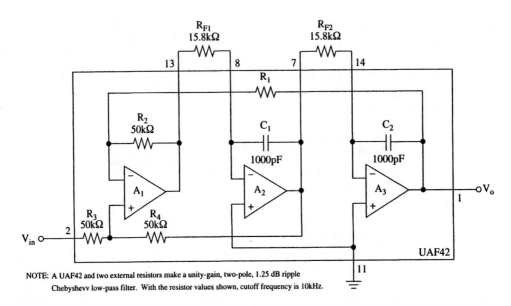

NOTE: A UAF42 and two external resistors make a unity-gain, two-pole, 1.25 dB ripple
Chebyshevv low-pass filter. With the resistor values shown, cutoff frequency is 10kHz.

Figure 7-14
Two-pole, 10-kHz low-pass filter using a one-chip circuit. (Courtesy of Burr-Brown under copyright 1991 Burr-Brown Corporation)

interference that contains frequencies above 500 kHz. Ten kHz is used to get good high-frequency attenuation while avoiding phase disturbance of the actual 100-Hz bandwidth ECG signal. Keeping the cutoff frequency way above the highest ECG frequency minimizes phase shifts in the ECG signal.

No biomedical filter discussion would be complete without considering the 60-Hz notch filter. Figure 7-15 depicts a circuit that rejects just 60 Hz. It passes frequencies below and above the 60-Hz center. Although the gain here is 101 V/V noninverting, it can be set using different feedback resistances. This type of filter is used in ECG and other biomedical equipment for cutting down on residual interference that is within the bandwidth of interest. For example, 60-Hz noise is undesirable inside the 100-Hz ECG spectrum. However, since the notch does cause some amplitude and phase distortion, biomedical equipment is often designed to take measurements with the notch switched out and switched in.

So far, active filters, which use an amplifier connected to a power supply, have been discussed. Passive or unpowered filters can also be used,

where appropriate. An example is shown in Figure 7-16. Here a pyroelectric infrared heat detector circuit uses a simple R-C or single-pole filter. It cuts off at 0.16 Hz to reduce noise. After filtering, the signal is gained up by 101 V/V. Pyroelectric detectors are used in applications that require high sensitivity. Heat radiating from an object, such as a person, can be sensed at a considerable distance. A

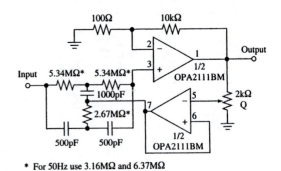

* For 50Hz use 3.16MΩ and 6.37MΩ
Gain = 101

Figure 7-15
High-impedance 60-Hz reject filter with gain. (Courtesy of Burr-Brown under copyright 1989 Burr-Brown Corporation)

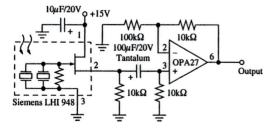

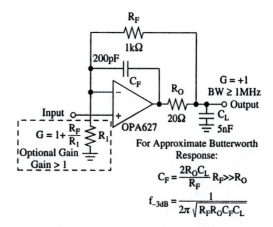

Figure 7-16
Balanced pyroelectric infrared (heat) detector. (Courtesy of Burr-Brown under copyright 1995 Burr-Brown Corporation)

concentration of body heat can reveal tumors, especially if infection is present.

It is often desirable to put bioelectronics as close to the sensor as possible. However, when this is done the amplifier may have to drive a voltage signal over a long electrical cable. Cables have capacitance and, if too large, tend to make op-amps oscillate. Figure 7-17 shows how a resistor in series with the op-amp output cures this problem. A small value, say 20 Ω, buffers the op-amp from the load, and since it is in the feedback path, it does not cause gain error. This circuit can drive a 5-nF or 5000-pF load. The 200-pF feedback capacitor also helps to maintain stability. Unstable bioelectric amplifier systems sometimes go undiagnosed.

Figure 7-17
Driving large capacitive loads. (Courtesy of Burr-Brown under copyright 1996 Burr-Brown Corporation)

One of the only ways to troubleshoot such instability, aside from observing erratic biomedical equipment operation, is to use an oscilloscope. Seeing a biophysical signal with high frequency riding on it indicates that the circuit is probably oscillating.

Op-amps, of course, can be used to create other bioelectronic circuits. The peak detector, shown in Figure 7-18, is frequently used to measure the peak of a biopotential, such as an ECG signal. The first stage is a noninverting amplifier with a diode in the

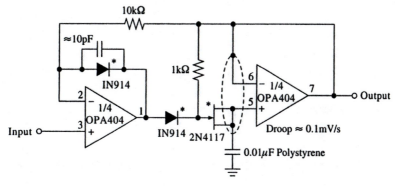

* Reverse polarity for negative peak detection

Figure 7-18
Low-droop positive peak detector. (Courtesy of Burr-Brown under copyright 1995 Burr-Brown Corporation)

feedback loop and a diode in series with the output. When the input voltage goes negative (below ground), the series diode blocks signal transfer to the second stage. The feedback diode ensures that the input stage is in low gain. But when the input goes positive, the series diode conducts into the FET transistor diode, which applies the signal peak to the 0.01-μF holding capacitor. A low-bias current FET op-amp is used for the second stage to ensure that the peak captured on the capacitor does not change very much. The droop, or amount of voltage decrease with time, is just 0.1 mV/s. The output, therefore, is a constant voltage that represents the positive peak of the input voltage. A greater understanding of biomedical instrumentation hinges on recognizing circuits and knowing how they work.

7-6 Multiple-input circuits

More than one input network may be used in an op-amp network, and the output voltage represents the summation of the respective input currents. An example of a multiple-input inverting follower is shown in Figure 7-19. Three input networks are used in this circuit, and there are three input sources: E_1 through E_3.

Again, the noninverting input is grounded, so we treat the inverting input as if it were also

grounded. From a course of reasoning exactly as before, we know that the transfer equation of a multiple-input circuit, such as the one in Figure 7-5, is

$$E_{out} = -R_4 \times \left(\frac{E_1}{R_1} + \frac{E_2}{R_2} + \frac{E_3}{R_3} + \cdots + \frac{E_n}{R_n} \right) \quad (7\text{-}12)$$

Example 7-3 —————

Find the output voltage in a circuit, such as the one in Figure 7-19, if $R_1 = R_2 = R_3 = 10$ kΩ, $R_4 = 22$ kΩ, $E_1 = 100$ mV, $E_2 = 500$ mV, and $E_3 = 75$ mV.

Solution

$$E_{out} = -R_4 \times \left(\frac{E_1}{R_1} + \frac{E_2}{R_2} + \frac{E_3}{R_3} \right) \quad (7\text{-}12)$$

$$E_{out} = -22\text{ kΩ}$$
$$\times \left(\frac{100\text{ mV}}{10\text{ kΩ}} + \frac{500\text{ mV}}{10\text{ kΩ}} + \frac{75\text{ mV}}{10\text{ kΩ}} \right)$$

$$E_{out} = -22\text{ kΩ}/10\text{ kΩ}\,(100\text{ mV} + 500\text{ mV} + 75\text{ mV})$$

$$E_{out} = -2.2 \times 675\text{ mV}$$
$$= -1490\text{ mV} = -1.49\text{ V}$$

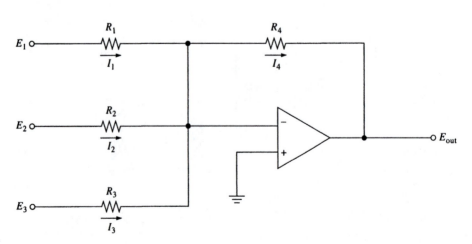

Figure 7-19
Multiple-input amplifier.

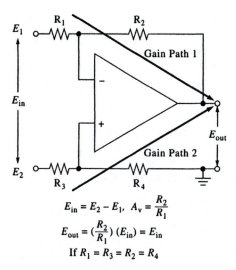

$$E_{in} = E_2 - E_1, \quad A_v = \frac{R_2}{R_1}$$

$$E_{out} = (\frac{R_2}{R_1}) (E_{in}) = E_{in}$$

If $R_1 = R_3 = R_2 = R_4$

Figure 7-20
Differential input amplifier basics (single-ended output).

Circuits such as Figure 7-19 are used in many medical instruments to *compute* a value (i.e., E_o) from several different input values (i.e., E_1 through E_3). It is also possible to use the noninverting input, in which case no polarity inversion takes place, and Equation 7-12 must be modified to reflect the contribution of signals applied to the noninverting input equation (Equation 7-11).

7-7 Differential amplifiers

A *differential amplifier* (diff-amp) produces an output voltage that is proportional to the *difference* between the voltage applied to the two input terminals. Since an operational amplifier has a pair of differential input terminals, it may be easily connected for use in a differential amplifier configuration.

In the most elementary form of dc differential amplifier (Figure 7-20) only a single IC operational amplifier is required. In this particular circuit, the voltage gain for differential signals is the same as for inverting followers (i.e., $A_v = R_2/R_1$), provided that the ratio equality $R_2/R_1 = R_4/R_3$ is maintained. It is standard practice to ensure this equality by stipulating that $R_1 = R_3$ and $R_2 = R_4$. Then gain path 1 is equal to gain path 2.

Figure 7-21 shows differential input amplifier circuit detail. Depicted is the external circuit and some internal "guts" of the diff-amp, which is really just an op-amp. All op-amps have plus and minus bias current (I_{b+} and I_{b-}), output load current (I_o), internal common-mode and differential resistance and capacitance, and output resistance, R_o. Of course, the ground reference is actually the point between the power supplies.

Examining Figure 7-21 reveals that the diff-amp is a combination of inverting and noninverting

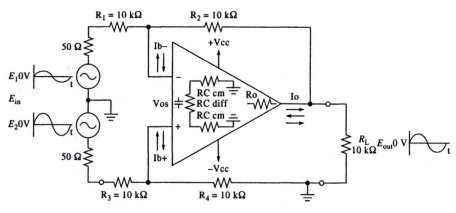

Figure 7-21
Differential input amplifier detail.

op-amp configurations. The external components interact with each other and with the op-amp to cause gain errors. For example, the external 50-Ω source resistance, R_s, in the inverting path causes a 0.5% gain error from the ideal of -1 V/V. Notice that the input resistance to the op-amp's inverting input is 10 kΩ. The input resistance ratio on the noninverting input also has a 0.5% error. This is why low input resistance diff-amps require very low source resistance to achieve high gain accuracy. The nice thing about the op-amp's positive (+) input is that it is high impedance (resistance and capacitive reactance). It therefore does not load or cause an error on the $R_3 - R_4$ resistor divider. We know that the internal op-amp resistance causes very little error, because R_{cm} is usually > 1000 MΩ. However, C_{cm}, usually < 5 pF, can cause a gain error at higher frequencies.

This discussion on op-amp circuit detail concludes that, although circuit gain is mostly dependent on external resistance, such as R_1, R_2, R_3, and R_4, certain dc and ac errors are always present. This information helps us understand how real-world diff-amp circuits work.

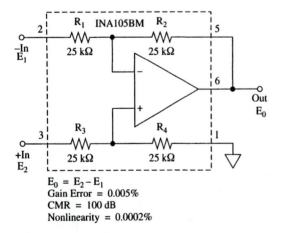

$E_0 = E_2 - E_1$
Gain Error = 0.005%
CMR = 100 dB
Nonlinearity = 0.0002%

Figure 7-22
One-chip (monolithic) precision unity gain difference amplifier. (Courtesy of Burr-Brown under copyright 1993 Burr-Brown Corporation)

Figure 7-22 shows a commercially available one-chip differential amplifier. It has internal thin-film resistors made of nichrome or nickel chromium. These resistors have been trimmed to high precision by cutting with a laser beam. The more the resistors are cut away by the automatic laser trimming machine, the higher the resistance because there is less conductive material). When precise resistor ratio accuracy is reached, cutting stops. In this component, the gain error is 0.005% and the common-mode rejection (CMR) is 100 dB. This means that the negative and positive gain paths are very nearly equal. Also, the gain and CMR temperature drift is very low—approximately five parts per million per degree centigrade (5 PPM/°C). It is really the resistor ratio that is changing slightly with temperature. This is much better than could be achieved by using separate external discrete resistors. Here the advantage of modern monolithic circuits becomes evident. All resistors on the same chip tend to behave exactly like one another. Their ratio stays constant.

The diff-amp is useful because it rejects common-mode voltages while amplifying the differential signal of interest. For example, suppose equal 60-Hz noise is present on each input, and one input is at 5 V dc and the other is at 2 V dc. The circuit in Figure 7-22 removes the noise and amplifies the 3-V dc differential signal. Remember, the CMR of this commercially available diff-amp is very high because on-chip resistors have been ratio-matched to make the + and − gain paths nearly equal. The unity gain diff-amp output is a 3-V dc signal in which 60-Hz noise interference is greatly reduced. The differential amplification removes noise, because equal common-mode noise is present on each input. The diff-amp just subtracts the equal noise voltage to give nearly zero while amplifying the difference in the unequal signals present on its inputs. How low noise becomes at the output depends on how high the diff-amp's CMR is.

The circuit shown in Figures 7-20 through 7-22 suffers from the same restrictions on input impedance as the inverting follower, because the input impedance is limited by R_1 and R_3. If a high gain is required, then a high R_2/R_1 ratio is required, yet practical circuit considerations limit the maximum and minimum values for these resistors.

The simple dc differential amplifier is used mostly in circuits where the source impedance is low. Strain gauge transducers, for example, typically have element resistances below 1 kΩ. Wheatstone bridge strain gauges with these resistor values have a resistance approximately equal to the resistance of each element arm (assuming all arms are equal). If the equivalent bridge resistance is as high as 1 kΩ, then the *minimum* value for R_1 and R_3 in the dc amplifier is 10 times as great, or 10 kΩ. Most low-cost IC operational amplifiers should not be used with feedback resistors greater than 1 MΩ. These limitations of real (as opposed to *ideal*) operational amplifiers limit the *practical* gain of a differential amplifier (Figure 7-20) to $10^6/10^4$, or 100.

The circuit of Figure 7-20, then, can be used with Wheatstone bridge strain gauge transducers

and other low-output impedance differential signal sources at gains up to 100. If higher gains are required, then a premium-cost amplifier (allowing feedback resistors greater than 10^6 Ω) must be used, or an additional stage of amplification is required. An alternate solution, one that provides a much higher input impedance, is to use the *instrumentation amplifier* circuit described in section 7-7-1.

7-7-1 Instrumentation amplifiers

The solution to both high-gain and high-input impedance problems is the *instrumentation amplifier* (IA) (Figure 7-23). This circuit uses *three* operational amplifiers, A_1 through A_3. The two input amplifiers (i.e., A_1 and A_2) are connected in the noninverting follower configuration, while the third amplifier is connected in the simple dc differential amplifier circuit shown in Figure 7-20. Let us initially simplify our circuit analysis by setting the gain of A_3 equal to unity (i.e., $R_4 = R_5 = R_6 = R_7$).

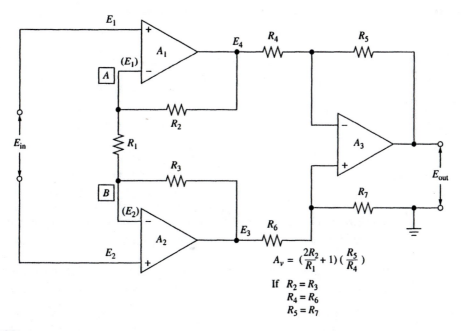

$$A_v = \left(\frac{2R_2}{R_1} + 1\right)\left(\frac{R_5}{R_4}\right)$$

If $R_2 = R_3$
$R_4 = R_6$
$R_5 = R_7$

Figure 7-23
Instrumentation amplifier.

Let us also assume that E_1 is applied to the non-inverting input of amplifier A_1 and that E_2 is applied to the noninverting input of amplifier A_2. Additionally, E_3 is the output of A_2, and E_4 is the output of A_1. Voltages E_1 and E_2 are also shown at the *inverting* inputs of A_1 and A_2, respectively, again reflecting property 6.

There are *two* contributing sources to E_3 and E_4. In the case of E_3:

$$E_3 = E_2 \times \left(\frac{R_3}{R_1} + 1 \right) - \left(E_1 \times \frac{R_3}{R_1} \right) \quad (7\text{-}13)$$

and for E_4:

$$E_4 = E_1 \times \left(\frac{R_2}{R_1} + 1 \right) - E_2 \times \left(\frac{R_2}{R_1} \right) \quad (7\text{-}14)$$

If we set $R_2 = R_3$ (not essential, but it simplifies the analysis), and then combine Equations 7-13 and 7-14, we may write

$$(E_3 - E_4) = (E_2 - E_1)\left(\frac{R_2}{R_1} + 1 \right)$$
$$+ (E_2 - E_1)\left(\frac{R_2}{R_1} \right)$$

$$(E_3 - E_4) = (E_2 - E_1)\left(\frac{R_2}{R_1} + 1 + \frac{R_2}{R_1} \right)$$

$$(E_3 - E_4) = (E_2 - E_1)\left(\frac{2R_2}{R_1} + 1 \right) \quad (7\text{-}15)$$

Therefore:

$$A_v = \frac{2R_2}{R_1} + 1 \quad (7\text{-}16)$$

The voltage gain of the A_1/A_2 section is given by Equation 7-16, but when the gain of A_3 is nonzero, we must also include a term that accounts for this extra gain. The gain of an IA such as the one in Figure 7-23 is given by the transfer function

$$A_v = \frac{E_{\text{out}}}{E_{\text{in}}} = \left(\frac{2R_2}{R_1} + 1 \right)\left(\frac{R_5}{R_4} \right) \quad (7\text{-}17)$$

Example 7-4

Find the gain of an IA (Figure 7-23) if the following resistor values are used: $R_2 = 10 \text{ k}\Omega$, $R_1 = 500 \text{ }\Omega$, $R_4 = 10 \text{ k}\Omega$, and $R_5 = 100 \text{ k}\Omega$.

Solution

$$A_v = \left(\frac{2R_2}{R_1} + 1 \right) \times \left(\frac{R_5}{R_4} \right) \quad (7\text{-}17)$$

$$A_v = \left(\frac{2 \times 10 \text{ k}\Omega}{0.5 \text{ k}\Omega} + \right) \times \left(\frac{100 \text{ k}\Omega}{10 \text{ k}\Omega} \right)$$

$$A_v = (40 + 1)(10) = \mathbf{410}$$

In ordinary practice the following equalities are observed: $R_2 = R_3$, $R_4 = R_6$, $R_5 = R_7$. Interestingly enough, a mismatch of R_2 and R_3 has little effect on the CMR ratio but does result in a differential gain error.

IAs are used in biomedical applications because of several factors: ability to obtain high gain with low resistor values, extremely high input impedance, and superior rejection of common-mode signals. Slight resistor mismatches in the circuit of A_3 can degrade CMR; therefore, many designers use a potentiometer for R_7. The potentiometer is adjusted (while a high-level, common-mode signal is applied) for *minimum* output signal.

The physical form taken by an IA might be a *discrete* op-amp circuit, such as Figure 7-23, in which three IC operational amplifier devices are used. It may also take the form of a *hybrid-function* module, in which chip-form IC operational amplifiers and the resistors are constructed on a thin ceramic substrate and then potted in a block of epoxy resin. The third form possible is a *monolithic* (IC) instrumentation amplifier. In both the hybrid and monolithic versions there may be a pair of external terminals for setting gain. These terminals are for an externally connected R_1 in Figure 7-23. The gain equation is usually a constant divided by the value of R_1 connected between the two terminals.

Modern IA design can be tailored to meet specific biomedical applications. The circuit in

Figure 7-24 shows how commercially available components are used to build IAs with specific front-end characteristics. Notice that the output stage is always a monolithic unity gain differential amplifier. Different IAs are designed by using different op-amps for the input stage. For example, a very low noise of 4 nV/$\sqrt{\text{Hz}}$ can be achieved with low noise bipolar op-amps. The bias current is 40 nA (40×10^{-9} A) in this first example. If a low-bias current of 1 pA (1×10^{-12} A) is needed, then the input op-amps are changed to the FET type. Notice that the voltage noise goes up 2.5 times to 10 nV/$\sqrt{\text{Hz}}$, because FET op-amps have inherently more voltage noise than bipolar input op-amps. If extremely low bias current, say 75 fA (75×10^{-15} A) is required, the input op-amps need to be the electrometer type. Notice again that the voltage noise

goes up almost four times to 38 nV/$\sqrt{\text{Hz}}$. By making the right trade-offs, one can build an IA to suit specific biomedical needs. Just like differential amplifiers, IAs reject equal noise on their inputs while amplifying unequal signal voltages on their inputs.

To refine the discussion on noise, a brief description of how to use the nanovolt per square root hertz specification will be reviewed here. The reason for this strange unit of measure is simple. It allows a designer to calculate noise in a specific bandwidth. If noise were given in, say, nV$_{rms}$ over, say, a 1-kHz bandwidth, it would be difficult to find the noise in, say, a 100-Hz bandwidth. Here's an example. Consider a noise density of 38 nV$_{rms}$/$\sqrt{\text{Hz}}$ at 1 kHz. It is easy to calculate the total noise: Just multiply 38 nV$_{rms}$/$\sqrt{\text{Hz}}$ by the square root of the bandwidth, namely 1000 Hz. The answer is 1.2 μV rms (38 nV/$\sqrt{\text{Hz}}$ × 32$\sqrt{\text{Hz}}$). The total noise is, therefore, a little more than 1 μV rms from, say, 10 Hz to 1 kHz. Since noise is made up of many uncorrelated sine wave frequencies, the peak-to-peak is statistically about six times higher than the rms. That is, it is about 7.2 μV peak-to-peak. In biomedical equipment, such as ECG machines, peak-to-peak noise is used to calculate dynamic range. In audio and video communications equipment, rms noise is often used.

Figure 7-25 shows a commercially available monolithic IA in which all three op-amps and resistors are one silicon chip. This particular component also has internal overvoltage protection diodes. It uses one external resistor to set the gain. You will see these types of single packaged parts used in modern compact biomedical equipment.

In fact, as discussed later, many biomedical systems are now being designed on one chip. All circuitry is contained on a single high-density integrated circuit. The name given to this newer approach is *application-specific integrated circuit* (ASIC). ASIC manufacturers make available standard design tools for manipulating standard cells or circuit functions. The advantage to the biomedical equipment designer is far-reaching. A

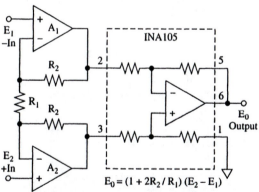

$$E_0 = (1 + 2R_2/R_1)(E_2 - E_1)$$

For low source impedance applications, an input stage using OPA37 op amps will give the best low noise, offset, and temperature drift performance. At source impedances above about 10kΩ, the bias current noise of the OPA37 reacting with the input impedance begins to dominate the noise performance. For these applications, using the OPA111 or Dual OPA2111 FET input op-amp will provide lower noise performance. For lower cost, use the OPA121 plastic. To construct an electrometer, use the OPA128.

A_1, A_2	$R_1(\Omega)$	$R_2(\Omega)$	Gain (V/V)	CMRR (dB)	Max I_s	Noise at 1kHz (nV/$\sqrt{\text{Hz}}$)
OPA37A	50.5	2.5k	100	128	40nA	4
OPA111B	202	10k	100	110	1pA	10
OPA128LM	202	10k	100	118	75fA	38

Figure 7-24

Building three op-amp precision instrumentation amplifiers with NPN and FET inputs. (Courtesy of Burr-Brown under copyright 1993 Burr-Brown Corporation)

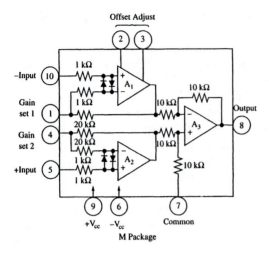

Figure 7-25
One-chip (monolithic) three op-amp precision instrumentation amplifier, INA101. (Courtesy of Burr-Brown under copyright 1993 Burr-Brown Corporation)

previously experienced printed circuit board engineer can now put together a complete system or subsystem on a chip, even though he or she is not an expert in monolithic semiconductor technology. Just as this text describes available bioelectric amplifiers, ASICs lay out available design and manufacturing technology.

Not only is the circuitry small, the packaging is becoming smaller as well. The small-outline integrated circuit (SOIC) and the leadless chip carrier (LCC) packages are becoming dominant. They mount on the surface of a printed circuit board (PCB) instead of in holes drilled through the PCB. It is easy to see how this construction technique saves cost and space by picturing dozens of SOICs mounted on both sides of a PCB.

No matter how sophisticated IAs become, they must still follow basic principles. Figure 7-26 shows an important consideration that readers should know about. In this chapter, we showed that real-world op-amps have bias current and that this current must flow somewhere for the circuit to work properly. Figure 7-26 indicates that a return path for bias current should always be provided.

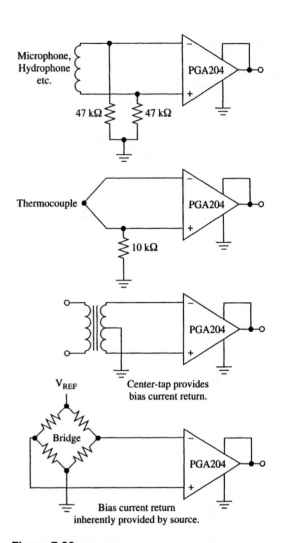

Figure 7-26
Important consideration: providing an input bias current path. (Courtesy of Burr-Brown under copyright 1992 Burr-Brown Corporation)

That is, if a floating source, such as a microphone, thermocouple, transformer, or the human body is used, resistors or some connection to ground or common must be present. If the return is disconnected, the output of the amplifier will slowly float up to the positive or down to the negative limit near the power supply voltage. The saturated output near the "rail" will no longer respond to the in-

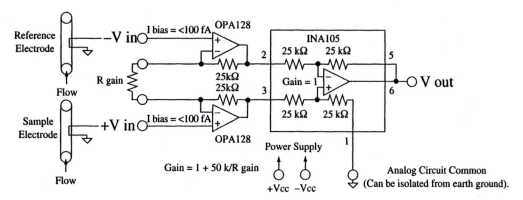

Figure 7-27
pH probe electrometer instrumentation amplifier.

put signal. If this condition is seen in an instrument, the bias current return path should be checked.

The following shows some IA applications to biomedical equipment. In older pH probes, one electrometer or femtoamp op-amp was used. Today, pH probes use electrometer IAs, as shown in Figure 7-27. Here, commercially available input-stage op-amps connect to the high-impedance reference and sample electrodes. pH is automatically measured as solutions flow through specially designed electrodes. Such circuits are often isolated from earth ground to prevent noise pickup. This circuit will be encountered frequently. For example, pH level is one of the measurements made in blood and body fluid analysis.

Instrumentation amplifiers are also used to amplify the differential voltage from Wheatstone bridges, as shown in Figure 7-28. Since the source resistance is relatively low at 300 Ω, a designer would usually use a bipolar input IA with moderate bias current of around 20 nA (20×10^{-9} A). But here, a commercially available monolithic FET IA is used. What is the advantage? Large resistors, say 75 kΩ, and a small value capacitor, say 1 μF, for passive filtering can be used. Filtering is achieved without loading the source very much. Low offset errors ($I_{bias} \times R_{source}$) are still being maintained, because the bias current is very low,

around 50 pA (50×10^{-12} A). The dc error is only 3.75 μV (50 pA $\times$ 75 kΩ). Commonly these chips achieve gain when two pins are strapped together where no external resistor is needed. Here the gain is 500 V/V. This example shows how modern components make biomedical instruments smaller and more reliable.

IAs usually amplify low-level signals in the range of tens of millivolts. Unfortunately, noise can ruin the measurement. Figures 7-29 and 7-30 show two important considerations that relate to noise. First, in Figure 7-29, CMR comes into play. Most commercially available IAs do a good job of rejecting low-frequency noise, say 50 or 60 Hz. However, when the CMR noise contains high frequencies, rejection can be poor. The typical product data sheet performance curve in Figure 7-29 shows that 60-Hz rejection is around 120 dB when the IA is in a gain of 500. Even when the interference is at 100 kHz, the graph shows rejection is still at 80 dB. Therefore, this particular component is useful in rejecting higher frequencies from sources such as switching power supplies.

Why does high-frequency interference disturb a low-frequency measurement? The answer is dc-offset caused by rectification through semiconductor junctions inside the IA and filtering by parasitic capacitance around the junctions. Therefore, rejecting high frequency outside the biomedical

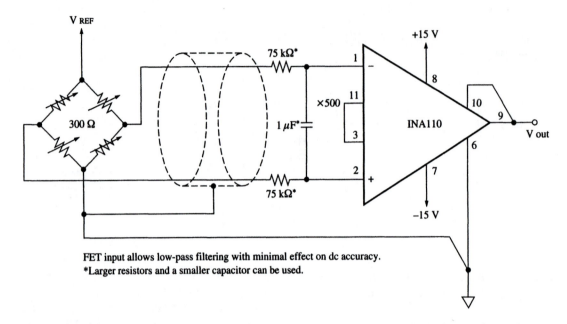

FET input allows low-pass filtering with minimal effect on dc accuracy.
*Larger resistors and a smaller capacitor can be used.

Figure 7-28
Bridge amplifier with 1-Hz low-pass filter. (Courtesy of Burr-Brown under copyright 1993 Burr-Brown Corporation)

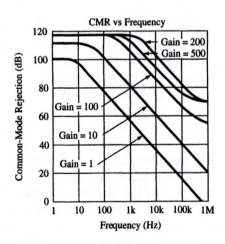

Figure 7-29
Important consideration: frequency effect on common-mode rejection (CMR), INA110. (Courtesy of Burr-Brown under copyright 1993 Burr-Brown Corporation)

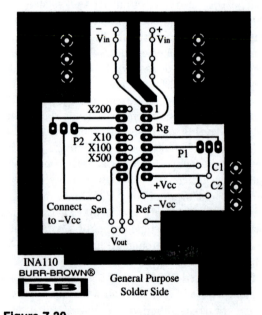

Figure 7-30
Important consideration: PC board layout for INA110. (Courtesy of Burr-Brown under copyright 1993 Burr-Brown Corporation)

bandwidth is important for maintaining baseline stability.

The second important consideration for IAs is printed circuit board layout. The electrical environment external to the IA can disturb performance. Figure 7-30 shows that good grounding keeps noise low. Also, care must be taken to reduce stray capacitance, because external *R-C* mismatch on the two inputs degrades CMR. Furthermore, care must be taken to separate the output from the input when a high-frequency IA is used. Notice that V_{out} is located at one end of the board and V_{in} is located at the other end. This prevents positive feedback that can cause oscillation. The reason for depicting good layout is to draw attention to proper construction practice. This is another important ingredient in achieving high bioelectronic amplifier performance.

Examining a few more biomedical applications will complete the important discussion of IAs. The hotwire anemometer shown in Figure 7-31 is used in industrial, scientific, and medical environments to indicate mass flow rate of gases and liquids. It is sometimes used in respiratory ventilators to measure patient breathing parameters. This allows the machine to provide just the right amount of assistance. (See the chapters on respiratory instrumentation and respiratory therapy equipment.)

The anemometer circuit in Figure 7-31 uses two IAs, one op-amp, and two voltage references. The first part of the circuit uses a thermistor temperature transducer. Its output is amplified by the noninverting op-amp to indicate air temperature of a patient's breath, usually 37°C. Accuracy is around ±1°C. The other part of the circuit produces an air flow voltage that is proportional to a patient's respiratory volume and rate. It works this way: A current, driven through the bridge by the power transistor, heats the tungsten wire or filament to a few hundred degrees centigrade. When the patient breathes, air flow increases and the wire cools off somewhat. This upsets the bridge balance and

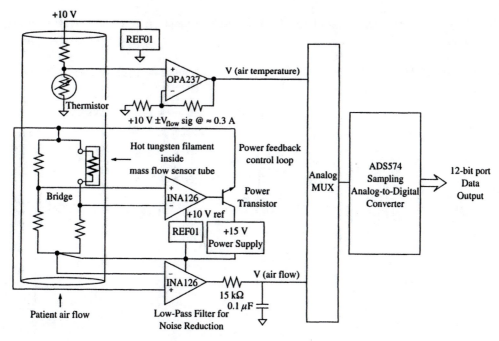

Figure 7-31
Hot-wire anemometer-thermistor circuit for measuring air flow.

causes a differential voltage to appear, which is amplified by IA. The increasing IA-output voltage causes more current to flow through the bridge, which reheats the filament. As the patient breathes, the power feedback loop tries to maintain the hot-wire at a constant temperature (also a constant resistance). As it does, the changing bridge voltage is amplified by the second IA. This signal, which is actually measuring air speed, is low-pass filtered at around 100 Hz for noise reduction. Both the air temperature and flow voltages are multiplexed into a sampling analog-to-digital converter, where they are digitized and fed to a computer for analysis.

Feedback loops are commonly used in biomedical instrumentation. To further understand the hot-wire power feedback loop, think of the loop having two voltages. One is the fixed $+10$ V reference. This goes through the loop IA and power transistor to apply a constant $+10$ V to the bridge. The second voltage is the varying bridge signal. It is picked up from the bridge and fed back to the bridge through the loop IA and power transistor. It causes the bridge voltage to vary in accordance with air speed and attempts to keep the hot wire at a constant temperature. In fact, it is this voltage that is amplified by the second IA at the bottom of the figure. Air speed is usually 0.1 to

200 L/s. It can be calibrated to about 0.1% of full scale. It is clear that IAs are the perfect companion to bridges, especially in biomedical equipment.

Another bridge amplifier is depicted in Figure 7-32. The clever technique shown here is how the amplified bridge signal is transmitted over a distance. If the IA output voltage were sent, say, 100 feet over twisted wire, it would pick up noise from the power lines before it reached the other end. An inexpensive technique for minimizing noise is to convert the voltage signal to a current and then transmit the current over the distance via a current loop. In Figure 7-32, an IA is used to drive a commercially available current transmitter. This monolithic component takes $+2$ V to $+10$ V and turns it into 4 mA to 20 mA, respectively. Why does the current signal in the loop pick up very little 60-Hz noise? The answer rests in how noise is picked up in the first place. EMI is an electromagnetic wave, pulsating at 60 Hz, which cuts across wires and induces noise voltages. These voltages add up along the wires as they traverse power lines. The total noise voltage tries to drive a noise current. However, it cannot drive much, because the loop is a high resistance. At one end of the loop is the current transmitter, which is actually a high-resistance current source, say 10 MΩ. At the other end is the

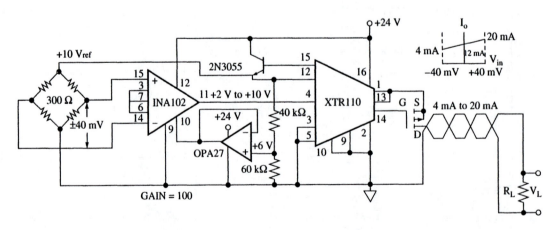

Figure 7-32
4 mA to 20 mA current loop bridge transmitter. (Courtesy of Burr-Brown under copyright 1988 Burr-Brown Corporation)

load resistor, say 250 Ω, which turns the signal current back into a signal voltage. Even if the noise voltage is 10 V_{rms} at 60 Hz, the noise current is only 1 μA rms (1.414 μA peak) at 60 Hz. Compared to the minimum-scale signal of 4 mA peak, this amounts to only a 0.04% peak error. This is a much lower error than you could achieve by sending a voltage over a 100-foot cable in an electrically noisy environment, such as a hospital.

Of course, nothing is perfect, not even precision IAs. For example, a medical or scientific weighing scale might have to measure milligrams out of several kilograms. The dynamic range required can be tens of thousands to one. To do this, you need to correct errors in the IA. Figure 7-33 shows how a precision +10 V voltage reference and ratio-matched resistors are used to automatically compensate for offset and gain errors. The zero (offset) calibration circuit derives 100 μV dc and differentially applies it to the IA through mechanical or electronic switches. Exactly 0 V dc could be used, but the 16-bit analog-to-digital converter shown

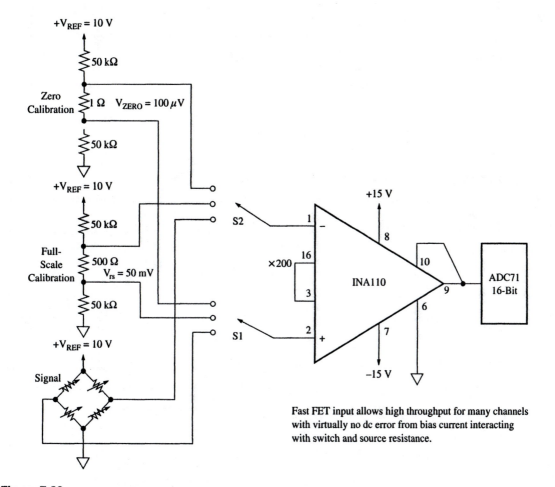

Fast FET input allows high throughput for many channels with virtually no dc error from bias current interacting with switch and source resistance.

Figure 7-33
Load cell weighing scale instrumentation amplifier. (Courtesy of Burr-Brown under copyright 1993 Burr-Brown Corporation)

has trouble digitizing 0 V absolutely. A voltage just above zero is acceptable. The full-scale (gain) calibration circuit derives 50 mV dc and applies it to the IA during a separate part of the calibration cycle. This technique allows IA and A/D converter errors to be stored in the computer. Then, when the bridge signal is applied to the IA, the computer stores the signal and subtracts out offset and gain errors associated with the electronic circuit. Such calibration cycles are used frequently in biomedical instrumentation.

It is usually desirable to locate an IA as close to a transducer as possible to minimize the chance of someone accidentally connecting overvoltages. However, when this is not practical, biomedical equipment designers include a front-end protection circuit like the one in Figure 7-34. Here two series resistors limit the input current that passes through clamp diodes. These diodes prevent the voltage on the IA input terminals from going more than one diode drop (about 0.7 V) above the positive or negative supply rail (V+ and V−). Therefore, should the common-mode input voltage (referenced to the common between power supplies) go above the IA's absolute maximum, no damage will occur. The external diodes clamp the overvoltage and take the current hit instead of the IA. How high is

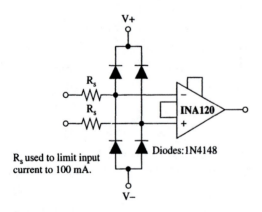

Figure 7-34
Important consideration: input protection circuit. (Courtesy of Burr-Brown under copyright 1990 Burr-Brown Corporation)

high? The answer depends on R_s. If R_s were 1 kΩ, for example, the overvoltage to the left of R_s could rise to plus or minus 100 V, if the limit were to be bounded at 100 mA. This diode clamp protection circuit is the one most commonly used in the IAs that amplify ECG signals. It is the second line of defense against the 5000-V defibrillation voltage, which is first clamped by gas tubes or special high-voltage semiconductor diodes.

7-8 Signal-processing circuits

Several special-purpose operational amplifier circuits are also used extensively in medical instrumentation. Among these are *integrators, differentiators, logarithmic amplifiers,* and *antilog amplifiers.*

Integrators and differentiators are analog circuits that perform the mathematical operations of integration and differentiation, respectively. If you are not familiar with these concepts, refer to appendix A.

7-8-1 Integrators

Integration is a mathematical process that allows us to find the area under the curve defined by a function. If the function is a time-dependent voltage, such as might be found in an instrumentation circuit, then a circuit such as Figure 7-35 may be used to integrate the voltage function. The transfer equation of the analog integrator (Figure 7-35) is

$$E_{\text{out}} = \frac{-1}{R_1 C_1} \int_0^t E_{\text{in}}\, dt + E_{ic} \qquad (7\text{-}18)$$

where

E_{out} is the output potential in volts (V)

E_{in} is the input signal potential in volts

R_1 is the input resistance in ohms (Ω)

C_1 is the feedback capacitance in farads (F)

t is the time in seconds (s)

E_{ic} is any initial condition output voltage already present at the integrator output when E_{in} begins (at $t = 0$)

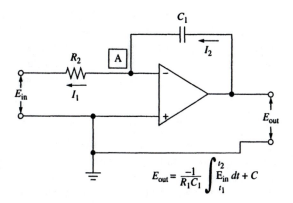

Figure 7-35
Integrator circuit.

$$E_{out} = \frac{-1}{R_1 C_1} \int_{t_1}^{t_2} E_{in}\, dt + C$$

Integrators also function as low-pass filters. This may be deduced by considering the frequency-dependent behavior of the capacitive reactance of C_1. In some medical instruments, integrators are labeled *low-pass filters*, even though integration may be their real function.

7-8-2 Differentiators

The differentiator circuit produces a voltage output proportional to the *time rate of change* of the input signal voltage. Differentiation is the inverse process of integration (which is the *time average* of the input signal). The circuit is similar to the integrator, except that the resistor R_1 and capacitor C_1 have changed places (see Figure 7-9). The transfer function of a differentiator is

$$E_{out} = -R_1 C_1 \frac{d(E_{in})}{dt} \qquad (7\text{-}19)$$

where

E_{out} is the differentiator output voltage in volts (V)

E_{in} is the input potential in volts

R_1 is the feedback resistor in ohms (Ω)

C_1 is the input capacitance in farads (F)

Example 7-6

Find the output voltage produced by an operational-amplifier differentiator (Figure 7-36) if R_1 = 100 kΩ, C_1 = 0.5 μF, and E_{in} has a constant slope (i.e., is a ramp function) of 400 V/s.

Solution

$$E_{out} = -R_1 C_1 \frac{dE_{in}}{dt}$$

$$E_{out} = -(10^5\ \Omega)(5 \times 10^{-7}\ \mu F)(400\ V/s)$$

$$E_{out} = -(5 \times 10^{-2}s)(400\ V/s)$$

$$= 2 \times 10^1\ V = \mathbf{20\ V} \qquad (7\text{-}19)$$

The $R_1 C_1$ time constant, in seconds, must be *very short* compared to the time constant or period of the input signal.

Example 7-5

An analog integrator (Figure 7-35) uses a 1-MΩ resistor and a 0.2-μF capacitor. Find the output voltage after 1 s if the input voltage is a *constant* 0.5 V.

Solution

$$E_{out} = -\frac{1}{R_1 C_1} \int_0^1 E_{in}\, dt + E_{ic} \qquad (7\text{-}18)$$

$$E_{out} = -\frac{1}{(10^6\Omega)(2 \times 10^{-7}\ F)} \int_0^1 (0.5)\, dt + 0$$

$$E_{out} = -\frac{1}{2 \times 10^{-1}} (.05)\Big|_0^1$$

$$= (-5)(0.5) = \mathbf{-2.5\ V}$$

The gain of the integrator is given by $-1/R_1 C_1$, and if R_1 is less than 10^6 Ω, and C_1 less than 0.001 μF, then the gain can become very large very quickly. For 10^5 Ω and 10^{-10} F, the gain is 10^5!

When a voltage is applied to the integrator input, current I_2 is generated and begins to charge C_1. The voltage at the output rises as C_1 charges (recall property 6 in section 7-4-1, the point A end of C_1 is effectively *grounded*). Charging continues in the manner dictated by E_{in}.

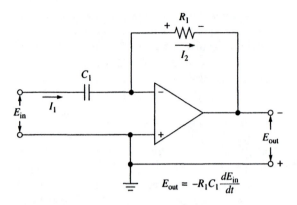

$$E_{out} = -R_1 C_1 \frac{dE_{in}}{dt}$$

Figure 7-36
Differentiator circuit.

The analog differentiator also functions as a *high-pass filter.* This feature follows from the same consideration of the reactance of C_1 that led us to the deduction that an integrator is a low-pass filter.

7-8-3 Log-antilog amplifiers

By now you should realize that many different transfer functions can be created using operational amplifiers. The designer need only know how to correctly manipulate the properties of the negative feedback network. Recall from our discussion of temperature transducers that the base-emitter voltage is proportional to the natural logarithm of the transistor collector current. The log dependence of I_c is used in circuits, such as the one in Figure 7-37a, to form an amplifier that has a *logarithmic* transfer function.

Similarly, an *antilog* amplifier (Figure 7-37b) is formed by placing the transistor in the input cir-

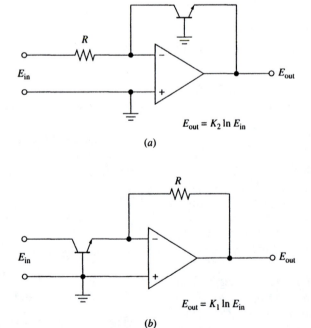

$$E_{out} = K_2 \ln E_{in}$$

(a)

$$E_{out} = K_1 \ln E_{in}$$

(b)

Figure 7-37
Log and antilog amplifiers. (*a*) Logarithmic amplifier. (*b*) Antilog amplifier.

cuit, between the input signal voltage and the inverting input of the operational amplifier.

The value of the logarithmic amplifier is best realized in applications in which the dynamic range of an input signal is very large (ranging over several orders of magnitude). If a nonlogarithmic operational amplifier circuit is used in the "front end" of an instrument in such a case, then it is often found that it can handle the higher amplitude signals only at the expense of weaker signals. Alternatively, if the gain is set high enough to accommodate weak signals, then large signals are clipped by the amplifier, which is driven into saturation.

If a logarithmic amplifier is used in the front end, however, then the gain of the circuit is lower for larger signals than it is for smaller signals. This results in a *range compression*. At the output of the instrument an *antilog amplifier* returns the voltage signals to their proper relationship. Most simple logarithmic amplifiers can handle four decades of dynamic range in the input signal, while some can handle up to seven decades (i.e., a range from zero to 120 dB).

From a practical point of view, how much accuracy can be obtained from commercially available logarithmic amplifiers? The answer depends on the range or number of decades of operation. For example, the log ratio component shown in Figure 7-38a is designed to handle six decades of input current (1 nA to 1 mA). Its output is $V_{out} = K \log_{10}(I_1/I_2)$. Laser trimming during manufacturing

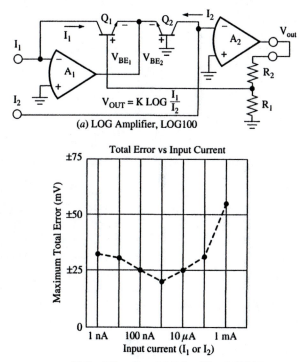

(a) LOG Amplifier, LOG100

(b) Total Error from LOG Amplifier, LOG100

Figure 7-38
Accuracy obtainable from analog logarithmic and log ratio amplifier, LOG100. (a) Logarithmic amplifier, LOG100. (b) Total error from logarithmic amplifier, LOG100. (Courtesy of Burr-Brown under copyright 1995 Burr-Brown Corporation)

guarantees total error in V_{out} to be around $\pm$ 25 mV, as shown in the typical performance curve of Figure 7-38b. This amounts to about 0.37% over five decades. However, if operated over six decades, the accuracy degrades to about 0.8%. Accuracy considerations for log ratio amplifiers are somewhat more complicated than for simple op-amp circuits. Errors include scale factor, bias current, log conformity, and offset voltage. The best a designer can hope for is something less than 0.5% at room temperature (25°C). At higher ambient temperatures, the log-amp becomes less accurate. This log-amp is very suitable for applications requiring, say, a few percentage points of accuracy. For higher precision, it is not. Most biomedical log functions are now done by computer software. But speed is sometimes an issue. It takes many machine cycles to get a log answer in hundreds of microseconds, unless a more expensive, high-speed computer is used. Clearly, the hardware log-amp is faster, giving an answer in 100 μs or so. However, the trend is unmistakable: software logging.

7-9 Practical op-amps: some problems reviewed

The practical operational amplifier does *not* possess the ideal properties that we have shown thus far. The approximations of the ideal properties, however, apply to most devices. "Infinite" open-loop gain, for example, translates as "very high." Even the low-cost economy op-amp models in the 741-class offer gain figures in the 20,000 to 50,000 range. Premium grade operational amplifiers have gain figures from around 100,000 to 1,000,000.

Similarly, "zero output impedance" translates as "very low." All commercially available operational amplifiers have an output impedance under 200 Ω, and most are under 100 Ω.

The input impedance of practical operational amplifiers, while not infinite, is about 10^5 Ω in low-cost types to over 10^{12} Ω in models that use a MOSFET for the input stage. The RCA CA3130 through CA3160 series, for example, boasts an input impedance of 1.5 TΩ (1.5×10^{12} Ω). Texas

Instruments LM-662 (dual) and LM-660 (quad) are CMOS op-amps operating from a single dc power supply.

Of course, the closer the operational amplifier specifications are to ideal, the nearer its performance is to ideal. In most cases, however, there may be several problems that must be recognized by circuit designers.

One problem is the existence of *input bias currents*. All operational amplifiers use some type of transistor in each side of the input stage, and these transistors will have bias currents. If bipolar NPN or PNP devices are used, then the bias current may be quite large. (For JFET and MOSFET stages it is much less.)

The input bias currents flow out of the respective input terminals to whatever resistances are connected to those inputs. In the inverting input circuit, this will be the parallel combination of feedback and input resistors. The bias current flowing in these resistors creates a *voltage drop* that is seen by the operational amplifier as a valid input signal.

The most obvious way to eliminate this voltage is placement of an equal *offset voltage* on the noninverting input. Since the same bias current flows in each input, we may cancel the voltage drop at the inverting input by placing a resistor to ground from the noninverting input that has a value equal to the parallel combination of the feedback and input resistors. The voltage drops applied to the two inputs have the same magnitude and phase, so by the basic properties of the operational amplifier, the resultant output voltage is zero.

Other forms of problems create output offset voltages. All may be solved by either of the offset null circuits shown in Figure 7-39. The circuit in Figure 7-39a uses a pair of *offset null* terminals found on many IC operational amplifiers. Each terminal is connected to one end of the null potentiometer. The wiper of the potentiometer is connected to the negative power supply (V_{ee}). The potentiometer is adjusted under zero input signal conditions so that the output voltage is also zero.

An alternative scheme is shown in Figure 7-39b. This circuit is used where there are no

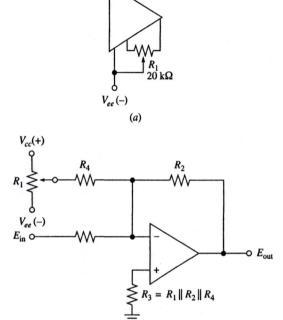

Figure 7-39
Offset null methods. (*a*) Using *offset adjust* terminals.
(*b*) Using a null circuit.

offset null terminals, or where a wider range than can be provided by the null terminals is required. The circuit of Figure 7-39*b* uses a potentiometer connected between V_{cc} and V_{ee}, with resistor R_4 connected between the potentiometer wiper and the inverting input of the operational amplifier. A current is set up in R_4 that cancels the offset voltage.

Op-amp offset voltage error can continuously be removed by using the adaptive circuit shown in Figure 7-40. It works this way: The op-amp configuration normally gives an inverting gain of -100 V/V. Automatic zeroing takes place when the input switch is placed in the zero mode and the feedback switch is closed on the op-amp's output. Any op-amp dc offset times the gain will be integrated by the feedback op-amp active integrator. It has a time constant of 0.1 seconds (100 kΩ

$\times$ 1 μF). After 10 time constants or so, the integrator's output, which is the inversion of the offset error, is present on the main op-amp's noninverting terminal. This error corrector voltage is amplified by a factor of 101 V/V and essentially cancels the error caused by the main op-amp. When the input switch is placed in the operate mode, and the feedback switch is opened, normal dc-coupled signal amplification takes place.

The feedback error integrator will accurately hold the offset error for some time. Any droop or rise is caused by the integrator's bias current charging or discharging the integrator capacitor. But since bias is low (e.g., 4 pA), it takes a long time to make any difference $V_o/t = I_b/C$. The main op-amp's offset can be continuously corrected if the feedback switch remains closed and the integrator time constant is set properly. But then the main amplifier will essentially be ac-coupled where it was dc-coupled before. This type of adaptive correction is commonly used in ac-coupled ECG systems to zero out the offset potential of body electrodes. It is called *dc restoration*.

Of course, another way to get rid of offset voltage is to measure it, store it in computer software, and then subtract it out when the actual measurement is made. However, this requires the use of an analog-to-digital converter and a computer. It is

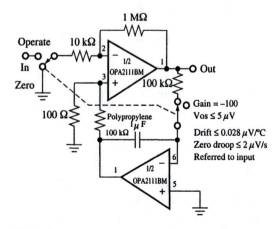

Figure 7-40
Auto-zero amplifier. (Courtesy of Burr-Brown under copyright 1989 Burr-Brown Corporation)

obvious that the analog hardware approach can be less expensive.

7-10 Bioelectric amplifiers reviewed

The simple bioelectric amplifiers may be constructed of discrete components, IC operational amplifiers, and other IC devices. The utility of the operational amplifier is great enough that even those models that use discrete components (rather than ICs) are actually discrete versions of an operational amplifier circuit.

In most cases the bioelectric amplifier is a differential input circuit. In those few cases in which a single-ended input is required, a differential amplifier may be used with one input grounded. However, many single-ended input noninverting buffers are used today ahead of the differential amplifier.

The properties desired in a bioelectric amplifier are:

1. Single-ended output, often differential input.

2. High common-mode rejection ratio (CMRR).

3. Extremely high-input impedance.

4. Variable gain adequate to do the job intended. The following categories are generally recognized: low gain ($\times 1$ to $\times 10$), medium gain ($\times 10$ to $\times 1000$), and high gain (over $\times 1000$).

5. Frequency response suitable for the application. In the case of a universal bioelectric amplifier, the response should be variable through switch selection.

6. *Zero suppression.* This is an optional feature that allows shift about the zero baseline by nulling offsets inherent in the signal. This feature permits small varying signals superimposed on a larger dc signal (or dc offset) to be processed in the amplifier, using the *full gain* of the amplifier for the small

varying signal only. For example, a 10-mV sinewave may be superimposed on a +1500-mV dc offset. This is seen as a 10-mV sinewave if a $\sum 1500$-mV zero-suppression signal is summed with the actual signal at the input.

The designations of front panel controls in bioelectric amplifiers often reflect the vocabulary and jargon of the user rather than standard electronic terms. For example, *gain* or *sensitivity* may be labeled *span* if the amplifier is designed for use by a life scientist or chemist. Similarly, the gain control may be divided into controls, *coarse* and *fine,* although the *fine* control might be labeled *span,* and the *coarse* control (usually a rotary switch) is labeled *range.*

On a specialized amplifier, the coarse control may be labeled with physical units peculiar to the application; on universal models, the labeling will be more generalized. Since many amplifiers are designed for connection to a CRO (or strip-chart recorder), the units may be labeled as a vertical deflection factor in millivots per millmeter or centimeter.

7-11 Isolation amplifiers

Some hospital patients are extraordinarily susceptible to electrical shock hazards. It is believed that 60-Hz ac currents small enough to be deemed harmless ordinarily may be lethal to a patient under certain circumstances.

To prevent accidental internal cardiac shock, the manufacturers of modern bioelectric amplifiers, especially those used in ECG recording, use *isolation amplifiers* (iso-amps) for the direct patient connection. These amplifiers provide as much as 10^{12} Ω of insulation (isolation) between the patient connector and the ac power mains line cord.

The basic design of an iso-amp is shown in Figure 7-41. It is usually composed of an input amplifier, some type of modulator, an isolation barrier, a demodulator, and an output amplifier. Modulation schemes include amplitude, voltage-to-frequency,

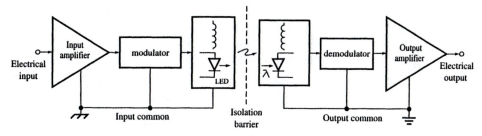

Figure 7-41
Basic design of an isolation amplifier.

duty cycle, pulse width, flyback loading, and others. Barriers can be optical, magnetic transformer, capacitive, or even heat transfer. Notice that there is an input common and an output common that are electrically isolated from one another to the tune of millions of ohms. The iso-amp is really an energy converter. Electrical energy on the modulator side is converted to some "nonelectrically conductive" energy in the barrier and then converted back to electrical energy on the demodulator side. That's all there is to it. But what function does an iso-amp really perform?

A circuit diagram symbol that is often used to represent the iso-amp is shown in Figure 7-42. This symbol has not been standardized, so some manufacturers use variations of their own on their circuit diagrams.

Isolation amplifiers actually operate on the principle of attenuation. The high barrier impedance ($>10^{12}$ Ω in parallel with <10 pF) acts in series between input and output as shown in Figure 7-43. Therefore, an interfering isolation-mode

voltage (IMV) referenced to the iso-amp's output must go through the large barrier resistance before it can mix with the input signal. Hence, most of the interfering voltage or noise is dropped across the barrier; very little adds to the input.

Since the barrier is not an infinite impedance, some error is created. We say that an IMV, shown as V_{im} across the barrier, causes an error to appear in the output voltage, V_{out}. Figure 7-44 shows how this error is calculated. The measure of how well the iso-amp attenuates or rejects the IMV is called isolation-mode rejection (IMR). The isolation-mode rejection ratio in V/V is called IMRR. IMRR in V/V = $\log^{-1}$ (IMR$_{dB}$/20). This is the reverse of the equation shown in Figure 7-44, IMR in dB = $20 \log_{10}$(IMRR$_{V/V}$). The error is gained up just like the input signal and results in some dc or ac voltage that adds to the normal signal. For example, from a commercially available product data sheet, if IMR were 120 dB, then IMRR would be 1,000,000 V/V. If V_{im} were 1,000 V dc, the error at the iso-amp's input would be 0.001 V or 1 mV dc. This would be 0.1% error if the input signal were 1 V dc. If the iso-amp had a gain of 10, then the output signal would be 10 V dc and the error would be 10 mV dc. The error would still be 0.1%. It is the same, provided that all voltages are taken with respect to the input (RTI) or with respect to the output (RTO). Note that the iso-amp rejects low-level dc or ac interfering voltages appearing across the barrier just as it rejects kilovolts. In fact, the iso-amp is just as good for attenuating noise as it is for attenuating high voltages.

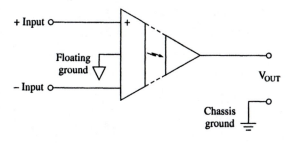

Figure 7-42
Symbol for an isolation amplifier.

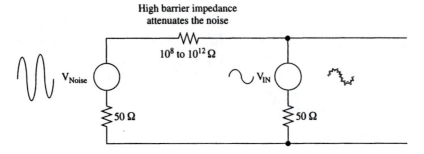

Figure 7-43
Reduction of interference in an IA is by cancellation. In an iso-amp, it can be thought of as attenuation.

In contrast, an IA cancels or rejects common-mode (CM) voltage present on each of its two input terminals. A comparison of CMR to IMR appears in Figure 7-45. CMR in an IA is a measure of how well it rejects interference or noise. It does this by cancellation through its balanced gain paths. IMR in an iso-amp is also a measure of how well it rejects interference or noise. It does this by attenuation through its high-barrier impedance. If one were clever enough to reconfigure the IA circuit at the top to make the CM voltage in the IA appear like isolation-mode (IM) voltage in the iso-amp, then one would get better rejection of noise. Why is this so? Because IMR in an iso-amp is usually higher (125 dB) than CMR in an IA (105 dB). It is just the way they are constructed that makes the difference.

Sometimes an iso-amp may have CM noise on its input as well as IM noise across its barrier. Figure 7-46 shows this. V_{cm} is noise on the two inputs with RTI common. V_{im} is noise on the input with RTO common. It is across the barrier. If an IA were inside the iso-amp shown, then CM as well as IM interference would be rejected. Here,

$$V_{out} = gain(V_{sig} + V_{cm}/CMRR$$
$$+ V_{im}/IMRR) \qquad (7\text{-}20)$$

In summary, modern isolation amplifiers serve three purposes: (1) They break ground loops to permit incompatible circuits to be interfaced to-

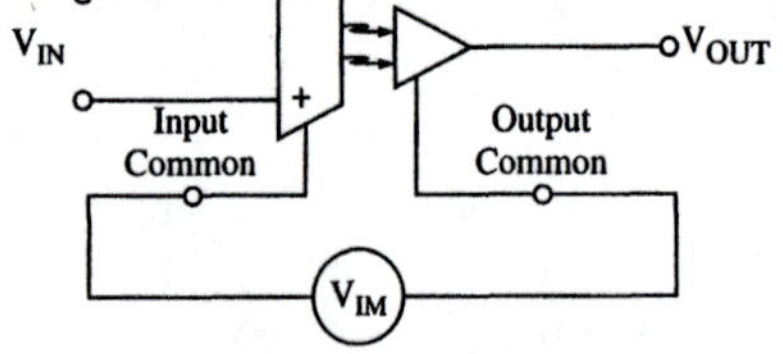

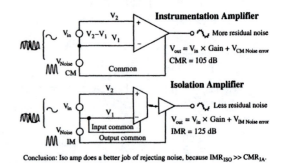

$$V_{OUT} = (V_{IN} + \frac{V_{IM}}{IMRR}) \times Gain = \underbrace{(V_{IN} \times Gain)}_{\text{Signal}} + \underbrace{(\frac{V_{IM}}{IMRR} \times Gain)}_{\text{Error}}$$

where $\underset{(dB)}{\underline{IMR}} = 20\, LOG_{10}\ \underset{(V/V\ Ratio)}{\underline{IMRR}}$

Figure 7-44
IMR error.

Conclusion: Iso amp does a better job of rejecting noise, because $IMR_{ISO} \gg CMR_{IA}$.

Figure 7-45
Comparison: CMR versus IMR.

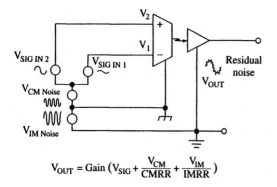

$$V_{OUT} = \text{Gain}\left(V_{SIG} + \frac{V_{CM}}{CMRR} + \frac{V_{IM}}{IMRR}\right)$$

Figure 7-46
An iso-amp may have common-mode (CM) noise on its input as well as isolation-mode (IM) noise across its barrier.

gether while reducing noise; (2) they amplify signals while passing only low leakage current to prevent shock to people or damage to equipment; and (3) they withstand high voltage to protect people, circuits, and equipment.

Several approaches to the design of isolation amplifiers are used: *battery powered, carrier, optically coupled,* and *current loading.*

7-11-1 Battery-powered

This approach is perhaps the simplest to implement, but it is not always the most suitable for the customer's convenience because of problems inherent in battery maintenance. A few products exist, however, that use a battery-powered, front-end amplifier, even though the remainder of the product is ac mains–powered. For cardiac output computers, this approach is almost universally used.

The bioelectric amplifier in this type of instrument is exactly like that in an ac-powered model. The sole difference is that it is powered from a battery pack.

This type of instrument must be totally self-contained. If any external instrument or device (e.g., oscilloscope, strip-chart recorder, rate meter, battery charger) is used, then a model employing

any one of the other isolation techniques must be used.

7-11-2 Carrier

Figure 7-47*a* shows an isolation amplifier using carrier technique. The circuitry inside the dashed line is isolated from the ac power mains and the rest of the circuitry that is powered from the ac mains. In most cases, the voltage gain of the isolated section is in the medium-gain range (e.g., ×10 to ×500).

The isolation is provided by separation of the ground, power, and signal paths in the two sections by transformers T_1 and T_2. These transformers have a core material that is very inefficient at 60 Hz but works well in the 20- to 250-kHz range. This feature allows the transformers to easily pass the carrier signal but impedes any 60-Hz energy that might be present.

Although most models use a carrier frequency in the 50- to 60-kHz range, there are several types that use almost any frequency in the 20- to 250-kHz range.

The carrier oscillator signal is coupled through transformer T_1 to the isolated stages. Part of the energy from the secondary of T_1 goes to the modular stage; the remainder is rectified and filtered and then used as an isolated dc power supply. The dc output of this power supply is used to power the input amplifiers and modulator stages.

An analog signal applied to the input is amplified by A_1 and is then applied to one input of the *modulator* stage. This stage modulates the amplitude of the signal onto the carrier.

Transformer T_2 couples the signal to the input of the *demodulator* stage on the nonisolated side of the circuit. Either envelop or synchronous demodulation may be used, although the latter is more common. Ordinary dc amplifiers following the demodulator complete the signal processing.

An example of a *synchronous demodulator* circuit is shown in Figure 7-47*b*. This type of circuit is based on switching action. Although the example shown uses *PNP* bipolar transistors as the

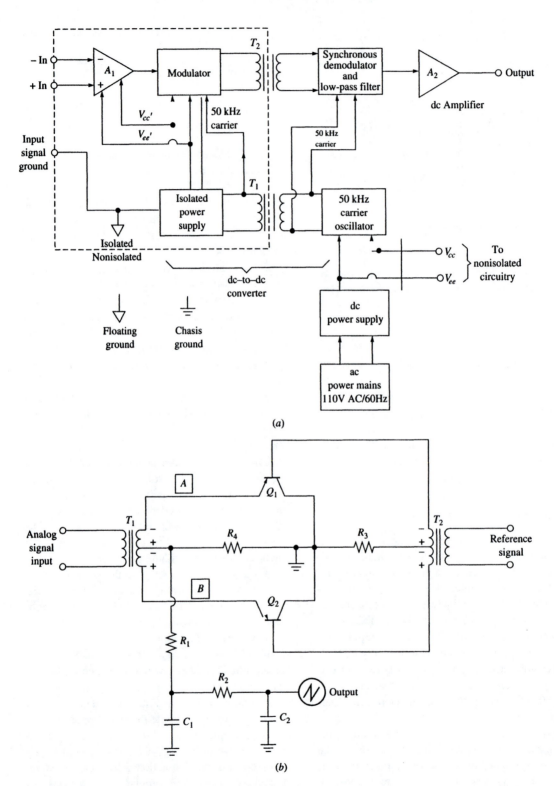

Figure 7-47
(a) Carrier-type isolation amplifier. (b) Synchronous demodulator.

electronic switches, others use CMOS analog switches or FET transistors.

The signal from the modulator has a frequency of 50 kHz (up to 250 kHz, or even 500 kHz) and is amplitude-modulated with the signal from the isolated amplifier. This signal is applied to the emitters of transistors Q_1 and Q_2 (via T_1) in *push-pull*. On one half of the cycle, therefore, the emitter of Q_1 will be positive with respect to the emitter of Q_2. On alternate half cycles, the opposite situation occurs: Q_2 is positive with respect to Q_1

The bases of Q_1 and Q_2 are also driven in push-pull, but by the 50-kHz carrier signal. This action causes Q_1 and Q_2 to switch on and off, but out of phase with each other.

On one half of the cycle, we will have the polarities shown in Figure 7-47b. Transistor Q_1 is turned on. In this condition point A on T_1 is *grounded*. The voltage developed across load resistor R_4 is positive with respect to ground.

On the alternate half cycle, Q_2 is turned on, so point B is grounded. But the polarities have reversed, so the polarity of the voltage developed across R_4 is *still positive*. This causes a full-wave output waveform across R_4, which, when filtered, becomes a dc voltage level proportional to the amplitude of the input signal. This same description of synchronous demodulators also applies to the circuits used in some carrier amplifiers.

A variation on this circuit replaces the modulator with a *voltage-controlled oscillator* (VCO) that allows the analog signal to frequency-modulate a carrier signal generated by the VCO. The power supply carrier signal is still required, however. A *phase detector, phase-locked loop* (PLL), or *pulse-counting detector* on the nonisolated side recovers the signal.

7-13-3 Optically coupled

Electronic *optocouplers* (also called *optoisolators*) are sometimes used to provide the desired isolation. In early designs of this class a *light-emitting diode* (LED) was sandwiched with a photoresistor or phototransistor. Modern designs, however, use

IC optoisolators that contain the LED and phototransistor inside of a DIP IC package.

There are actually several approaches to optical coupling. Two very popular methods are the *carrier* and *direct* methods. The carrier method is the same as discussed in section 7-11-2, except that an optoisolator replaces transformer T_2.

The carrier method is not the most widespread in optically coupled amplifiers because of frequency response limitations of IC optoisolators. Only recently have these problems been resolved.

A more common approach is shown in Figure 7-48. This circuit uses the same dc-to-dc converter to power the isolated states as was used in other designs. This will keep A_1 isolated from the ac power mains but is not used in the signal coupling process.

The LED in the optoisolator is driven by the output of isolated amplifier A_1. Transistor Q_1 serves as a series switch to vary the light output of the LED proportional to the analog signal from A_1. Transistor Q_1 normally passes sufficient collector current to bias the LED into a linear portion of its operating curve. The output of the phototransistor is ac-coupled to the remaining amplifiers on the nonisolated side of the circuit, so that the offset condition created by LED bias is eliminated.

7-11-4 Current loading

A *current loading* isolation technique was used by Tektronix in their portable medical ECG monitors. A simplified schematic is shown in Figure 7-49. Notice that there is no *obvious* coupling path for the signal between the isolated and nonisolated sides of the circuit.

The gain-of-24 isolated input amplifier in Figure 7-49 consists of a dual JFET (Q_1) and an operational amplifier. This circuit illustrates use of JFETs to improve the input impedance of an operational amplifier.

The output of A_1 is connected to the isolated $V_{ee'}$ (i.e., -10 V dc power supply through resistor R_7). This power supply is a dc-to-dc converter operating at 250 kHz. Transformer T_1 provides

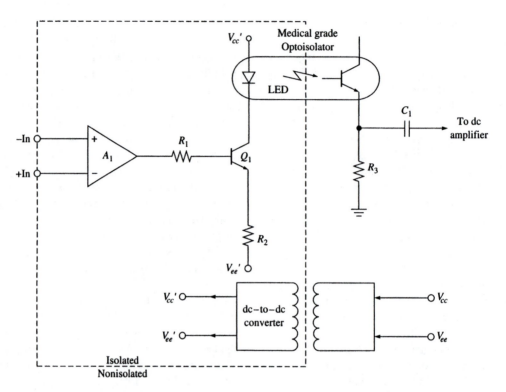

Figure 7-48
Optically coupled isolation amplifier.

isolation between the floating power supplies on the isolated side and the normal mains-powered supplies on the nonisolated side.

An input signal (i.e., an ECG waveform) causes the output of A_1 to vary the loading on the floating power supply ($B_1/C_1/C_2$), through resistor R_7.

Changing the loading on the floating power supply proportional to the analog signal causes variation of the T_1 primary current that is *also* proportional to the analog signal. This current variation is converted to a voltage waveform by amplifier A_2. An *offset null* control (R_{11}) is provided in the A_2 circuit to eliminate the offset at the output caused by quiescent current flowing when the analog input signal is zero. In that case, the loading on T_1 is constant.

Having discussed the basic principles of isolation, let's look at how it is implemented in some commercially available components. An optically coupled iso-amp in a single-wide, 18-pin dip package appears in Figure 7-50. This component accepts an input current, generated by a voltage source through R_{in}, and produces an output voltage across an isolation barrier. Notice that there are two optical paths. One is feed-forward across the isolation barrier from the LED to the output photodiode light detector. The other is negative feedback from the LED back to the input photodiode. The latter linearizes the response of the LED in the input stage, which normally has quite a curve. That is, light output from the LED on its own does not exactly double when the voltage applied to it doubles. Interestingly, the two paths actually operate in a ratio fashion. This technique preserves accuracy as the LED slowly loses light intensity over its lifetime. The transfer function (V_{out}/I_{in}) depends

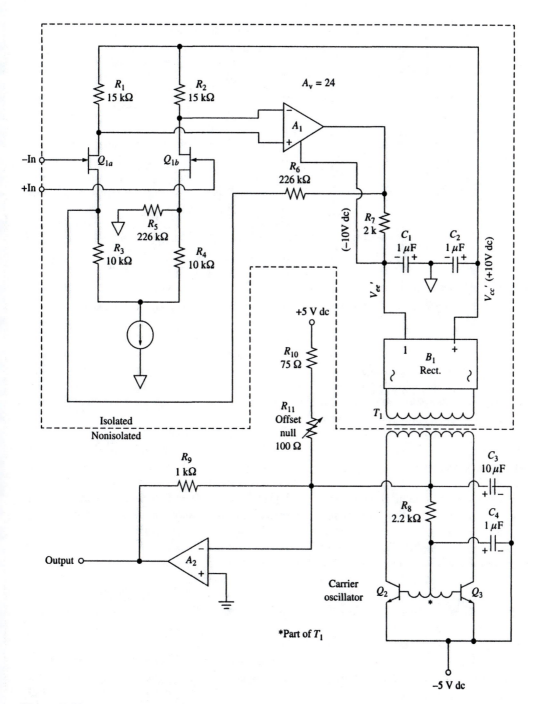

Figure 7-49
Current-loading type of isolation amplifier.

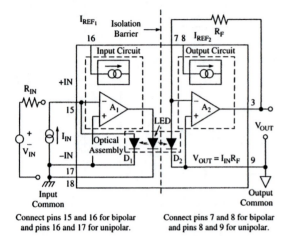

Connect pins 15 and 16 for bipolar
and pins 16 and 17 for unipolar.

Connect pins 7 and 8 for bipolar
and pins 8 and 9 for unipolar.

Figure 7-50
Single-package optically-coupled isolation amplifier,
ISO100. (Courtesy of Burr-Brown under copyright
1992 Burr-Brown Corporation)

on optical match rather than on absolute optical performance (LED to output photodiode). Laser-trimming improves matching and enhances accuracy. Discrete designs often struggle to achieve the good performance obtained from the single-packaged component.

Input and output current sources are used to provide offsetting for bipolar operation (plus and minus voltage swing around ground or common). This is necessary because LEDs and photodiodes are inherently unipolar. That is, there is no such thing as a "dark-emitting diode." The barrier of this device is tested at 2500 V dc and rated at 750 V dc. Many standards, such as AAMI (Association for the Advancement of Medical Instrumentation), UL (Underwriters Laboratories), and IEC (International Electrotechnical Commission) recommend this type of testing at two times rated voltage plus 1000 in volts.

Some biomedical applications, like defibrillator-protected ECG machines, require very high voltage ratings (e.g., 5000 V dc). However, some can live with a much lower rating, as in EEG (brain waves) or industrial/home heart rate moni-

toring. The low leakage current of about 0.15 μA at 120 Vrms provided by the optically coupled component shown in Figure 7-50 works well in such applications, even though the barrier rating is only 750 V dc. AAMI, UL544, and IEC601 standards require that leakage be limited to less than 10 μA through the patient at all times.

Another commercially available iso-amp is shown in Figure 7-51. This is a transformer-coupled device containing a signal path and internal isolated power. It is housed in a low-profile single in-line (SIL) package. We say that this iso-amp is self-powered because it has its own 25-KHz oscillator, rectifier bridge, and filter capacitors. It also provides some external power on the isolated side. Signals get across the barrier as follows: The input op-amp drives an amplitude modulator (AM) which, on the other side of the barrier, is synchronously demodulated to minimize noise and interference. This iso-amp is rated at 750 Vrms continuous at 60 Hz and has 1-μA leakage at 120 Vrms. It is suitable for low-barrier voltage medical and industrial applications, in which low-leakage current is necessary for patient or operator safety.

When medical circuits must withstand high defibrillation voltages, iso-amp barriers need to be specially designed. The barrier of the modern iso-amp shown in Figure 7-52 is constructed with high-voltage, differential ceramic capacitors. It is tested at 7900 Vpeak and rated for 5000 Vpeak continuous. It uses two 1-pF caps formed by firing tungsten on green ceramic. Hence, the barrier becomes part of the package. In fact, the barrier and the electronics located on the ends of the 40-pin DIP are hermetically sealed. This makes the iso-amp internally immune to moisture, which improves reliability. The input is first duty-cycle modulated, then formed into opposite phase pulses, and transmitted digitally across the barrier. The small barrier caps essentially differentiate the edges of the digital signal to form spikes. The trick in recovering the digital signal is to differentially amplify the tiny spikes. This is done by the sense amp, which drives the output demodulator. The

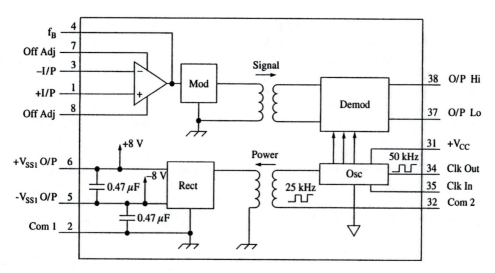

Figure 7-51
Single-package transformer-coupled isolation amplifier, ISO212. (Courtesy of Burr-Brown under copyright 1995 Burr-Brown Corporation)

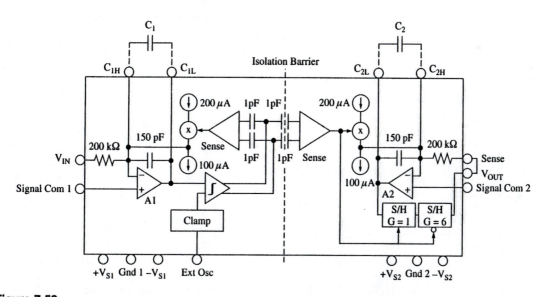

Figure 7-52
Single-package differential-capacitive isolation amplifier, ISO121. (Courtesy of Burr-Brown under copyright 1992 Burr-Brown Corporation)

demodulator is just a low-pass filter with a sample-hold amplifier in the feedback to further remove ripple. Because the modulation is digital, the barrier characteristics do not affect signal integrity. This results in good high-frequency transient immunity across the barrier, which is important in rejecting high-frequency iso-mode noise.

An important consideration in isolation amplifiers is the frequency effect on isolation-mode rejection. Figure 7-53 shows that, for the iso-amp in Figure 7-52, the 1-Hz IMR is 150 dB, and at 60 Hz it is 115 dB. This means that a 60-Hz sine wave appearing across the barrier will be attenuated at the output by 562,000 times ($1/\log^{-1}$ $(115/20)$). Remember, IMR = $20 \log_{10} (V_{iso(60\ Hz)}/ V_{out(60\ Hz)})$ or IMR = $-20 \log_{10} (V_{out\ (60\ Hz)}/ V_{iso(60\ Hz)})$. Only 0.0002% of 60-Hz residual gets through. But what happens at higher frequencies? Most iso-amps leak heavily at high frequency due to barrier capacitance. This is why the component in Figure 7-52 is built with such low barrier capacitance (2 pF total). From the typical performance curve in Figure 7-53, it appears that the IMR at 10 kHz is 70 dB. At 300 kHz it is still 40 dB. While this is relatively good, it may not be high enough to reject electrosurgery unit (ESU) interference, which contains frequencies from several MHz up to 10 MHz. Other modern rejection techniques must be used to get rid of ESU noise, including fancy input and barrier filtering.

Noise rejection is obviously important in isolation amplifiers. However, even more important is *high-voltage testing.* An isolation voltage rating describes the voltage a device can reliably withstand for long periods. Some iso-amps are stress tested first at a high voltage for short periods and then functionally tested at their rated voltage for a longer fixed period of time. If the iso-amp survives, it is good. A new method has been established in the industry to ensure higher barrier reliability. It is called *partial discharge testing.* It tests for internal microscopic voids in the barrier. Such defects display localized ionization when exposed to high voltage (HV). That is, intense electric fields build up across the voids, and at some point, called *inception voltage,* charges flow. At this point the void shorts itself out. As the barrier voltage decreases, charge flow stops. This is called the *extinction voltage.* This action redistributes charge within the barrier and is known as *partial discharge.* Today, specialized production equipment can test for discharge under HV conditions. First, a 1-s rated voltage test is conducted to check for leakage current. Second, another 1-s test checks for partial discharge at 1.6 times rated voltage per the VDE 0884 German standard. This takes into account the ratio of transient voltage to continuous rating. If partial discharge is less than 5 pC, the barrier has high integrity. In fact, this is the best test of all, because it ensures that the barrier is not being damaged by excessive partial discharge. The iso-amp shown in Figure 7-52 is 100% partial-discharge tested.

Another important consideration in isolated systems is power supply feed through noise and carrier ripple reduction. Figure 7-54 shows how an L-C π filter on the iso-amp's power supply pins attenuates the noise before it gets into the iso-amp. The noise is actually coming from the switching power supply oscillator, which is part of the isolated dc-to-dc converter. While the frequency is much higher than, say, a 100-Hz physiological signal, it can be rectified and filtered inside the iso-

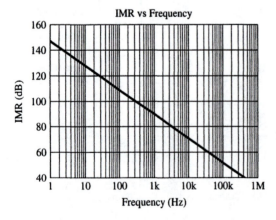

Figure 7-53

Important consideration: frequency effect on isolation-mode rejection (IMR), ISO121. (Courtesy of Burr-Brown under copyright 1992 Burr-Brown Corporation)

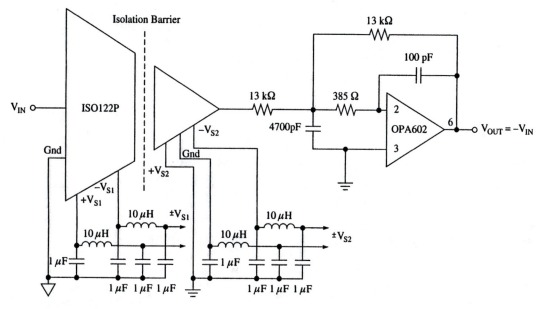

Figure 7-54
Important consideration: π filter to minimize power supply feedthrough noise and output two-pole filter to remove 500-kHz carrier ripple. (Courtesy of Burr-Brown under copyright 1993 Burr-Brown Corporation)

amp to cause a dc offset. What about carrier noise? Notice the active op-amp filter at the output. It removes noise associated with the carrier frequency, which is part of the modulation scheme inside the iso-amp. Keeping noise low in isolated bioelectric amplifiers is a never-ending battle.

So far we have looked at single-component optical, magnetic, and capacitive isolation amplifiers. There is one more isolation technique, which is actually the best. It is fiber-optic isolation, as shown in Figure 7-55. Here a transducer, or perhaps a human body signal, is first amplified by an IA. It is then applied to a voltage-to-frequency converter (VFC). The signal information is now contained in frequency-modulated form, and the actual voltage levels are digital. This is perfect for optical transmission. But this time the fiber-optic transmitter (FOT) energizes an LED and drives light down a fiber-optic cable. Since the glass or plastic cable responds only to light, it is not subject to EMI. It can also withstand hundreds of kilovolts to provide

the best isolation imaginable. It also makes a wonderfully secure system, because fiber-optic cables cannot easily be tapped into. The fiber-optic receiver (FOR) recovers the electrical digital signal and feeds it to a counter, where it is turned into a clocked digital word of, say, 12 bits. This system is actually an analog-to-digital (A/D) converter that has been partitioned into a transmitter portion and digital recovery portion with isolation in between. Its drawback is that the VFC runs relatively slowly (< 100kHz), and hence, it takes some milliseconds to complete an A/D conversion.

Another way to transmit an isolated signal after it has been digitized is to use a fiber-optic limited distance modem like the one shown in Figure 7-56. A modem (modulation-demodulation device) uses standard protocol to send and receive digital data. Transmit *(T)* and receive *(R)* connectors accept fiber-optic cables. This particular modem is powered by the host RS-232 port and provides complete EMI/RFI rejection, elimination of

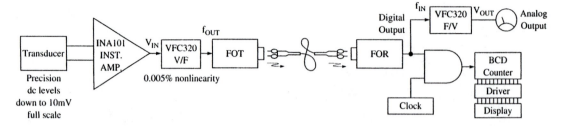

Figure 7-55
Fiber-optic isolation amplifier using voltage-to-frequency converter eliminates power supply feedthrough and noise coupling. (Courtesy of Burr-Brown under copyright 1993 Burr-Brown Corporation)

ground loops, reduced error rate, and data security against tampering.

As we have shown, isolation applications can take many forms. Many bioelectric amplifiers use isolation to protect the patient. Other amplifiers use isolation in the hospital/medical environment to protect operators and expensive equipment.

Figure 7-57 shows an isolated bioelectric ECG amplifier. Notice that the NE2H gas-filled neon tubes, series resistors, and clamp diodes protect the IA from defibrillation voltages up to 5000 Vpeak. This protection is not part of the isolation. It prevents high voltages from destroying the electronics only on the patient side. It clamps to the input common, not the output common. Before look-

ing at how the isolation works, we will briefly discuss ECG front-end characteristics.

The commercially available IA shown derives the CM 60-Hz voltage internally and applies it to an inverting amplifier that drives the patient's right leg. This acts in a feedback loop (patient and electronics) to servo or drive the CM noise on the patient to a low level. While the 60-Hz noise on the left or right arm may become bigger with respect to the right leg, the 60-Hz noise on the IA input terminals (pins 15 and 14) with respect to the IA common (pin 10) becomes smaller. Hence, the IA does not have to reject as much 60-Hz noise. The IA's CMR then reduces noise even further. The isolation amplifier's IMR also reduces noise by establishing 10^{12} Ω and 9 pF between the patient (pin 37) and earth ground (pin 17), as shown in Figure 7-57. Remember, barrier impedance is the parallel combination of the isolation amplifier and the isolated dc-to-dc converter. Isolation acts to attenuate noise (say, 1 V_{p-p}) that is trying to mix with the low-level ECG input signal (say 1 mV_{p-p}). Three actions reduce 60-Hz interference dramatically: right leg drive, IA CMR, and iso-amp IMR. A low-pass filter and/or 60-Hz notch filter following the iso-amp will further shrink noise. This circuit is dc-coupled and is in high gain = 1000 V/V. It works only when the electrode offset potentials are low (< 10 mV) to avoid IA output satuation. Restoration, covered in chapter 8, allows much larger offsets to be tolerated.

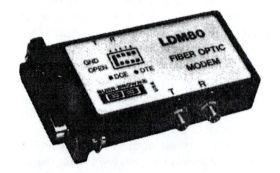

Figure 7-56
Fiber-optic isolated limited-distance modem. (Courtesy of Burr-Brown under copyright 1986 Burr-Brown Corporation)

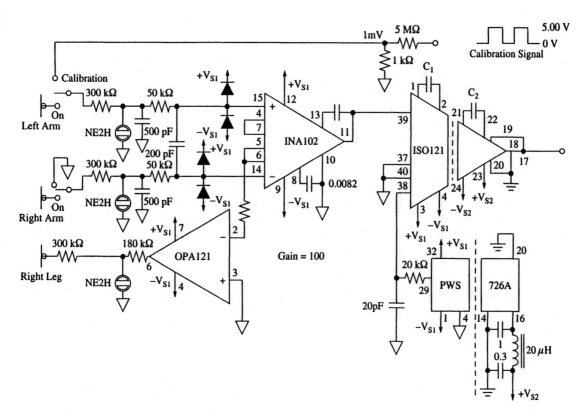

Figure 7-57
Right-leg-driven ECG amplifier with defibrillator protection and calibrator. (All capacitor values
in μF unless otherwise noted. Diodes are IN4148.) (Courtesy of Burr-Brown under copyright
1992 Burr-Brown Corporation)

Remember, this discussion is dedicated to explaining the uses of isolation in health care environments, so let's ask an interesting question. Is
the only purpose of isolation to reduce 60-Hz
noise pickup in the ECG example of Figure 7-57?
The answer is no. The iso-amp also stands ready to
protect semiconductor circuitry on the iso-amp's
output when a HV defibrillation pulse is applied to
the patient. Actually, most of the time HV does not
appear across the iso-amp's barrier. It only appears
when, say, the patient accidentally comes in contact with earth ground. For example, if a patient lying on an electrically controlled bed is being de-
fibrillated, and the patient's arm touches the metal
bed rail, the "defib" pulse will be impressed di-

rectly across the iso-amp. In this situation, the barrier must be able to withstand about 5000 V peak.
Fortunately, the barrier is very high impedance
compared to the source or load impedance, and it
drops nearly all the voltage. Very little is felt on
the output stage, which shares a common with
other circuitry hooked to it. Isolation in this case
saves the electronics. It has nothing to do with protecting the patient from shock. After all, defibrillation is used to intentionally shock the patient to
restart the heart.

What about other amplifiers that use isolation
in the hospital/medical environment? They may
not strictly be called bioelectric amplifiers, but
they do amplify signals while protecting operators,

medical staff, and expensive machines, such as computers. One such isolated circuit is shown in Figure 7-58. It is an isolated power line monitor. An IA measures the small voltage across a 5-mΩ power resistor. This voltage represents the current in the Y-connected power transformer often used in hospitals. The low-bias current FET IA shown makes low-pass filtering with large resistors and a small value capacitor easy.

Why is isolation used for this application? The answer is: noise reduction and protection under fault conditions. The iso-amp isolates (attenuates) the noisy transformer power ground form, say, an instrumentation or computer ground. If the iso-amp's output were digitized, a computer could accurately monitor transformer load current on a continuous basis. Should the power resistor burn open, the 120-V ac line voltage would not be impressed on the computer circuitry or a person touching the output. Isolation reduces noise to maintain clean measurements and protects humans from shock and equipment from damage, should a fault occur.

A few more example applications will solidify our understanding of isolation. In Figure 7-59, the thermocouple could be used to take a temperature measurement in a medical oven, autoclave, or boiler, for instance. First let's discuss the front end and then examine why isolation is used. A thermocouple is a device made of two dissimilar metal wires spot-welded together at one end. It produces a small voltage of, say, 5 mV in response to a temperature gradient across the wires. Table 7-1 shows materials used and how much voltage they produce for E, J, K, and T thermocouples. Again the classical IA is used to amplify the difference between the thermocouple voltage and a diode voltage that is mounted to an isothermal block. This technique is called *cold junction compensation.* The diode establishes a reference to the ice point or 0°C. The diode voltage changes with ambient temperature and, hence, compensates for changes in ambient temperature of the electronic amplifier. No matter what the ambient temperature goes to, within reason, the thermocouple always takes the measurement relative to 0°C.

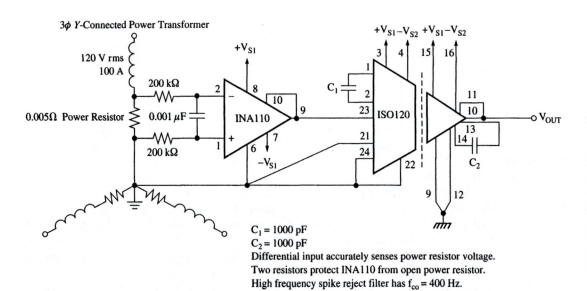

$C_1 = 1000$ pF
$C_2 = 1000$ pF
Differential input accurately senses power resistor voltage.
Two resistors protect INA110 from open power resistor.
High frequency spike reject filter has $f_{co} = 400$ Hz.

Figure 7-58
Isolated power line monitor. (Courtesy of Burr-Brown under copyright 1992 Burr-Brown Corporation)

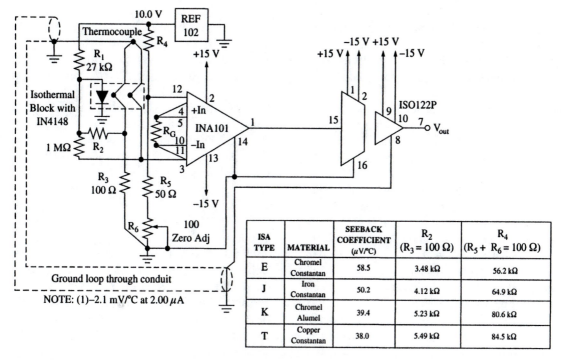

ISA TYPE	MATERIAL	SEEBACK COEFFICIENT (μV/°C)	R_2 ($R_3 = 100 \ \Omega$)	R_4 ($R_5 + R_6 = 100 \ \Omega$)
E	Chromel Constantan	58.5	3.48 kΩ	56.2 kΩ
J	Iron Constantan	50.2	4.12 kΩ	64.9 kΩ
K	Chromel Alumel	39.4	5.23 kΩ	80.6 kΩ
T	Copper Constantan	38.0	5.49 kΩ	84.5 kΩ

NOTE: (1)–2.1 mV/°C at 2.00 μA

Figure 7-59
Thermocouple (temperature) amplifier with ground loop elimination, cold junction compensation, and upscale burnout indication. (Courtesy of Burr-Brown under copyright 1995 Burr-Brown Corporation)

Now what purpose does isolation serve in Figure 7-59? It simply breaks the ground loop to reduce noise interference that can ruin the low-level sensitive temperature measurement. Although high voltage may not be present here, the thermocouple can be attached to a grounded metal heater or heated surface. This ground may be very "dirty" with respect to the instrumentation amplifier ground. That is, there may be large power or spike currents passing through the point where the thermocouple is attached. Therefore, a ground loop is created through a conduit that eventually gets back to the input amplifier, as shown in Figure 7-59. Noise can then mix with the small temperature signal. So it should be obvious that the isolation amplifier with its high impedance prevents noise from

TABLE 7-1 THERMOCOUPLE MATERIALS

Thermocouple type	ISA type	Sensitivity @ 20°C (μV/°C)	Useful range (°C)
Chromel/Constantan	(E)	59	0 to +500
Iron/Constantan	(J)	50	−150 to +1000
Chromel/Alumel	(K)	40	−200 to +1200
Copper/Constantan	(T)	38	−150 to +350

interfering with the 1-mV differential input signal. Should the thermocouple become open, the IA's output will go to its positive P/S rail, around +12 V dc. This is called *up-scale burnout*. Isolation really has nothing to do with burnout, but the iso-amp must pass the overranged signal to allow, say, a computer to detect the fault condition.

An example will show a special way to transmit isolated temperature measurements over long distance. It is known as an isolated 4-mA to 20-mA current loop, as shown in Figure 7-60. These current loops pick up much less noise than sending voltages over long wires. Loops may be used without isolation, but when isolation is added, the noise pickup drops even lower. In an electrically noisy hospital environment, this may be the only way to cost-effectively monitor a temperature remotely. Otherwise, special shielded wires and conduits must be installed.

In Figure 7-60, the resistor temperature device (RTD) measures the temperature at its surface of,

say, a medical incubator or perhaps a hospital room. The commercially available two-wire transmitter shown turns the temperature voltage into a current that circulates through a twisted-pair, two-wire loop on its way to the receiver. Here the current, 4 mA representing the minimum temperature and 20 mA the high temperature, is converted back into a voltage and applied to the iso-amp. The transmitter has two 1-mA current sources. One excites the transducer and creates a voltage drop across the RTD resistance. When temperature varies, RTD resistance varies, and the IA inside the two-wire transmitter amplifies it. The other 1-mA current source provides a differential reference for the RTD. Notice that there is no power supply at the remote site of the RTD. Power is applied through the two-wire loop. In fact, the loop accepts power in one direction and delivers the signal in the other direction over the same wires. It is actually the power supply current in the loop that is changing in response to a changing temperature signal. Such isolated circuits

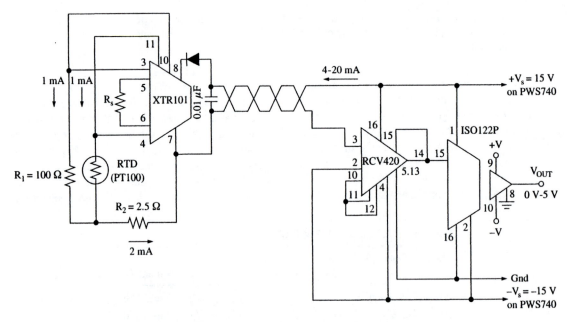

Figure 7-60
Isolated 4-mA to 20-mA resistor temperature device (RTD) instrumentation current loop.
(Courtesy of Burr-Brown under copyright 1993 Burr-Brown Corporation)

allow modern biomedical systems to do a better job of measuring important temperatures.

The final example of isolation is one that does not really break a ground loop; it just adds a moderate resistance in series. We say that when a very large resistance is provided between two points in a circuit, they are isolated. But this is a matter of degree. The circuits shown in Figure 7-61 make the point. Here, a commercially available component takes a differential measurement, but its reference points (pins 1 and 5) are only about 400 kΩ away from either input (pin 2 or 3). Since typical semiconductors can handle around 10 to 20 V before breakdown, something special must be done to withstand 200 V. Here is what is done: The circuits in Figure 7-61 first attenuate the common-mode voltage on each input by a factor of 20. Two hundred volts are reduced to an acceptable 10 V. Then the reduced voltage is gained up by a factor of 20. The result is a unity gain differential amplifier with a unique characteristic. With 400 kΩ of input resistance, this circuit handles 10-V differential signals riding on as much as 200 V maximum.

Do the circuits in Figure 7-61 replace classical isolation amplifiers? The answer is: sometimes. There is not enough isolation resistance to make such circuits suitable for ECG applications, but they are excellent for applications such as monitoring battery cells. Here +200-V and −200-V power supplies are employed to charge, say, 30 12-V lead-acid batteries. Uses range from supplies in portable X-ray equipment to emergency power backup in hospitals, for example. Battery cells near ground do not need a 200-V breakdown diff-amp, but cells near the maximum supplies require some similar type of amplifier. The multiplexer can select any channel, representing any battery cell, which can be sent to an A/D converter, digitized, and stored in a computer.

7-12 Chopper-stabilized amplifiers

Two problems arise when one tries to record low-level biopotentials (i.e., EEG recording of brainwaves): *noise* and *dc drift*. Both of these problems

are made worse by the high-gain amplifiers needed to increase the very weak biopotentials to a readable level.

Noise is generated by almost every part of the recording apparatus, including the patient's body, but the worst offender is the noise contribution of the amplifier itself.

Drift is the change in gain or dc offset (i.e., baseline) caused by thermal effects on the amplifier components. Drift may be substantially reduced through the use of large amounts of negative feedback in an ac-coupled amplifier. The problem to be solved is to convert a dc (or near-dc, low-frequency analog) signal to an ac signal that will pass through the amplifier.

The solution is to sample, or *chop,* the analog signal at a frequency that *will* pass through the ac-coupled amplifier. Although most biomedical chopper amplifiers use a 400-Hz excitation signal for the chopper, some models use 60-, 100-, or 1000-Hz chopper frequencies.

An example of a simple chopper amplifier is shown in Figure 7-62a. The chopper is a vibrator-driven single-pole, double-throw (SPDT) switch that grounds the amplifier input and output terminals on alternate swings of the switch.

The chopper vibrator coil is excited by a 400-Hz ac carrier signal. Figure 7-62b shows the analog waveforms for both the original and chopped versions. Only the chopped version of the signal will pass through the ac amplifier.

The chopper technique not only gains stability from the ac-coupled amplifier but also provides low-noise operation. The sampling rate, by itself, tends to act as a *low-pass* filter for externally generated noise, although it puts some noise of its own on the system. Most manufacturers further limit the noise by making the ac-coupled amplifier a *band-pass amplifier* that passes only the narrow range of frequencies around 400 Hz. The rms value of the noise signal in any given system is proportional to (among other factors) the square root of the circuit bandwidth. By limiting the bandwidth, we also limit the noise amplitude.

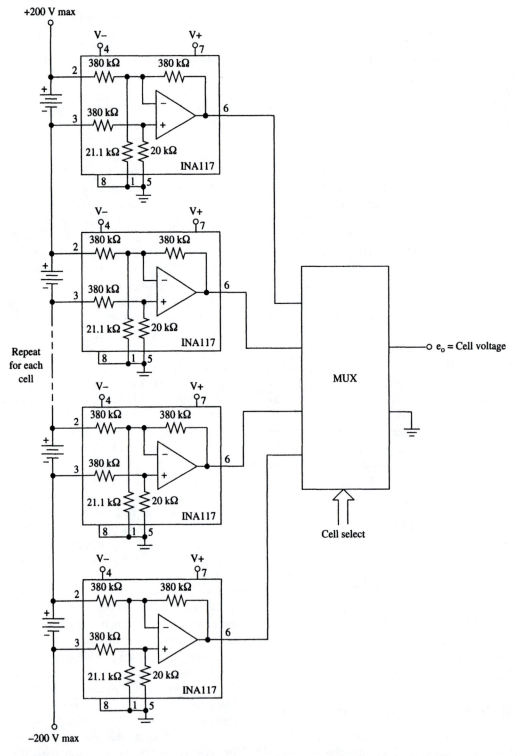

Figure 7-61
Battery cell voltage monitor. (Courtesy of Burr-Brown under copyright 1995 Burr-Brown
Corporation)

176

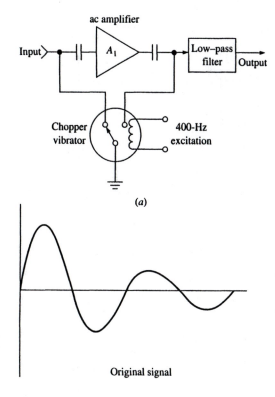

Original signal

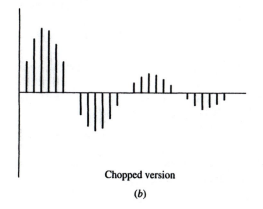

Chopped version

(b)

Figure 7-62

Chopper amplifier. (*a*) Simplified circuit. (*b*) Comparison of original and chopped waveforms.

A differential-input chopper amplifier is shown in Figure 7-63. In this circuit, the chopper is on the input circuit only. Input transformer T_1 is connected so that its center tap becomes one terminal of the input connector, while the two winding extremities are connected to the chopper. The pole of the chopper switch becomes the other terminal of the input connector.

Most of the gain in this circuit is provided by ac-coupled amplifier A_1. The signal remains a chopped version of the input waveform until it is applied to the synchronous demodulator, where it is detected and filtered to recover the original waveform.

The chopper amplifier technique of Figure 7-63 is typically used in EEG amplifiers and those universal bioelectric amplifiers that have gains in the range of $\times 1000$ and over.

7-13 Input guarding

Physiological signals tend to have low-level amplitudes. The -80-mV action potential is a powerhouse compared to the 1 mV of the ECG waveform and the 50 μV of the EEG waveforms.

In most cases, the physiological signal of interest is accompanied by large CM signals. Frequently, several hundred millivolts of 60-Hz signal will be coupled into the input cables of a bioelectric amplifier designed to sense and amplify low-level physiological signals.

This situation is shown in Figure 7-64. The circuit is shown in Figure 7-64*a,* in which a differential amplifier is connected to a differential signal source through a shielded cable. Both differential (E) and common-mode (E_{cm}) signals are present. If the usual practice of grounding the shield is followed, then the equivalent circuit of Figure 7-64*b* is obtained. Resistances R_1 and R_2 are the sum of the cable resistances and the signal source output impedance. Capacitors C_1 and C_2 represent the capacitance of the shielded cable.

The networks R_1/C_1 and R_2/C_2 are of little consequence, provided that $R_1 = R_2$ and $C_1 = C_2$, but if these equalities are not maintained, the inputs

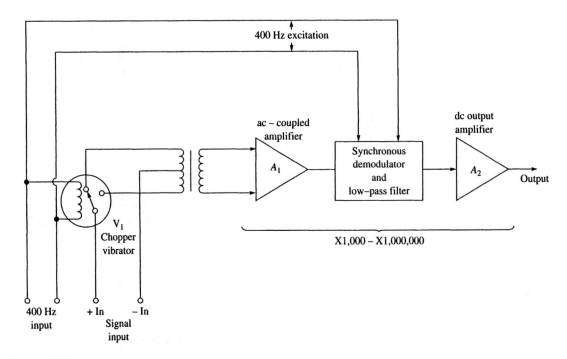

Figure 7-63
Differential chopper amplifier.

become unbalanced to ground. Under that condition the circuit may *manufacture* a differential component from a CM signal. The amplifier will be unable to distinguish the artifact from the real signal because *both* are differential signals.

The solution to this problem is to use *input guarding,* as shown in Figure 7-65. The main concept here is to place the *shield* at the CM signal potential, which in effect places both sides of C_1 and C_2 at the same potential for CM signals.

Most bioelectric amplifiers use only single-shielded input cables, but Hewlett-Packard uses a double-shielded input, as shown in the example. The H-P series 8800 bioelectric amplifiers are equipped with an input connector that separates guard and chassis grounds so that the circuit of Figure 7-65 can be used. The outer shield is especially useful when high-intensity CM interference is expected.

The drive source for the guard shield is derived by summing the +IN and −IN signals in the R_1/R_2

resistor network. In some cases, the summation junction is connected directly to the guard shield; in others, it is passed through a unity gain buffer amplifier (A_2).

In ECG amplifiers the right leg of the patient is designated as the *common,* so the guard shield may be connected to the right leg.

Figure 7-66 depicts a commercially available instrumentation amplifier and single-ended op-amp used as the shield driver. Here the transformer-coupled signal is brought to the IA over two-wire shielded cable. The 60-Hz noise, equally cutting across each wire through the shield, tends to induce voltages. In fact, the distributed cable capacitance tries to charge and discharge in response to 60 Hz. This allows interference to take place. To minimize this effect, the shield is driven with the common-mode voltage. The capacitance is actually made up of metal wires as one plate, insulation as the dielectric, and metal shield as the other plate. By driving the shield with the same noise

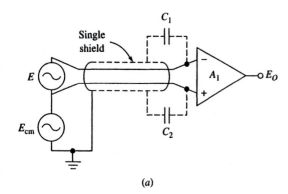

(a)

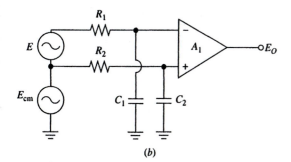

(b)

Figure 7-64
Bioelectric amplifier input circuitry. (*a*) Actual circuit.
(*b*) Equivalent circuit.

voltage that is induced on the wires, this parasitic capacitance cannot charge or discharge. It is effectively nulled out. This technique goes a long way toward reducing noise pickup in cables. It is better than just grounding the shield. Isolation would not help here, because the noise is on the input with respect to the input common. The shield cannot be isolated. The shield and wires it surrounds are intended to be part of the same circuit.

So far we have examined many types of bioelectric amplifiers handling signals from a variety of transducers. Some signals were biophysical, arising directly from the human body. Others were from temperature and pressure Wheatstone bridges. Still others were from separate temperature, optical, and chemical devices. We have looked at filters and peak detectors and flow and

weighing scale transducers. We have also discussed log amplifiers, instrumentation, and isolation amplifiers. With this working knowledge, it is easy to see how powerful these modern circuits have become in medical equipment.

The remaining circuits shown in this chapter are also commonly used in biomedical instrumentation. Understanding them will expand one's view of how medical instrumentation works and how to troubleshoot problems.

First is the current source. Figure 7-67*a* shows the basic constant current source, consisting of a low-resistance voltage source in series with a large resistor. The current is constant because, as the load varies from, say, 0 Ω to 10 kΩ, the current does not vary much. This is because 10 kΩ is very small compared to 10 MΩ. The constant current source in Figure 7-67*b* is better because the transistor makes the series resistance 100 MΩ instead of 10 MΩ.

Figure 7-68 shows how a current source is made from monolithic commercially available components. Notice the +10-V reference which, through R_1, produces a constant current into the load. The load, of course, is a much smaller resistance than R_1. The voltage follower forces the reference ground to be equal to the load voltage. This results in an accurate 10 V across R_1. Output current is easily calculated, $I_{out} = 10$ V/R_1.

Figure 7-69 shows a voltage-controlled current source with differential inputs. It can accept a differential voltage and drive a proportional current. It is also very versatile, since grounding one input gives a noninverting or inverting transfer function. Notice that it is actually built from the basic diff-amp—that is, an op-amp plus four ratio-matched resistors. With the output connected as shown, this represents the modified Howland current pump.

Figure 7-70 shows a single-chip (monolithic) dual 100-μA current source component that is commercially available. It also has a current mirror, which is a two-transistor circuit. A current, injected into one collector (pin 5), is reproduced on the other collector (pin 4). This occurs because the

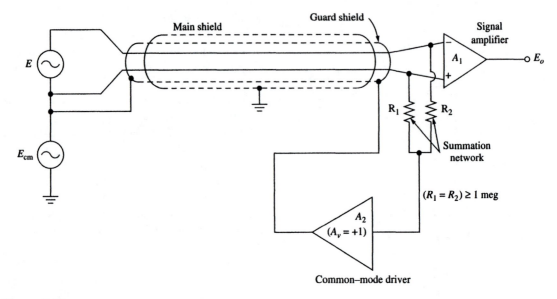

Figure 7-65
Guarded input circuit.

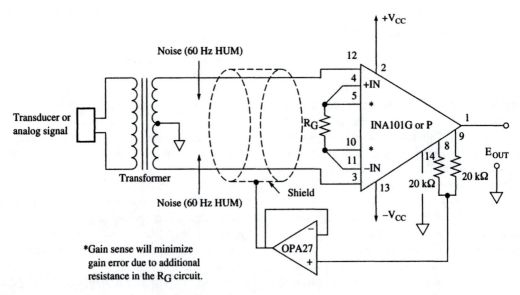

Figure 7-66
Amplification of transformer-coupled signal with shield driver. (Courtesy of Burr-Brown under copyright 1993 Burr-Brown Corporation)

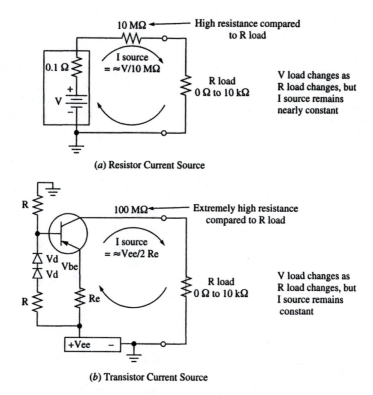

(a) Resistor Current Source

(b) Transistor Current Source

Figure 7-67
Basic current source. (a) Resistor current source. (b) Transistor current source.

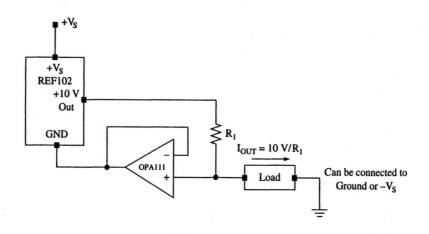

Figure 7-68
Current source using voltage reference and op-amp. (Courtesy of Burr-Brown under copyright 1993 Burr-Brown Corporation)

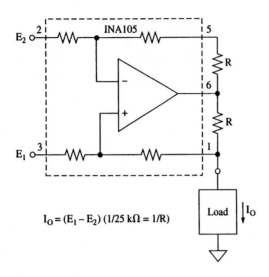

Figure 7-69
Voltage-controlled current source with differential inputs and bipolar output. (Courtesy of Burr-Brown under copyright 1993 Burr-Brown Corporation)

base and emitter currents are nearly equal (tied together), and the NPN transistors are matched. If I_b's and I_e's are equal, then I_c's must be equal. A current mirror is used extensively inside op-amps to reproduce biasing currents, which move together as the temperature changes. It can also be used in test equipment in which the current from one circuit must be connected to several places, but loading effects must be eliminated. it delivers the same current while being impedance-isolated from the original source.

How can current sources be used in biomedical equipment? One example is the slew rate limiter shown in Figure 7-71. Here a constant 100-μA current drives a diode bridge. The 10-kΩ input and feedback resistors drive the left side of the bridge. The right side is connected to the inverting op-amp terminal. Virtual ground is maintained by the flow of current through the capacitor, C. But when that current exceeds 100 μA, the bridge reverses, thus limiting the output slew rate (V/sec) to a value equal to 100 μA/C in farads. These types of circuits are very useful in ECG systems, in which the slew rate of an artificial pacer pulse riding on the

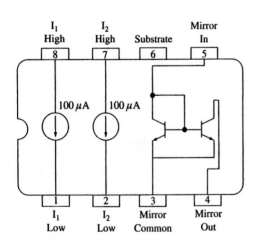

Figure 7-70
Single-chip (monolithic) dual current source with current mirror. (Courtesy of Burr-Brown under copyright 1994 Burr-Brown Corporation)

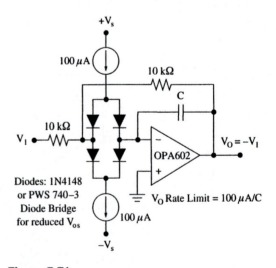

Figure 7-71
Slew rate limiter using current sources (REF200) and diode bridge. (Courtesy of Burr-Brown under copyright 1994 Burr-Brown Corporation)

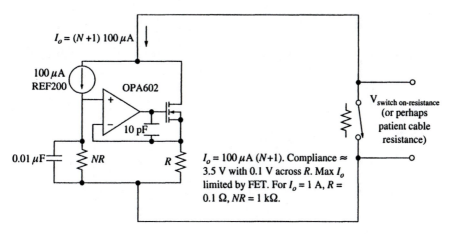

Figure 7-72
Switch on-resistance measurement using accurate current source.

ECG signal must be limited and essentially removed. This is necessary to prevent successive amplifiers from saturating.

Another use of current sources is the measurement of switch on-resistance (or perhaps patient cable resistance). In Figure 7-72, a floating current source is made of a commercially available current source (100 μA), op-amp, and N-channel enhancement MOSFET (metal oxide semiconductor field effect transistor). This circuit can be used to test a switch. The on-resistance equals the voltage across the switch divided by I_o, which can be made as large as desirable [$I_o = (N + 1)$ times 100 μA] to test the switch under actual current load conditions. Switches that are going bad change their on-resistance as current through them increases. The floating current source makes it easier to test switches while they are in the circuit. Sometimes, during troubleshooting, it is highly desirable to test switches in biomedical circuits.

Another circuit commonly used in biomedical systems is the sample-and-hold (S/H) amplifier, sometimes called track-and-hold. Figure 7-73 shows that it is composed of an input FET switch followed by a holding capacitor and noninverting amplifier. It works this way: When the sampling signal is at the ON-state (10 V), the input signal, V_{in}, charges the capacitor, C, through the on-

resistance of the solid-state FET switch. When the sampling signal is taken to the OFF-state (-7.5 V), the input signal stops charging the capacitor. Whatever voltage was on the capacitor at that time will be held there. The only change will be the result of the op-amp's bias current. This can cause droop or rise, depending on whether the bias current is plus or minus. Biomedical instrumentation incorporates S/H amplifiers to make sure bioelectric signals remain constant during A/D conversion.

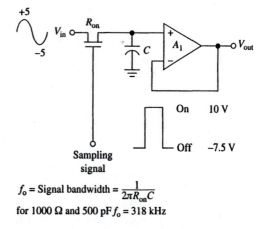

f_o = Signal bandwidth = $\dfrac{1}{2\pi R_{on}C}$

for 1000 Ω and 500 pF f_o = 318 kHz

Figure 7-73
Basic sample-and-hold (S/H) amplifier.

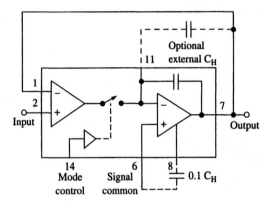

Figure 7-74
Single-chip (monolithic) noninverting unity-gain
sample/hold, SHC5320. (Courtesy of Burr-Brown
under copyright 1993 Burr-Brown Corporation)

Modern S/H amplifiers use monolithic circuits.
Figure 7-74 depicts a component very common in
the industry. It has the holding capacitor in the feedback loop of the output amplifier. An external holding capacitor can be added to reduce output voltage
droop rate: Droop [V/s = $I_{discharge}$(pA)/ C_{hold}(pF)].
This also reduces noise, because it provides
greater filtering. Notice that this component has an
input buffer amplifier to provide high-input impedance through a noninverting terminal. The S/H amplifier can also be connected in the inverting configuration by grounding the + input and feeding a
signal into the − input through a resistor.

S/H function and timing are shown in Figure
7-75. The S/H has four phases: (1) acquisition
time, (2) aperture delay time, (3) aperture uncertainty time, and (4) output amplifier settling time.
The control signal, at the top, with its two states,
sample and hold, starts and stops the process.
When n the sample or track state, the input voltage, shown in the second graph, is continuously
charging the hold capacitor, also called the tracing
capacitor, at this point. This first phase is called
the *acquisition time,* because the capacitor is acquiring the signal. Of course, there are imperfec-
tions in the S/H that cause offset and gain errors.

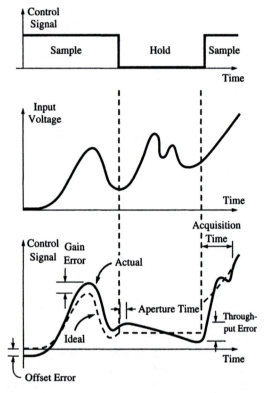

Figure 7-75
Sample/hold function and timing. (Courtesy of Burr-
Brown under copyright 1991 Burr-Brown Corporation)

This makes the acquired signal other than ideal,
but the difference is usually small. When the control signal goes to the hold state, the second phase
begins. This is the *aperture delay time.* It occurs
because the S/H switch does not respond instantly.
It starts to open after a small delay, say 25 ns for
the component shown in Figure 7-74. The third
phase, *aperture uncertainty,* automatically follows.
It occurs because of noise around the switching
threshold. In other words, the exact time when the
switch opens is statistically uncertain, with about a
300-picosecond variation. When many samples are
taken, this single uncertain event turns into aperture jitter. When input signals are moving fast, this
time jitter turns into amplitude noise at the S/H

output. The fourth phase is the setting of the output amplifier, often called sample-to-hold transient settling time. S/H amplifiers are used extensively throughout medical instrumentation.

Not all amplifiers used in medicine are slow. The next example application involves video. Figure 7-76 shows a commercially available high-speed amplifier in a noninverting gain of 2, acting as a video distribution amplifier. This component can drive 6 V peak to peak into a 50-Ω load. Three back-terminated lines, so called because they are loaded, represent one-third of 150 Ω, or 50 Ω. These types of amplifiers are used to transfer bioelectric signals that have been modulated or translated into the video bandwidth.

As discussed earlier, many bioelectric signals are modulated on a carrier and then transmitted across an optical sensor, magnetic transformer, or capacitive barrier. Modern components, like the one shown in Figure 7-77, are actually high-

speed analog multipliers. In this example, the multiplier is used as a single-chip balanced amplitude modulator. Notice the 120-kHz signal modulated on the 2-MHz carrier frequency. This circuit uses very few external components to accomplish its job.

The last application area to be discussed in this chapter is the data acquisition system (DAS). It is usually a multichannel system with some type of input signal amplification, followed by a sample-hold amplifier that feeds into an analog-to-digital converter. Most biomedical systems are DASs. Figure 7-78 shows a rapid scanning rate DAS with 5 μs settling time. The front-end differential input/differential output multiplexer steers a differential signal to the input of a fast settling time IA. Its output drives a familiar S/H. This system can quickly scan many channels. This is sometimes a requirement in medical instrumentation when a large number of channels are included in a big

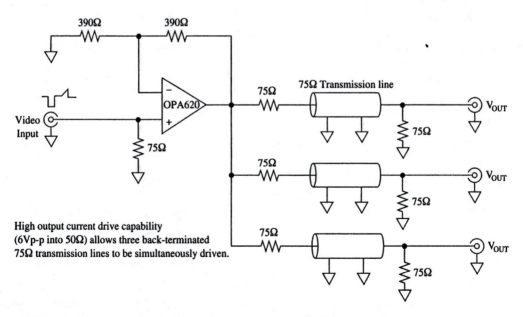

Figure 7-76
Video distribution amplifier. (Courtesy of Burr-Brown under copyright 1992 Burr-Brown Corporation)

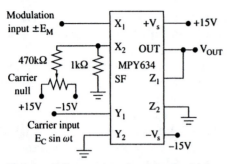

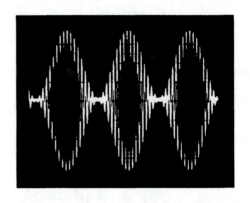

The basic multiplier connection performs balanced modulation. Carrier rejection can be improved by trimming the offset voltage of the modulation input. Better carrier rejection above 2MHz is typically achieved by interchanging the X and Y inputs (carrier applied to the X input).

CARRIER: f_c = 2MHz, AMPLITUDE = 1Vrms
SIGNAL: f_s = 120kHz, AMPLITUDE = 10V peak

Figure 7-77
Single-chip (monolithic) balanced amplitude modulator. (Courtesy of Burr-Brown under copyright 1995 Burr-Brown Corporation)

system. Otherwise, a scanning time of 50 to 100 μs per channel is acceptable.

The input IA in a DAS often has to be put into different gains depending on the level of the input signal being amplified at the time. Figure 7-79 shows a commercially available one-chip, programmable-gain IA (PGIA). Although this PGIA is capable of higher frequencies, the input common-

mode filter limits the response to 0.16 Hz. Under digital gain control, this component can be set to gains of 1, 10, 100, and 1000. When placed, for example, in front of an A/D converter, the PGIA essentially increases the system's dynamic range. That is, the system can digitize smaller input voltages with the PGIA than without. PGIAs are frequently used in biomedical equipment to

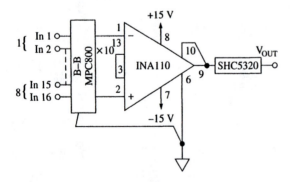

Figure 7-78
Rapid scanning rate data acquisition with 5-μs setting time to 0.01%, 1/2 LSB for 12-bit system. (Courtesy of Burr-Brown under copyright 1993 Burr-Brown Corporation)

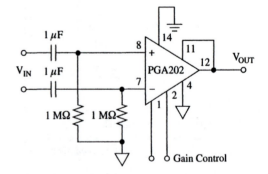

Figure 7-79
One-chip (monolithic) ac-coupled programmable-gain instrumentation amplifier (PGIA) for frequencies above 0.16 Hz. (Courtesy of Burr-Brown under copyright 1993 Burr-Brown Corporation)

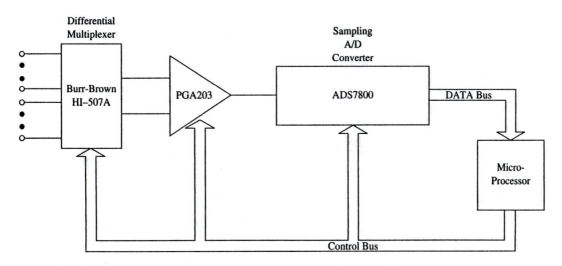

Figure 7-80

Eight-channel differential input data acquisition system with programmable-gain front end.
(Courtesy of Burr-Brown under copyright 1993 Burr-Brown Corporation)

automatically gain range under computer or software control.

The application shown in Figure 7-80 is a block diagram of an eight-channel differential input data acquisition system with programmable-gain front end. It contains an input multiplexer, PGIA, and sampling A/D converter. This particular A/D converter represents a trend in the industry. It has an internal S/H amplifier to capture and hold any channel's signal constant during the conversion time. Also, the A/D is the modern complementary metal oxide semiconductor (CMOS) type, which requires very low quiescent power to operate. The parallel output data is composed of 12-bit digital words, each word representing each channel as it is selected through the multiplexer. Output 12-bit information on the data bus is analyzed by the microprocessor. Understanding medical instrumentation hinges on one's knowledge of modern data acquisition systems.

Another application diagram of this chapter is shown in Figure 7-81. It is a schematic of an eight-channel differential input DAS with channel-to-channel isolation. Notice that all the commercially available IAs are on the input side. These are low-cost, eight-pin mini-DIP precision IAs that use one external resistor to set their gain. They drive eight low-cost isolation amplifiers in 16-pin single-wide plastic DIPs, also on the input side. That is why this system has channel-to-channel isolation. Each channel can accept a low-level input signal with respect to its own common, which is isolated from all the other commons, including the output ground. Also, the eight isolated power supplies or dc-to-dc converters supply $\pm$ 15 V separately to each channel. After crossing the eight isolation barriers, the power supply becomes the same. That is, $\pm$ 15-V, nonisolated, is supplied to the output stages of each iso-amp and to the analog multiplexer. Remember that isolation resistance and capacitance is made up of eight iso-amp barriers and eight iso-P/S barriers, all in parallel. The isolation is specified for 750 V dc continuous rating. The sampling A/D converter in Figure 7-81 accepts each channel as it is selected, samples it in a S/H amplifier inside the A/D

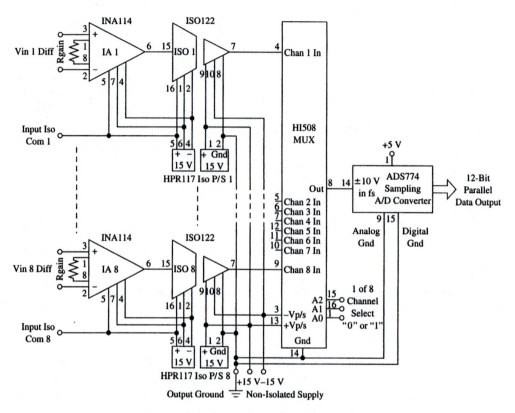

Figure 7-81
Eight-channel differential input DAS with analog channel-to-channel isolation.

converter, and digitizes it into 12-bit digital words. The A/D converter shown is capable of sampling at a 117-kHz rate. This means that the system can switch to a new channel about every 8.5 µs. Also, the A/D converter shown is the modern low quiescent power CMOS type, operating from a single +5-V digital power supply. Notice that A/D grounds are returned separately to the power supply point where ground enters the system. This ensures that the analog signal at the output of the multiplexer is referenced to a "clean" ground. Mixing analog and digital ground currents too close to the A/D converter can cause digital noise

to mix with the analog signal unless a ground plane is used.

The type of channel-to-channel isolated DAS depicted in Figure 7-81 is used in some medical and many industrial systems. Although isolation is necessary for most ECG monitoring, it does not require channel-to-channel isolation. That is, all channels on the input share the same isolated common (right-leg patient signal return), which is isolated from the output ground. This appears as follows. Some multi-channel medical diagnostic systems use the analog isolation approach, shown in Figure 7-82, while some use

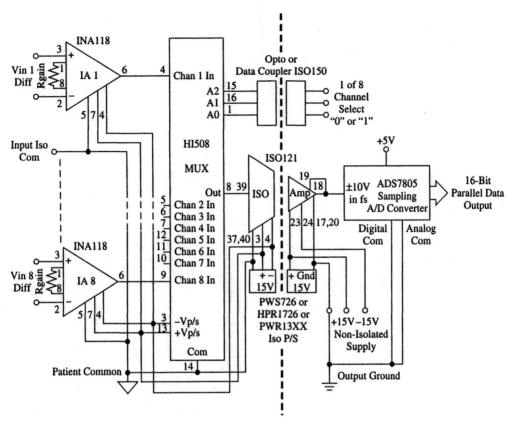

Figure 7-82
Eight-channel differential-input medical diagnostic system, analog isolation.

the digital isolation opto or data coupler, shown in Figure 7-83.

Many of the semiconductors described in this chapter have, to one degree or another, some static sensitivity, especially CMOS chips. Special care in handling these types of components is necessary to avoid catastrophic failure (burnout) and latent failure (works but is erratic and eventually drifts out of specification and then fails). Body and machine models have been established to try to quantify how static charge buildup and discharge occurs through semiconductors. Keeping humidity high enough and using special insulation with antistatic sprays can help prevent static buildup, which can

reach levels of thousands of volts. Using conductive wrist straps, standing on conductive floors, and grounding metal surfaces can drain off charge before it reaches dangerous levels. Static discharge damages semiconductors but rarely hurts humans, even though it can feel like a sharp pin prick. Knowing how to deal with static is very helpful in troubleshooting and repairing medical electronic equipment. A lack of adherence to static rules can introduce new failures.

The remaining chapters of this textbook discuss medical systems that use the bioelectric amplifier circuits and DASs described in this chapter.

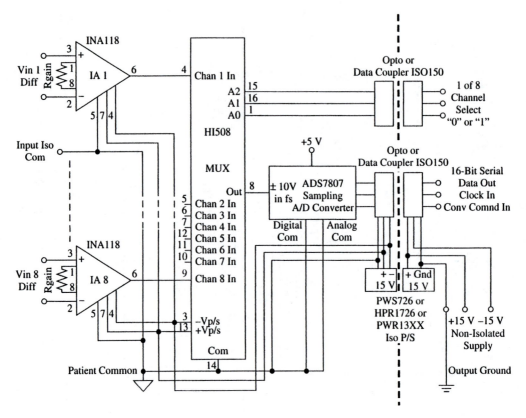

Figure 7-83
Eight-channel differential-input medical diagnostic system, digital isolation.

7-14 Summary

1. The properties of operational amplifier circuits can be set by manipulating the negative feedback loop.

2. Operational amplifier voltage gain is set by the ratio of two external resistors.

3. Isolation amplifiers provide up to $10^{12} \, \Omega$ of insulation between the patient connectors and the 120-V ac power mains.

4. Chopper amplifiers are used to process low-level signals because they possess superior noise and drift characteristics.

5. Input guarding is used to prevent formation of differential signals from common-mode signals.

6. There is no actual ground pin on a typical bipolar-supply, general-purpose op-amp. The ground is located between the power supplies, which is the point where the minus portion of plus supply and plus portion of minus supply are connected together. If a single supply op-amp is used, the ground is usually the negative supply pin on the op-amp itself.

7. Internal detail of a real-world op-amp shows nonideal parameters, such as bias current,

common-mode (one terminal to ground) resistance and capacitance, differential (across the two plus and minus inputs) resistance and capacitance, and output resistance.

8. Nonideal parameters of op-amps cause errors in the circuit to which they are connected. Errors in dc are caused by resistance and ac errors are caused by capacitance. Although electronics causes errors that are not part of bioelectric signals, modern commercially available components accurately amplify these signals.

9. A transimpedance (voltage output/current input) amplifier is a configuration of an inverting op-amp circuit, in which an input current is converted to an output voltage. In real-world op-amps, bias current causes an error in the output voltage.

10. A photodiode amplifier usually employs a transimpedance amplifier to convert the photodiode current into an output voltage.

11. Noninverting op-amp circuits are used to provide a high input impedance that does not load down the signal source very much.

12. A pH probe amplifier usually employs a very high input impedance noninverting op-amp circuit to avoid loading down the high-resistance pH probe. This allows amplification of the probe voltage without significant errors and degradation of the probe.

13. Three important considerations in pH probe op-amp circuits are (1) bias current over temperature, (2) noise at high source resistance, and (3) PCB layout and shielding.

14. Electronic filter circuits are very important in achieving good biomedical instrumentation performance. They reduce noise outside the bioelectric signal bandwidth. Low-pass filters with very low frequency cutoff, such as a few hertz, are used when dc signals are measured to reduce noise. Moderate frequency low-pass filters are used to reduce noise in the 50 to 60 Hz range. Low-pass filters of higher frequency, such as 10 kHz, are used to reduce wideband noise. Notch or band reject filters are used to selectively reduce specific interference, such as noise in the 50 to 60 Hz range. Some filters are active and use amplifiers, others are passive and use only resistors and capacitors.

15. Peak detector circuits are used to selectively measure maximum voltage excursions in bioelectric signals, such as ECG waveforms.

16. Differential amplifiers are among those most commonly found in biomedical equipment. They amplify the input voltage difference while rejecting noise common to both inputs.

17. The basic diff-amp has two gain paths, one inverting and the other noninverting. Errors associated with real-world op-amps also influence the accuracy of diff-amps.

18. Instrumentation amplifiers often employ two stages, one noninverting with high input impedance, followed by a basic diff-amp. The advantage is minimal loading on the signal source and versatility in setting the gain.

19. Two important considerations in IA circuits are (1) CMR at higher frequency and (2) PCB layout to prevent noise pickup and possible oscillation of high-frequency amplifiers.

20. A special 4- to 20-mA current loop technique is sometimes used after an IA to transmit low-level signals through electrically noisy environments. This works better than transmitting a voltage, because noise pickup affects current signals less than voltage signals.

21. Integrators are used in biomedical equipment to measure the area under a curve, such as a pulse, and differentiators are used to measure a slope, such as the rising *QR* portion of an ECG *QRS* complex waveform.

22. A log-amp is used in biomedical equipment to derive the absorbance number in laboratory measurements or to compress the range of wide dynamic range signals.

23. Isolation amplifiers consist of an input amplifier, a modulator, some type of barrier energy converter (such as magnetic or optical), a demodulator, and an output amplifier.

24. Isolation amplifiers (1) prevent shock to patients, (2) prevent damage to equipment and operators, and (3) reduce interfering noise.

25. Isolation amplifiers reduce noise by attenuation of interference (or IMR) across its iso-barrier, and IAs reduce noise by cancellation of interference on its two inputs.

26. An important consideration in iso-amp circuits is IMR at high frequency.

27. Modern isolation amplifiers use magnetic, optical, and capacitive barriers.

28. A fiber-optic isolation link has the highest IMR.

29. Current sources, as well as voltage sources, are used in biomedical equipment. For example, a current can be circulated through a switch to determine whether it is faulty.

30. S/H amplifiers are used in front of A/D converters to ensure that bioelectric signals remain constant during conversion time. Modern A/D converters have internal S/H converters.

31. Not all amplifiers used in biomedical equipment have low bandwidth. Video distribution amplifiers, for example, handle signals of a few megahertz up to hundreds of megahertz.

32. An analog multiplier can be used as an amplitude modulator, in which a bioelectric signal is superimposed on a high-frequency carrier. This allows transmission across an isolation barrier, for example.

33. Biomedical equipment systems employ the principles of data acquisition systems. These use an input multiplexer, a programmable-gain amplifier (to adjust to varying input signal level), an A/D converter, and a microprocessor or full computer.

7-15 Recapitulation

Now return to the objectives and self-evaluation questions at the beginning of the chapter and see how well you can answer them. If you cannot answer certain questions, place a check mark next to each and review appropriate parts of the text. Next, try to answer the following questions using the same procedure. When you have answered all of the questions, solve the problems.

Questions

1. List the properties desired in a bioelectric amplifier.

2. It is not possible to accurately measure biophysical signals with op-amps because of the errors created by the electronic circuit. True or false.

3. Noninverting op-amp circuits usually cause less loading of the signal source than inverting op-amp circuits because of high input impedance. True or false.

4. What type of error is caused by a real-world op-amp's finite input impedance, especially at high frequencies? (a) offset, (b) gain, (c) both offset and gain.

5. In a real-world transimpedance amplifier circuit, such as a photodiode amplifier, the op-amp's input _____ current causes an error in the output voltage.

6. Photodetector circuits appear commonly in what three types of biomedical equipment?

7. Name three important amplifier and circuit considerations in pH probe applications: higher temperature _____ current, total

_____ at high source resistance, and PCB _____ .

8. What is the purpose of a 60-Hz notch filter?

9. Differential-input amplifiers work on the principle of how many gain paths?

10. Op-amp internal common-mode and differential input _____ and _____ cause errors in a differential amplifier circuit just as they do in inverting and noninverting circuits.

11. In a three op-amp, two-stage instrumentation amplifier, the input stage noninverting amplifiers serve to provide _____ input impedance.

12. Name two important considerations in keeping high-frequency noise interference from ruining a biomedical measurement: high-frequency _____ and PCB _____ .

13. An important consideration in protecting instrumentation amplifiers is to use series resistors and _____ diodes.

14. 4- to 20-mA current loop transmitters are better at rejecting _____ pickup than voltage transmitters.

15. Where is the ground on an operational amplifier?

16. List the terminals you would ordinarily expect to find on an operational amplifier.

17. Give the three types of signal voltage applied to operational amplifier input terminals.

18. List the six basic properties of an ideal operational amplifier and give a brief definition or implication of each.

19. The _____ input produces an output signal that is out of phase with the input signal.

20. What is a "virtual ground"? From which basic operational amplifier property does it follow? (see question 7-18)

21. What is a "summing junction" and how does it differ from a virtual ground?

22. List the three basic classes of operational amplifier voltage follower configuration.

23. Write the transfer equations for (a) inverting follower, (b) noninverting follower with gain, (c) instrumentation amplifier.

24. Write the transfer equation for (a) an integrator, (b) a differentiator.

25. What property of transistors gives us the logarithmic and antilog amplifiers?

26. Can a modern logarithmic amplifier achieve < 1% accuracy? Yes or no.

27. Draw two different types of offset null circuit.

28. Define zero suppression and describe how it is used.

29. A span control sets the _____ of the amplifier.

30. What is an isolation amplifier? Why is it used?

31. List four different types of isolation amplifier circuit.

32. Describe current-loading coupling.

33. Draw the block diagram for, and describe the operation of, a carrier-type isolation amplifier.

34. What problems are encountered when low-amplitude signals are processed in high-gain dc amplifiers?

35. How does a chopper amplifier work, and how does it solve the problems discussed in question 4-34?

36. Draw the simplified schematic for a chopper amplifier.

37. How can a differential component be formed from a common-mode signal in a shielded input cable?

38. Describe input guarding. How does it work and why is it sometimes needed?

39. What is a common-mode amplifier? How is it different from a right-leg amplifier?

40. Isolation amplifiers are usually composed of an input _____, _____ barrier, _____, and output _____.

41. Isolation amplifiers reject interference by _____ compared to instrumentation amplifiers, which reject interference by cancellation.

42. _____-mode voltage is applied to the input terminals of an instrumentation amplifier, and _____-mode voltage is applied across the barrier in an isolation amplifier.

43. _____-mode rejection is an instrumentation amplifier term, and _____-mode rejection is an isolation amplifier term.

44. An important consideration in isolation amplifiers, especially when switching power supplies are used, is power supply _____, which can be accomplished by filtering.

45. Fiber-optic links eliminate power supply _____ and _____ coupling.

46. Chopper amplifier techniques provide dc _____ and low _____ operation, which are useful in EEG measurements in which signal levels are very low.

47. Two applications of current sources are slew-rate _____ and switch _____.

48. Biomedical instrumentation incorporates S/H amplifiers to ensure that bioelectric signals remain _____ during A/D conversion.

49. Analog multipliers can be used as _____ modulators to provide a suitable signal for transmission across an isolation _____.

50. Medical instrumentation is basically a DAS, which stands for _____ _____ system.

51. A multichannel DAS consists of an input multiplexer and/or amplifier, followed by an _____/_____ converter, which feeds a _____ processor.

Problems

1. Find the voltage gain of an inverting follower (Figure 7-3) if $R_1 = 10$ kΩ and $R_2 = 220$ kΩ.

2. Calculate the voltage gain of an inverting follower if $R_1 = 500$ Ω and $R_2 = 5000$ Ω.

3. Calculate the voltage gain of an inverting follower if (a) $R_1 = 1$ kΩ and $R_2 = 1$ Ω, and (b) $R_1 = 1$ kΩ and $R_2 = 100$ Ω.

4. What is the voltage gain of a noninverting follower (Figure 7-7a) if $R_1 = 10$ kΩ and $R_2 = 100$ kΩ?

5. Compute the gain of a noninverting follower if $R_1 = 1.2$ kΩ and $R_2 = 100$ kΩ.

6. Select resistors for an inverting follower with a gain of $\times 75$ if the source impedance looking into the amplifier input is 200 Ω.

7. Compute the output voltage of a multiple-input circuit, such as the one in Figure 7-20, if $R_4 = 10$ kΩ, $R_1 = 10$ kΩ, $R_2 = 5$ kΩ, $R_3 = 5$ kΩ, and $E_1 = E_2 = E_3 = 620$ mV.

8. Find I_4 in Figure 7-20, using the parameters given in problem 7-7.

9. Computer the gain of a simple dc differential amplifier, such as the one in Figure 7-21, if $R_1 = R_3$, $R_2 = R_4$, $R_4 = 100$ kΩ and $R_1 = 9.1$ kΩ.

10. Compute the gain of an instrumentation amplifier (Figure 7-23) if $R_2 = 47$ kΩ, $R_1 = 1.8$ kΩ, $R_5 = 10$ kΩ, and $R_4 = 3.9$ kΩ. Assume that $R_2 = R_3$, $R_4 = R_6$, and $R_5 = R_7$.

Suggested reading

1. Stout, David F. and Milton Kaufman (eds.), *Handbook of Operational Amplifier Circuit Design,* McGraw-Hill (New York, 1976).

2. Smith, John I., *Modern Operational Circuit Design,* Wiley-Interscience (New York, 1971).

3. Carr, Joseph J., *Op-Amp Circuit Design & Applications,* TAB Books (Blue Ridge Summit Pa., 1976).

4. Faulkenberry, L. M., *An Introduction to Operational Amplifiers,* Wiley (New York, 1976.

5. Graeme, Jerald G., Gene E. Tobey, and Lawrence P. Huelsman, *Operational Amplifiers: Design and Applications,* McGraw-Hill (New York, 1971).

6. Strong, Peter, *Biophysical Measurements,* Measurements Concepts Series, Tektronix, Inc. (Beaverton, Ore., 1976).

7. *A Miniature Anemometer for Ultrafast Response,* H. Thurman Henderson and Walter Hsieh, University of Cincinnati, December, 1989, *Sensors* Magazine, 174 Concord St., Peterborough, N.H. 03458.

8. Product data sheets for components shown in this chapter. Burr-Brown Corp., P.O. Box 11400, Tucson, Ariz., 85734, 1-800-548-6132.

9. Application Bulletins, AB-001 through AB-035, Burr-Brown Corp., 1991.

10. Application Notes, AN-163 (Partial Discharge Testing, 1989), AN-165 (Current Sources and Receivers, 1990), Burr-Brown Corp.

11. *Design Update,* Volume 2, Number 3 (Filters and Temperature Sensor Circuit, 1991), Burr-Brown Corp.

12. "Test Methods for Static Control Products," chapter by James R. Huntsman and Donald M. Yenni, 1982; and *Basic Electrical Considerations in the Design of a Static-Safe Work Environment,* by Don Yenni, 1979, 3M, Static Control Systems, 223-2SW, 3M Center, St. Paul, Minn. 55101.

13. Standards and Organizations.

Consensus standards (not law) referenced by legal organizations

Specifications can be obtained from the particular association or from the following company, which specializes in acquiring and selling standards: Global Engineering Documents, Division of Information Handling Services, 2805 McGraw Ave, P.O. Box 19539, Irvine, CA 92713, Tel: 714-261-1455.

1. Association for the Advancement of Medical Instrumentation (AAMI), 3330 Washington Blvd., Suite 400, Arlington, VA 22201, Tel: 703-525-4890.

   a. *Standards and Recommended Practices, Volume 1: Biomedical Equipment.* Safe current limits for electromedical apparatus.
   b. *Standards and Recommended Practices/American National Standard.* Safe current limits for electromedical apparatus.
   c. *Biomedical Safety and Standards,* periodically issued.

2. Underwriters Laboratories (UL), 333 Pfingsten Road, Northbrook, IL 60062.

   a. UL544, *Standard for Medical and Dental Equipment,* 1985.
   b. UL508, *Standard for Industrial Control Equipment,* 1984.
   c. UL1244, *Electrical and Electronic Measuring and Testing Equipment,* 1980.
   d. UL1577, *Standard for Optical Isolators,* 1986.

3. International Electrotechnical Commission (IEC), France.

   a. IEC601-1, *Medical Electrical Equipment, Part 1: General Requirements for Safety,* 1988.

4. Verband Deutscher Elektroteckniker (VDE), Germany.

   a. DIN VDE 0884, UDC 621.372.2, 621.391.63, 620.1, 614.8, *Optocouplers for Safe Electrical Isolation—Requirements and Tests,* 1987.

5. National Electrical Code (NEC).

6. National Fire Protection Association (NFPA), Publication 70, Article 517, and Publication 99 from NEC.

7. Joint Commission on the Accreditation of Healthcare Organizations (JCAHO).

    a. Accreditation Manual for Hospitals, Requirements for 1992.

8. U.S. Public Health Service (PHS).

9. U.S. Occupational Safety and Health Administration (OSHA).

10. State and local government and public health service departments.

CHAPTER 8
Electrocardiography

8-1 Objectives

1. Be able to describe the fundamentals of an electrocardiographic ECG recording.
2. Be able to describe the basic ECG machine.
3. Be able to draw and describe the basic *lead system* and ECG *amplifiers*.

4. Be able to list the causes and cures for most common ECG recording malfunctions.
5. Be able to list the basic *maintenance* procedures for the ECG machine.

8-2 Self-evaluation questions

These questions test your prior knowledge of the material in this chapter. Look for the answers as you read the text. After you have finished studying the chapter, try answering these questions and those at the end of the chapter.

1. Which leads form the *Einthoven triangle?* Which limb electrodes are used?

2. How does a bioelectric amplifier *differ* from an ECG amplifier?

3. Which leads form the *unipolar limb leads?*

4. How do the unipolar limb leads differ from bipolar limb leads?

5. What is the standard speed in millimeters per second of the basic ECG machine?

6. Which limb signals are summed to form the through V_1 through V_6 leads?

8-3 The heart as a potential source

The heart is a muscle formed in a way that allows it to act as a pump for blood. In section 2-6 we learned that the heart contracts (i.e., pumps) under command from an electrical stimulus in the *electroconduction system.*

The heart pumps blood when the muscle cells making up the heart wall contract, generating their *action potential.* This potential creates electrical currents that spread from the heart throughout the body.

The spreading electrical currents create differences in electrical potential between various locations in the body, and these potentials can be detected and recorded through surface electrodes attached to the skin.

The waveform produced by these biopotentials is called the electrocardiogram (ECG), that is, a written record (graph) of the cardiac electrical potential waveform.

8-4 The ECG waveform

An example of a typical ECG waveform is shown in Figure 8-1. This particular waveform is typical of a measurement from right arm to left arm. In Figure 8-1a we see the various time intervals that are often measured by physicians examining the waveform, while Figure 8-1b shows the voltage amplitude relationships. A 1-mV *calibration pulse* isalso shown in Figure 8-1b.

The low-level amplitudes normally encountered in ECG recording cause several problems that are dealt with in section 8-10.

8-5 The standard lead system

In standard ECG recording there are *five* electrodes connected to the patient: *right arm* (RA), *left arm* (LA), *left leg* (LL), *right leg* (RL), and *chest* (C). These electrodes are connected to the inputs of a differential buffer amplifier through a *lead selector switch*.

The recording obtained across different pairs of electrodes results in different waveform shapes and amplitudes; these different views are called *leads*. Each lead conveys a certain amount of unique information that is not available in the other leads. Figure 8-2 shows the electrical axis of the heart that is examined by six of the standard leads: I, II,III, aVR, aVF, and aVL. The physician is often able to diagnose the *type* and *site* of heart disease by examining these different views because waveform anomalies have been correlated with disease conditions in the past.

The electrical connections, for the 12 standard leads are shown in Figure 8-3a. The ECG machine uses the patient's *right leg* as the *common* electrode, and the lead selector switch (deleted for sake of simplicity) connects the proper limb or chest electrodes to the differential amplifier input.

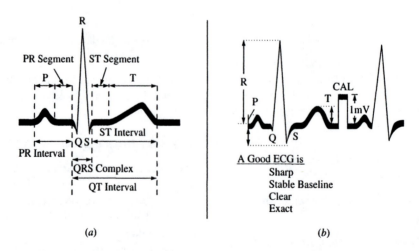

(a)   *(b)*

Figure 8-1
ECG time and amplitude measurements. (*a*) Time measurements. (*b*) Amplitude measurements. (Reprinted courtesy of Hewlett-Packard)

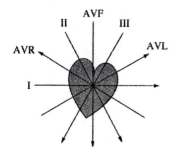

Figure 8-2
Cardiac axis viewed by different leads. (Reprinted courtesy of Hewlett-Packard.)

The *bipolar limb leads* are those designated lead I, lead II, and lead III and form what is called the *Einthoven triangle* (Figure 8-3b).

1. *Lead I:* LA is connected to the amplifier's *noninverting* input, while RA is connected to the *inverting* input.

2. *Lead II:* The LL electrode is connected to the amplifier's *noninverting* input, while the RA is connected to the *inverting* input (LA is shorted to RL).

3. *Lead III:* The LL is connected to the *noninverting* input while LA is connected to the *inverting* input (RA is shorted to RL).

The *unipolar limb leads,* also known as the *augmented limb leads,* examine the composite potential from all three limbs simultaneously. In all three augmented leads, the signals from *two* limbs are summed in a resistor network and then applied to the amplifier's inverting input, while the signal from the remaining limb electrode is applied to the noninverting input.

1. *Lead aVR:* RA is connected to the *noninverting* input, while LA and LL are summed at the *inverting* input.

2. *Lead aVL:* LA is connected to the *noninverting* input, while RA and LL are summed at the *inverting* input.

3. *Lead aVF:* LL is connected to the *noninverting* input, while RA and LA are summed at the *inverting* input.

The *unipolar chest leads* (V_1 through V_6) are measured with the signals from certain specified locations on the chest applied to the amplifier's *noninverting* input, while the RA, LA, and LL signals are *summed* in a resistor Wilson network at the amplifier's *inverting* inputs (called the "indifferent electrode").

Figure 8-3a shows the locations for V_1 through V_6, plus some other locations that are also frequently used.

Figure 8-4 shows the waveforms from a single patient taken in the 12 different lead positions. The square pulse shown in some of the waveforms is a 1-mV calibration signal supplied by the ECG machine. Note the differences in shape and amplitude of the ECG signals.

8-6 Other ECG signals

In addition to the conventional ECG signals discussed earlier, there are certain specific signals that are sometimes acquired. While the use of these is rare, the biomedical equipment technician or clinical engineer should be aware of them (see item 3 in the suggested reading list).

8-6-1 Interdigital ECG

This signal is taken between any two fingers. The interdigital ECG is used primarily in home monitoring of patients (especially those with implanted pacemakers—reduced heart rate often precedes battery failure). One common technique is to use the index finger of each hand as the signal source.

8-6-2 Esophageal ECG

In this type of ECG recording, an electrode is set placed in the esophagus close to the heart. A special ECG catheter containing a "pill electrode," an external bipolar pacing electrode, or a special

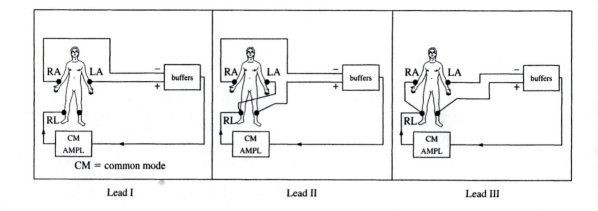

Lead I   Lead II   Lead III

Unipolar limb leads

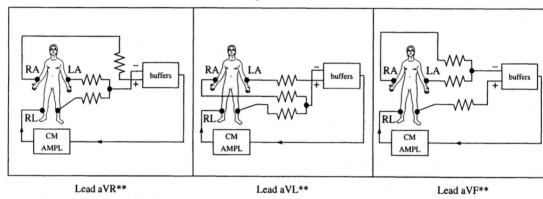

Lead aVR**   Lead aVL**   Lead aVF**

** Also known as "augmented" leads

Unipolar chest leads

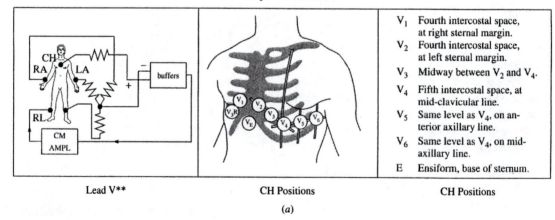

Lead V**   CH Positions   CH Positions

(*a*)

Figure 8-3

Standard leads and Einthoven triangle. (*a*) Limb and chest leads. (Reprinted courtesy of Hewlett-Packard)

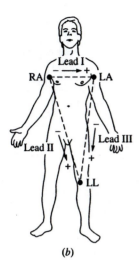

(b)

Figure 8-3
(continued) *(b)* Einthoven triangle.

electrode-equipped nasogastric tube is used to acquire the electrical signal. A principal application of the esophageal ECG is to examine atrial activity of the heart. The relative amplitudes of the *P* and *R* waves are used to establish the position for atrial sensing.

8-6-3 Toilet seat ECG

This type of recording uses two electrodes placed on either side of a toilet seat. The acquired signal is often connected to a computer in which arrhythmia detection software is running. The purpose is to detect cardiac arrhythmias that sometimes occur when the patient is straining during defecation.

8-7 The ECG preamplifier

An ECG preamplifier is a differential bioelectric amplifier (chapter 7). The input circuitry consists of the high-impedance input of the bioelectric amplifier, a lead selector switch, a 1-mV calibration source, and a means for protecting the amplifier against high-voltage discharges from defibrillators used on the patient.

The amplifier may be the bioelectric instrumentation amplifiers discussed in chapter 7, although, in all modern machines, one of the *isolation amplifier* designs will be used for patient safety.

The simplest limited type of ECG amplifier is shown in Figure 8-5. Here a one-chip (monolithic) ECG amplifier with right-leg drive indicates that an instrumentation amplifier (IA) can be connected directly to a person through body electrodes. In this particular commercially available three op-amp IA, the output of the internal input amplifiers appears as V_G. By connecting two 2.8-kΩ resistors to a single point, the common-mode voltage (CMV) can be derived. The CMV in the ECG case is composed of two components: (1) dc electrode offset potential and (2) 50- or 60-Hz ac-induced interference. Hum interference is caused by magnetic and electric fields from power lines and transformers cutting across ECG electrodes and patients. Hum currents flow in signal, common, and ground wires via capacitive coupling between the fields and the system. This type of noise seems to be ever-present, and the battle to get rid of it seems to be never-ending. Fortunately, modern noise reduction schemes are successful at minimizing hum in the ECG recordings.

The technique in Figure 8-5 works as follows. First the common-mode rejection (CMR) of the commercially available IA is very high and cancels some of the noise. The IA output is an ECG signal that has the 60-Hz noise greatly reduced. How does the IA do this? The differential amplification nature of the IA removes it, because equal common-mode (CM) noise is present on each IA input. The IA just subtracts equal noise voltages to give nearly zero while amplifying the difference in the unequal ECG signals present on its inputs. ECG signals on the left arm and right arm are different levels, because they come from different points on the body. How small the noise becomes at the output depends on how high the IA's CMR is.

The other noise reduction technique is right-leg drive. The CMV is inverted by the right-leg amplifier in Figure 8-5 and the resultant voltage is

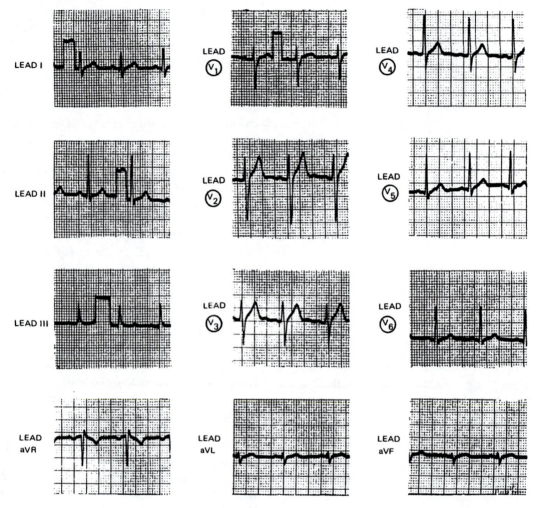

Figure 8-4
Typical tracings from the various ECG leads. (Reprinted courtesy of Hewlett-Packard)

applied to the patient's right leg. Just several microamperes or less are actually driven into the patient. This is quite safe, since UL544 and VDE-0884 require a limit of 10-µA maximum to prevent internal cardiac shock. Why is a noise-cancelling voltage applied to the patient in Figure 8-5? It is done to reduce 50- or 60-Hz noise. This circuit acts in a feedback loop (patient and electronics) to servo or drive the CM noise on the pa-

tient to a low level. Since the right-leg drive voltage is the inversion of the CMV (opposite phase), the right leg goes in the opposite direction compared to the CMV on the patient leads. While the 60-Hz noise on the left or right arm may become bigger with respect to the right leg, the 60-Hz noise on the IA input terminals with respect to IA common or ref becomes smaller. Hence, the IA does not have to reject as much 60-Hz noise. The

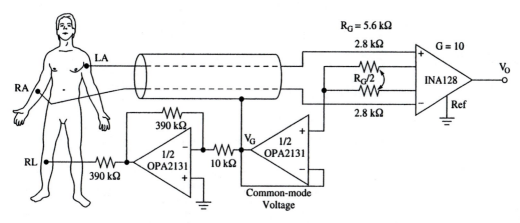

Figure 8-5
One-chip (monolithic) ECG amplifier with right-leg and shield drive. (Courtesy of Burr-Brown under copyright 1996, Burr-Brown Corporation.)

IA's CMR then reduces noise even further. Right-leg drive feedback circuits can oscillate if the phase shift through the patient flips the phase of the signal being fed back to the electronics. If high-frequency oscillation is present on the ECG signal, positive feedback may be the problem.

Usually an isolation amplifier would follow the IA in Figure 8-5. The iso-amp's isolation-mode rejection (IMR) also reduces noise by establishing 10^{12} Ω and 9 pF between the patient and earth ground. Isolation acts to attenuate noise (say, 1 V_{p-p} at 60 Hz) that is trying to mix with the low-level ECG input signal (say, 1 mV_{p-p}). Actually, four actions reduce 60-Hz interference dramatically: right-leg drive, IA CMR, shield drive, and iso-amp IMR. A low-pass filter and/or 60-Hz notch filter following the iso-amp will further shrink noise. This circuit is dc-coupled and is in high gain (1000 V/V). It only works when the electrode offset potentials are low (< 10 mV) to avoid IA output saturation. Restoration of dc allows much larger offsets to be tolerated.

The standard −3 dB frequency response of the amplifier used in making *diagnostic* grade recordings is 0.05 to 100 Hz, while *monitoring* instruments have a response of about 0.05 to 45 Hz (varies from manufacturer to manufacturer).

ECG preamplifiers must be ac-coupled so that artifacts from the electrode offset potential are eliminated. The low-frequency response of the amplifier, then, must not extend down to dc, but since certain features of the ECG waveform have a very-low-frequency component, the response is very nearly dc (0.05 Hz).

Figure 8-6 shows how to overcome patient electrode offset potentials, which can rise as high as 300 mV, according to Association for the Advancement of Medical Instrumentation (AAMI) standards. Sometimes they can go to ± 500 mV. If high gain, say 500 or 1000 V/V, were provided immediately, the input amplifiers would saturate and be unable to amplify the ECG signal. To cure this problem, three things are done. First, the input stage buffer amplifiers (A_1 and A_2) are placed in low gain, such as 10 V/V. Even if the electrode offset were 0.5 V, the output of the input amplifiers wouldonly go to 5 V. This leaves plenty of "head room" or voltage to the plus-or minus-power supply "rails" for the amplified ECG signal.

Second, the next stage (A_3) in Figure 8-6 is a unity gain differential amplifier, so there are no worries here about head room. Third, a dc restorator amplifier is used in a feedback arrangement to

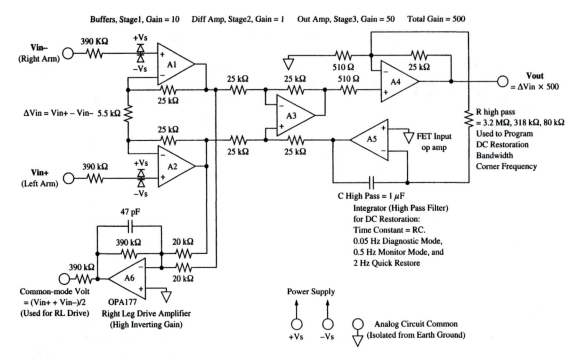

Figure 8-6
ECG amplifier schematic: Three-patient electrode (1-lead) ECG front end.

null out the dc offset. It works this way: Assume the left arm electrode offset to be +300 mV dc, although it can be plus or minus. Also assume that the right arm electrode is 0 V dc. The dc differential input voltage is then 300 mV. This results in +3 V at the output of A_3 (remember the gain of 10). Now the output of A_4 would try to go to +150 V dc, because the A_4 is in a gain of 50. However, the circuit will not allow 150 V. Actually, it does not go very high, because as soon as it goes in the positive direction, the feedback integrator, A_5, applies a negative voltage to A_3 through the reference point (right side of 25-kΩ resistor). The gain from this point to A_3's output is unity (one). Therefore, we have what amounts to a linear summing effect. The positive 3-V offset goes through A_3 at the same time a negative correction voltage goes through A_3. This reduces the offset voltage that appears at A_3's output and hence A_4's output. In turn, this reduces the error fed to the integrator, which reduces the er-

ror correction voltage fed back. This negative feedback loop continues for about 10 RC time constants, until it stops at the point where the offset at A_4's output is zero. Even the small offset contributed by A_4 as an op-amp error is removed. Since the feedback circuit in Figure 8-6 is an integrator or high-pass filter, it responds only to ac signals above its cutoff frequency. It can be set by R and C in the high pass filter for 0.05 Hz (diagnostic quality ECG), 0.5 Hz (monitoring), or 2 Hz (quick offset restore). The result of this dc restorator is to turn the original dc-coupled amplifier into an ac-coupled amplifier just as if a coupling capacitor were placed in series with the signal path. All frequencies below the cutoff are removed with either approach, but in the feedback dc restorator, the signal does not actually go through the capacitor. The only advantage is that the feedback approach uses an active integrator, which is linear and more easily controlled than a passive RC-coupling circuit.

Since the dc electrode offset voltage has been removed, the output amplifier (A_4) in Figure 8-6 can now gain up the signal by 50 V/V without becoming saturated. It is just amplifying the ac components of the ECG waveform. The dc component is gone. If the signal level from the left arm minus the right arm were 1 mV_{p-p}, then the output of A_3 would be 10 mV_{p-p}. The output of A_4, which is the output of the ECG amplifier V_{out}, becomes 0.5 V_{p-p}.

The significant ECG signal high frequencies extend to 100 Hz, but interfering skeletal muscle signals also have significant components in this range and will generate *somatic artifact* in the ECG tracing.

It is usually easy to obtain the patient's cooperation for the few minutes required to make a diagnostic ECG recording; he or she will lie still, reducing the muscle artifact to a minimum. But during long-term *monitoring* of the ECG the patient will be unwilling or unable to cooperate, so there will be substantial amounts of somantic artifact in the ECG signal. Instruments used for monitoring, then, are designed to have a frequency response that extends only from 30 to 50 Hz. The lower frequency response limit used in monitoring instruments *distorts* the waveform (by elimination of harmonics) too much for diagnostic purposes but is sufficient to allow detection of the life-threatening arrhythmias that make monitoring a necessity.

The *lead selector* switch is a front-panel control that permits the operator to select the waveform to be displayed. It will be a rotary or multilevel push-button switch in manually selectable machines, and complementary metal oxide semiconductor (CMOS) or junction field effect transistor (JFET) electronic switches in automatic machines. Some monitors do not have a lead switch, and in those instruments only the *common* and two *limb* electrodes are connected to the patient.

The *gain* of the ECG amplifier must be *standardized* when recording a waveform for diagnostic purposes. A 1-mV calibration pulse circuit is provided for this purpose.

In ECG machines, or other ECG systems using a strip-chart recorder as the display device, it is standard practice to adjust the gain to produce a tracing that is 10 mm high when the 1-mV button is pressed. The calibration pulse is also a powerful troubleshooting tool.

The *defibrillator* is a high-voltage electrical heart stimulator used to resuscitate heart attack victims. It is necessary to have an ECG monitor connected to the patient when using the defibrillator, so the ECG preamplifier input must be designed to withstand high voltages and high peak currents, even though the *normal* ECG waveforms are on the order of millivolts. The high-voltage (over a kilovolt) burst from the defibrillator will last 5 to 20 ms.

In some ECG preamplifiers the protection circuits are quite elaborate, while others—principally older machines—have little protection. An example of various types of protection is given in Figure 8-7. This figure shows many forms of protection circuits, but most equipment uses only a few of them.

Most ECG preamplifiers use from two to nine neon glow lamps (i.e., type NE-2) across the input lines. Those shown in Figure 8-7 are representative of the most common configuration. Most preamplifiers also use series resistors R_1 through R_6, although in some models the input resistors are physically located inside of the patient cable or its connector.

The resistors serve to limit the current flow, while the glow lamps serve a voltage *bypass* function. These lamps consist of a pair of electrodes mounted in a glass envelope in an atmosphere of low-pressure neon gas, or a mixture of inert gases. Normally, the impedance across the electrodes is very *high*, but if the voltage across the electrodes exceeds the ionization potential of the gas, then the impedance drops suddenly to a very low value. For most lamps in the NE-2 class used in medical monitors, the firing potential is between 45 and 70 V.

Potentials normally encountered in ECG recording will not ionize the gas inside of the glow

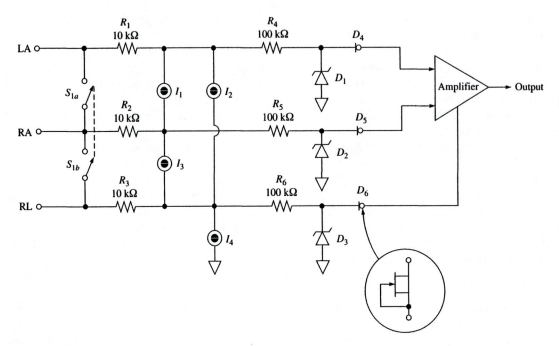

Figure 8-7
Defibrillator protection circuit.

lamps, but the potentials from defibrillators *will* fire the lamps, bypassing most of the charge harmlessly to the ground.

Some monitors also use *zener diodes* (D_1 through D_3) shunted across the amplifier inputs to ground. These diodes serve a function that is similar to the job performed by the neon lamps, but at a lower voltage.

Diodes D_4 through D_6 are called *current-limiting diodes,* even though they are not really diodes in the normal sense of the word, but are JFETs with the source and gate terminals tied together (see inset, Figure 8-7). Although the same current-limiting behavior is exhibited by an ordinary three-terminal JFET that is connected in the aforementioned manner, many manufacturers offer two-terminal JFET current-limiting diodes, in which the connection is made internally. These diodes are usually rated as to the limiting current.

The current-limiting diode acts as a resistor (i.e., the JFET channel resistance) as long as the

current level remains below the limiting point. If the current attempts to increase above that level, however, it is clamped and limited.

In some machines, *metal oxide variable resistors (varistors)* are used in place of the shunt zener diodes. These devices are similar to the surge protectors used on computers. They maintain a high resistance until the voltage exceeds a critical threshold, but above that point the resistance drops. These devices thereby clip the high-voltage spike.

8-7-1 Types of defibrillator damage

The protection circuits available to an ECG preamplifier are never totally effective in all cases; after all, the voltage from the defibrillator is more than six orders of magnitude greater than the normal working voltages. Some damage will occur.

Two forms of damage from defibrillator discharge are common, and they tend to produce different symptoms. If both amplifier inputs are blown out, then the readout device will show a *flat baseline* (i.e., no output signal and little noise). If, on the other hand, only *one* of the two inputs is affected, then the output waveform may be merely distorted. Typically, when this occurs, the output waveform will be unable to deflect above or below the baseline, depending on which input is damaged. This type of problem may very well be occult, that is, hidden, and not noticed by the medical staff unless they compare the display with an ECG taken from the same patient on another instrument.

The most common mechanisms for such failures are defective glow lamps and open zener diodes. The glow lamps eventually lose their ability to protect the amplifier because the firing potential rises due to airleaks, recombination or absorption of the gases, and other defects. Some manufacturers recommend replacement of the glow lamps every one or two years, or more frequently if the machine is used in emergency rooms or intensive or critical care units.

If a defibrillator discharge opens a zener diode, as is sometimes the case, then a subsequent discharge may destroy the preamplifier input transistors.

8-7-2 Electrosurgery unit filtering

Preamplifier damage from defibrillator high-voltage pulses is prevented by special clamping circuits. Likewise, preamplifiers must be protected from electrosurgery unit (ESU) high voltages. The ESU interference can range from hundreds of kilohertz to 100 MHz and up to several kilovolts. It can greatly disrupt the ECG signal. Why does this occur when the ECG bandwidth is only 100 Hz? The answers are (1) dc offsets and (2) obscuring the signal. ECG-type IAs may be relatively low bandwidth, but the junctions inside are capable of rectifying high frequency, such as the ESU waveform. Then, parasitic capacitance around the junctions filters the high frequency, resulting in dc offsets. The ECG baseline can actually move around when the ESU is triggered.

Also, the high frequency goes right through amplifier stages, low-pass filters, and isolation stages to obscure the ECG as displayed on a cathode ray tube (CRT).

In the past, an ECG system had to tolerate the ESU interference without being damaged. Then the requirement was to operate in some fashion. That is, the displayed ECG waveform had to be recognizable. Now medical professionals are requiring that ECG diagnostic quality remain in the presence of ESU noise.

Figure 8-8 shows a technique for reducing ESU noise in the front end of an ECG amplifier. It is composed of a three-stage *RC* filter arranged in a pi (π) configuration. An *LC* filter can also be used, but it is more difficult to maintain an *LC* match compared to *RC* match to common on one lead compared to the other lead. The common-mode effect results from series *R* or *L* and parasitic capacitance to patient common. Why does the common-mode time constant need to be matched? Because a mismatch in effect causes a 60-Hz differential error to appear. The effort in trying to reduce hundreds of kilohertz of ESU interferences unfortunately results in degraded total CMR at 60 Hz. However, one can tolerate a little additional 60-Hz noise, because the right-leg drive still reduces 60 Hz, the IA still has its high CMR, and the isolation amplifier still has its high IMR to 60 Hz. It is worth it to get rid of ESU noise. Also, some systems tune the isolation barrier to form a band reject filter around the ESU frequencies to further reduce ESU interference. The input filter shown has a cutoff frequency of 10 kHz. This is low enough to reduce ESU noise but high enough to prevent phase distortion of the ECG signal.

Wouldn't it be nice to get rid of ESU interference and retain as much 60-Hz rejection as possible? The circuit in Figure 8-9 can help to do this. It is a high-speed IA designed with commercially available video op-amps. The gain is set to 5 V/V for the ECG signal, but the CMR is not only fairly good at 60 Hz, it is also good at very high frequency.

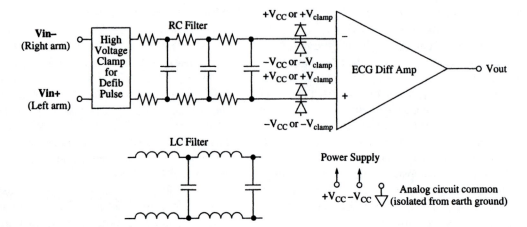

Figure 8-8
Electrosurgery unit interference filter.

The typical product data sheet shown in Figure 8-10 reveals that the CMR is about 75 dB at 60 Hz. This is not extremely high, but the op-amp CMR is still 40 dB at 100 MHz. Since two input op-amps are used to make the IA, their match might result in, say, 30-dB CMR for the complete instrumentation amplifier at 100 MHz and 60 dB at 1 MHz. That is high enough to reject ESU interference rather effectively. There is only one problem with the IA shown in Figure 8-9, aside from having to pay careful attention to printed circuit board (PCB) and system front-end layout: It

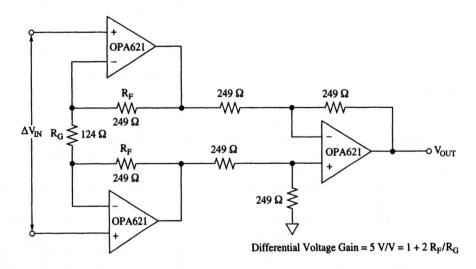

Figure 8-9
Wideband, fast-settling instrumentation amplifier with high common-mode rejection at high frequency. (Courtesy of Burr-Brown under copyright 1992 Burr-Brown Corporation)

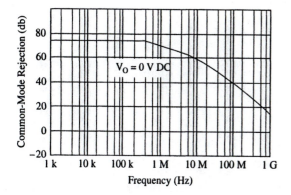

Figure 8-10
Important consideration: frequency effect on common-mode rejection, OPA621. (Courtesy of Burr-Brown under copyright 1992 Burr-Brown Corporation)

has high bias current. The bias current of the high-speed op-amp shown is about 30 μA. This exceeds the 10-μA limit set by AAMI and UL544 standards. Also, the op-amp's input resistance is less than 1 MΩ. This component was chosen to show that although it is possible, it is hard to find commercially available components that will have low bias current and high CMR at very high frequencies. To make the circuit shown in Figure 8-9 work for ECG systems, two high-speed, high-impedance, low-bias current input buffers would have to be added to the IA front end. Again, PCB layout and parasitic capacitance to common is critical in making the circuit function properly. This increases cost, but it may be worth it to get rid of ESU interference.

As we have seen, the ECG front-end amplifier is critical in achieving good performance. How does the ECG IA fit into the electronics of the entire monitoring channel? Figure 8-11 shows a block diagram of a multichannel phsyiological monitoring system. It accepts ECG, several channels of blood pressure (BP), body temperature, oxygen saturation, and perhaps other gases or body parameters. Notice the stray capacitance from the person to patient common and to earth ground. As mentioned earlier, this capacitance

passes 60 Hz and other interference currents. These noise currents circulate in the patient and cables connected to the patient. Some efforts have been made to electronically model this phenomenon and predict how to minimize its effect. Stray capacitance should always be minimized to extract clean ECG signals from the human body. This involves connecting as little equipment to the patient as possible.

The system in Figure 8-11 is composed of input buffers, an analog multiplexer (mux) plus Wilson network, programmable-gain instrumentation amplifier (PGIA), and sampling analog-to-digital (A/D) converter with internal sample hold (S/H) amplifier. Notice that the digitized signals are in the form of serial data at the output. This allows isolation with just a few opto or isolated data couplers (e.g., one for data, one for clock, one for start conversion [convert/command], one for data framing). If a 12-bit parallel output A/D converter were used, many more couplers would be needed (maybe 15).

The next few figures concentrate on how the ECG front end is implemented today. Although the complete ECG system uses 10 to perhaps 14 patient electrodes, some more basic schemes use just three patient electrodes. These are right arm, left arm, and right leg. For this a simpler ECG amplifier composed of an IA, right-leg driver, and dc restorer can be used. Other ECG machines use five patient electrodes, as shown in Figure 8-12. Notice that all electrodes are buffered by a unity gain amplifier. These buffers have series protection resistors, on the order of tens to hundreds of kΩ, somewhere in the circuit and clamping diodes. This ensures that amplifier inputs (from high defibrillation voltage) do not go more than one diode drop (about 0.7 V) above or below the plus and minus clamping voltage (sometimes just the power supply rails). Interestingly, modern AAMI and UL standards require that two or more faults occur before any current is driven through the patient. The fault current from the electronics is required not to exceed 50 μA. Therefore, a monolithic circuit front end that has the series resistors on the chip

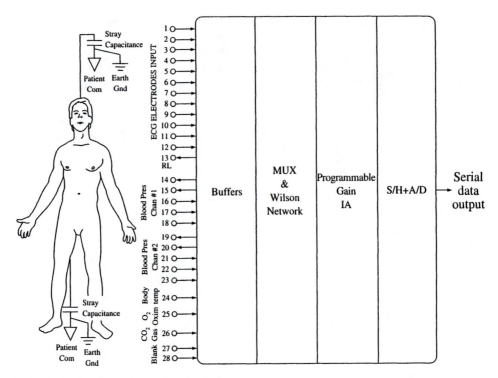

Figure 8-11
Multichannel physiological monitoring system.

might not qualify. One allowable fault on the chip could be the + input to the RA amplifier shorting to plus power supply of, say, 5 V. If patient resistance were 10 kΩ, 500 μA would flow, if it were not for the series protection resistors. If these resistors were on the chip, and the one fault occurred on the left side of a resistor to +5-V power supply, then 500 μA would flow through the patient. This is not permitted. Off-chip resistors qualify as a separate fault condition. Therefore, series protection resistors should not be part of the monolithic semiconductor ECG front end shown in Figure 8-12. The only alternative is to make the clamp voltage so low that <50 μA would flow, should one fault occur on the integrated circuit. It would have to be 25 mV to limit current if patient electrode impedance were 500 Ω. This is less than a one-diode drop (700 mV), which means the clamp

will never turn on. So it may not be practical to put resistors on the chip after all.

Another part of the circuit in Figure 8-12 is the Wilson network, which is a passive resistor array that is used in deriving the six basic leads (I, II, III, aVR, aVL, and aVF). The tap points shown drive the bank of six differential input amplifiers each set to a gain of, say, 5 or 10 V/V. Gain must be low to prevent electrode offset voltage from saturating the amplifiers. Each diff-amp amplifies a tap or combinations of taps with respect to another tap, as shown. For example, lead I from the top diff-amp has left arm (LA) on its + input and right arm (RA) on its − input. Lead I, therefore, is (LA − RA). Other leads are derived similarly, as shown. The output leads are ECG signals that have the 60-Hz noise greatly reduced. How does the circuit do this? The diff-amps remove it,

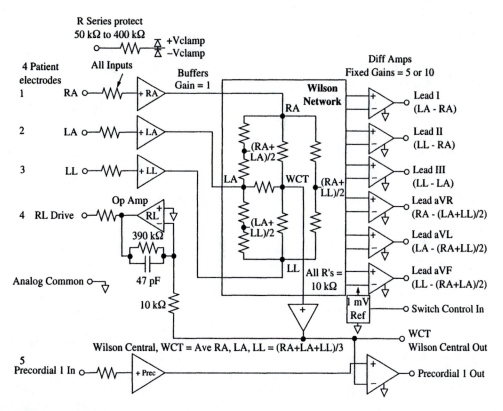

Figure 8-12
Five-patient electrode (6-lead) ECG front end.

because equal CM noise is present on each input of each diff-amp. The diff-amp just subtracts the equal noise voltage to give nearly zero while amplifying the difference in the unequal ECG signals (from different body locations) present on its inputs.

The Wilson central represents ECG zero and common-mode interference. It is derived from patient electrodes RA, LA, and LL and is actually the average of these (sum divided by 3). This is equal to the dc and 60-Hz common-mode voltage. The ECG signal from the Einthoven triangle is presumed to sum to zero. Of course, the right-leg drive is the inversion of the common-mode interference. The gain of the right-leg driver, RL, is usually set at around 30 to 50 V/V, but it could be higher. Actually, the higher the better, but care

must be taken to ensure that the RL driver does not saturate. The 47-pF capacitor in the feedback loop limits the high-frequency gain and helps to prevent oscillation. How can oscillation occur? It breaks out if the patient's stray capacitance is such that the CM phase shift is enough to flip the total phase 180 degrees around what was a negative RL-drive feedback loop. When this takes place, positive feedback occurs, and high frequency may appear on the ECG signal. The Wilson central is shown as a buffered output in Figure 8-12 because it is used as one input to precordial diff-amps for removing 60-Hz interference. Phase shift through this buffer should be kept low.

No ECG front end would be complete without a 1-mV reference. The circuit shown in Figure 8-12 has a 1-mV reference connected to the input of the diff-amps. On manual switch or computer software command, this reference will be applied and appear on all output leads.

ECG systems often use the *QRS* configuration (left ventricular contraction) and pacer pulse (artificial pacemaker) detectors. Figure 8-13 shows a block diagram of such a circuit. Any of the six derived ECG leads or any of the precordial signals can be used. Sometimes by examination, the best one is chosen and used. The *QRS* configuration detector is really just a differentiator. It measures how fast the ECG waveform is rising. If it is faster than, say, the *P*-wave but slower than, say, a pacer pulse, the circuit outputs a voltage transition to indicate that the *QRS* was present. The pacer pulse detector is also a differentiator set to detect faster-moving voltages. It outputs a voltage transition when the pacer pulse comes along during the ECG waveform. Actually, the pacer pulse is removed before further amplification is undertaken and is reinstalled when the ECG signal is displayed. Amplitude accuracy is not necessary, because the pacer pulse is much bigger than the *QRS* complex. However, the time it occurred should be detected accurately. In Figure 8-13, both the *QRS* complex and pacer pulse detect transitions are applied to comparators to make sure they really occurred. Then through output logic, digital levels indicate the presence of the respective signal. It is often very difficult to detect these signals correctly, because high noise may be present as well as ECG abnormalities like large *T*-waves or even muscle artifacts. *AAMI Standard for Cardiac Monitors, Heart Rate Meters and Alarms, EC13,* June, 1983, *Revised* June, 1991, sets forth the amount of detection precision that is required.

How much circuitry is involved in a 10-patient electrode (12-lead) ECG system? Figure 8-14 shows the block diagram. Notice that the four top patient electrodes involve buffers, Wilson network, and output diff-amps as described previously. The Wilson central, derived from the average of RA, LA, and LL signals, supplies a voltage to the negative inputs of the lower bank of six diff-amps set to a gain of 10. This acts to differentially cancel out the 60-Hz noise in the precordial signals. The upper bank of diff-amps remove 60-Hz noise and produce the six standard ECG leads, I, II, III, aVR, aVL, and aVF. These leads are applied to an analog multiplexer and selected one at a time for the *QRS* and pacer pulse detectors. They are also fed to a bank of 60-Hz notch filters, which can be switched in or out. Remember, notches remove residual 60-Hz noise but can cause phase shifts that disturb the normal ECG signal. That is why provisions for switching them out should be made.

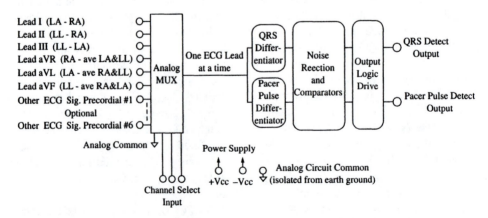

Figure 8-13
QRS complex and pacer pulse detector block diagram.

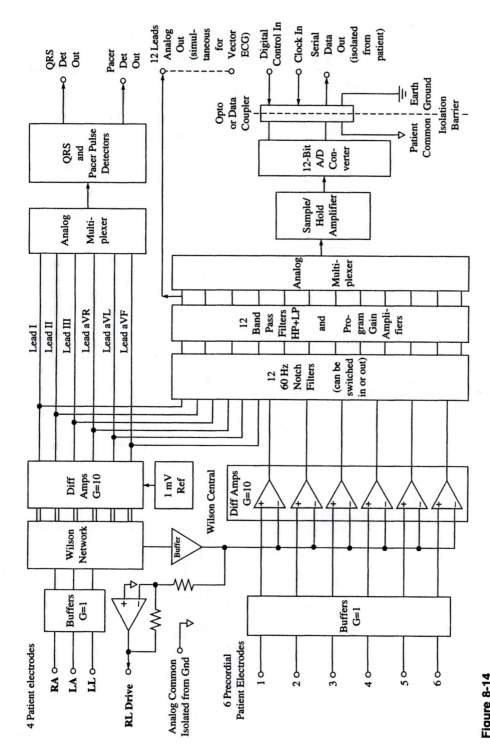

Figure 8-14
Ten-patient electrode (12-lead) ECG block diagram.

213

The buffered precordial signals are also fed to the notch filters in Figure 8-14. Following the notches is a bank of 12 band-pass filters composed of high pass and low pass. The high-pass filters are selectable for 0.05 Hz (diagnostic quality ECG), 0.5 Hz (monitoring), and 2 Hz (quick dc restore). If just one high-pass filter were used, there would be a long time constant for it to charge to the new offset potential of a newly selected lead. Following the high-pass filters are programmable-gain amplifiers selectable for gains of 10, 20, 50, and 100 V/V. Then come low-pass filters, selectable to roll off at 40, 100, 150, and perhaps 3000 Hz. The bandpass filtered, amplified ECG signal is then applied to an S/H amplifierECG signal is then applied to an S/H amplifier that holds the ECG signal constant for the A/D conversion time period. The serial data output from the A/D can be optically coupled for isolation to the computer. Also,

the analog output from several of the 12 ECG signals can be simultaneously used for vector ECG. During transition between leads, the 1-mV reference can be switched in for calibration. The preceding discussion basically shows how a modern ECG system is constructed. New electronics available in the industry make the performance better and better with each passing year.

The diagrams in Figures 8-15 through 8-18 show trends in physiological monitoring, especially in ECG systems. The most significant change emerging is high-resolution digitization. Figure 8-15 shows the older approach, although it will still be used for some years to come. Basically, the ECG signal has to be digitized to the 10-bit to 12-bit level. That is, the resolution is one step out of 2^{10} or 1024 total steps. Each step is 0.1% of the total ($1/2^{10} \times 100\%$.) If the differential ECG input signal is 1 mV peak to peak, then

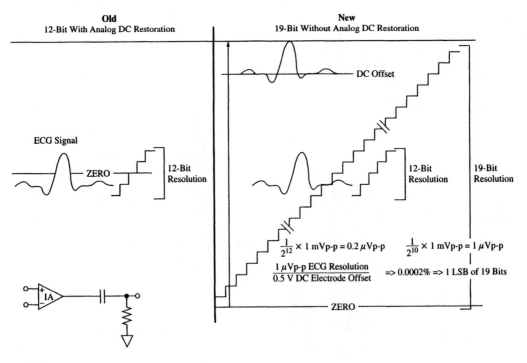

Figure 8-15
Digitization trend in physiological monitoring.

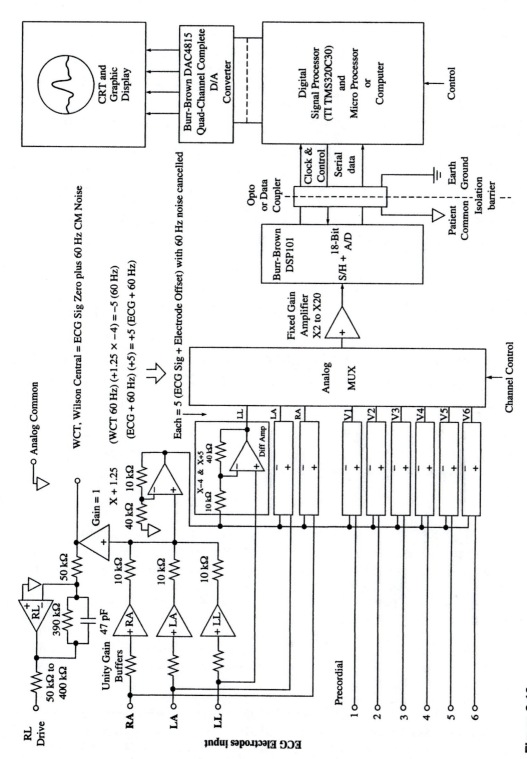

Figure 8-16
ECG system with high-resolution digitization.

215

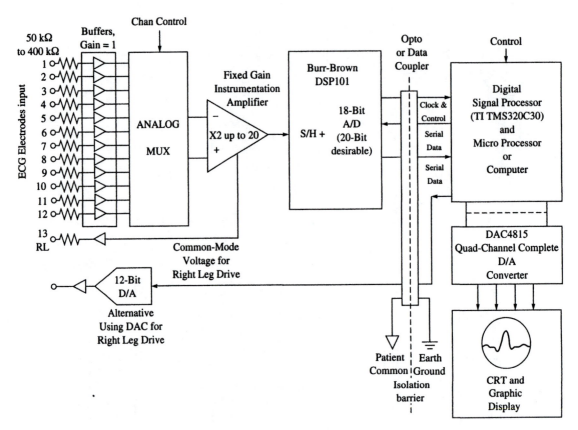

Figure 8-17
ECG system with high-resolution high-speed digitization: a possibility.

one step must be 1 μV peak to peak, if it is digitized to 10 bits. This means that the input analog amplifiers must have noise that is somewhat lower, say 0.9 μV peak to peak. Since the rms noise is statistically about six times lower, the total rms noise of the input amplifiers in the 100-Hz ECG bandwidth must be about 0.15 μV rms. That is small but achievable with commercially available components.

The one difficulty in all this is the high gain required to get the ECG signal to a reasonable level, such as 1 V peak to peak. As discussed earlier, electrode dc offset potentials must be removed or dc restored to zero before such high gain can be

used. Figure 8-15 shows that 12-bit digitization can be done when analog hardware dc restoration is used. However, the trend is toward forgoing hardware dc restoration and using a high-resolution digitization as shown on the right. Here the 1-mV (or even as small as 0.25-mV) ECG signal rides on a 300-mV (or even as big as 500-mV) electrode offset. How many bits of resolution are necessary to do the job under the worse-case condition? The answer is around 19 bits. Remember, the smallest ECG signal step for 10 bits on 1 mV is about 1 μV and this is the least significant bit (LSB). Therefore, 1-μV ECG step/500 mV dc offset equals 0.0002%. This means that there must be

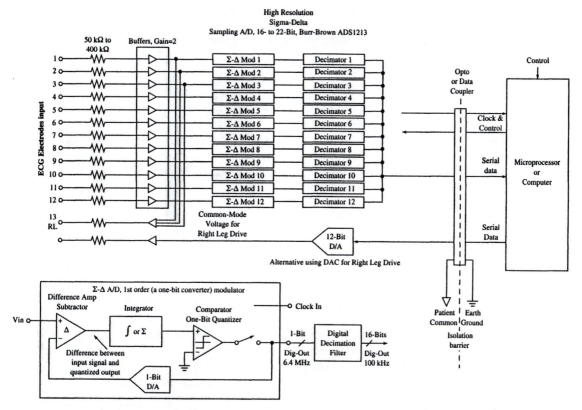

Figure 8-18
ECG system with high-resolution digitization per channel: a possibility.

500,000 steps (1/0.000002). The nearest digital count is 19 bits, which is 2^{19} or 524,000 steps.

Some designers are even trying for 22 bits. The high-resolution digitization shown in Figure 8-15 allows, say, a 1-mV ECG signal to be digitized to 10 to 12 bits while riding on a 500-mV electrode offset voltage. Once in the computer, the offset can be removed by the software, and the ECG signal can be analyzed. This technique makes the analog front end simpler, although it places heavy demands on the A/D converter. This approach is used in industrial DASs also. One clear advantage is that no hardware dc restorer or high-pass filter bank is necessary. Digital offset subtraction and digital filtering take the place of hardware. There

are no electronic high-pass filters with low cutoff frequencies that have long time constants. Therefore, one can switch from one channel to another without having to wait for the filter to charge to a new offset value.

How can this high-resolution digitization be implemented with commercially available components? Figure 8-16 shows an ECG system with 18-bit resolution. Notice how simple the analog front end is. It takes just three buffers, RA, LA, LL, a Wilson central resistor network, an amplifier with a gain of -1.25, and a bank of diff-amps to remove 60-Hz CM noise. The reason for this is clear when one examines how the RA, LA, LL, and V_1 through V_6 ECG signals are amplified. The object is to amplify these signals of interest while rejecting the 60-Hz noise interference. The bank of nine very simple diff-amps does the job. The Wilson central 60-Hz CM noise times $+1.25$ V/V is gained up by -4 V/V to make it an inverted gain of -5 V/V at the output of the diff-amps. The signal with original phase 60 Hz riding on it is also gained up by $+5$ V/V ($1 + 40$ kΩ/10 kΩ) when it goes through the simple diff-amp. Hence, the original phase 60-Hz and inverted phase 60-Hz noise is cancelled at the diff-amp's output. Then all ECG signals are amplified by a factor of 5 V/V with CM noise greatly reduced at the diff-amp's output. Through a CM multiplexer (mux) these signals can be further gained up by 2 V/V or perhaps as high as 20 V/V. The patient electrode offset potential, however, has not been removed. Hence the ECG signals plus electrode offset will be digitized by the high-resolution A/D.

The commercially available integrated circuit A/D converter shown in Figure 8-16 has an internal S/H amplifier, an 18-bit A/D converter, and glue logic to make it easily interfaceable to a digital signal processor (DSP). Its serial output, representing ECG signals riding on electrode offset voltages, is isolated through an opto or isolated data coupler and presented to the DSP and computer. The ECG waveforms, after software has removed electrode offset, can be analyzed by the computer. ECG signals can be reconstructed into analog again through the commercially available quad-channel digital-to-analog (D/A) converter shown. The analog ECG signal can be presented on a CRT or strip-chart recorder.

Since we are on the subject of high-resolution digitization, it would be interesting to discuss some future possibilities. Commercially available components are hard to come by to accomplish these system requirements. The block diagram shown in Figure 8-17 depicts the simplest analog hardware front end of all. It is just unity gain buffers. Through the analog mux, these voltages, representing ECG electrode signals, can be amplified in a fixed-gain amplifier by a factor of 2 up to 20 V/V. The signals could be digitized by a high-resolution, high-speed sampling A/D converter and then fed to a microprocessor through opto isolation. If the A/D were fast enough, the 60-Hz noise interference could be digitized instantaneously along with the ECG signal. The software could then remove dc electrode offsets and 60-Hz noise and derive all the leads. If the system were fast enough, it could even provide an analog signal through a D/A converter for the right-leg drive. Of course, right-leg drive could be done in hardware without looping through the computer.

This is all somewhat hypothetical, since low cost, super-speed, super-high-resolution converters are not readily available. However, it is interesting to contemplate such a marvelous DAS.

The last futuristic ECG system, shown in Figure 8-18, might be a little closer to realization. It uses simple analog circuitry for the front end, followed by a bank of high resolution sigma-delta A/D converters (sometimes called delta-sigma converters), one for each channel. The sigma-delta converter is really a one-bit digitizer that samples at a very high rate. The output is then decimated to reduce the data. *Sigma-delta* means that summing (integration) and difference take place. One input is the analog signal, and the other is a feedback signal from the quantizer output of the integrator circuit. The object is to force the D/A output to equal the input signal level. The digital word, necessary to do this, is the sigma-delta A/D output. By going around the loop many times, the converter accumulates counts. The decimation filter produces the final digital word. This technique heavily oversamples the input analog signal; therefore, the input antialiasing filter can be very simple. No brick wall or sharp cutoff filters are necessary. The digital output from each A/D can be digitally multiplexed into an opto coupler and then into the microprocessor.

Sigma-delta A/D and D/A converters are becoming very popular today, not just for ECG systems but for EEG systems as well. If the A/Ds in Figure 8-18 become less expensive and perhaps compact, with several in one package, then this scheme could become reality.

8-8 ECG readout devices

Two forms of ECG readout device are commonly employed: oscilloscopes and stripchart recorders.

Medical oscilloscopes are very much like any other cathode ray oscilloscope (CRO), except that the vertical amplifier bandwidth is severely limited, and the CRT *persistence* is very long. Most oscilloscopes made for ECG display use a horizontal sweep speed of 25 mm/s, while some also offer speeds of 50 mm/s and 100 mm/s.

Medical strip-chart recorders offer the same speeds; the 25-mm/s speed is standard, while the others are optional. Medical chart recorders may also offer 1 mm/s or 5 mm/s if they are to be used to make *trend* recordings of the arterial blood pressure waveform (Chapter 9).

Standard ECG paper (Figure 8-19) has a grid pattern that is 50 mm wide. The small grid divisions are 1 mm apart, while the large grid divisions are 5 mm apart. These lines are used for making time and voltage measurements on the waveform. The vertical scale is calibrated at 0.1 mV/mm (i.e., 1 mV represented by two large divisions).

At 25 mm/s, the standard paper speed, the time interval between two small lines is 0.04 s (40 ms), and between two heavy lines it is 0.2 s (200 ms). The time intervals normally measured on the ECG waveform are shown in Figure 8-1*a*.

Heart rate in beats per minute can be measured on ECG paper because the rate *(frequency)* is the reciprocal of the *period,* which is measured on the

recording using the aforementioned time intervals. Some ECG paper will have 3- or 6-s marks printed on the top margin, and on any paper 3-, 6-, or 10-s intervals can be selected by counting heavy lines. Several methods for measuring the patient's heart rate are given next. Remember, however, that these are *sampling* methods that are only valid on patients with a regular heart rate (i.e., a constant *R* to *R* interval.)

1. Count the number of *R* waves in 3 s (15 large divisions) and multiply by 20.

2. Count the number of *R* waves in 6 s (30 large divisions) and multiply by 10.

3. Count the number of *R* waves in 10 s (50 large divisions) and multiply by 6.

4. Measure the time *(t)* between two *R* waves, and divide 1500 by that number.

5. Use a millimeter ruler, or count the small divisions, to measure the distance between two adjacent *R* waves. Find the heart rate on the standard chart (usually supplied free by medical suppliers, sales representatives, and pharmaceutical representatives).

6. Use a *heart rate ruler* (usually given away free by medical suppliers' sales representatives).

Some medical oscilloscopes use triggered sweep; the sweep cycle is initiated by the occurrence of an *R* wave. In those oscilloscopes, it is possible to read heart rate accurately by noting the distance between the left edge of the screen and the position of the first visible *R* wave. Tektronix prints a heart rate scale on the upper margin of the screen to facilitate this measurement.

8-9 ECG machines

8-9-1 A typical ECG machine

A number of ECG machines are available today. At one time, single-channel portable and roll-aroundmodels predominated. Today, most ma-

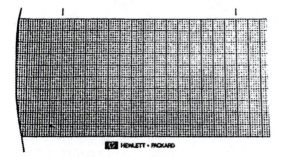

Figure 8-19
Standard ECG paper. (Photo reprinted courtesy Hewlett-Packard.)

chines sold are multichannel devices, such as the one in Figure 8-20. Regardless of the specific configuration, however, there are certain elements common to all regular ECG machines.

The block diagram for a typical ECG machine is shown in Figure 8-21a. The electronics section is an ECG preamplifier (see Section 8-6) and a power amplifier to drive the pen assembly, or *galvanometer.*

A galvanometer is a *permanent magnet moving coil* (PMMC) assembly (Figure 8-21b) that is similar in operation to the D'Arsonval meter movement.

A small bobbin wound with many turns of wire is mounted on a jewel bearing in the field of

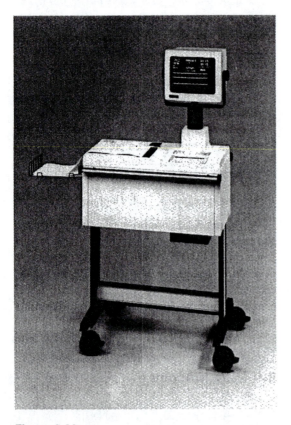

Figure 8-20
Portable ECG machine. (Reprinted courtesy Hewlett-Packard.)

a permanent magnet. The writing pen is mounted, like a meter pointer, to the moving coil.

The PMMC assembly is constructed so that the pen will be at rest in the center of its travel when no current flows in the coil, but the pen will *deflect* in one direction when a current flows in the coil; the *direction* of the pen deflection is determined by the *polarity* of the current in the coil, while the *amount* of deflection is determined by the *amplitude* of the current. The deflection is caused by the tiny magnetic field generated by the coil current interacting with the field of the permanent magnet.

Several different writing methods are used in strip-chart recorders, but most ECG recorders use *hot-tip,* or *thermal,* writing. The writing tip is not a pen but a *stylus* heated by a *resistance wire.* Early recorders fashioned the tip of the stylus from the heater wire, while most modern types place the heater inside a hollow cylindrical metal tube.

The paper used in thermal recorders is specially treated so that it turns black when heated. The hot tip of the stylus, then, will turn the paper black wherever it touches, thus recording the analog waveform applied to the galvanometer.

Very few ECG recorders actually use pens and pressurized ink to make the recording, and most of those that do use ink are in research applications.

The mechanical part of the ECG machine is also shown in Figure 8-21a. Not surprisingly, the mechanics cause the largest share of faults in most models.

The ECG recording paper comes in either roll or Z-fold (folded flat) and is stored in a compartment just below the paper tray. A button release is usually found along one edge of the tray and allows the tray to swing up to give access to the paper storage compartment.

The paper is passed over the *writing edge* and the *paper tray* and between the drive roller and idler roller. Two forces act on the paper, and both are essential to the proper operation of the machine: a *forward* tension, provided by the drive/idler roller assembly, and a *reverse* tension. These

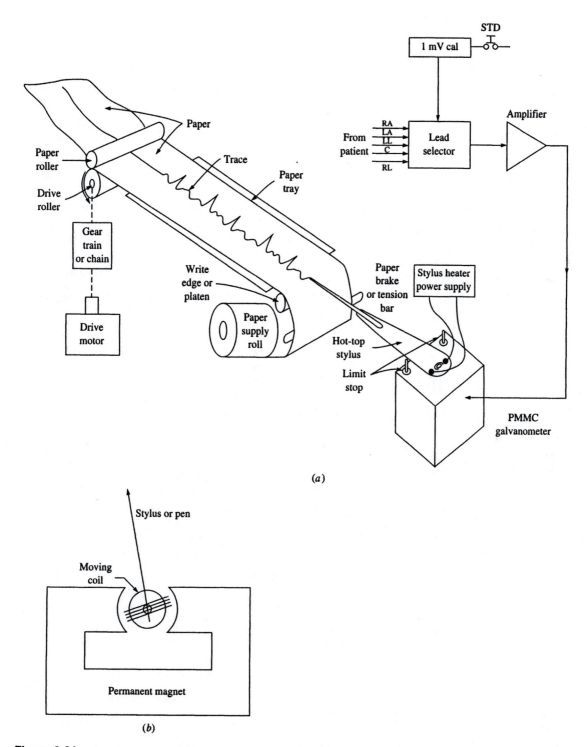

Figure 8-21
ECG machine mechanism. (*a*) Block diagram. (*b*) PMMC galvanometer. (Reprinted courtesy of Hewlett-Packard)

forces act together to stretch the paper taut across the writing edge.

The reverse force is weaker than the forward force and may be provided in any of several ways. In some machines a *paper brake* is used, while in others *tension bars* or *tension rollers* are used. These structures are located between the paper supply and the writing edge.

The writing (knife) edge in the thermal recorder is essential to producing an undistorted recording. The tip of a pen or stylus travels in an *arc,* so fast-rise-time waveforms such as a square-wave or an ECG *R* wave will appear to be curved, or, as an ECG machine user is likely to claim, "It writes backwards." But in ECG recorders using a thermal stylus, the trace is made on the write edge and will appear *rectilinear,* as opposed to *curvilinear,* which is how noncorrected traces would appear. This type of recording is not truly rectilinear but is known as a *pseudorectilinear* recording. The secret to the pseudorectilinear recorder is that different portions of the stylus touch the paper over the write edge in different portions of the paper.

The motor is connected to the drive roller through either a drive chain or a gear train. Most machines use ac motors, with tapped windings to select drive speed. Some ac motors provide very accurate drive speeds that are synchronized to the ac power main's frequency—60 Hz in the United States.

Only a few models use dc motors, and those regulate speed by using a regulated dc power supply, and in some cases an alternator/tachometer on the motor shaft to provide negative feedback.

A large number of modern ECG recorders are based on the same principle as the dot-matrix printer used with computers. Even a 27-pin printer can make good-quality recordings of the waveform and print out numerical data, such as heart rate, patient ID number, date, time, and numerical data from other sensors (e.g., blood pressure, temperature). These recorders will be discussed more fully when we discuss mechanical recorders.

8-9-2 Multichannel machines

Some hospitals use multichannel ECG machines to make diagnostic recordings or in the exercise ECG laboratory. The example shown in Figure 8-22 is the Hewlett-Packard Model 1505A. This machine examines three of the 12 leads at a time and automatically sequences through four groups of three leads each until the entire set of 12 leads are displayed. Each group is displayed on the paper for several seconds.

A few multichannel models are equipped with a transmitter device that converts the analog waveform and digitally encoded numerical data, such as the date, time, and patient ID number, to audio tones that can be sent to a central station in another part of the hospital or even to another hospital. Tone-encoded systems allow a tentative diagnosis to be made by computer, followed by a manual reading by a trained physician.

The analog or digital-to-audio converter that allows communication of the analog ECG data to audio tones for transmission over phone lines is called a *modulator-demodulator,* although its acronym, MODEM, is sufficiently widespread that it is considered a noun in its own right (*modem* instead of *MODEM*). (Just as *laser* and *radar* became nouns, the computer culture is making *modem* a noun.) The modem allows thephysician to transmit the ECG signal to either a physician with superior knowledge of ECG reading or to a central computer, where one of several validated diagnostic programs will evaluate it. Indeed, some of the computer diagnostics are superior to the abilities of most physicians, except those specially trained in electrocardiography. At one time, the modem-equipped ECG machines were rare and expensive, but currently it is possible to obtain portable ECG instruments with a modem option at only slightly higher cost than stand-alone machines.

8-9-3 Stress-testing ECG

Some potentially dangerous cardiac arrhythmias and other anomalies show up only under stress

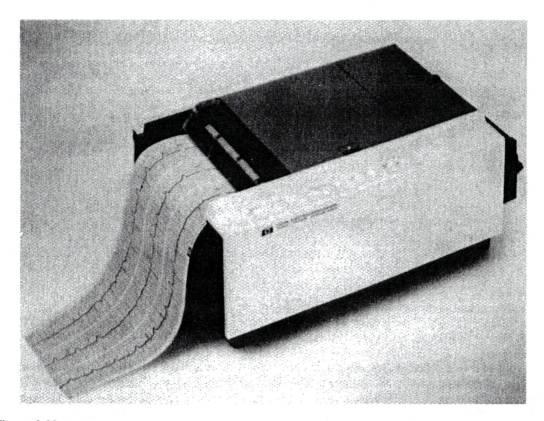

Figure 8-22
Hewlett-Packard Model 1505A automatic three-channel electrocardiograph. (Photo courtesy of
Hewlett-Packard)

conditions. Physicians examine the stress condition by placing the patient on a treadmill or stairstepper while monitoring the patient's ECG waveform on both an oscilloscope monitor and a paper chart recorder (Figure 8-20). Modern stress-testing ECG machines are usually equipped with a microcomputer that analyzes the waveform and highlights specific arrhythmias.

A common method is to perform the stress test, recording the ECG waveform, and then follow the stress test with a thallium scan. The radioactive thallium is taken up by healthy cardiac cells, so areas of the heart where blood flow is insufficient appear darker on a gamma camera display than healthy areas. These two tests allow the physician to evaluate the existence, location, and extent of cardiac disease.

8-9-4 Patient cables

In one respect, the patient cable (Figure 8-23) is the most important part of the system; it is most frequently at fault when the machine fails to operate properly.

Several different patient cable configurations are used in ECG recording. Some are constructed of two pieces that plug together (Figure 8-23), while others are one piece. Two-piece units are generally more expensive initially but often prove more economical in the long run because breakage most frequently occurs at the electrode connector end of the cable. This end can be replaced at a cost that is somewhat lower than the cost of a one-piece cable. Additionally, a two-piece cable allows the

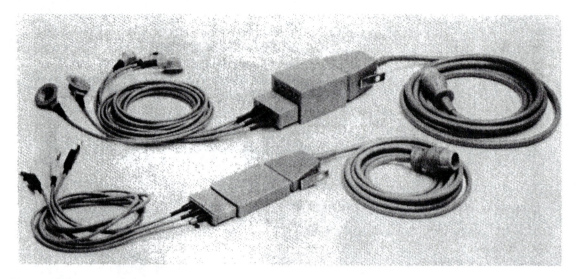

Figure 8-23
ECG patient cables. (Photo courtesy of Hewlett-Packard)

use of different types of electrodes. A single main cable (i.e., the machine end) and several adapters allow for the different electrode types.

There are three basic types of electrode connectors on the patient end, and these occur in various configurations; some are unique to one manufacturer's electrodes.

A *tip-end* cable is used to connect temporary, or short-term, electrodes, such as the plate or suction cup. These are available with standard *banana plug* ends or a special end that closely resembles a slightly oversized telephone tip plug (i.e., *pin tip*).

Another type of cable (the upper cable in Figure 8-23) has a silver-silver chloride cup electrode already attached. The cup is filled with electrode jelly every time that it is used and is secured to the patient's skin with adhesive tape or with adhesive patches intended specifically for this application.

The last type of cable uses a special *clip,* or *buttonsnap,* fastener that connects to the standard monitoring electrode. This is the type of cable most often used in intensive or cardiac care unit monitoring.

Notice in Figure 8-23 that one of the cables has five patient electrode leaders, while the other has only three leads. A cable for a diagnostic machine would need all five electrodes to record all 12 leads, but in monitoring, often only the existence of the ECG and certain gross arrhythmias are required, and these can be obtained through any lead. For those cases, a three-electrode cable is sufficient. In most cases, the three-electrode system is configured to produce lead I, although the nurse or physician can select any lead by proper electrode placement.

The upper cable in Figure 8-23 has a large block between the two halves of the cable. This device is a special *filter* to reduce the effects of *electrosurgery* equipment; that is, high-power rf generators. The filter is optional, and if not used, the two halves of the cable simply plug together as in the other cable shown.

Most ECG cables are made of shielded wire, so an ohmmeter connected between each electrode connector and the appropriate terminal on the main plug will read a short circuit. But some cables have a 1- to 10-kΩ resistor in series with each electrode to provide defibrillator protection. These resistors are usually located inside the molded plastic connector that joins the two halves of the cable on the machine end.

There is no universal standard ECG input plug, and machines by the same manufacturer may have different input connectors. The plug shown on the cables in Figure 8-23, however, is the most widely encountered. Several companies claim credit for developing this plug, but most people seem to call it the *Sanborn* configuration after the company that popularized and possibly invented it. Sanborn was bought by, and became the medical division of, Hewlett-Packard some years ago.

The semistandard Sanborn plug uses a five-pin, size 14, AN/MS military plug. Table 8-1 shows the pinouts for the plug and the color code used to identify the electrode leaders.

8-10 ECG machine maintenance

The typical hospital ECG machine is a rugged instrument and must be reliable under very difficult circumstances. In many hospitals the machines receive little care from operating personnel, but many hospitals now delegate an ECG technician or biomedical equipment technician to periodically inspect and perform minor repairs to the ECG machines.

A reasonable procedure for daily or weekly operational checks is as follows:

1. Turn machine on and allow it to warm up for a minute or so (longer on vacuum-tube models).

2. Place the *function* switch in RUN and the *lead selector* switch in STD. Observe whether a trace is present.

3. Press the *1-mV cal* button several times. Take note of (a) whether vertical edges of the pulse are visible and (b) whether the *sensitivity* control can be adjusted to provide at least 10 mm of deflection. (c) Is the pulse reasonably square?

4. Adjust the *position* control through its entire range and note whether the stylus travels to the limits or stops at the top and bottom margins of the paper.

5. Short together all electrode connectors at the patient end of the cable, and then turn the *lead selector* switch through all 12 positions. You should see a quiet, stable baseline on the paper in all positions of the switch. This test allows you to spot an open wire in the cable. If you note which leads are not "quiet," then you can determine which wire in the cable is open by noting which electrode is uniquely common to all affected leads.

6. Adjust the *sensitivity* for exactly 10-mm deflection when the *lead selector* is in STD and the *1-mV cal* button is pressed.

7. Press and *hold* the *1-mV cal* button. The stylus should deflect 10 mm and then slowly drop back to its original position (Figure 8-24). The decay rate should be

TABLE 8-1 STANDARD CABLE COLOR CODE AND CONNECTOR PINOUTS

AN/MS Plug pins	Goes to	Electrode color code
A	RA	White
B	LA	Black
C	LL	Red
D	C	Brown
E	RL	Green

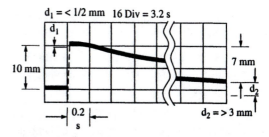

Figure 8-24
Self-check decay curve. (Reprinted courtesy of Hewlett-Packard)

slower than 7 mm in 16 large divisions (i.e., 3.2 s). This checks the *low-frequency response* of the machine.

ECG machine manufacturers may specify a more elaborate procedure for half-yearly or yearly checks, but the foregoing procedure will allow you to locate and correct the most commonly found faults, and it can be performed in only a few minutes per machine.

Additional safety inspections involving electrical leakage to the patient from the power mains are also specified.

8-11 ECG faults and troubleshooting

Internal electrical or mechanical faults occur only occasionally in ECG machines, yet incidents of malfunction occur often enough that many hospital personnel become convinced that ECG machines "are always on the blink." In most cases, however, the malfunction is an operator error or can be corrected by a simple adjustment or repair. The problems discussed in the following examples are common enough to occur daily in many large hospitals.

Example 8-1

Symptom: Machine runs, but the thermal-tip stylus does not write or writes very lightly.

Possible Causes: (1) Too little heat on the stylus tip and (2) insufficient stylus pressure on the paper.

Troubleshooting (machine running):

1. Using an insulated probe, such as a screwdriver, gently press the stylus onto the paper.

2. If a dark line appears on the paper, the problem is too little pressure, but if no dark line appears, the problem is not enough heat.

(Note: Some people use their finger to quickly touch the stylus to see if there is plenty of heat, but this is potentially painful. If the heat is sufficient to write on the paper, then it is also sufficient to cause second-degree burns.)

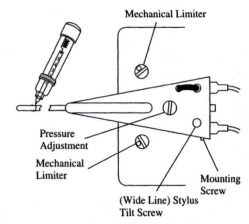

a. Calibrate stylus pressure tester by holding vertically at eye level with 2-g calibration cap on hook, slide knurled ring to read 2 g.

b. Measure stylus pressure by hooking tester under writing arm tip near where it makes contact with the paper. Read gauge just as stylus loses contact with paper.

Figure 8-25
Measuring stylus pressure. (Reprinted courtesy of Hewlett-Packard)

Solutions

1. For no heat, check the heater voltage at the stylus wires. If the voltage is correct, then change the stylus. If the voltage is not correct, then refer to the service manual for troubleshooting.

2. Adjust the stylus pressure (Figure 8-25). DO NOT GUESS at the proper pressure, as different models may require between 2 and 20 g. Use a stylus pressure gauge and refer to the manufacturer's service manual for the correct value. On some models, the pressure must be made at a specific heater voltage.

Example 8-2

Symptom: Smeared trace (Figure 8-26*a*).
Possible Causes: Worn stylus or incorrectly loaded paper.

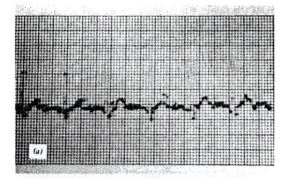

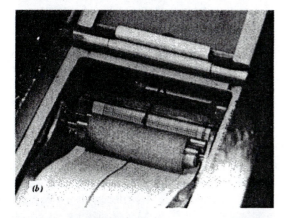

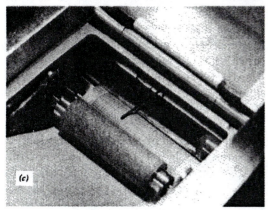

Figure 8-26
(a) Smeared trace. *(b)* Paper correctly loaded. *(c)* Paper incorrectly loaded.

Troubleshooting: Check paper loading and, if proper, check stylus for wear, pitting, or other irregularities.

Discussion: Incorrectly loaded paper is one of the most common faults, and in most cases the error resulted from bypassing the paper brake or tension bars (see Figures 8-26*b* and 8-26*c*).

Example 8-3 _____

Symptom: Poor recording.

Possible Causes: Electronic or mechanical problems, bad lead switch or input connector, bad patient cable, or improper connection to patient.

Troubleshooting

1. Place *lead selector* switch in STD, short all electrodes together, and press the *1-mV cal* button.

2. If normal calibration pulses appear, then the problem is the connection to the patient.

3. If problem persists, repeat step 1 using a patient cable that is known to be functional or a *deadhead plug* (i.e., ECG connector with all pins shorted together). If the problem clears up, then replace the bad patient cable, but if it persists, the fault is inside the machine. Refer to the service manual for troubleshooting.

The approximately 1-mV ECG biopotential must be recorded in a hostile environment; 60-Hz interference may exist, in addition to muscle potentials and other bioelectric artifacts. Figure 8-27 shows four common artifacts encountered in ECG recordings.

Figure 8-27*a* shows 60-Hz interference from nearby power mains. Ordinarily, the 60-Hz signals induced into the electrode wires form a CM signal because all electrodes and wires are affected equally; these signals usually do not interfere because the ECG preamplifier has differential inputs. But electrode defects, open patient cable wires, or poor contact to the patient result in an unbalanced input to the preamplifier and will thereby manufacture a differential signal from the CM 60-Hz signal.

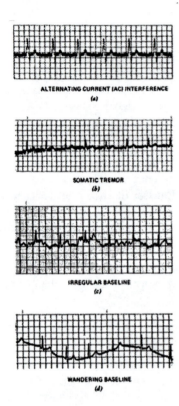

Figure 8-27
ECG recording irregularities. (*a*) Alternating current
(ac) interference. (*b*) Somatic tremor. (*c*) Irregular
baseline. (*d*) Wandering baseline. (Reprinted courtesy of Hewlett-Packard)

This type of interference often results from a
lack of electrode jelly or loose contact to the patient. This problem is especially prevalent on patients with moist or sweaty skin.

Another cause of 60-Hz interference is a loose
or broken power mains ground on the ECG machine, or certain other instruments that may be
connected to the patient. Additionally, certain dc-
power supply problems (i.e., an open filter or
shorted voltage regulator) produce a similar artifact from 120-Hz ripple from the rectifiers.

The problem can be isolated by shorting together all electrodes of the patient cable and then
checking each position of the *lead selector*
switch.

1. If the interference ceases, then the problem is a
   bad electrode, no electrolytic jelly, poor skin
   preparation, and so forth.

2. If the interference exists on all positions of the
   lead selector switch, then the problem is
   probably internal to the machine.

3. If the problem exists only in certain lead
   positions of the selector switch, then suspect an
   open wire in the patient cable. Use an
   ohmmeter or conductance checker, or analyze
   the situation to determine which electrode is
   uniquely common to the affected leads.

Muscle jitter, also called *somatic tremor,* is
shown in Figure 8-27*b*. It is distinguishable from
60-Hz interference by its lack of regularity in both
amplitude and *frequency* components and is
caused by muscle bioelectric potential.

In some cases the symptoms can be eliminated
by having the patient lie still, but if the patient has
a tremor, or is being monitored on a long-term basis, then electronic *filtering* must be used. Most
bedside monitors are designed with a frequency
response of only 30 to 50 Hz to reduce the effects
of somatic tremor signals.

Figure 8-27*c* shows an irregular baseline, resulting from dirty electrodes caused by dried jelly
on the surface or metal particles on the patient's
skin, for example. Both are cured by cleaning, in
the former case of the electrodes and in the latter
of the skin.

The wandering baseline in Figure 8-27*d* is almost always caused by movement of the electrode
with respect to the surface of the skin. In theory,
there are also electronic problems that could cause
this problem, but these are very rarely encountered. In most cases, the wandering baseline is
caused by changes in electrode contact impedance
creating a varying electrode offset potential. Three
reasons for wandering baseline are commonplace:

1. Loose or poorly fitted electrodes (may also
   create a 60-Hz artifact).

2. Patient cable dangling toward the floor, placing
   a tension force on the electrode.

3. Electrode or cable moving with the patient's respiration.

Securing the electrode will cure the first problem, and dressing the cable properly will cure the others.

8-12 Summary

1. The electrocardiograph machine takes 12 leads (I, II, III, aVF, aVR, aVL, and V_1 through V_6) to give the physician different views of the heart's activity.

2. There are three basic lead configurations: *bipolar limb leads* (I through III), *unipolar limb leads* (aVR, aVL, aVF), and *unipolar chest leads* (V_1 through V_6).

3. *Diagnostic* ECG recordings require a bandwidth of 0.05 to 100 Hz; *monitoring* requires a bandwidth of 0.05 to about 40 Hz.

4. An ECG preamplifier is a bioelectric amplifier with a *lead* selector switch, 1-mV calibration source, and defibrillator protection.

5. Five techniques used to reduce 50- to 60-Hz noise in ECG machines include (1) CMR of the instrumentation amplifier, (2) right-leg drive, (3) shield drive, (4) notch filter, and (5) IMR of the isolation amplifier.

6. In a three-patient electrode ECG front end, the +V input of the instrumentation amplifier is connected to the patient's left arm and the −V input is connected to the right arm. The amplifier then subtracts these electrode signals and produces lead I at its output.

7. Three techniques can be used to remove the 300-mV electrode offset potential. These are (1) a series coupling capacitor, (2) a feedback integrator that stores the offset and sums it back into the bioelectric amplifier, and (3) digitization with a high-resolution A/D converter that allows the offset to be removed in software.

8. Front-end electronics must be protected from defibrillation pulses that exceed the breakdown voltage of semiconductor amplifiers. Two stages are often used, the first consisting of series resistors and neon bulbs, and the second of series resistors and clamp diodes.

9. ESU signals create considerable noise at high frequency when they are applied to a patient's body. These get into the front-end electronics of ECG systems and either go directly through the amplifiers or are rectified and filtered by semiconductor junction inside the amplifiers to cause a base line offset. Such interference can be reduced by using multistage πRC or LC filters.

10. A multichannel physiological monitoring system is actually a DAS. It consists of input buffers followed by an analog mux connected to a Wilson network. A PGIA amplifies the derived standard leads and passes them to an A/D converter, the output of which is fed to a microprocessor or larger computer.

11. In a five–patient electrode ECG front end, a bank of differential amplifiers is often used to derive the six standard leads from the Wilson network.

12. It is very challenging for electronic circuits to detect a pacer pulse in the presence of the normal *QRS* complex, 50- to 60-Hz noise, and patient muscle artifacts. The AAMI specifies requirements for ECG machines regarding accuracy detection of the pacer pulse will cause diagnostic problems in patients with implanted or external pacemakers.

13. In a 10–patient electrode ECG system, four electrodes are amplified to derive the standard six leads, with the precordial electrodes being amplified separately. Notch filters may be used to remove 50- to 60-Hz, and bandpass filters are used to limit the ECG signal to standard bandwidths. A sampling A/D converter then digitizes the ECG signal and is

applied to a computer across an opto or data coupler.

14. Some modern ECG systems now use a high-resolution A/D converter to digitize 300-mV electrode offset potentials. Once in the computer, offsets can be removed in software. If one A/D converter is used to digitize many electrodes, its speed has to be relatively high along with the high-resolution requirement. If one A/D converter is used per channel, its cost has to be relatively low to keep the system from becoming too costly.

15. Strip-chart recorders and oscilloscopes are used as ECG readout devices. The standard speed is 25 mm/s; some machines also offer 50 mm/s and 100 mm/s.

16. ECG strip-chart recorders must present both forward and reverse tension on the paper so that it is stretched taut across the *write edge*.

8-13 Recapitulation

Now return to the objectives and self-evaluation questions at the beginning of the chapter and see how well you can answer them. If you cannot answer certain questions, place a check mark next to each and review appropriate parts of the text. Next, try to answer the following questions using the same procedure. When you have answered all of the questions, solve the problems.

Questions

1. The ECG waveform is created by _____, generated in the heart spreading throughout the body.

2. The peak amplitude on the ECG waveform is approximately _____ mV.

3. The five electrodes used to make 12-lead ECG recordings are connected to the patient's _____, _____, _____, _____, and _____.

4. The _____ electrode is used as the common terminal in ECG recording.

5. Leads I, II, and III form the _____.

6. Leads I, II, and III are called the _____ limb leads.

7. Leads aVF, aVR, and aVL are called the _____ limb leads or _____ leads.

8. In leads aVF, aVR, and aVL, the signals from two limbs are summed in a resistance network and applied to the _____ input of the preamplifier.

9. Leads V_1 through V_6 are called the _____ leads.

10. State the principal features of an ECG amplifier. How does it differ from a bioelectric amplifier?

11. The frequency response of a diagnostic ECG machine is from 0.05 to _____ Hz.

12. An ECG monitor usually has a frequency response of 0.05 to about _____ Hz.

13. Noise reduction in an ECG system is accomplished by the _____-mode rejection of an instrumentation amplifier, the _____-leg drive, and the _____-mode rejection of an isolation amplifier.

14. In a three-patient electrode front end, a technique used to remove patient electrode offset potential of 300 mV is to place a coupling _____ in series with the signal following the first stage gain, or to put an _____ in the feedback loop of the second stage.

15. An alternative technique for removing patient electrode offset potentials is to digitize it with a _____ resolution _____/_____ converter, which then eliminates it in software.

16. ESU noise can be kept out of front-end ECG electronics by either an _____ C or an _____ C pi filter.

17. Defibrillator protection in the input of bioelectric amplifiers uses _____ lamps, fol-

lowed by series resistors and _____ diodes.

18. The typical multichannel physiological monitoring system includes input _____, mux, _____ network, instrumentation _____, and sampling _____/_____

19. A five–patient electrode ECG front-end can use the _____ central for the right-leg drive, which is the average among the *RA* and *LA*, and _____ and represents _____ zero.

20. Precordial number 1 signal is derived from the first precordial patient _____ subtracted from the _____ central.

21. A pacer pulse detector circuit must discriminate between a _____ complex, 50- to 60-Hz _____, and muscle _____.

22. A 10–patient electrode ECG system can use a bank of differential _____ to derive the standard six _____, called I, II, III, aVF, aVR, and aVL.

23. In a 13–patient electrode ECG system, a _____ resolution _____, _____ speed, _____/_____ converter could be used to quickly scan all channels, thus eliminating considerable front-end circuitry.

24. In a 13–patient electrode ECG system, a multichannel sigma-_____ converter could be used to simultaneously capture all 13 patient electrode signals.

25. The chief artifact rejected by limiting the bandwidth of an ECG monitor is _____.

26. Most ECG preamplifiers have an internal calibrator that injects a _____-mV pulse into the preamplifier input.

27. ECG preamplifiers require protection circuits against electrical potentials from a machine called a _____.

28. A protection device (question 8-17) used in most ECG preamplifiers is a _____ lamp.

29. List two types of damage that can result from the phenomenon in question 8-17.

30. List two types of ECG readout devices.

31. Name (a) standard speed and (b) two optional speeds on an ECG machine.

32. Describe how heart rate is determined on a triggered sweep oscilloscope.

33. Most ECG machines write using a _____ stylus.

34. Both _____ and _____ tensions must be applied to the paper in an ECG recorder to pull it taut across the _____.

35. List three types of electrode connector used in patient cables.

36. Why do some ECG patient cables use resistors in series with each electrode? What is the approximate range of values used for these resistors?

37. List the pinouts of the standard, or nearly standard, ECG connector.

38. Describe how the input circuitry and patient cable may be checked using only the machine itself.

39. What are the probable causes of no-trace conditions on an ECG machine?

40. What is the principal cause of a smeared trace from an ECG machine? What are other possible causes?

41. What are the principal causes of 60-Hz interference?

42. What are the principal causes of erratic baseline recordings?

43. What are the principal causes of wandering baseline?

44. Give the quick method for isolating the cause of 60-Hz interference.

45. What can be done to reduce the effects of somatic tremor in ECG recordings?

46. Give a probable cure for (a) irregular baseline and (b) wandering baseline.

Problems

1. What is the heart rate in beats per minute of a patient with an R to R interval of 856 ms?

2. What is the heart rate of the patients whose ECG is shown in Figure 8-27a? Assume that the recording speed was standard.

Suggested reading

1. Strong, Peter, *Biophysical Measurements,* Measurement Concepts Series, Tektronix, Inc. (Beaverton, Ore., 1977).

2. *Technician's Guide to Electrocardiography,* 3rd ed. Hewlett-Packard applications note (Waltham, Mass., 1972).

3. Rawlings, Charles A., *Electrocardiography,* Spacelabs, Inc. (Redmond, Wash., 1991).

4. Service manual for the H-P model 1500B/1511B (Waltham, Mass., 1971).

5. *ECG Techniques,* Hewlett-Packard applications note AN721 (Waltham, Mass., 1972).

6. *ECG Measurement,* Hewlett-Packard applications note AN711 (Waltham, Mass., 1972).

7. *High Fidelity ECG Measurement,* unnumbered Hewlett-Packard applications note (Waltham, Mass., 1971).

8. Clinica, *World Medical Device and Diagnostic News,* Issue 464, July 31, 1991 (consistent ECGs possible with new standardizer device), 18/20 Hill Rise, Richmond, Surrey TW10 6UA, U.K., Tel: 081-948-3262; or 1775 Broadway, Suite 511, New York, NY 10019, Tel: 212-262-8230; also Dialog Information Services, Inc., 3640 Hillview Ave., Palo Alto, CA 94304, Tel: 1-800-334-2564 or 415-858-3810.

9. *Biomedical Instrumentation and Technology* magazine, January/February, 1991 (and "A BMET Study Program Should Ask Why," "Creating a Quality Measurement System for Clinical Engineering," "Biomedical Information Management for the Next Generation," "The Safe Medical Devices Act of 1989: A Burden on Medical Facilities, Device Manufacturers, and the FDA?"), publication of Association for the Advancement of Medical Instrumentation (AAMI), 3330 Washington Blvd., Suite 400, Arlington, VA 22201, Tel: 703-525-4890.

10. *AAMI News,* Volume 26, Number 5, September-October, 1991 (Information: "Patient Monitors in High Demand"; Standards, government, and European EC activities), publication of Association for the Advancement of Medical Instrumentation (AAMI), 3330 Washington Blvd., Suite 400, Arlington, VA 22201, Tel: 703-525-4890.

11. AAMI 1991 Resource Catalog, Publications & Services, publication of Association for the Advancement of Medical Instrumentation (AAMI), 3330 Washington Blvd., Suite 400, Arlington, VA 22201, Tel: 703-525-4890.

12. ANSI (American National Standards Institute)/AAMI (Association for the Advancement of Medical Instrumentation), *Standard for Cardiac Monitors, Heart Rate Meters, and Alarms,* EC13-June, 1983, Revision—June 1991, 3330 Washington Blvd., Suite 400, Arlington, VA 22201, Tel: 703-525-4890.

13. *Biomedical Technology,* Issue 7 ("Integrating Monitoring: Better Event Detection & Alarm Accuracy?"), 1991, Quest Publishing Company, 1351 Titan Way, Brea, CA 92621, Tel: 714-738-6400.

14. *Biomedical Safety & Standards,* Issue 7 ("Safe Medical Devices Law: Hospitals Must Report Incidents to FDA," "Power Failure

Leads to New Emergency Power Policies"),
1991, Quest Publishing Company, 1351 Titan
Way, Brea, CA 92621, Tel: 714-738-6400.

15. *Occupational Biohazards Affecting Clinical
Engineers & BMETs,* 1989, Quest Publishing
Company, 1351 Titan Way, Brea, CA 92621,
Tel: 714-738-6400.

16. *Hewlett-Packard Journal,* October, 1991,
Hewlett-Packard Company, P.O. Box 51827,
Palo Alto, CA 94303-0724; subscriptions to
editor, *HP Journal,* 3200 Hillview Avenue,
Palo Alto, CA 94304 (Articles on
physiological monitoring: HP Component
Monitoring System: medical expectations for
patient monitors, hardware architecture,
software, parameter module interface;
measuring the ECG signal with a mixed A/D
ASIC; small noninvasive blood pressure
measurement device; patient monitor two-
channel stripchart recorder and human
interface design; globalization tools and
processes, physiological calculation
application, mechanical implementation, an
automated test environment, production and
final test; calculating the real cost of software
defects.)

17. *IEEE Transactions on Biomedical
Engineering,* Vol. BME-20, No. 2, March,
1973 ("60-Hz Interference in
Electrocardiography," James Huhta and John
G. Webster).

18. *IEEE Transactions on Biomedical
Engineering,* Vol. BME-30, No. 1, January,
1983, ("Reduction of Interference Due to
Common Mode Voltage in Biopotential
Amplifiers," Bruce B. Winter and John G.
Webster).

19. *IEEE Transactions on Biomedical
Engineering,* Vol. BME-30, No. 1, January,
1983, ("Driven-Right-Leg Circuit Design,"
Bruce Winter and John G. Webster).

20. *International Medical Device & Diagnostic
Industry,* September/October, 1990 ("Surface
Biomedical Electrode Technology," E.
McAdams).

21. *Spectra,* February, 1991, Laurin Publishing
Co., Inc., Berkshire Common, P.O. Box 4949,
Pittsfield, MA 01202, Tel: 413-499-0514,
Section in Medicine & Surgery. ("The
Evolution of the Endoscope").

22. Henderson Electronic Market Forecast for
Medical Electronics, July, 1990, and August,
1991, Henderson Ventures, 101 First Street,
Suite 444, Los Altos, CA 94022, Tel: 415-
961-2900.

23. Product data sheets for components shown in
this chapter, Burr-Brown Corp., 1997, P.O.
Box 11400, Tucson, AZ 85734, 1-800-548-
6132.

CHAPTER 9
Physiological Pressure and Other Cardiovascular Measurements and Devices

9-1 Objectives

1. Be able to describe how *pressure* is measured.
2. Be able to describe the operation of a *cardiac output computer.*
3. Be able to describe how a cardiac *pacemaker* works.
4. Be able to describe the operation of *defibrillators* and *cardioverters.*

9-2 Self-evaluation questions

These questions test your prior knowledge of the material in this chapter. Look for the answers as you read the text. After you have finished studying the chapter, try answering these questions and those at the end of the chapter.

1. Define *pressure* in your own words.

2. How does *hydrostatic pressure* affect the accuracy of transducer readings?

3. Describethe *auscultation* technique of measuring arterial blood pressure. Describe both the apparatus and the technique.

4. What is a *sphygmomanometer* and how is it used?

5. Describe the proper *placement* of an arterial blood pressure transducer when using an *intracardiac catheter.*

6. A *defibrillator* _____ the heart with an electrical shock so that all cells in the heart can reenter their refractory periods at the same time.

7. What is heart *block?*

8. A _____-_____ catheter may be used directly to measure pressures in the pulmonary artery.

9-3 Physiological pressures

The measurement of physiological *fluid* pressures is of interest to both biomedical researchers and medical clinicians. Given a rigorous definition of *fluid,* we would have to include both *liquids* and *gases,* but in this chapter our discussions center around liquids. The difference between liquids and gases is that the latter are *compressible,* while the former are not; compressibility affects the measurement technique. Gas pressure measurement is discussed more fully in section 10-6 (pulmonary instrumentation).

The most common pressure measurement is *arterial blood pressure,* which is almost routinely monitored by electronic instruments in intensive care units (ICUs), coronary care units (CCUs), and other critical care areas. Also of interest, however, are the *central venous pressure* (CVP), *intracardiac blood pressure,* special pressures in the *pulmonary artery, spinal fluid pressures,* and *intraventricular* (brain) *pressures.*

9-4 What is pressure?

A group of students were asked to give definitions of *pressure.* Several gave the correct answer, but most wrote hazy, ambiguous statements that indicated they did not really understand what is meant by that concept. Some students came close, indicating that pressure is a *force;* but this is still not correct. The correct definition is that *pressure is force per unit area.*

$$P = \frac{F}{A} \qquad (9\text{-}1)$$

where

> P is the pressure in newtons per square meter (N/m^2), or pascals (Pa); $1 \ N/m^2 = 1 \ Pa$
> F is the force in newtons (N)
> A is the area in square meters (m^2)

Example 9-1 _____

A small coin has a diameter of 1 cm and a mass of 1.5 g. Find (a) the gravitational force (weight of coin) in dynes and millinewtons and (b) the pressure this coin exerts lying horizontally on a flat table top in dynes per square centimeter and newtons per square meter (or pascals).

Solution

$f = 1.5 \ g(a) \ f = ma$ (Newton's second law) $\times 980$ $cm/s^2 = 1470 \ g\text{-}cm/s^2 = 1470 \ dyn$

(a) $f = 1470 \ dyn \times \dfrac{1 \ N}{10^5 \ dyn}$

$\quad = 1.47 \times 10^{-2} \ N$

$\quad = \mathbf{14.7 \ mN}$

(b) $P = \dfrac{F}{A} \qquad (9\text{-}1)$

$P = \dfrac{1470}{\pi(1 \ cm/2)^2} = \mathbf{1872 \ dyn/cm^2}$

$P = 1872 \ dyn/cm^2 \times 10^{-5} \ N/dyn$
$\qquad \times (10^2 \ cm/m)^2$

$P = \mathbf{187.2 \ N/m^2} = \mathbf{187.2 \ Pa}$

Note that *pressure* can be *increased* by either *increasing* the applied *force* or by decreasing the area on which the force acts. Alternate units for pressure, as shown in Example 9-1, are dynes per square centimeter (dyn/cm^2) in the centimeter-gram-second *(cgs)* system and pounds per square inch (psi) in the British engineering system.

When the force in a system under pressure is constant or static (i.e., unvarying), the pressure is said to be *hydrostatic.* If the force is *varying,* on the other hand, the pressure is said to be *hydrodynamic.* Most human physiological pressures are hydrodynamic, of which the most easily recognized is the pulsatile flow of arterial blood.

Pressure in a closed system obeys a physical law known as Pascal's principle (after French scientist Blaise Pascal, 1623-1662), which states that:

Pressure applied to an enclosed fluid is transmitted undiminished to every portion of the fluid and the walls of the containing vessel.*

_____

*David Halliday and Robert Resnick, Physics Parts I and II, 3rd ed., Wiley (New York, 1978), p. 430. Reprinted by permission of publisher.

If a pressure is applied to the stoppered syringe in Figure 9-1, then, the *same* pressure is felt throughout the interior of the syringe. *Changing the pressure applied to the plunger causes the same change to be reflected at every point inside of the syringe.*

Pascal's principle holds true in hydrostatic systems and also in *quasistatic* systems, in which a *small* change is made and the turbulence is al-

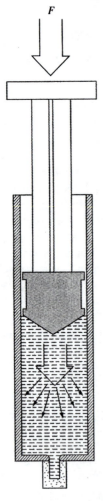

Figure 9-1
Sectioned view of a syringe. A pressure exerted by the plunger is transmitted through the fluid to all parts of the system.

lowed to die down before subsequent measurements are made. Pascal's principle holds *approximately* true in hydrodynamic systems in which the flow is nonturbulent and the vessel lumen is small (except at the vessel wall boundaries). The study of pressure in turbulent or large lumen systems, or near the vessel wall, is a subject for engineering mechanics and physics courses. In this text, we assume that Pascal's principle holds generally true but recognize that it results only in approximations when applied to the turbulent human circulatory system.

Pressure is exerted in the human circulatory system by the force created by the pumping heart, which is transmitted through the fluid (i.e., blood) against the vessel walls. The circulatory system regulates blood pressure by constricting and dilating vessels, which causes changes in vessel surface area by changing vessel diameter. The pressure, as a result, is never constant, and our measurements always assume an *average* value.

9-5 Pressure measurements

The air forming our atmosphere exerts a pressure on the surface of the earth. This pressure is usually expressed as being 1 atmosphere (atm) or approximately 14.7 psi, 1.013×10^6 dyn/cm², or 1.013×10^5 Pa at mean sea level.

Example 9-2 _____

A barometer measures a pressure of 750 mm Hg during a snowstorm. Convert this pressure to (a) atmospheres, (b) psi, (c) pascals, (d) dynes per square centimeter, and (e) newtons per square meter.

Solution

(a) $750 \text{ mm Hg} \times \dfrac{1 \text{ atm}}{760 \text{ mm Hg}} = \textbf{0.987 atm}$

(b) $0.987 \text{ atm} \times \dfrac{14.7 \text{ psi}}{1 \text{ atm}} = \textbf{14.5 psi}$

(c) $0.987 \text{ atm} \times \dfrac{1.013 \times 10^5 \text{ Pa}}{1 \text{ atm}}$

$= \textbf{1.00} \times \textbf{10}^{\textbf{5}} \textbf{ Pa}$

(d) $0.987 \text{ atm} \times \dfrac{1.013 \times 10^6 \text{ dyn/cm}^2}{1 \text{ atm}}$

  $= \mathbf{1.00 \times 10^6 \text{ dyn/cm}^2}$

(e) $1 \times 10^5 \text{ Pa} \times \dfrac{1 \text{ N/m}^2}{1 \text{ Pa}} = \mathbf{1 \times 10^5 \text{ N/m}^2}$

If a pressure is measured with respect to a vacuum (0 atm), then it is called an *absolute pressure,* and if measured against 1 atm it is called a *gauge pressure.* Two gauge pressures may be compared with each other in the form of a single number called *relative pressure* or *differential pressure* (i.e., the *difference* between two gauge pressures).

Pressures in the human circulatory system are measured against atmospheric pressure and are gage pressures. In the pulmonary system, some pressures are gauge pressures, while others are relative pressures.

Figure 9-2a shows the Torricelli *manometer* (after Evangelista Torricelli, Italian scientist, 1608-1647) used to measure atmospheric pressure. An evacuated glass tube with a small lumen stands vertically, with the open end immersed in a pool of mercury (Hg). The pressure exerted by the atmosphere on the surface of the mercury pool forces mercury into the tube, forming a column. The mercury column rises in the tube until its weight

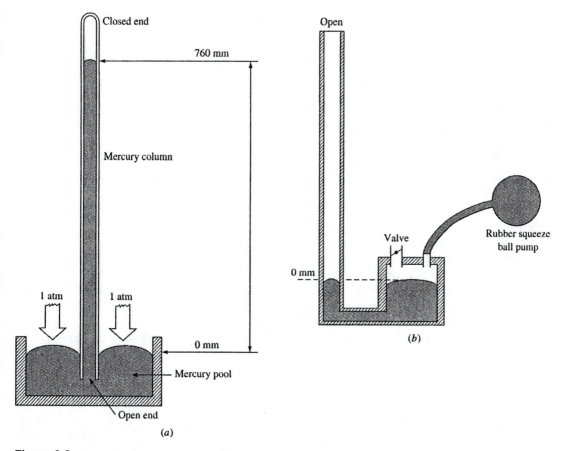

(a)

(b)

Figure 9-2
Mercury manometer. (*a*) Torricelli manometer for measuring atmospheric pressure. (*b*) Gauge pressure manometer.

(i.e., a gravitational force) exactly balances the force of the atmospheric pressure. Torricelli found that the height of the mercury column that can be supported by atmospheric pressure is approximately 0.76 m, or 760 mm. Atmospheric pressure, then, is frequently given in units of millimeters of mercury and 1 atm is 760 mm Hg.[†]

The *proper* unit of pressure, as established by scientists and adopted by the *National Bureau of Standards,* is the torr (after Torricelli), in which 1 torr is equal to 1 mm Hg (1 torr = 1 mm Hg).[‡]

Gauge pressures are usually given in millimeters of mercury above or below atmospheric pressure. A manometer is any device that measures gauge pressure, although in commonly accepted jargon, gauge pressures below 1 atm are said to be measured on a *vacuum gauge,* and pressures above 1 atm are said to be measured on a *pressure gauge.* Both instruments are, however, examples of manometers. Some manometers, including most of the electronic instruments discussed in this chapter, measure both positive pressures (i.e., above 1 atm) and negative pressures (i.e., vacuums).

The *zero reference* in gauge pressure measurements, therefore, is a pressure of 1 atm. Even though atmospheric pressure varies from one place to another, and in the same location over the course of a few hours, zero can be established at each measurement by setting the zero scale with the manometer open to atmospheric pressure. Figure 9-2b shows a mercury manometer similar to those used to make blood pressure measurements. The open tube is connected to a mercury reservoir that is fitted with a rubber squeeze-ball pump that can be used to increase pressure; a valve is used to either open the chamber to atmosphere or close it off.

If the valve is open to atmosphere, then the pressure on the mercury in the chamber is equal to the pressure on the column (i.e., 1 atm). The mercury in the column will have the same height as the mercury in the chamber, and this point is designated as a pressure of 0 mm Hg. If the valve is *closed,* and the pressure inside of the chamber is *increased* by operating the pump, then the mercury in the column will *rise* an amount *proportional* to the increased pressure.

Example 9-3 _____

The mercury in a manometer, such as the one in Figure 9-2b, rises to a height of 120 mm Hg. Find (a) the gauge pressure and (b) the absolute pressure.

Solution

(a) **120 mm Hg** (by definition)

(b) 120 mm Hg + 760 mm Hg = **880 mm Hg**

_____

We use gauge pressure because it is more easily referenced at zero and can be easily recalibrated at each use, and the absolute pressure confers no special advantage as to information content. The variation of atmospheric pressure from one location to another (dependent upon mean sea level) and over the course of a single day makes the use of gauge pressures more advantageous.

9-6 Blood pressure measurements

The earliest recorded attempt at the measurement of arterial blood pressure was performed in 1773 by English scientist Stephen Hales, who used an open-ended tube inserted directly into an artery in the neck of an *un*anesthetized horse (presumably tied down securely). The tube was long enough that blood rose to a height at which the weight of the blood exactly balanced the horse's arterial pressure.

According to Hales's observation, the blood pulsed its way up the tube, attaining a height of approximately 4 ft on the first pulse but requiring an additional 40 or 50 pulses to attain a final height of just over 8 ft. After the blood in the

_____

[†]The *barometer* reading given in English units is usually inches of mercury *(in. Hg).* 760 mm Hg = 29.92 in. Hg

[‡]If convention were followed, we would quote physiological pressures in torr, but it is common practice in medicine to use the unit mm Hg. To avoid confusion, we will follow this practice, but keep in mind that it is no longer accepted outside the medical world.

manometer tube had stabilized to about the final height, it rose and fell approximately 2 or 3 in. on each pulse because of the diastolic and systolic pressures.

Hales's technique is an example of *direct* measurement of blood pressure. *Routine* clinical measurements of blood pressure in humans, however, required the development of suitable *indirect* techniques without the painful and potentially hazardous surgical procedures performed by Hales.

Today, both indirect and direct methods are used to measure blood pressure in humans. The most popular indirect method, familiar to almost everybody whose blood pressure has been checked by a physician or nurse, involves *sphygmomanometry*. Currently used direct methods usually involve *electronic amplifiers* that process a signal from a *pressure transducer* that is coupled to the patient's artery or vein through a saline-filled *catheter* or *needle*. Hales's two-century-old method is still used in modern hospitals to measure *spinal fluid* pressure and CVP. Almost every hospital stocks CVP and spinal-tap kits that contain a water (H_2O) manometer not dissimilar to Hales's crude apparatus of the eighteenth century.

The indirect method routinely used by physicians requires a device called a *sphygmomanometer* (Figure 9-3), consisting of an inflatable rubber bladder called the *cuff*, a rubber squeeze-ball pump-and-valve assembly, and a manometer. The manometer might be a mercury column (as shown), or a dial gauge. Professional-grade sphygmomanometers are based on an aneroid assembly or structure similar to the Bourdon tube, while many cheaper varieties offered as part of "blood pressure kits" to the general public use spring-loaded pressure gauges. The spring-loaded types are usually just as accurate as more costly types initially, but substantial errors develop as the spring wears out.

The procedure for using this apparatus is as follows:

1. The cuff is wrapped around the patient's upper arm at a point about midway between the

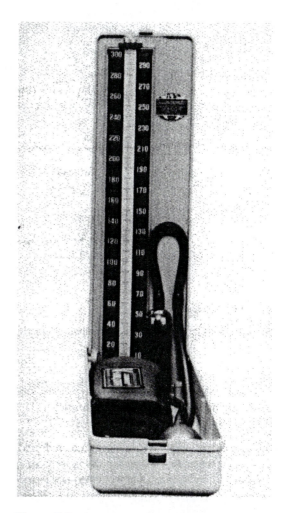

Figure 9-3
Mercury column sphygmomanometer. (Photo courtesy of E. Baum Co., Inc.)

elbow and shoulder. The stethoscope is placed over an artery distal (i.e., downstream) to the cuff. This placement (Figure 9-4) is preferred because the *brachial artery* comes close to the surface near the *antecubital space* (i.e., inside the elbow) and so is easily accessible.

2. The cuff is inflated so that the pressure inside the inflated bladder is increased to a point greater than the anticipated systolic pressure.

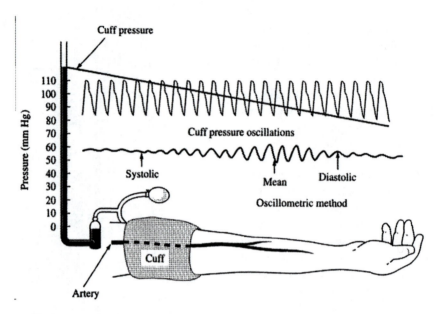

Figure 9-4
Cuff placement for the auscultatory method of blood pressure measurement.

This pressure compresses the artery against the underlying bone, causing an *occlusion* that shuts off the flow of blood in the vessel.

3. The operator then *slowly* releases (i.e., reduces) the pressure in the cuff, shown in Figure 9-5a (about 3 mm Hg/s is usually deemed best) and watches the pressure gauge or mercury column. When the systolic pressure first exceeds the cuff pressure, the operator begins to hear some crashing, snapping sounds in the stethoscope that are caused by the first jets of blood pushing through the occlusion. These sounds, called *Korotkoff sounds* (Figure 9-5b), continue as the cuff pressure diminishes, becoming less loud as the blood flow through the occlusion becomes smoother. Korotkoff sounds disappear or become muffled when the cuff pressure drops *below* the patient's *diastolic* pressure. To read the blood pressure, the operator notes both the gauge pressure at the *onset* of Korotkoff sounds (systolic) and when the sounds become muffled (or disappear) altogether (diastolic). These pressures are usually recorded in the ratio of systolic over diastolic (i.e., 120/80 mm Hg).

The first use of sphygmomanometry for the measurement of blood pressure was reported by Korotkoff in 1905, but the technique was not verified for correlation between indirect and direct measurements in animals until 1912. It was not until 1931 that a similar correlation was established for humans—that is, that variations of less than 10 mm Hg existed between direct and indirect methods. More recently it has been shown that indirect diastolic pressures are less in error if the reading is taken at the point where the Korotkoff sounds disappear. Yet most clinicians prefer to use the point where the sounds become muffled because this point can be recognized more consistently. The American Heart Association recommended in 1967 that muffling be used as the criterion for diastolic pressure but that *both* pressures (i.e., muffling and the cessation of Korotkoff sounds) be indicated if a significant difference between them exists. This measurement is recorded as a double-diastolic pressure (i.e., 120/80/77 mm Hg).

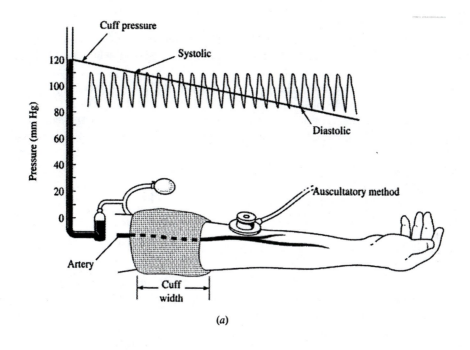

(a)

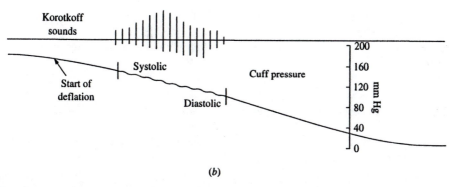

(b)

Figure 9-5
Diagram of the auscultatory method of blood pressure measurement. (a) Cuff placement.
(b) Korotkoff sounds.

The use of Korotkoff sounds as the indirect indicator of blood pressure is also called *auscultation* (i.e., use of hearing) and is by far the most common indirect method used. It is accurate enough for ordinary clinical use and is simple enough so that even nonprofessional personnel can be rapidly trained to "take blood pressures."

Limitations on the auscultatory method include the hearing acuity of the operator and how accu-

rately the operator is able to read a *changing* pressure gauge when the Korotkoff sound features are heard. In *hypotensive* (i.e., *low* blood pressure) patients, the event chosen to indicate the diastolic pressure may be either obscured or nonexistent.

Several modern instruments are available for the indirect measurement of blood pressure in hypotensive patients by replacement of the stethoscope with an electronic transducer. Some devices that use ultrasound are discussed in section 17-10. Other devices that use *infrasound* (i.e., frequencies lower than 50 Hz) are merely low-frequency microphones. The instrument will amplify and filter the microphone output signal and use it to turn on a beeper or lamp when the systolic and diastolic features are recognized. These instruments are also used in emergency rooms, ICUs, and CCUs where high ambient noise levels often obscure the Korotkoff sounds on nonhypotensive patients.

There are two other major indirect methods of blood pressure measurement: *palpation* and *flush*. Both use the cuff but differ in the respective methods used to detect the pressure points.

The palpation method uses the sense of *touch* to detect the patient's pulse in the radial artery (wrist). The cuff is inflated until the radial pulse *disappears.* The operator then slowly releases the pressure in the cuff until a pulse becomes palpable in the radial artery. The pressure at which this occurs is the *systolic* blood pressure.

Palpation can detect *only* the *systolic* pressure because no known palpable change occurs at the diastolic pressure. Also, palpable changes tend to disappear below 75 or 80 mm Hg of systolic pressure, so the technique is often not useful on the hypotensive patient.

The flush technique requires *two cuffs* and *two operators*. The cuffs are placed on the arm and are inflated. The blood in the section *between* the two cuffs is massaged out, leaving the lower arm pale and blanched. The pressure in the upper cuff is then released slowly. The pressure at which a sudden red flush is noted in the blanched skin is recorded as the *mean arterial pressure* (MAP).

9-7 Oscillometric and ultrasonic noninvasive pressure measurements

The aforementioned auscultatory measurement method is the most widely used procedure for measuring blood pressures. It suffers, however,

from at least two problems. First, the measurement is intermittent because it takes time to accomplish. A medical person who constantly takes blood pressure readings has little time for anything else. Second, the Korotkoff sounds are normally in the range (less than 200 Hz) where human hearing is not very acute. If long-term monitoring in intensive care is done, or if the ambient noise level is high, then either *oscillometric* or *ultrasonic* blood pressure measurement may be used.

9-7-1 Oscillometric blood pressure measurement

The oscillometric method of blood pressure measurement is similar to ordinary sphygmomanometry, except that we measure small fluctuations (i.e., *oscillations*) in the cuff pressure rather than direct pressure (Figure 9-6).

When blood breaks through the occlusion created by the inflated cuff, which occurs when the cuff pressure drops below the systolic blood pressure, the walls of the artery begin to vibrate slightly. The vibrations are related to the fact that the blood flow at this point is turbulent, rather than laminar, although the physiological basis is not well understood.

The fluctuating walls of the blood vessel slightly alter the blood pressure, giving rise to oscillations in the cuff pressure (Figure 9-6). The onset of the pressure oscillations correlates well with the systolic pressure, while the amplitude peak of the oscillations corresponds to the MAP, which is the *time average* of blood pressure. The diastolic pressure event on the oscillation curve is somewhat less well-defined than the systolic event but corresponds to the point where the rate of amplitude decrease suddenly changes slope.

Oscillometric blood pressure monitors are used extensively when monitoring is needed, but it is not desirable for invasive procedures where *direct pressure measurements* are needed (section 9-8). A typical oscillometric blood pressure monitor is microprocessor-controlled and is designed to pe-

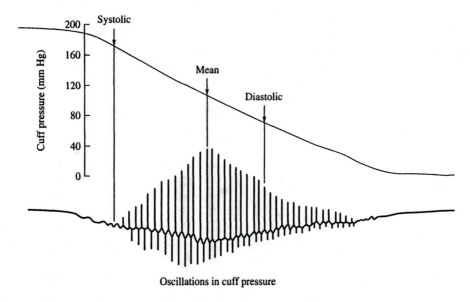

Figure 9-6
Illustration of oscillometric method of blood pressure measurement.

riodically inflate and slowly deflate the cuff. The pressure sensor is designed to maximize *variations* in pressure rather than read the static pressure heads.

9-7-2 Ultrasonic pressure measurements

Ultrasonic waves are acoustical waves (like regular sound waves, 30 Hz to 20 KHz) in the range above human hearing (more than 20 KHz). Like all acoustical waves, ultrasonic waves are subject to *Doppler shift*—that is, a slight alteration of frequency (ΔF) when reflected from a moving object. If piezoelectric ultrasound sensors are placed over the artery, under the cuff, then they can perform Doppler detection of the blood flowing in the artery.

The principle of operation is a bit like radar. A transmit crystal sends a sine-wave beam into the tissue. When it encounters a fluctuating vessel wall (see section 9-7-1), some of its energy is reflected back ("backscattered") to the receive crystal, which is located close to the transmit crystal. If ΔF is the Doppler shift, $F \pm \Delta F$ describes the fre-

quency content of the backscattered wave. The existence of the ΔF component alerts the circuit to the turbulent flow that corresponds to Korotkoff sounds, and it diminishes when near-laminar flow resumes ($P < P_{\text{diastolic}}$).

9-8 Direct methods: H₂O manometers

Hales's method is still used in the measurement of spinal fluid pressures and CVP. Most hospitals stock standard kits containing plastic tubes calibrated in centimeters of water (cm H_2O). Water rather than mercury is used for two reasons. One is that the thin manometer tube is introduced directly into the patient's body, so the use of a poisonous material like mercury as the pressure indicator must be avoided. Water is physiologically compatible with the patient's body and thus is less hazardous. Second, the pressure in either CVP or spinal fluid is low (only a few millimeters of mercury). If a material (e.g., water), that is less dense than mercury is used, then the column with a weight equal to the pressure force will be higher.

This will greatly improve resolution. Water has a specific gravity of 1 (by definition), and mercury has a specific gravity of approximately 13.5. The column of water produced by a given pressure will be 13.5 times higher than the column of mercury at the same pressure. CVP and spinal manometers are usually calibrated in cm H_2O, but a millimeters-of-mercury value is easily found by dividing the H_2O value by 13.5 to yield a centimeters-of-mercury.

9-8-1 Direct methods: electronic manometry

An electronic pressure transducer can be connected to the patient through a thin piece of tubing called a *catheter*. The catheter is introduced into the vessel through a thin, hollow tube called a *cannula*. The transducer's pressure diaphragm is coupled to the patient's bloodstream by a column of saline solution that fills the catheter.

The catheter to the patient must be placed inside a peripheral artery. There are two general methods for inserting the catheter: *percutaneous puncture* and *arterial cutdown*. The percutaneous methods involve puncturing the skin over an artery and then using a needle and catheter assembly to insert the catheter into the artery. When the catheter is in place, the needle is withdrawn. The arterial cutdown method is a surgical procedure in which the tissue overlying the artery is cut and laid out of the way, revealing the artery. A puncture is then made, and a catheter is put into place.

Figure 9-7a shows a typical apparatus used for measuring blood pressure with an electronic transducer. The transducer is mounted to a pole or support at bedside. There are two ports into the transducer's *pressure dome;* one is "deadheaded" and the other is connected to a hydraulic fitting called a *three-way stopcock*. One terminal of the stopcock goes to the catheter from the patient, while the other goes to a small syringe that is used to administer medications directly to the patient through the catheter, or to withdraw arterial blood samples for laboratory analysis.

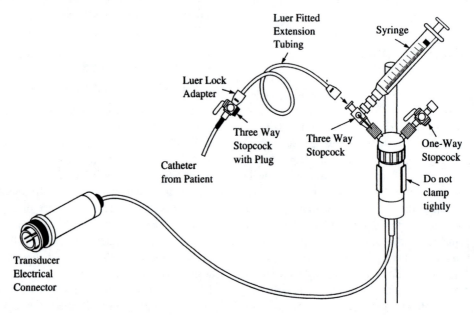

Figure 9-7
Infusion system. Arterial monitoring setup.

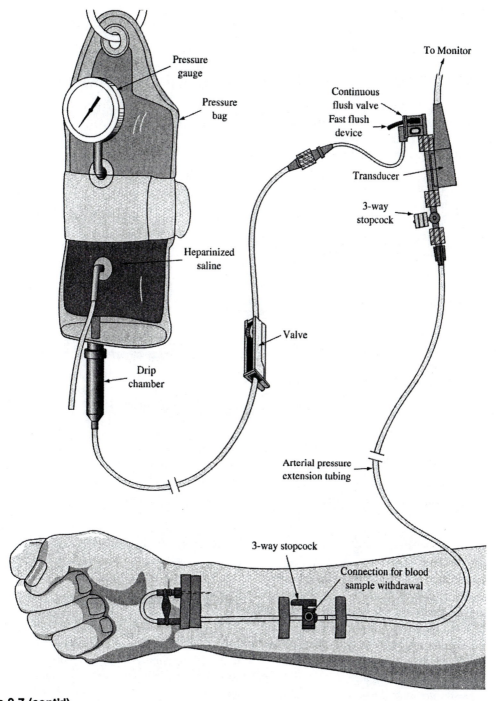

Figure 9-7 (cont'd)
(*b*) Constant flush infusion system. (Courtesy of Spacelabs)

9-8-2 Constant flush infusion system

When direct pressure measurements are made over a long time (e.g., several hours), as they are in ICUs, there is a danger of coagulated blood stopping up the pressure catheter. In those cases, medical personnel may opt to use a *constant flush infusion system* (CFIS), such as the one in Figure 9-7b.

The CFIS consists of a special valve connected to a bag of intravenous (IV) solution, usually 0.9% saline with 1 or 2 U of aqueous heparin (a drug that prevents blood clotting) per milliliter, or cubic centimeter, of IV fluid. A constant low-flow rate of about 3 mL/hr is set. Pressure is applied to the bag of IV solution by a standard IV pressure bag (a bladder) that is pumped to a pressure of about 300 mm Hg.

A *fast flush lever* is used to inject a sudden bolus of heparinized saline into the system to fill the transducer dome and clear blood clots. It can also be used to provide a square-wave stimulus to test the frequency response of the total system (see section 9-18).

9-9 Pressure transducers

Figures 9-8 and 9-9 show typical blood pressure transducers. A transducer is an electrical device that converts the pressure transmitted through the fluid-filled catheter to an electrical signal (recall Pascal's principle).

The basic components of a blood pressure transducer are shown in Figure 9-8. A thin, flexible metal diaphragm is stretched across an opening at one end of the transducer body. This diaphragm is connected to an inductive bridge strain gauge and will flex the strain gauge an amount proportional to the applied pressure. Other models use a resistive Wheatstone bridge strain gauge.

A clear plastic *pressure dome* fits over the diaphragm to contain the fluid and provide hydraulic connection to the catheter. The electrical connector is a little larger in the model shown because it houses part of the bridge circuit (i.e., two resistors)

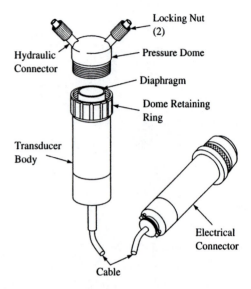

Figure 9-8
Components of a blood pressure transducer.
(Reprinted courtesy of Hewlett-Packard)

and a sensitivity control. This transducer is the Hewlett-Packard model 1280 and, since it is inductive, requires an ac excitation potential.

The Statham model P23Id blood pressure transducer, shown in Figure 9-9, is also very common in medical monitoring systems. This particular version of the P23 series is insulated to prevent damage to itself and injury to the patient during defibrillator discharge. The P23Id is an unbonded piezoresistive strain gauge Wheatstone bridge of the type discussed in chapter 6.

9-10 Pressure amplifiers

There are four basic types of pressure amplifiers in common use: *dc, isolated dc, pulsed excitation,* and *ac carrier amplifiers.* The dc amplifiers work with resistance strain gauges only, while the ac carrier amplifiers work with either resistive or inductive transducers. The pulsed excitation amplifiers may work with some inductive transducers but are generally used only with resistive transducers.

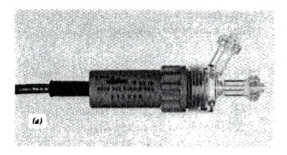

(a)

Figure 9-9
Arterial blood pressure transducer. (a) Photo. (b) Cross-sectional view. (Photo courtesy of Statham Instruments Division, Gould, Inc., Oxnard, Calif.)

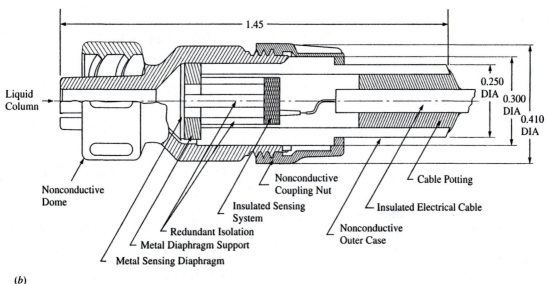

1.45

0.250 DIA
0.300 DIA
0.410 DIA

Liquid
Column

Nonconductive
Dome

Metal Sensing Diaphragm

Metal Diaphragm Support

Redundant Isolation

Insulated Sensing
System

Nonconductive
Coupling Nut

Nonconductive
Outer Case

Insulated Electrical Cable

Cable Potting

(b)

Regardless of the design, there are certain features common to all pressure amplifiers. Instruments intended for use in catheterization laboratories or research facilities should be capable of measuring a wide range of pressure values, and they must be very accurate and stable. Instruments in this class are generally more complex than clinical instruments and thus are not often found in bedside monitoring applications.

The pressure amplifier used for bedside applications is less complex and thus is less flexible and often somewhat less accurate. While its simplicity allows less-trained personnel to successfully operate the instrument, it is more accurate than most indirect methods. In the ICU, CCU, or operating room

(OR), the operator is usually a physician, nurse, or monitoring technician who has duties other than equipment operation and has limited time to calibrate pressure equipment. For these busy people, it is a valid trade-off to sacrifice a small amount of accuracy for simpler operation. As a result, clinical pressure amplifiers tend to have fewer front-panel controls and a simplified calibration procedure.

In applications in which superior accuracy is needed, a mercury or aneroid manometer is used to calibrate pressure equipment every time it is used. Clinical pressure monitors have an internal calibration signal that is used for day-to-day operation and is checked periodically (usually monthly) against a manometer.

9-11 Typical calibration methods

The typical clinical pressure monitor has the following controls: *zero,* or *balance; sensitivity,* or *gain;* and *calibrate,* or a control yielding some specific pressure in mm Hg.

The zero control is used to adjust the amplifier output to zero volts under zero pressure conditions (i.e., 1 atm).

The sensitivity control adjusts the gain of the amplifier to produce the correct amplifier output voltage to represent a specific calibration pressure that is generated with a manometer/pump or supplied as a simulated pressure signal by an external transducer substitute or internal calibration control.

The best accuracy is obtained when a manometer and squeeze-ball pump are used to calibrate the system. A mercury sphygmomanometer can be disconnected at the cuff and the loose end fitted with an appropriate Luer-lock hydraulic connector so that it can couple to the transducer. It is essential that the transducer be disconnected from the patient when calibrating with a manometer, because we are going to introduce *air* into the system. An air bubble in the circulatory system can kill a patient.

1. When the manometer is correctly connected to the transducer (Figure 9-10), open the stopcock to atmosphere and adjust the amplifier zero balance control for an indication of zero on the meter (Figure 9-7).

2. Next, close the stopcock and pump a standard pressure on the manometer, say, 100 mm Hg.

3. Adjust the sensitivity control for an indication of 100 mm Hg on the meter (Figure 9-7). It is prudent to check the agreement between the manometer and the meter at several points above and below the test pressure. If a transducer diaphragm has been strained beyond its safe limits, it may become *nonlinear.* Check for agreement at 50% and 200% of the test pressure, assuming that the transducer upper limit is not exceeded.

The same general procedure just described also works when an internal calibration signal is used to simulate a standard pressure. Some adjustment is necessary, however, to account for differences between several normal transducers. Even two transducers with the same model designation exhibit different sensitivity figures. One popular model, for example, has a *nominal* sensitivity specification of 5 μV/V/mm Hg. But calibration certificates supplied with each unit by the manufacturer attest that actual sensitivity figures range from 3.7 to 6.5 μV/V/mm Hg.

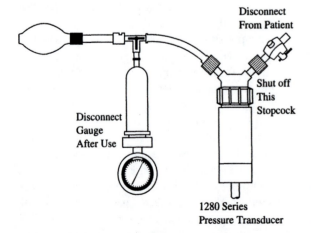

Figure 9-10
A manometer is used to calibrate the transducer.
(Reprinted courtesy of Hewlett-Packard)

There are three approaches to standardizing the adjustment procedure to accommodate different transducers: tight specification by the manufacturer, use of an internal transducer sensitivity adjustment, and use of a *calibration factor* unique to each individual transducer used with a given pressure amplifier.

Some manufacturers of pressure-monitoring equipment solve the problem by requiring the transducer manufacturer to supply them with units that fall within very tight limits for sensitivity and *zero-stimulus offset error.* This approach works well in some situations, but it does not allow for changes in offset and sensitivity caused by abuse and aging. It also forces the consumer to buy transducers at a premium price from the equipment manufacturer rather than directly from the transducer manufacturer at a lower price.

Other manufacturers, notably Hewlett-Packard, use a potentiometer inside the transducer electrical connector to *trim out* differences in sensitivity. The *actual* transducer sensitivity is always higher than that seen by the amplifier, but the effect of adjustment is that the amplifier always sees the *same* sensitivity regardless of which individual transducer is in use.

Some companies use a *calibration factor* for each transducer. The simplified circuit is shown in Figure 9-11. Each transducer must have its own calibration (cal) factor. Record the *cal factor* number or mark it on the transducer body. When that transducer is used again, the operator need only dial in the correct calibration factor.

Subsequent calibrations do not require a manometer test. The calibration factor for any given transducer remains valid for several months unless the transducer is physically abused. Of course, any transducer that is suspect should be checked out more frequently, and immediately after an incident of abuse has been reported. Between periodical checks however, the following procedure is used:

1. Open the transducer stopcock to air; place switch S_1 in the 0-mm Hg position. Adjust

balance for a 0-V output indication (i.e., 0 mm Hg on the meter).

2. Set switch selector to the position that is most convenient for the range being calibrated. In general, a setting that would put the meter pointer at mid-scale or above is best.

3. Set the *cal factor* knob to the figure recorded previously (use a manometer if the calibration date is more than 6 months old).

4. Adjust the gain control until the meter reads the standard pressure used in the original calibration.

In general, it is preferable to settle on a single standard pressure for all calibrations. This avoids problems that could occur if one "standard" is used by one person making the initial calibration and another standard is selected by subsequent people performing the same job. For arterial monitors, 100 or 200 mm Hg are good choices.

9-12 Pressure amplifier designs

The four basic types of pressure amplifier design (i.e., dc, isolated dc, pulsed excitation, and ac carrier) are implemented using transistors, operational amplifiers, special linear integrated circuits (LICs), or (in older equipment) vacuum tubes. The basic difference between the four classes is in the type of excitation applied to the transducer.

9-12-1 dc pressure amplifiers

Figure 9-11 shows the simplified circuit of a dc pressure amplifier that uses the calibration factor method. The pressure amplifier ($A1$) is a dc amplifier, so the pressure transducer is a resistive Wheatstone bridge strain gauge. Diode $D1$ provides the 7.5-V dc excitation to the transducer, and the potentials for the *balance* and *cal factor* controls. The calibration factor for the transducer sometimes changes, so it is necessary to provide a procedure for measuring the new factor. The dc

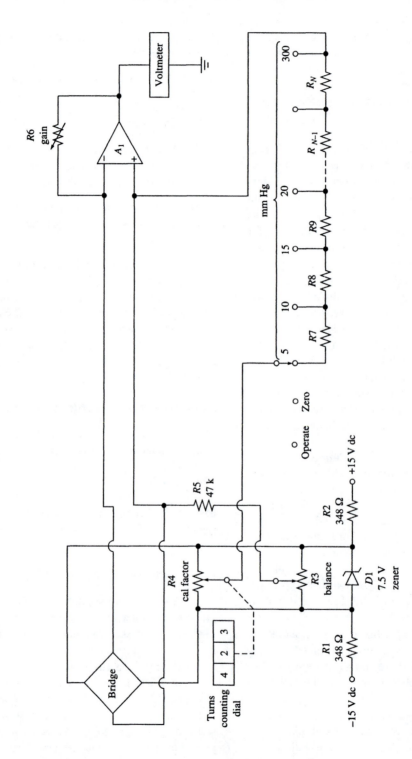

Figure 9-11
Calibration factor circuit.

pressure amplifier is first calibrated with an accurate mercury manometer:

1. Set switch $S1$ to the *operate* position, open the transducer stopcock to atmosphere, and adjust $R3$ for zero volts output (i.e., 0 torr reading on the display).

2. Close the transducer stopcock and then pump a standard pressure (e.g., 100 torr, or at least half-scale). Adjust gain control $R6$ until the meter reads the correct (standard) pressure. Check for agreement between the meter and the manometer at several standard pressures throughout the range (e.g., 50, 100, 150, 200, 250, and 300 torr). This last step is necessary to ensure that the transducer is reasonably linear—that is, that the diaphragm was not strained by out-of-range pressures or vacuums.

3. Turn switch $S1$ to the position corresponding to the applied standard pressure, and then adjust *cal factor* control ($R4$) until the same standard pressure is obtained on the meter. The *cal factor* control is ganged to a turns-counting dial. The number appearing on the dial at the position of $R4$ that creates the same standard pressure signal is the calibration factor for that transducer. Record the turns-counter reading for future reference.

For a time (usually 6 months) the calibration factor need not be redetermined unless damage to the transducer occurs. The calibration factor is entered into the amplifier by turning $R4$ (or digitally in modern instruments). The following procedure is normally used:

1. Open the transducer stopcock to atmosphere, place switch $S1$ in the 0 torr (0 mm Hg) position, and adjust $R3$ for a 0-V output indication (0 torr on the display).

2. Set switch $S1$ to the position that is most convenient for the range of pressures to be measured. In general, select a scale that places the reading mid-scale or higher.

3. Set the *cal factor* knob to the figure recorded previously. Adjust the gain control ($R6$) until the meter reads the standard pressure used in the original calibration.

The circuit in Figure 9-11 is an example of a dc pressure amplifier; Figure 9-12 is a more detailed version of the actual amplifier block. Note that there are only two operational amplifiers in this circuit—little about the simple dc amplifier is complex. Amplifier $A1$ is the input amplifier, and it should be a low-drift, premium model. Both gain and zero controls are provided, so the amplifier will work with a wide variety of transducers.

The excitation voltage of the transducer is determined (as a maximum) by the transducer manufacturer, with a value of 10 V being common. In general, it is best to operate the transducer at a voltage lower than the maximum to prevent drift caused by self-heating. Pressure amplifier manufacturers typically specify either 5 or 7.5 V for a 10-V transducer (maximum).

The required amplifier gain can be calculated from the required output voltage that is used to represent any given pressure. Because digital voltmeters are used extensively for readout displays, the common practice is to use an output voltage scale factor that is numerically the same as the full-scale pressure. For example, 1 or 10 mV/mm Hg is common. Let's assume a maximum pressure range of 400 mm Hg (common on arterial monitors), if we use a scale factor of 1 mV/mm Hg, when 400 mm Hg is represented by 400 mV, or 0.40 V. No further scaling of the meter output is needed.

9-12-2 Isolated dc amplifiers

Patient safety considerations identified in the past few years have caused many manufacturers to redesign their pressure monitors to improve electrical isolation of the patient from the ac power mains supply. These amplifiers are built along the same lines as the isolated amplifiers discussed in Section 7-11.

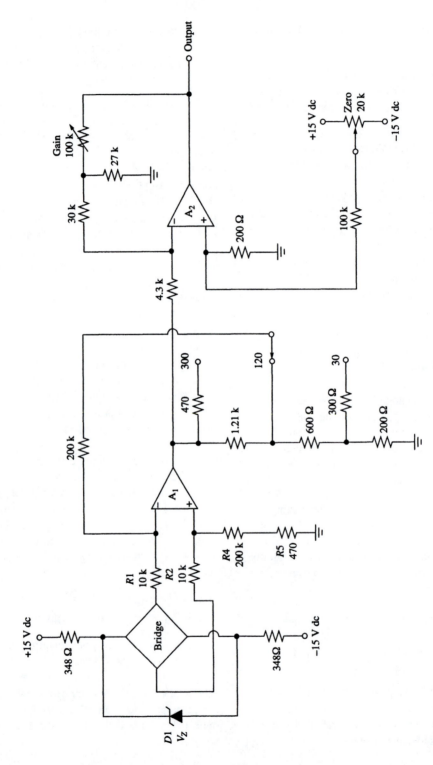

Figure 9-12
Detailed version of actual amplifier block.

9-12-3 Pulsed-excitation amplifiers

Figure 9-13 shows the block diagram for a pulsed-excitation pressure amplifier. This amplifier uses a Wheatstone bridge strain gauge transducer, although inductive types can be accommodated in some models. The excitation signal is a biphasic short-duration pulse. In one model, the pulse (Figure 9-13b) has a duration of 1 ms and a 25% duty cycle.

Amplifier A_1 is a dc pressure amplifier, and amplifier A_2 is a unity gain summation stage. The output indicator is a digital voltmeter that will update the display only when the *strobe* line is high. Switches S_1 through S_5 are CMOS *electronic switches,* which *close* when the control line *(C)* is

high. All circuit action is controlled by a four-phase clock. Phases ϕ_1 and ϕ_2 excite the transducer and operate the amplifier *drift cancellation* circuit. Phase ϕ_3 updates the display meter, and phase ϕ_4 resets the circuit following update.

All dc amplifiers tend to drift (i.e., create spurious offset voltages resulting from thermal changes). Switches S_2 and S_3, capacitor C_1, and amplifier A_2 serve as a drift cancellation circuit (Figure 9-13a).

The transducer is excited *only* when ϕ_1 is *high* and ϕ_2 is *low;* at all other times the transducer is *not* excited, which keeps transducer self-heating to a minimum. Amplifier A_1 will drift, however, because of its high gain and inherent offset voltages.

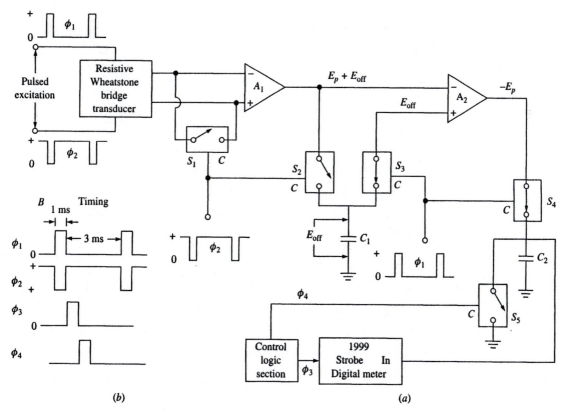

(b)   (a)

Figure 9-13
Pulsed excitation system. (a) Circuit diagram. (b) Timing diagram.

9-13 ac carrier amplifiers

The carrier amplifier requires ac excitation for the transducer, so it operatesequally well with both inductive and resistive strain gauges. Carrier frequencies are typically between 400 and 5000 Hz, with amplitudes ranging between 5 and 12 V rms. Hewlett-Packard equipment, for example, once was standardized on a frequency of 2400 Hz and an amplitude of 5 V rms.

Self-contained pressure monitors *will* contain their own carrier oscillator signal sources, while many *central* monitoring systems and rack-mounted catheterization laboratory instruments tend to use a *common* carrier source powerful enough to drive several carrier amplifiers.

Figure 9-14 shows the block diagram of a typical carrier amplifier. The carrier signal to the transducer is supplied through a push-pull transformer, so a 180-degree phase difference exists, allowing ground-referenced operation of the transducer.

1. Amplifier A_1 is a single-ended ac amplifier that is stabilized by heavy negative feedback. It is the stability of the ac amplifier that confers so much flexibility and quality on the carrier amplifier.

2. A calibration signal is supplied by switch S_1 and the voltage divider consisting of R_1 and R_2. This circuit introduces a small signal, equal to the output of the transducer at some standard pressure, into the ac amplifier. Calibration is performed with the transducer open to atmosphere, and the amplifier is prezeroed.

3. The balance control is a potentiometer connected to another pair of carrier signal lines that are also 180 degrees out of phase. The wiper of the potentiometer is connected to an amplifier input, where it is *summed* with the transducer signal.

4. The *balance* control nulls the system by injecting a signal of *equal magnitude,* but *opposite phase,* into the system to algebraically sum with the offset signal to produce a net result of zero output.

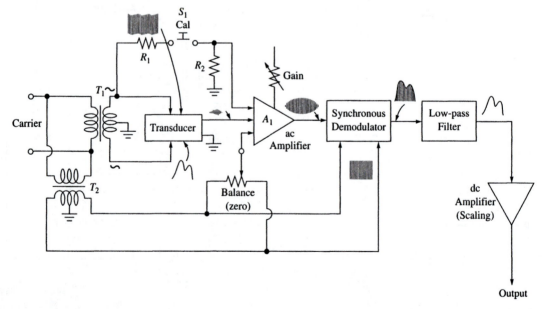

Figure 9-14
Carrier amplifier.

5. The same carrier signal that is applied to the balance control is also sent to a synchronous demodulator, where it converts the ac amplifier output signal to a varying dc signal. A low-pass filter following the demodulator removes any residual carrier signal, and a final dc amplifier buffers the output and provides any needed final scaling.

In many pressure amplifiers, the designers find it convenient to *scale* the output voltage so that it is *numerically* the same as the pressure it represents. Hewlett-Packard, for example, uses a scale of 0 to 3.0 V to represent 0 to 30 mm Hg or 0 to 300 mm Hg. The scale factor is 10 mV/mm Hg. Using a numerically equal scale factor allows the use of simple 3 V dc voltmeters (scaled in mm Hg, or so labeled if digital) as the output indicator. In the case of a digital display instrument, it is necessary to use numerically equal scale factors because it is not possible to have an appropriate scale printed, as is often done in analog voltmeters. A digital voltmeter may be scaled by shifting the decimal point.

9-14 Systolic, diastolic, and mean detector circuits

The pressure amplifier produces an analog waveform with a peak amplitude representing the systolic pressure, and a minimum, or "valley," that represents the diastolic pressure. Additional circuitry is required that recognizes these points, and from them produces a steady dc voltage or current that can be used to drive a display meter.

The partial schematic of a pressure detector is shown in Figure 9-15a; the timing diagram is shown in Figure 9-15b. Amplifiers A_1 through A_3 are operational amplifiers; switches S_1 through S_4 are CMOS electronic switches. Note that the operational amplifiers may be integrated types, as shown, or may be constructed of discrete components in older models.

1. This circuit operates from a two-phase clock created by flip-flop FF_1. The Q and not-Q ($\overline{Q}$) outputs are complementary, so one will be *high* when the other is *low*.

2. Switches S_1 and S_4 are turned on when the Q is high, and switches S_2 and S_3 are turned on when the $\overline{Q}$ is high.

3. The analog waveform from the output of the pressure amplifier is applied simultaneously (i.e., in parallel) to the inputs of A_1 and A_2. The waveform, therefore, appears simultaneously at the outputs of A_1 and A_2.

4. During period T_1 (Figure 9-15b), the Q output of FF_1 is high, so switches S_1 and S_4 are closed. When S_4 is closed, capacitor C_2 is discharged, so it has no effect on the output. Closing switch S_1 allows the signal appearing at the output of A_1 to charge capacitor C_1 to the peak voltage, representing the *systolic pressure*.

5. The voltage across capacitor C_1 forward biases diode D_3, which then conducts and applies the voltage to the input of amplifier A_3. The output of amplifier A_3 goes to the *systolic* output meter.

6. The situation reverses during the time T_2: The $\overline{Q}$ of FF_1 becomes high and the Q is low. This turns on switches S_2 and S_3 and turns off S_1 and S_4. Closing S_2 causes capacitor C_2 to rapidly charge to the peak voltage of the input signal. This occurs within less than a second in most cases.

7. Switch S_3 closes to allow capacitor C_1 to discharge slowly through resistor R_3. The charge on C_2 will reach peak before any appreciable decay of the C_1 charge takes place. In some models each charge switch is operated directly from FF_1, while the discharge switch is operated by the same signal after it has passed through an R-C network delay line (Figure 9-15c). This network ensures that one capacitor is fully charged before the other begins to decay.

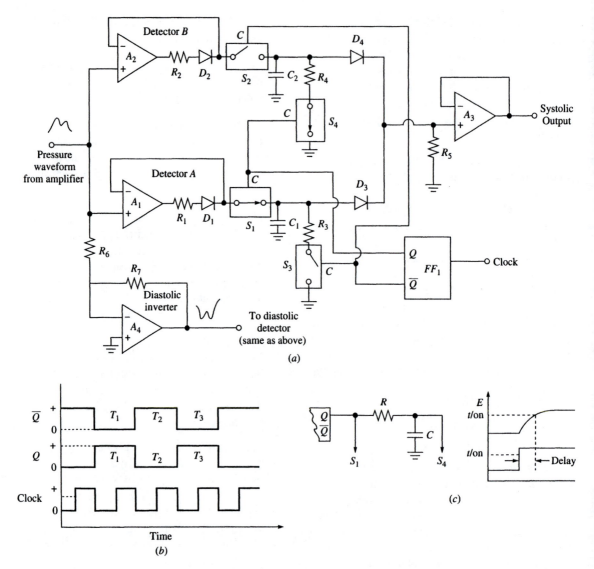

Figure 9-15
(a) Systolic detector circuit. (b) Timing diagram. (c) Turn-on delay circuit for S_4 and waveform.

8. The voltage at the output of Figure 9-15a represents the *peak* of the waveform, which corresponds to the *systolic* pressure. The same circuit may be used to detect the diastolic voltage by inverting the waveform so that the diastolic feature becomes the peak.

The MAP is found by taking the time average (i.e., *integrating*) of the pressure waveform (Figure 9-16a). An example of a simple mean value integrator is shown in Figure 9-16b. Most pressure monitors use a simple R-C integrator with buffering amplifiers rather than regular operational amplifier integrators.

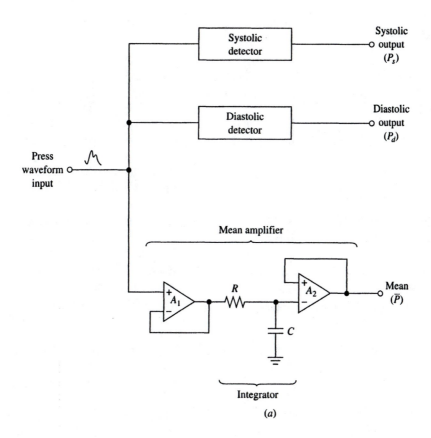

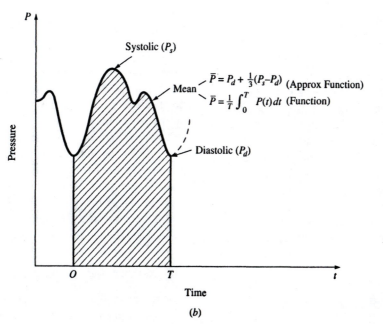

$$\bar{P} = P_d + \frac{1}{3}(P_s - P_d) \text{ (Approx Function)}$$

$$\bar{P} = \frac{1}{T}\int_0^T P(t)\,dt \text{ (Function)}$$

Figure 9-16

(a) Mean arterial pressure (MAP) detector. (b) Graphical and mathematical meaning of MAP.

The mean reading may confuse some medical and nursing personnel who were taught the *functional* definition of MAP, which is

$$\overline{P} = P_d + \frac{P_s - P_d}{3} \qquad (9\text{-}2)$$

where

   $\overline{P}$ is the *mean* arterial pressure in mm Hg

   P_d is the diastolic pressure in mm Hg

   P_s is the systolic pressure in mm Hg

Example 9-4

A patient's blood pressure is measured as 120 mm Hg systolic and 80 mm Hg diastolic. What is the mean arterial pressure?

Solution

$$\overline{P} = P_d + \frac{P_s - P_d}{3} \qquad (9\text{-}2)$$

$$\overline{P} = (80 \text{ mm Hg}) + \frac{(120 - 80)}{3} \text{ mm Hg}$$

$$\overline{P} = (80 \text{ mm Hg}) + \left(\frac{40}{3}\right) \text{ mm Hg}$$

$$\cong \textbf{93 mm Hg}$$

Equation 9-2 is only an *approximation* of the correct integral. It is used to find the *functional mean pressure,* which is accurate only when the patient's arterial waveform has approximately the correct *shape.* Although a wide latitude exists, a significant error results if the waveform is not normal. Some problems (see section 9-17) will *distort* the arterial waveform, so the mean displayed by the *meter* is in *error.* In other cases, however, the patient's correct (actual) waveform is atypical, resulting in a discrepancy between the meter and functional values. In that case, however, the *meter* reading is *correct.*

9-15 Pressure differentiation (*dP/dT*) circuits

Most pressure amplifiers designed for research applications, and many clinical instruments, are equipped with a special output producing a signal representing the *derivative* (i.e., the *time rate of change*) of the pressure waveform. In calculus notation this is *dP/dT;* it marks the derivative signal output jack on the pressure amplifier case or front panel.

Figure 9-17a shows a typical operational-amplifier *differentiator* used to differentiate physiological pressure signals. Resistor R_1 and capacitor C_1 are the actual differentiator components, while C_2 and R_2 are used to improve the stability of the circuit.

The *time constant* of a true differentiator must be very short compared with the *period* of the input signal. In the case of waveforms such as arterial pressure, it must be very short compared with the rise time of the waveform's *leading edge.* The *R-C* time constant of the circuit in Figure 9-17a is 10 ms, which is appropriate in *dP/dT* circuits. The same circuit principle is used in other physiological instruments with time constants as low as 25 μs.

Figure 9-17b shows the standard method for calibrating a differentiator. A *sawtooth,* or *ramp* signal, is applied to the input. The derivative of a signal quantifies its rate of change or *slope,* so the derivative of a ramp (i.e., *constant* rate of change) is a constant voltage.

The derivative of a ramp can be found from computation of its slope, which is defined as the ratio of *rise* over *run* (*Y* over *X,* or simply *Y/X*). On a strip-chart recorder or oscilloscope display, we may count the number of divisions the signal rises and divide by the number of horizontal divisions that were required for the signal to rise to that height. The vertical divisions represent the pressure in mm Hg, while the horizontal divisions represent time in seconds. The unit for *dP/dT* output, then, is mm Hg/s.

9-16 Automatic zero circuits

Many recent models of blood pressure monitors incorporate circuitry that automatically balances the amplifier to zero null. There is usually a front-panel pushbutton marked "zero." The operator opens the transducer stopcock to atmosphere,

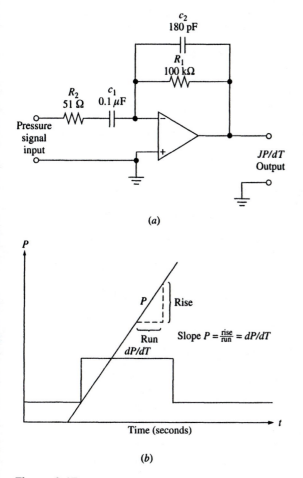

(a)

(b)

Figure 9-17
Differentiator to generate the *dP/dT* waveform. (*a*)
Differentiator circuit. (*b*) Calibration with a linear
ramp.

which is the zero pressure reference, and then
presses the *zero* button. Any voltage existing at the
output of the amplifier when the button is pressed
is assumed to be an offset or error voltage, so it is
nulled out.

Figure 9-18 shows the block diagram for an
auto-zero circuit. The three major sections are
summation amplifier, ramp generator, and *control
logic.*

The summation amplifier receives the output of
the pressure amplifier and the output of the ramp

generator. Its output will be the *algebraic sum* of
these two input signals.

The ramp generator produces a voltage that begins at zero and rises to a maximum voltage in a
linear manner. The circuit shown in Figure 9-18
uses a digital-to-analog converter (DAC) to generate the ramp. A few obsolete instruments are still
found that use a glass dielectric (i.e., low-leakage)
capacitor charged from a constant current source
to do substantially the same job.

The DAC produces an output voltage proportional to the binary word applied to its digital inputs. The binary word is created by a binary
counter that is incremented by a 2.5-kHz clock. In
this case the counter starts at 00000000_2 and
moves one increment for each clock pulse until a
count of 11111111_2 (i.e., 256_{10}) is reached, or the
counter is halted by an external gate.

The control logic section consists of two monostable multivibrators (i.e., one-shots), a three-input
not-and (NAND) gate, and a ground-referenced
voltage comparator. As long as any *one* input of
the NAND gate is *low* (i.e., zero volts), its output
will remain *high.* If *both* inputs 1 and 3 are high,
then the clock pulses will pass through the gate
to the input of the binary counter. The output of
the voltage comparator will remain high as long
as the summation amplifier output voltage E_o is
greater than zero. Operation of the circuit is as
follows:

1. The operator opens the transducer stopcock to
atmosphere and presses the *zero* button. This
action triggers the first one-shot (OS_1), which
produces a 1-ms pulse.

2. The pulse from OS_1 resets the binary counter
to zero and triggers the second one-shot
(OS_2).

3. The output of OS_2 goes high, forcing input 3 of
the NAND gate to go high also, for a period of
500 ms.

4. If voltage E_o is greater than zero, then the
output of the voltage comparator turns gate 1 of
the NAND gate also high, allowing clock
pulses to pass through to the binary counter.

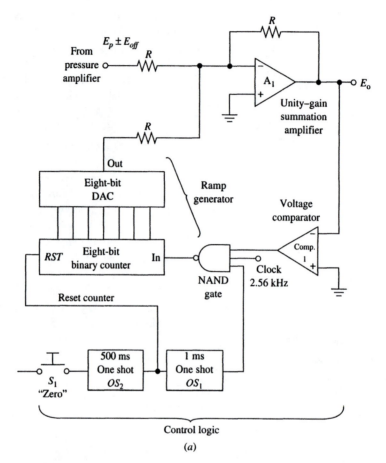

Figure 9-18
Automatic zero circuit (*a*) Circuit diagram.

5. The counter begins incrementing immediately, and this forces the DAC output voltage to rise. This voltage is applied to the input of the summation amplifier.

6. Output E_o will now be a summation of the error offset voltage and the ramp voltage. Since the ramp voltage has a polarity opposite that of the error voltage, it begins to cancel the offset component of E_o.

7. When E_o drops to zero, the voltage comparator output goes low, closing the NAND gate. The counter will stop, and its output digital word is that which existed at the instant E_o reached zero, plus or minus the usual one count.

8. The amplifier is now zeroed, so the transducer stopcock is closed. From now on, the voltage appearing at the output of the summation amplifier will represent *only* the pressure signal.

The capacitor-type circuits work in substantially the same manner but suffer from a type of zero drift caused by *droop* of the capacitor charge voltage (i.e., discharge of the capacitor through leak-

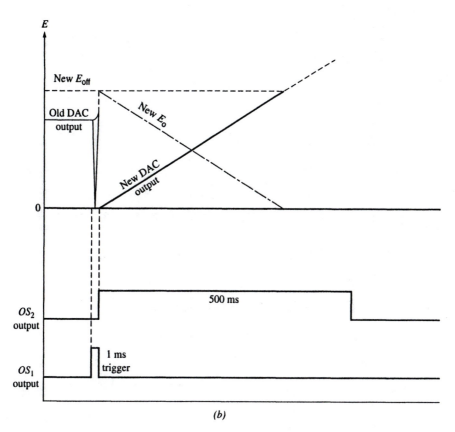

(b)

Figure 9-18 (cont'd)
(b) Timing and waveform diagram.

age and ordinary circuit impedances). The DAC method is preferred by most manufacturers because it holds the zero longer, and the cost of modern (IC) DACs is actually *lower* than the large glass capacitors formerly used in auto-zero circuits.

9-17 Practical problems in pressure monitoring

In practical monitoring situations, there are a few problems that must be solved by either operating personnel or the people who deal exclusively with medical instrumentation (i.e., biomedical equipment technicians, clinical engineers, or monitoring/cardiovascular technicians).

9-17-1 Hydrostatic pressure

The liquid in the transducer plumbing system has mass, so its weight can apply a force to the transducer diaphragm that is also interpreted as a pressure. This force creates an offset voltage at the transducer output.

Figure 9-19a shows a transducer with a *positive* hydrostatic pressure head caused by the weight of the fluid in the tubing brought to the transducer from *above*.

Similarly, a *negative* pressure head is obtained when the tubing is predominantly *below* the level of the transducer diaphragm (Figure 9-19b). The solution to this offset problem is shown in Figure 9-19c; the tubing has approximately equal lengths

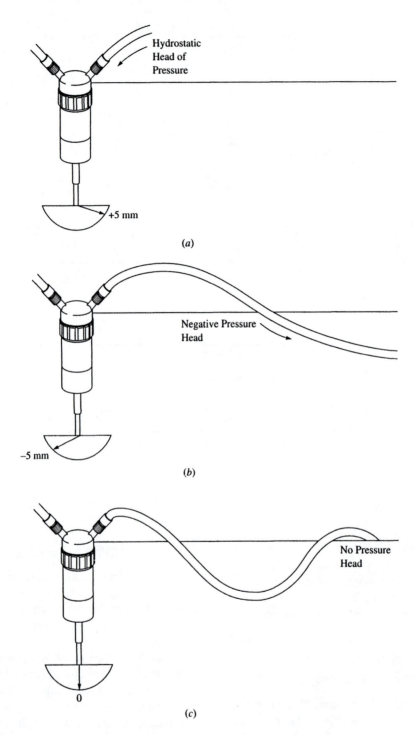

Figure 9-19
Hydrostatic pressure. (*a*) Positive pressure head. (*b*) Negative pressure head. (*c*) Balancing positive and negative pressure heads. (Reprinted courtesy of Hewlett-Packard)

above and below the level of the diaphragm. The transducer diaphragm serves as the guide point for positioning one end of the plumbing system, while the catheter tip inside the patient serves as the reference for the other end.

The transducer is usually physically mounted on a special stand, or standard IV pole, next to the patient's bed. The transducer will be on a special mount that allows it to be moved up and down on the pole to adjust for different hydrostatic pressure situations. The diaphragm should be level and at a height equal to the height from the floor to the catheter *tip,* not the point on the patient's body where the catheter is inserted. In any given case, the catheter tip may be several centimeters above the insertion point.

Figure 9-20 shows the correct point for locating the transducer when intracardiac catheters are used: the midline of the chest as viewed from the side. Most authorities agree that a good approximation on most patients is 10 cm above the bed, when the patient is in the *supine* position. Earlier advice (referencing the midline to an anatomical point on the patient's chest) is used less often because it more frequently results in erroneous readings.

Hydrostatic pressure accounts for many *apparent* errors in pressure measurement systems. But these can be minimized by correct positioning of

the transducer and need not affect a properly configured system.

9-17-2 Plumbing system distortion

It is possible for mechanical problems in the transducer plumbing system to adversely affect the waveform and meter readings that are obtained. The properties of the system can create mechanical resonances and damping that distort the waveform. The arterial pressure waveform is *nonsinusoidal,* containing a fundamental frequency plus a number of *harmonics* (whole number multiples) of that fundamental frequency. If the plumbing system were perfect (which it never is), then the fundamental frequency and all its harmonics would be transmitted through the system unattenuated in *amplitude* and *unchanged* in phase.

Figure 9-21*a* shows a good reproduction of the arterial waveform at the output of the transducer. This situation occurs when the plumbing system and the transducer have a frequency response high enough so that no significant harmonics of the arterial waveform are attenuated. The systolic and diastolic values determined by the peak holder circuits (see section 9-15) are then correct.

The lower waveform in Figure 9-21*b* shows a slightly *damped* waveform. It is essentially a good representation of the original, although some loss

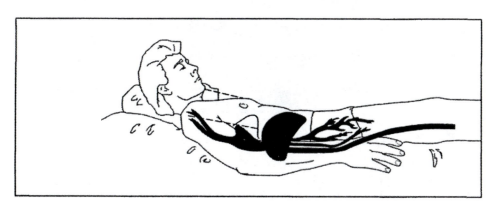

Figure 9-20
Proper transducer placement for measuring intracardiac pressures is along the midchest line.
(Reprinted courtesy of Hewlett-Packard)

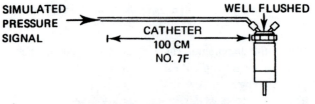

TO PRESSURE MONITOR

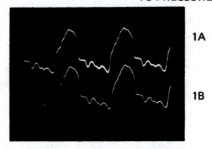

1A

1B

WAVEFORM 1A – SIMULATED ARTERIAL WAVEFORM

WAVEFORM 1B – A GOOD REPRODUCTION THROUGH PLUMBING

(a)

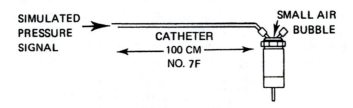

TO PRESSURE MONITOR

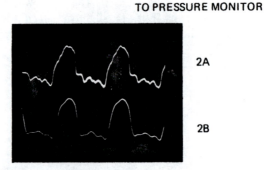

2A

2B

WAVEFORM 2A – SIMULATED ARTERIAL WAVEFORM

WAVEFORM 2B – SLIGHTLY DAMPED WAVEFORM
PRESSURE VALUES PROBABLY NOT LOST

(b)

Figure 9-21
Waveforms associated with several pressure monitoring system faults. (a) Proper reproduction
of the waveform. (b) Mildly damped waveform. (Reprinted courtesyof Hewlett-Packard)

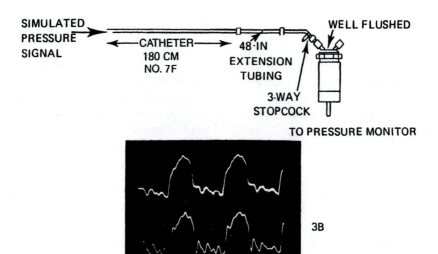

WAVEFORM 3A – SIMULATED ARTERIAL WAVEFORM

WAVEFORM 3B – ARTIFACT CAUSED BY RESONANCE
PRESSURE VALUES TOO HIGH

(c)

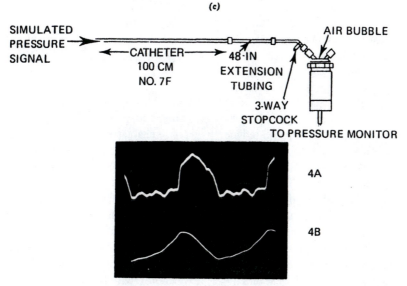

WAVEFORM 4A -- SIMULATED ARTERIAL WAVEFORM

WAVEFORM 4B – BADLY DAMPED WAVEFORM
SYSTOLIC PRESSURE VALUES VERY LOW

(d)

Figure 9-21 (cont'd)
(*c*) Ringing in the waveform due to resonance in the system. (*d*) Badly damped waveform.
(Reprinted courtesy of Hewlett-Packard)

of the high-frequency components occurs. This waveform is close to those ordinarily found in clinical pressure-monitoring situations. Most important to consider, however, is that the diastolic and systolic values are still very accurate and essentially as good as those obtained from the waveform in Figure 9-21a.

An example of *ringing* in the waveform caused by *system resonances* is shown in Figure 9-21c. This problem inevitably causes systolic and diastolic readings that are *too high.*

The opposite problem, *excessive damping* of the waveform, is shown in Figure 9-21d. In the lower tracing all high-frequency components are obliterated, and the overall amplitude of the waveform is seriously *reduced.* The diastolic value obtained by the peak detectors will probably fall within reasonable bounds, but the systolic reading will probably be *very low.* A similar waveform is obtained *normally* from hypotensive patients, even though there is no fault in the system. (In such cases, however, measuring the patient's pressure by auscultation reveals the low pressures.)

The example in Figure 9-21b shows slight damping of the waveform caused by the introduction of a *small* air bubble into the dome. Fluid is not compressible, but air (being a gas) is very compressible. As a result, an air bubble will reduce the frequency response of the system, attenuating the high-frequency components of the arterial waveform. The plumbing system, therefore, must be assembled in a way that reduces the chance of air bubble formation. A reasonable rule of thumb is that less complex systems are less prone to air bubble formation. It is also true that *metal* hydraulic fittings are *more* prone to such problems; metal fittings tend to leak because of wear and the effects of ethylene oxide gas used in sterilization on the rubber washers and lubricant. These washers must be replaced periodically, and the internal mechanism of the fittings must be relubricated using a product such as Dow-Corning High-Vac grease.

The waveform in Figure 9-21c resulted from extending the catheter tubing, which modifies the system resonance to a point closer to the frequency components of the arterial waveform. The higher harmonics are therefore transmitted to the dome *faster* than the lower harmonics, and this *enhances* the high-frequency features of the waveform.

The last waveform, Figure 9-21d, resulted from the formation of a *large* air bubble in the system. The cure is to purge the system of bubbles properly. This waveform can also result from the formation of the products of blood coagulation in the catheter line.

It is advisable to be careful as to the dimensions and properties of the tubing used in pressure-measuring systems. The catheter should have a large diameter, not less than the standard No. 7 French or 18-gauge sizes, and should be stiff and noncompliant. Teflon tubing is preferred, while standard flexible IV tubing should *never* be used. The tubing should be less than 100 cm long, and the system should be as simple as possible (i.e., fewest number of fittings).

9-18 Step-function frequency response test

The ability of a pressure system to respond to *changes* in pressure depends on its *dynamic response* characteristics, which are also its *frequency response.* All waveforms other than a perfect sine wave are composed of a *Fourier series* of sine and cosine harmonics of the fundamental frequency. The specific harmonics present, and their respective amplitude and phase shifts, determine the actual shape of the wave. If the harmonics are removed by any kind of filtering action, including damping (as in fluid pressure systems), then the waveform will be distorted. The electronic circuitry and fluid "plumbing" of the pressure measurement system, as well as the characteristics of the transducer, must be selected to pass frequencies from near-dc to about 20 Hz, or distortion of the blood pressure waveform will result.

Figure 9-22a shows a test apparatus that can be used to square-wave test the system. A water-filled catheter or needle to the system terminates in a

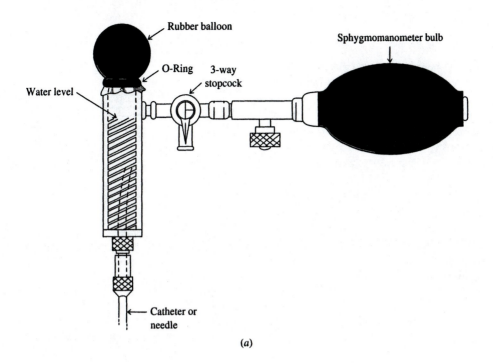

Rubber balloon

O-Ring

3-way
stopcock

Sphygmomanometer bulb

Water level

Catheter or
needle

(a)

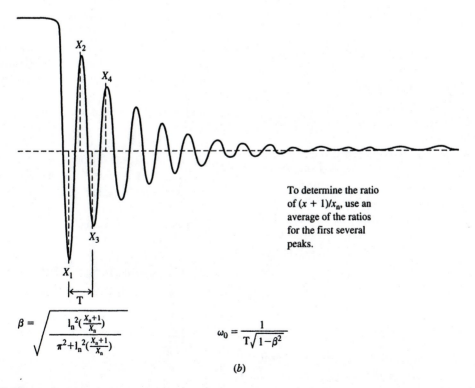

X_2

X_4

To determine the ratio
of $(x + 1)/x_n$, use an
average of the ratios
for the first several
peaks.

X_3

X_1

T

$$\beta = \sqrt{\frac{l_n^2(\frac{X_n+1}{X_n})}{\pi^2 + l_n^2(\frac{X_n+1}{X_n})}}$$

$$\omega_0 = \frac{1}{T\sqrt{1-\beta^2}}$$

(b)

Figure 9-22
(a) An assembly used in testing the transient oscillatory response of the catheter-transducer
system. (b) The transient oscillatory response of a catheter transducer system on application
of a pressure square wave. (Courtesy of Spacelabs)

syringe body just below a port that accommodates a standard three-way stopcock. A small balloon is attached to the open end of the assembly with an O-ring. A sphygmomanometer squeeze-bulb pump is used to apply pressure to the system, inflating the balloon. Once a static pressure head is registering on the electronic pressure meter, a flame is used to pop the balloon, resulting in a sudden decrease in pressure that nearly simulates an actual negative-going square wave. The result is a *free oscillation* of the pressure in the system with a frequency ω_o (Figure 9-22b) that dies out at an exponential rate determined by the *damping factor* (β). The oscillation frequency is given by:

$$\omega_o = \frac{1}{T\sqrt{1 - \beta^2}} \tag{9-3}$$

while the damping factor is given by:

$$\beta = \sqrt{\frac{\ln^2\left(\dfrac{X_{n+1}}{X_n}\right)}{\pi^2 + \ln^2\left(\dfrac{X_{n+1}}{X_n}\right)}} \tag{9-4}$$

It is usually desirable for β to be on the order of 0.7 for a frequency response of 20 Hz. This number provides *critical damping*. If the number is very much less then the system is *subcritically damped* and may *ring* (i.e., provide unnaturally high systolic readings resulting from a sharpening of the waveform caused by excess high-frequency components). Similarly, an *undercritically damped* system, with $\beta \gg 0.7$, results in attenuation of high-frequency components, causing an unnaturally low systolic reading. The output of the system will correlate closely to actual pressure when β is about 0.7.

9-19 Transducer care

Blood pressure transducers are delicate instruments. Physical abuse *will* damage a transducer. The diaphragm is especially sensitive and should *never be touched*. It may be cleaned by using a

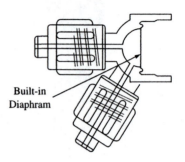

Built-in
Diaphram

Figure 9-23
Disposable transducer dome. (Courtesy of Statham Instruments Division, Gould, Inc., Oxnard, Calif.)

gentle solvent and a cotton ball or swab. Do not apply any pressure to the diaphragm while cleaning; if the dirt cannot be wiped off with the cotton, then leave it on.

Transducers are often sterilized after use on each patient to prevent spread of disease. Steam sterilization in the autoclave must *never* be used because it destroys the transducer. Only *gas sterilization* may be used unless a disposable dome (Figure 9-23) is used. The disposable dome is discarded after each use, so the transducer may be disinfected using a liquid disinfectant agent (such as Cydex).

The disposable dome uses a thin membrane to couple pressure inside the dome to the diaphragm. Most designs require that a single drop of fluid be placed on the diaphragm before the dome is secured to the transducer body. The water or fluid drop ensures good coupling.

9-19-1 Transducer calibration and balance procedure

Most arterial blood pressure transducers and amplifiers have two basic controls: *zero* and *calibration*. The procedure for adjusting the amplifiers is as follows:

1. Open the stopcocks on the transducer to atmosphere.

2. Adjust the *height* of the transducer to the level of the catheter tip inside of the patient's arm.

3. Adjust the *zero* control on the amplifier for a zero reading on the meter or for a zero baseline on the oscilloscope.

4. Press the *calibrate* button (this injects a simulated pressure signal into the amplifier, usually 100, 150, or 200 mm Hg. This button is often labeled with the pressure level simulated).

5. Adjust the *calibration* control (also called *span* or *sensitivity* control on many models) so that the meter readout, or oscilloscope, reads the indicated pressure level.

6. Close the transducer stopcock. The system should now be ready to use.

If there is any doubt as to the accuracy of the system, or if the transducer has been abused or is old, then it may be necessary to check the calibration. Also, in many cases the amplifier does not have a calibration signal built in. In those cases, modify the aforementioned procedure to allow the use of a mercury, or aneroid-assembly, *manometer* to check the calibration. Most biomedical equipment technicians use a modified blood pressure gauge for this purpose (mercury manometers are sometimes preferred to the aneroid types). Take an ordinary blood pressure set and remove the cuff (there is sometimes a hose connector at the site where the hose enters the cuff; otherwise, *cut the line*). Install a Luer-lock connector (usually available in most hospital central supply departments or the anesthesiology department) in the end of the hose removed from the cuff. When this setup is used, we can check and adjust the amplifier. Once the zero is set, close the stopcocks and pump a pressure onto the system. Then adjust amplifier to indicate this pressure level. Check the linearity of the system by comparing manometer pressure against indicated pressure.

There are two ways to pressurize the transducer for this test. One is to place a fluid-filled blood transfusion bag on the system and pump it up to the required pressure level. The other is to use air. The former is preferred in clinical settings, while the latter may be used in bench-testing pressure systems. One word of warning, however: Always disconnect the catheter from the patient; *it is not acceptable to pump air into the patient.*

9-20 Cardiac output measurement

Cardiac output (CO) is defined as the volume rate at which the heart pumps blood. CO is measured in *liters per minute* (L/min). In adults, CO reaches a value between approximately 3 and 5 L/min.

One quantitative definition of cardiac output is that it is the product of *stroke volume* and *heart rate*. The stroke volume is the volume of blood ejected from the ventricle during a single contraction of the heart. Cardiac output, then, is

$$CO = V \times R \qquad (9\text{-}5)$$

where

CO is the cardiac output in *liters per minute* (L/min)

V is the stroke volume in *liters per beat* (L/beat)

R is the heart rate in *beats per minute* (beats/min)

Example 9-5

Calculate the cardiac output for a patient with a heart rate of 86 beats/min if the stroke volume is 42 mL/beat.

Solution

$CO = V \times R$
$CO = 42 \text{ mL/beat} \times 1\ 1/1000 \text{ mL}$
       $\times 86 \text{ beats/min}$
     $= 3612/1000 \text{ L/min}$
$CO = \textbf{3.61 L/min}$

It is difficult, and usually impossible, to measure CO using a technique based on Equation 9-5 in practical situations because of the difficulty in obtaining adequate stroke volume data.

9-20-1 Blood flow measurements

Blood flow measurements can yield CO data. Such instruments measure the blood flow rate, and the CO is determined by *integrating* the blood flow signal over a known period of time.

The problem with this method, however, is that most blood-flow transducers capable of delivering meaningful quantitative data must be applied directly to the blood vessel being measured. It is not possible to obtain valid CO data from blood vessels taken far downstream in the arterial system; thus none of the easily accessible peripheral arteries (i.e., in an arm or a leg) can be used. The measurement must be done either in the pulmonary artery or in the aorta immediately after these vessels leave the heart. This requirement limits CO measurement via blood flow measurement to thoracic surgery procedures, when the vessels are normally exposed anyway (see section 9-24 for a more detailed discussion of blood-flow measurement).

9-20-2 Dilution techniques

Most modern cardiac output measurement systems use a *dilution* technique in which a known concentration of some tracer material is injected into the bloodstream just before the heart. The diluted concentration is measured downstream, past the heart, thus yielding the cardiac output.

Different types of tracer materials are used in CO measurement (the most common is indiocyanine green, discussed in section 9-21-2). These are used almost routinely on certain patients in special hospital laboratories or even at bedside in ICUs and CCUs.

All dilution techniques used to obtain CO information use an injectate that enters the heart at the atria in concentration. The diluted concentra-

tion is measured distal to the heart (on the output side), and the flow is given by

$$CO = \frac{\text{Injection rate (mg/min)}}{\text{Concentration (mg/L)}} \text{ (L/min)} \qquad (9\text{-}6)$$

9-21 Dilution methods

9-21-1 The Fick method

An early—but still used—technique called the *Fick method* uses room oxygen inhaled by the patient during normal respiration as the indicator substance. The oxygen is injected into the system during respiration by the lungs.

The infusion rate is determined by the measurement of respiratory gases. It is necessary to subtract the oxygen concentration of the patient's exhaled air from the room air concentration, normally taken to be 21%.

Concentration is determined by measuring the oxygen concentration of arterial blood as it leaves the lungs. But the term *arterial blood* contains an error term because returning venous blood contains some oxygen. This amount must be determined and subtracted from the arterial oxygen concentration. Repeated measurements made over several minutes are averaged for the final result.

The Fick method has been automated and is still used, but for the most part it has been supplanted by other methods.

9-21-2 Dye dilution

Dye dilution uses either an *optical* dye, such as indocyanine green, or a *radioactive* tracer dye. In the optical case the dilution curve is measured by a *light densitometer* and in the latter case by a *scintillation counter,* or *gamma camera.*

Figure 9-24 shows the concentration at the point of measurement distal to the injection site. Shortly after injection, the concentration at the measurement site rises abruptly to a maximum value and then falls off exponentially as the injec-

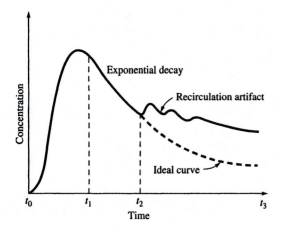

Figure 9-24
Dilution curve showing recirculation artifact.

tate bolus passes the point. This exponential decay is caused by the injectate bolus not remaining as a lump but spreading out (diluting) over a long path as blood flows.

CO is then measured by integrating the concentration curve. This information is used in an equation of the general form of Equation 9-7:

$$\text{Blood flow rate} = \frac{k \times M}{\displaystyle\int C\,dt}\,(\text{mL/min}) \qquad (9\text{-}7)$$

where

k is a constant, usually 20 to 150 depending on injectate

M is the volume of injectate, in mL

C is the concentration, in mg/mL

A problem arises, however, in the form of a *recirculation artifact* (at time t_2 in Figure 9-24). The artifact changes the shape of the exponential decay curve between times t_2 and t_3 from the expected ideal shape.

In most early instruments, the curve was traced out by a chart recorder. Graphical means were then used to extrapolate, and then integrate, the area under the curve in the exponential region. This pro-

cedure could be done with a mechanical graphics integrator device or by counting (i.e., summing) the number of squares under the idealized curve on the graph paper.

9-21-3 Thermodilution

Thermodilution has become one of the most common methods for measurement of cardiac output and forms the basis for most of the modern cardiac output computers on the market. The injectate used is ordinary IV solutions, such as saline or 5% dextrose in water (D_5W).

Most thermodilution CO computers operate on a version of the following equation:

$$\text{CO} = \frac{K G_B G_I V_I (T_B - T_I)}{U_B U_I \displaystyle\int T'_B\,dt}\,(L/min) \qquad (9\text{-}8)$$

where

CO is the cardiacoutput in *liters per minute* (L/min)

K is a constant, approximately 20 to 150

G_B is the density of human blood, in kg/m³

G_I is the density of the injectate, in kg/m³

V_I is the injectate volume, in liters (L)

U_B is the heat energy content of the blood in joules (J)

U_I is the heat energy content of the injectate in joules (J)

T_I is the preinjection temperature of the injectate in degrees Celsius (°C) (Note: either *iced* or *room temperature* injectate may be used)

T_B is the preinjection temperature of the blood in degrees Celsius

T'_B is the postinjection temperature of the blood at the measurement site

Equation 9-8 looks rather formidable, but we find that it becomes a lot simpler once it is recognized that most of the terms are constants.

Furthermore, many of the constants need not be measured, but assumptions can be made. Edwards Laboratories, for example, manufactures a CO computer in which the following simplified version of Equation 9-8 is used:

$$CO = \frac{(60)(1.08)(C_t)(V_I)(T_B - T_I)}{\int T'_B \, dt} \qquad (9\text{-}9)$$

where

CO   is the cardiac output in *liters per minute* (L/min)

60   is the conversion factor for seconds to minutes

1.08   is a composite of other constants, dimensionless

C_t is a dimensionless correction factor for the injectate temperature rise in the catheter and is published by the catheter manufacturer specific to each different type

Example 9-6 _____

A special cardiac output test fixture enters a thermistor signal that represents a temperature change of 7°C. Find the expected cardiac output reading if the instrument is set to measure the following parameters: injectate volume of 10 mL, body temperature of 37°C, and an injectate temperature of 25°C. The catheter correction factor C_t is 52.5 and the computation time is 10 s.

Solution

$$CO = \frac{(60)(1.08)C_t V_I (V_B - T_I)}{\int T'_B \, dt}$$

$$CO = \frac{60 \text{ s/min } (1.08)(52.5)[10 \text{ mL} \times 1 \, 1/1000 \text{ mL}](37 - 25)°C}{(7°C)(10 \text{ s})}$$

$$CO = (60)(1.08)(52.5)(0.01)(12)$$

$$= (1/70 \text{ min}) = \mathbf{5.81 \text{ L/min}}$$

The excitation of the Wheatstone bridge used to make the temperature measurement is done by a dc source and must be very stable, at least over the short term. Batteries usually meet this requirement because they maintain the same voltage level over the short term, even though they deteriorate over the long term. In many cases, however, the isolated front-end dc power supply is dropped to a low level and then regulated by the drop across a germanium diode. This is an unusual procedure but is justified because it limits the transducer excitation potential to approximately 200 mV, a value consistent with the electrical safety requirement of the design.

The recirculation artifact is small in thermodilution, so it is often the case that computers designed specifically for use in this technique may not have a means for compensating for the artifact.

Figure 9-25 shows the block diagram of one popular CO computer. The bridge produces zero output when the thermistor is at normal blood temperature, and the balance adjustment is made. After injection of the saline or D_5W, however, the bridge produces an output potential of 1.8 mV/°C. This signal is amplified in the preamplifier stage to a level of 1 V/°C. The high-level output signal is passed through an isolator to the remainder of the circuit. Part of the signal goes to an output jack so that it may be recorded on a strip-chart recorder while it is simultaneously applied to the input of an operational amplifier electronic integrator stage. The integrator output, which supplies the denominator of Equation 9-9, changes by a factor of 1 V/°C-s. This stage provides the integral of temperature required by the instrument. The integrator output signal is applied to the denominator (i.e., V_y) input of an analog divider circuit.

9-21-4 Some sample computers

Most thermodilution CO computers use a special catheter that has a *thermistor* in the tip to make the measurement. The catheter is introduced into the right side of the heart via a venous cutdown. It is threaded through the right atrium and right ventri-

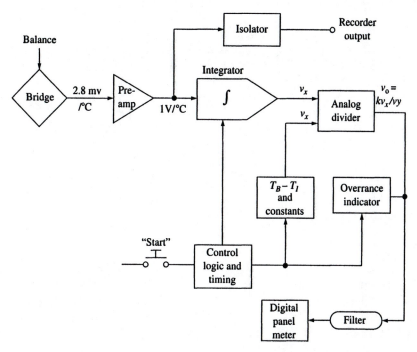

Figure 9-25
Block diagram for a cardiac output computer.

cle to the pulmonary artery. One lumen of the catheter carries the injectate, which is injected into the bloodstream just prior to the right atrium.

As the injectate bolus passes the thermistor tip of the catheter, the thermistor resistance changes an amount proportional to the temperature change. A Wheatstone bridge and an isolated preamplifier are used to actually acquire the temperature signal.

Figure 9-26 shows a typical front-end circuit for a thermodilution CO computer. Resistors R_1 through R_4 form a Wheatstone bridge and may be either fixed or variable to allow the operator to compensate for differences between catheters. In the circuit shown, resistor R_4 is the thermistor in the catheter tip, and R_2 is the potentiometer used to adjust the circuit for null condition. This potentiometer should be adjusted only after the thermistor in the catheter tip has been in place for several minutes so that it has time to come into thermal

equilibrium with the blood. At that time, R_2 is adjusted to produce a null or zero output from the preamplifier.

It is absolutely necessary to isolate the patient from any electrical hazards during any medical procedure, and in the case of a cardiac output computer special precautions are required because the catheter is introduced directly into the patient's heart (see chapter 19). Any electrical defects could potentially be very serious. That is why it is standard procedure to operate the CO computer from rechargeable batteries rather than the ac power mains. It is also why isolated input preamplifiers are universally used in these machines. A typical CO computer operates as follows:

1. The numerator input of the divider is obtained from a stage that multiplies together the constants and a signal entered by the operator or, in more sophisticated models, taken from

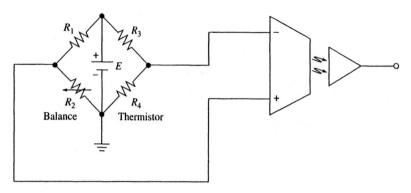

Figure 9-26
Input circuit for a thermodilution cardiac output computer.

another electronic temperature measurement circuit that indicates the differences between blood and injectate temperatures. The output of the circuit is scaled at 10 mV/°C. The analog divided output signal is filtered and scaled before being applied to a digital panel meter that serves as the cardiac output indicator.

2. A control logic circuit is required to time the operation of the CO measurement cycle. When the operator has the external controls (i.e., *balance* and *temperature difference*) adjusted and is ready to inject the solution, it is then necessary to press the *start* button. This action clears the integrator and resets the circuit to zero. Most computers have a beeper or audio tone that sounds as soon as the integrator is cleared, and this is the signal to immediately begin infusing the injectate. A short time later the cardiac output reading will appear on the digital panel meter. If the integration runs to overrange, then a panel light comes on to let the operator know that the data obtained is invalid. This problem is usually caused by too short a time selected for the measurement, a front-panel adjustment easily made on the CO computer. Skilled operators can spot this problem easily if the thermistor output curve is displayed on a strip-chart recorder. In any event,

the data obtained during the measurement that caused the lamp to turn on is invalid and must be discarded; another measurement must be made to obtain valid data.

3. CO computers that are used in both dye and thermal dilution must have a circuit to compensate for the recirculation artifact during dye procedures. Most circuits that do this are based on the time constant of the exponential decay portion of the temperature curve. The time constant of any exponential decay curve is the time required for it to drop from its maximum value to 36.7% of the maximum value.

4. Two different techniques are commonly used in predicting the path of the ideal exponential decay curve in the presence of the recirculation artifact.

   (a) The time period before the appearance of the artifact is used to predict the path of the ideal curve, and this is used to approximate the true integral.

   (b) The technique of *geometric integration* (Figure 9-27) is used to approximate the ideal curve.

Figure 9-27 shows the dilution curve. The curve is *assumed* to enter the exponential decay portion

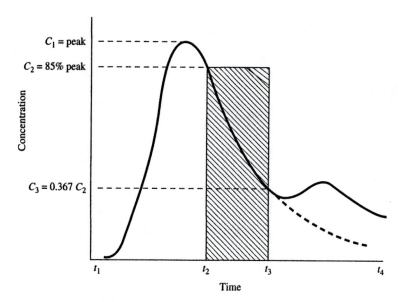

Figure 9-27
Geometric integration for determining the area under the exponential decay portion of the dilution curve.

when the dilution signal has passed the peak and then fallen to a value of 85% of the peak value. A voltage comparator is used to compare the concentration signal with the peak value stored in a peak holder circuit. The input of the electronic integrator stage will be connected to the thermistor or dye transducer from time t_1, when the computation begins, until the curve enters the exponential portion at time t_2.

At time t_2 the input of the integrator is switched to another source and receives a signal equal to 85% of the peak value for a time period t_3 to t_2. A very good approximation of the area under the exponential decay portion of the dilution curve is obtained by creating a rectangle with a height equal to the maximum value of the exponential curve, in this case 85% of the thermodilution curve, and a base equal to the time constant of the decay curve, defined as the time required for the curve to drop from its maximum value to 0.367 of its maximum. If the area of this rectangle is known, then the approximate area under the exponential portion of the curve is also known. In the case of the elec-

tronic CO computer, the area under the rectangle is determined by connecting the integrator to a source equal to 85% of the peak for a period of time t_3 to t_2. The mathematical expression for the area under the curve, in calculus notation, is

$$\int_{t1}^{t4} C\, dt \approx \int_{t1}^{t2} C_1\, dt + \int_{t2}^{t3} C_2\, dt \qquad (9\text{-}10)$$

The Edwards Laboratories Model 9520 bedside CO computer is shown in Figure 9-28. This model uses a liquid-crystal readout display to reduce battery drain to a bare minimum. Previous models required the operator to manually enter the temperature of the injectate and the patient's blood temperature, but this model measures those parameters automatically using thermistor probes. Additionally, this CO computer is equipped with a self-test feature that allows the operator to check the instrument. A thumbwheel switch on the side of the unit allows the operator to enter the computation constant, which is a function of which particular catheter is selected.

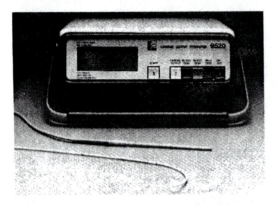

Figure 9-28
Cardiac output computer. (Courtesy of Edwards Laboratories, Inc.)

Almost any CO computer can be checked by constructing a *dummy thermistor.* Some biomedical equipment technicians build a tester using the electrical fittings salvaged from a used thermistor, described in the following procedure.

1. Select a resistor with a value equal to the nominal value of the catheter thermistor at 37°C. Connect a second resistor of 100 to 500 Ω in series with the first resistor. The exact values depend upon the specific computer being tested, but 12 kΩ and 200 Ω work for many popular models.

2. A *normally closed* switch is connected across the low-value resistor, shorting it out. This assembly is connected to the computer as if it were a thermistor.

3. Once the computer is adjusted for normal operation according to the manufacturer's instructions, the technician presses the computer's *start* button and opens the switch on the tester simultaneously. After about 5 to 8 s, the tester switch is closed, and a few seconds later a CO measurement appears. This value will vary from one test to another because of differences in the technician's

perception of 5 to 8 seconds but indicates that the circuits are working. In practice, one of the authors found it consistently possible to produce readings between 4 and 5 L/min using a stopwatch as the timer. Undoubtedly, an electronic timer and switch to automate the tester would yield more reproducible results.

9-22 Right-side heart pressures

The measurement of CVP and the other pressures on the right side of the heart are performed with a catheter such as the *Swan-Ganz,* shown in Figure 9-29a and 9-29b. This catheter is a multilumen model with a thermistor tip, so it may also be used for CO measurements by thermodilution.

To measure CVP the catheter tip is introduced into the right atrium of the heart (Figure 9-30), so this measurement is sometimes called the *right atrial pressure* (RAP). The catheter is inserted into the patient's body through one of the major peripheral veins (e.g., *jugular, brachial, subclavian*).

The pressure-measuring instrument may be an electronic model (described earlier in this chapter), or it may be a water manometer, calibrated in centimeters of water, not too dissimilar from Hales's eighteenth-century method. The modern CVP manometer, however, is made of plastic and is disposable.

The *pulmonary artery wedge pressure* (PAWP) can serve as an indicator of *left ventricular function,* the pumping efficiency of the heart. A flow-directed catheter with a balloon tip (Figure 9-29b) is passed from a peripheral vein through the *vena cava, right atrium, right ventricle,* and the *pulmonary valve* to the *pulmonary artery.* If one of the lumens of the balloon-tipped catheter has an end (or tip) hole, and the balloon is *inflated* (Figure 9-31a), the catheter sees only the pressure ahead (i.e., distal) to the catheter tip. This pressure is called the *pulmonary artery wedge pressure* and is strongly correlated to *left* atrial pressure; this pressure is considered a good indicator of left ventricular function.

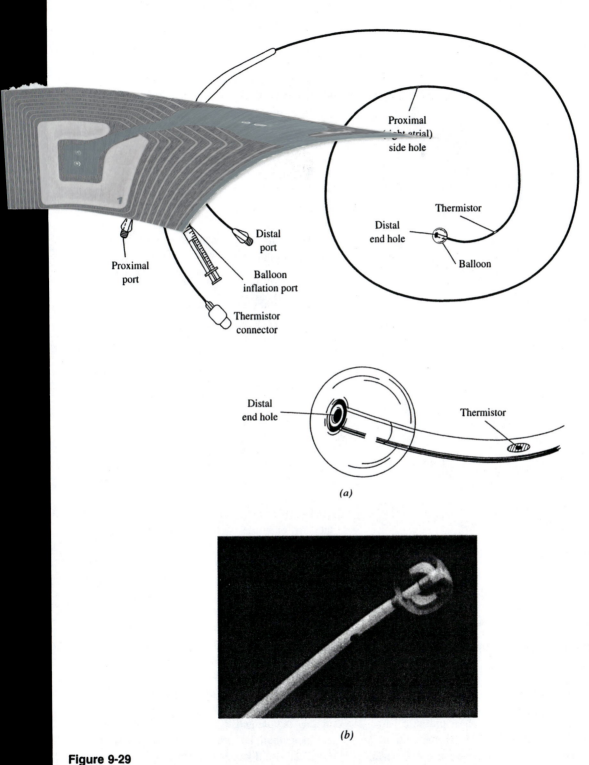

Proximal
(right atrial)
side hole

Thermistor

Distal
end hole

Balloon

Proximal
port

Distal
port

Balloon
inflation port

Thermistor
connector

Distal
end hole

Thermistor

(a)

(b)

Figure 9-29
(*a*) The No. 7 French quadruple-lumen thermodilution pulmonary artery catheter illustrated in both drawings. (*b*) Balloon-tipped catheter. (Courtesy of Edwards Laboratories, Inc.)

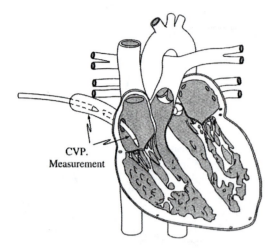

Figure 9-30
Catheter placement for measurement of CVP.
(Reprinted courtesy of Hewlett-Packard)

Inserting the catheter is a surgical procedure performed under sterile conditions but may be done at bedside in the ICU or CCU. An X-ray fluoroscope can be used to follow the progress of the catheter through the body. Alternatively, an oscilloscope or strip-chart recording of the pressure waveform will also indicate the progress of the catheter through the heart. Figure 9-31*b* shows typical waveforms at various points in the heart. There are also coded distance markings on the body of the catheter. (In jargon, this procedure is often called "inserting a Swan-Ganz" or, simply, a "swan.")

9-23 Plethysmography

Plethysmography is the determination of blood flow in a limb by measurement of *volume changes* of the limb. The plethysmograph produces a waveform that is similar to the arterial pressure waveform. To date, however, it has not proven possible to calibrate the plethysmograph waveform in terms of pressure units. The waveform is useful in measuring *pulse velocity* and indicating arterial obstructions.

The photoplethysmograph (PPG), also called the pseudoplethysmograph, is constructed from a *photocell* and a *light source*. The circuit for the PPG is shown in Figure 9-32*a;* the mechanical arrangement is shown in Figure 9-32*b*. In this example the light source is a light-emitting diode (LED), although in earlier models an incandescent lamp was used for the light source. The detector is a photoresistor (PC_1) excited by a constant current source. Changes in light intensity cause proportional changes in the resistance of PC_1. Since the current through the photoresistor is constant, the resistance changes produce voltage changes (E_o) at the output terminal.

The arterial pulse in the thumb causes the blood volume to change, changing the optical density of the blood. Therefore, the arterial pulse modulates the intensity of the light passing through the blood. Light from the LED is reflected into PC_1 by scattering and by direct reflection from the underlying bone structures.

The PPG does *not* indicate "calibratable" volume changes. Its usefulness is limited to pulse-velocity measurements, determination of heart rate, and an indication of the existence of a pulse in the finger.

A "true" plethysmograph is a little more difficult to construct and operate but yields quantitative data. An example is shown in Figure 9-33*a*. This device uses a sealed chamber surrounding the limb or digit being measured. The chamber is designed to have a constant volume, so volume changes in the limb are recorded as pressure variations inside of the chamber. The chamber pressure is measured electronically by a transducer and amplifier in the manner discussed earlier in this chapter.

A small syringe is connected to the chamber and serves as a volume calibrator. Once the zero baseline has been established on the pressure amplifier readout device, the position of the syringe's plunger is changed to vary the volume of the system by a small, but precise, amount. The span control of an oscilloscope or strip-chart recorder used to display the output waveform may then be adjusted to properly represent the unit volume change. Note that most small syringes are already

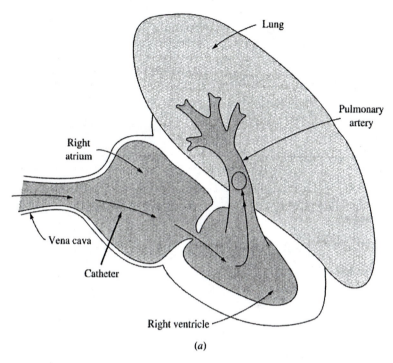

(a)

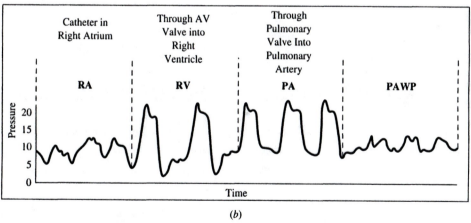

(b)

Figure 9-31
Placement of catheter for measurement of wedge pressure. (a) Placement in heart. (b)
Pressure waveforms during insertion of catheter. (From R. S. C. Cobbold, *Transducers for
Biomedical Measurements*, John Wiley & Sons, New York, 1974. Used by permission.)

calibrated in cubic centimeters (cc or cm^3), which
are units of volume equal to 1 mL.

The blood pressure cuff placed proximal to the
chamber seal is inflated to a pressure slightly
higher than the venous pressure. This condition

permits the flow of arterial blood into the limb
while preventing the outflow of venous blood,
allowing the limb volume to increase slightly
following each systole. These changes (Figure
9-33b) are recorded on the strip-chart recorder.

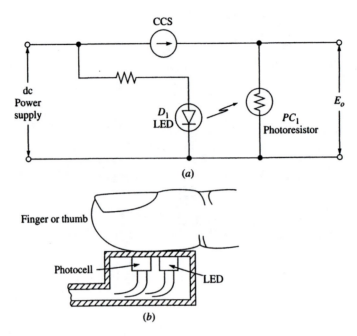

Figure 9-32
Photoplethysmograph. (*a*) Circuit. (*b*) Cutaway view.

Note, however, that a saturation point is reached and the curve flattens out at a specific level. This phenomenon is caused by the trapped venous blood distal to the cuff; that is, the system "fills up."

Capacitance, mercury strain gauges, and impedance plethysmographs are also used occasionally but mostly in research applications. In fact, most clinical plethysmography is done using the PPG despite its limitations.

9-24 Blood flow measurements

The measurement of *blood flow* is almost as important in many instances as the measurement of blood pressure. Although several techniques have been described,* the *electromagnetic* and *ultra-*

sonic methods have found the widest acceptance, although the latter is used less often clinically than the former. In this section we discuss the electromagnetic type, reserving the ultrasonic discussion for chapter 17.

The popularity of the magnetic flowmeter is the result of the following factors:

1. It measures volume flow rate independent of velocity.

2. It produces accuracies up to ±5%.

3. The technique can accommodate blood vessels of diameters from 1 mm to approximately 20 mm.

9-24-1 Theory

We know from basic electrical theory that a voltage is created when a moving conductor "cuts" the flux of a magnetic field. If that conductor is a

---

*Richard S. C. Cobbold, *Transducers for Biomedical Measurements,* Wiley-Interscience (New York, 1974).

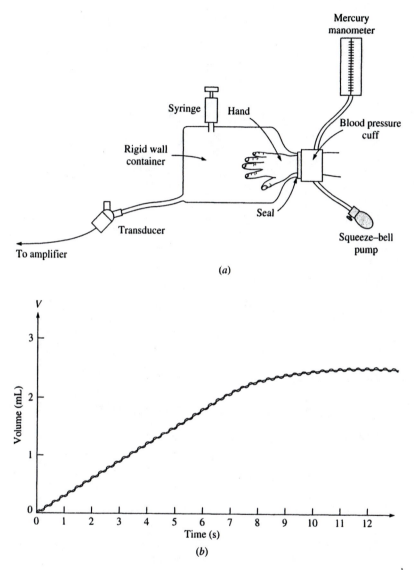

(a)

(b)

Figure 9-33
True plethysmograph. (a) Apparatus. (b) Output function.

blood-carrying vessel of diameter EE' (see Figure 9-34), the voltage generated will be

$$E = \frac{QB}{50\pi a}\,(\mu V) \qquad (9\text{-}11)$$

where

E is the potential in *microvolts* (μV)

Q is the volumetric flow rate in *cubic centimeters per second* (cm³/s) ($Q = \pi \bar{v} a^2$, where $\bar{v}$ is the average flow velocity over

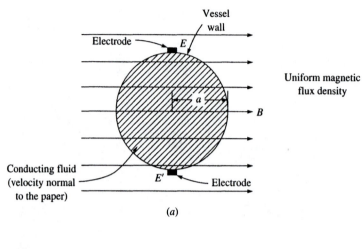

(a)

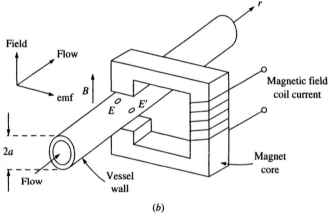

(b)

Figure 9-34
Electromagnetic flowmeter (a) Cross-sectional view. (b) Block diagram. (From R. S. C. Cobbold, *Transducers for Biomedical Measurements*, John Wiley & Sons, New York, 1974. Used by permission.)

the region from the center of the vessel to the vessel wall)

- *B* is the magnetic flux density in *gauss* (G)

- *a* is the vessel radius in *centimeters* (cm)

Example 9-7

Find the potential generated if blood flowing in a vessel with a radius of 0.9 cm cuts a magnetic field of 250 G. Assume a volume flow rate of 175 cm³/s.

Solution

$$E = \frac{QB}{50\pi a}$$

$$E = \frac{(175 \text{ cm}^3/\text{s})(250 \text{ G})}{(50)(3.14)(0.9 \text{ cm})}$$

$$E = 309 \text{ G-cm}^2/\text{s} = \textbf{309 } \boldsymbol{\mu}\textbf{V}$$

Figure 9-34 shows the typical transducer construction for magnetic flow measurements, while Figures 9-35a and 9-35b show commercially pro-

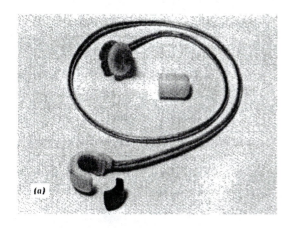

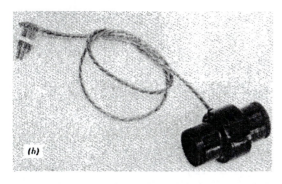

Figure 9-35
Electromagnetic flowmeter transducers. (*a*) Clip-on type. (*b*) In-line type. (Photo courtesy of Biotronix Laboratory)

duced models for in vivo and *extracorporeal* use, respectively.

Most magnetic blood flow amplifiers use ac to excite the electromagnet coil in the probe. The electrode potential that exists in dc-excited systems introduces an offset artifact that proves difficult to discriminate from the actual voltage signal. The ac carrier usually has a frequency between 200 and 2000 Hz.

The block diagram for a magnetic flowmeter is shown in Figure 9-36a, with the associated waveforms shown in Figure 9-36b. This circuit uses a full-wave synchronous phase-sensitive demodulator circuit to extract the flow rate information from the amplified electrode signal. This technique is used because the ac excitation produces an artifact in the electrodes by transformer coupling action. This signal has an amplitude that is several orders of magnitude *greater* than the desired flow signal and thus creates a tremendous level of interference if other types of detectors (i.e., simple envelope detectors) are used.

The detection system in Figure 9-36 is able to eliminate artifacts because of two factors: It is a *sampled* system, and the transformer electromotive force (emf) is in *quadrature* (i.e., 90 degrees out of phase with the excitation signal). The phase difference means that the artifact transformer emf signal is *zero* when the excitation signal is *maximum*. If a *short* sample of the waveform is taken when the transformer signal is near zero, then the magnitude of the artifact is reduced considerably. As with many pulse-sampling instruments, an *integrator* is used to extract the analog signal from the sampled ac signal.

9-25 Phonocardiography

Phonocardiography is the recording of *heart sounds*. The heart, like any mechanical pump, produces characteristic sounds as it beats. These are the sounds the physician hears with a stethoscope. Basic heart sounds occur mostly in the frequency range of 20 to 200 Hz. Certain heart murmurs produce sounds in the 1000-Hz range, and some frequency components exist down to 4 or 5 Hz.

The *first* heart sound (Figure 9-37) is generated at the end of atrial contraction, just at the onset of ventricular contraction. This sound is generally attributed to movement of blood into the ventricles, the atrioventricular (AV) valves closing, and the abrupt cessation of blood flow in the atria.

The *second* heart sound corresponds to the closing of the aortic and pulmonary valves, the *third* sound corresponds to the cessation of ventricular filling, and the *fourth* sound is correlated to the atrial contraction. This last sound has a very low amplitude and a low-frequency component (Figure 9-37).

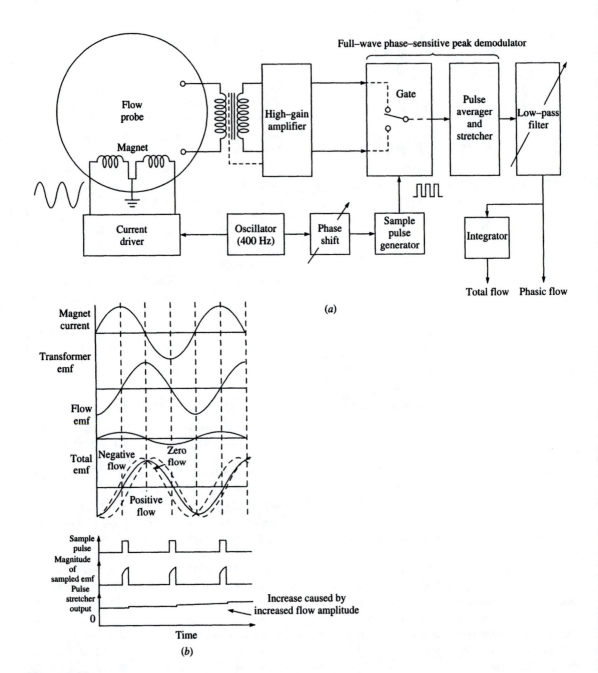

Figure 9-36
Electromagnetic flowmeter circuit. (*a*) Block diagram. (*b*) Timing waveform. (Courtesy of
Biotronix Laboratory)

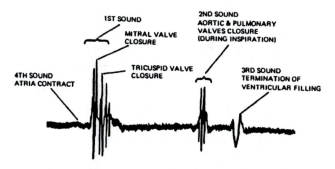

Figure 9-37
Basic heart sounds. (Reprinted courtesy of Hewlett-Packard)

The phonocardiograph transducer is a contact or air-coupled acoustical microphone held against the patient's chest (Figure 9-38). Various types of microphones are used, but most are the piezoelectric *crystal* or *dynamic* type of construction.

The crystal microphone generally costs less and is more rugged than the dynamic type. Also, the crystal microphone produces a larger output signal for a given level of stimulus.

The dynamic microphone uses a moving coil coupled to the acoustical diaphragm. The coil encircles a permanent magnet loudspeaker. The dynamic microphone is used when it is desirable to have a signal frequency response similar to that of the medical stethoscope.

An *air-coupled* microphone with a 2-s *time constant* is often used in *apex phonocardiography*

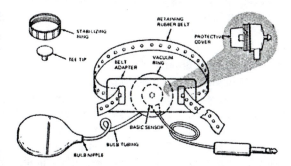

Figure 9-38
21050A sensor and accessories. (Reprinted courtesy of Hewlett-Packard)

recordings. These microphones are generally crystal types and are coupled to the patient's chest through a column of air.

Although oscilloscopes are used to visualize heart sounds while they are being taken, hardcopy recordings are usually made on a stripchart recorder. The frequency response of ink-pen and thermal stylus recorders such as those used in ECG recording is only 100 to 200 Hz. Direct recording of the phonocardiogram requires a frequency response to 1000 Hz, so either an optical or a high-velocity ink-jet model recorder is used.

Not all frequency components are important in phonocardiography, so some models use an *envelope recording* technique. In one commercial product, the frequency components below 80 Hz are recorded directly, but the frequency components above 80 Hz are integrated (i.e., averaged) before recording. This technique allows the use of an ordinary low-frequency thermal or ink-pen type of strip-chart recorder.

A technique used in the Hewlett-Packard 1514 phonocardiograph is to *sample and hold* the positive and negative envelopes of the complex input signal from the microphone at an 85-Hz rate. This system is capable of detecting the shape, timing, duration, and intensity of the heart sounds plotted against time (50 or 100 mm/s). The sampled envelope signal can also be recorded on a low-frequency machine.

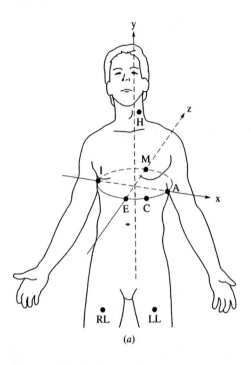

(a)

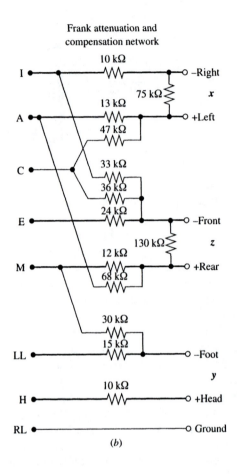

Frank attenuation and
compensation network

(b)

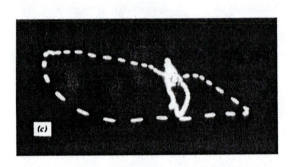

(c)

Figure 9-39
Vectorcardiography. (a) XYZ planes. (b) Frank lead
network. (c) Vectorcardiogram. (a and b reprinted
courtesy of Hewlett-Packard)

9-26 Vectorcardiography

The vectorcardiograph (VCG) examines the ECG
potentials generated along the three-dimensional
axes of the body; that is, the *x*, *y*, and *z* planes. The
x vector is taken as the potential between two
points under the arms (Figure 9-39*a*), the *y* vector
is between the head and right leg, and the *z* vector
is from the front to the back of the body.

These vectors are not exactly orthogonal, and
the amplitudes of the signals from the three planes

are considerably different. The *Frank electrode system* in Figure 9-39*b* is used to normalize the input
signals before applying them to the oscilloscope.

The oscilloscope must be an *x-y* model instead
of the more common *y*-time type of display. A
switching network at the output of the Frank lead
system circuit will select the proper signal combinations for making a recording of *frontal, transverse,* or *sagittal* vectorcardiograms.

Figure 9-39*c* shows an oscilloscope VCG tracing. There are three individual loops corresponding

to the *P* wave, *QRS* complex, and *T* wave on the ECG waveform. These are joined at a single iso-electric point where all three vector components are zero. The dotted line effect is from *intensity* (*z*-axis) *modulation* of the CRT beam.

9-27 Catheterization laboratories

Assessing the condition of a patient's heart may require data obtained from inside of the heart it-self. The data is obtained by a process called *catheterization* and is used to make preoperative judgments on the need for surgery.

The catheter is inserted into the heart via the peripheral vascular system. It can record intracar-diac pressures and allow withdrawal of blood from the heart chambers to measure oxygen and carbon dioxide levels.

In *right catheterization* the catheter is intro-duced through a peripheral *vein* to the vena cava and into the right side of the heart.

A *retrograde catheterization* requires introduc-tion of the catheter via an artery, usually the *brachial* or *femoral* artery. The catheter is threaded through the arterial system and enters the left ven-tricle via the aorta.

In *transseptal catheterization,* a special large-diameter catheter is introduced through the femo-ral vein into the right atrium, where a special nee-dle in the end of the catheter is used to puncture the septum wall dividing the right and left sides of the heart. A smaller catheter is then threaded through the large catheter and the needle to enter the left ventricle via the left atrium. This technique is used primarily when aortic stenosis prevents use of the retrograde technique.

The electronic equipment used in catheteriza-tion includes several channels of pressure ampli-fiers and ECG monitors; a chart recorder is used to make a permanent record of the pressure and ECG waveforms. Figures 9-40*a* and 9-40*b* show two types of catheterization laboratory equipment.

In addition to the measuring instruments, it is necessary to keep a *defibrillator* and other resus-citation equipment in the catheterization labora-

tory. In some cases, cardiac arrhythmias are gen-erated when the catheter tip hits the ventricle wall. For this reason, the ECG waveform is monitored continuously during the catheterization procedure.

The equipment must be designed for very low ac (power mains) leakage operation. Because of the sensitivity of the heart to 25 to 60 Hz (60 Hz in the United States) power mains current, leak-age from that source must be kept to a minimum. This requirement mandates the use of isolated equipment.

9-28 The heart revisited

In chapter 2 we discussed the heart and its pump-ing operation. The heart is able to pump blood through the circulatory system only because the fibers that make up the heart muscle contract in a synchronous manner. A group of cells called the sinoatrial (SA) node is located on the rear wall of the right atrium. The SA node serves as a natural *pacemaker* for the heart by producing an electrical pulse output that stimulates contraction of the heart muscle fibers. The pacemaker pulse spreads across the atria, causing them to contract and force blood into the ventricles. The pulse spreading across the atrial tissue also flows to the electro-conduction system of the heart to the ventricles. To be effective, ventricular contraction must fol-low atrial contraction by a fraction of a second so that atrial blood can fill the ventricular spaces. The heart's electroconduction system provides this de-lay. Part of the delay is caused by the speed of propagation of the pulse down the electroconduc-tion system, and part is the result of the biological "delay line" called the *AV node.* The AV node is to the electroconduction system what a monostable multivibrator is to certain electronic circuits (i.e., pulse delay).

As long as the muscle fibers of the heart con-tract synchronously, the heart will function as an efficient blood pump. But certain problems can de-velop that disturb synchrony. One of these prob-lems, called *arrhythmias,* is *fibrillation,* in which the muscle fibers of the heart quiver randomly and

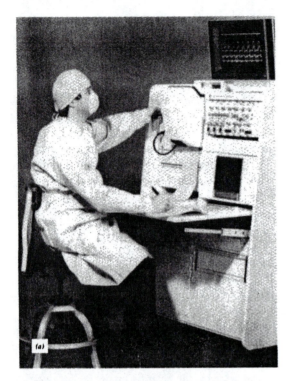

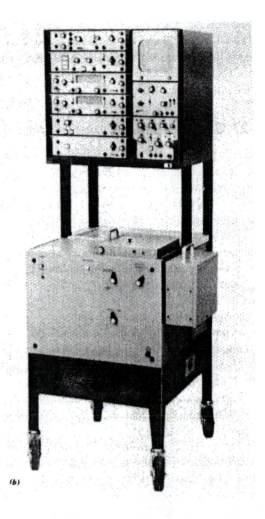

Figure 9-40
(*a*) H-P 8890B catheterization laboratory system. (Courtesy of Hewlett-Packard) (*b*) E-for-M VR-6 Simultrace Recorder. (Courtesy of Electronics for Medicine)

erratically instead of contracting together. If the atrial portion of the heart is in fibrillation, then it is called *atrial fibrillation,* and if the ventricles are involved, *ventricular fibrillation.*

When the heart is in atrial fibrillation it will still pump some blood because the ventricles are still able to contract, and the ventricular contraction maintains the system pressure. But when ventricular fibrillation occurs, the heart cannot pump, and death will occur within minutes unless the condition is corrected.

Figure 9-41 shows several ECG waveforms, including two arrhythmias and a normal waveform for comparison. The normal waveform is shown in Figure 9-41*a*. In this context, "normal" refers not necessarily to the total absence of any disease

process but to the fact that all salient features of the waveform are present. Ventricular fibrillation is shown in Figure 9-41*b*. Notice the low amplitude and erratic aspects of the waveform, caused by the quivering heart muscle. The large sinusoidal-like waveform in Figure 9-41*c* is ventricular tachycardia.

These waveforms can often be corrected by application of an *electric shock* to the heart. The electric shock causes all of the heart muscle fibers to contract simultaneously, so they all enter their refractory periods together, after which their normal rhythm should return.

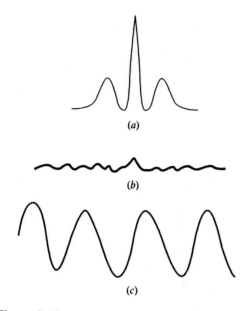

Figure 9-41
(*a*) Normal waveform. (*b*) Ventricular fibrillation.
(*c*) Ventricular tachycardia.

9-29 Defibrillators

A *defibrillator* is a device that delivers electric shock to the heart muscle undergoing a fatal arrhythmia. Defibrillators before about 1960 were ac models. These machines applied 5 to 6 A of 60 Hz ac across the patient's chest for 250 to 1000 ms. The success rate for ac defibrillators was rather low, however, and the technique was useless for correcting atrial fibrillation. In fact, attempting to correct atrial fibrillation using ac often results in producing ventricular fibrillation, a much more serious arrhythmia.

Since 1960, several different dc defibrillators have been devised. These machines store a dc charge that can be delivered to the patient. The principal difference between dc defibrillators is in the waveshape of the charge delivered to the patient. The most common forms are the *Lown, monopulse, tapered (dc) delay,* and *trapezoidal* waveforms.

In 1962, Dr. Bernard Lown of Harvard University introduced the waveform that bears his name. The Lown waveform, shown in Figure 9-42, shows

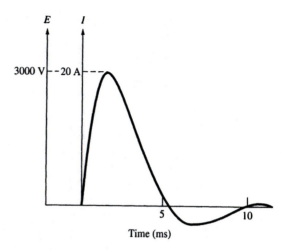

Figure 9-42
Lown defibrillator waveform.

the voltage and current applied to the patient's chest plotted against time. The current will rise very rapidly to about 20 A under the influence of slightly less than 3 kV. The waveform then decays back to zero within 5 ms, and then produces a smaller negative pulse, also of about 5 ms.

Figure 9-43 shows a simplified diagram of a Lown defibrillator. The charge delivered to the patient is stored in a capacitor and is produced by a high-voltage dc power supply. The operator can set the charge level using the *set energy* knob on the front panel. The knob controls the dc voltage produced by the high-voltage power supply and so can set the maximum charge on the capacitor. The energy stored in the capacitor is given by:

$$U = \frac{1}{2} CV^2 \qquad (9\text{-}12)$$

where

U is the energy in *joules* (J)

C is the capacitance of C_1 in *farads* (F)

V is the voltage across C_1 (V)

Example 9-8 _____

Calculate the energy stored in a 16-μF capacitor that is charged to a potential of 5000 V dc.

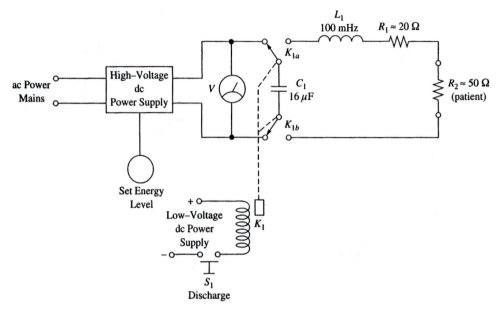

Figure 9-43
Typical circuit for a Lown waveform defibrillator.

Solution

$$U = \frac{1}{2} CV^2$$

$$U = \frac{1}{2} (1.6 \times 10^{-5} \text{ F})(5 \times 10^3 \text{ V})^2$$

$$U = \frac{1}{2} (400) = \textbf{200 J}$$

The stored energy is indicated by a voltmeter connected across the capacitor. The scale of the voltmeter is calibrated in energy units. It is common practice to use *watt-seconds* as the unit of energy instead of joules, but this is no problem because (by definition) 1 J is equal to 1 W-s. Older dc defibrillators had energy meters calibrated in *stored* energy, but present regulations require that the *delivered* energy be indicated. Some energy is lost in the relay switching contacts and in the ohmic resistance of inductor L_1.

The capacitor charge is controlled by a relay switch, K_1. In early models single pole–double throw (SPDT) relays were used, but in all recent

models double pole–double throw (DPDT) relays are used so that isolation of the patient circuit from ground is maintained. Although there are a few portable defibrillators that use open-air high-voltage relays, most use special sealed vacuum relays such as the Torr Laboratories type TMR-10. The vacuum relay is justified because of the high voltages used to charge capacitor C_1. If 16 µF is used (a common value) and 400 J are stored, the potential across the capacitor will be greater than 7000 V dc.

The patient circuit of the Lown defibrillator consists of a 100-mH inductor (L_1), the ohmic resistance of L_1 (i.e., R_1), and the patient's ohmic resistance (i.e., R_2). It is the energy stored in the magnetic field of coil L_1 that produces the negative excursion of the Lown waveform during the last 5 ms. When the capacitor has discharged, the coil's field collapses, dumping energy back into the circuit. The sequence of events is described as follows:

1. The operator turns the *set energy* control to the desired level and presses the *charge* button (i.e., closes S_2).

2. Capacitor C_1 begins charging and will continue to charge until the voltage across the capacitor is equal to the supply voltage.

3. The operator positions paddle electrodes on the patient's chest and presses the *discharge* button (i.e., S_1).

4. Relay K_1 disconnects the capacitor from the power supply and then connects it to the output circuit.

5. Capacitor C_1 discharges its energy into the patient through L_1, R_1, and the paddle electrodes. This action occurs in the first 4 to 6 ms and gives rise to the high-voltage positive excursion of the waveform in Figure 9-42.

6. The magnetic field built up around L_1 collapses during the last 5 ms of the waveform, producing the negative excursion of the waveform in Figure 9-42.

The *monopulse* waveform shown in Figure 9-44 is a modified Lown waveform and is commonly found in certain portable defibrillators. It is created by a circuit such as the one in Figure 9-43 but without inductor L_1 to create the negative second pulse. Consequently, the waveform decays to zero in the exponential manner expected of an *R-C* network.

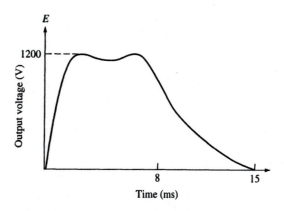

Figure 9-45
Tapered dc delay defibrillator waveform.

Another form of dc defibrillator waveshape is the *tapered delay* shown in Figure 9-45. This waveform differs from the two previous pulses in that it uses a lower amplitude and longer duration to achieve the energy level. The energy transferred is proportional to the area under the square of the curve, so we may attain the same energy as in other waveforms. The double-humped waveform characteristic of tapered delay machines is achieved by placing two *L-C* sections, such as L_1/C_1 in Figure 9-43, in cascade with each other.

The trapezoidal waveform shown in Figure 9-46 is another low-voltage, long-duration shape. The initial output potential is about 800 V, which

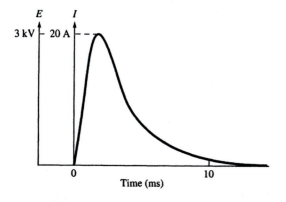

Figure 9-44
Monopulse defibrillator waveform.

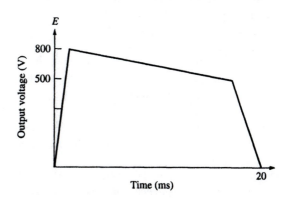

Figure 9-46
Trapezoidal defibrillator waveform.

drops continuously for about 20 ms until it reaches 500 V, where it is terminated.

The energy from a defibrillator is delivered through a set of high-voltage paddle electrodes. Several popular styles are shown in Figure 9-47. The type shown in Figure 9-47*a* is called an *anterior* paddle. In this design the insulated handgrip is perpendicular to the metal electrode surface. The high-voltage cable enters from the side. A thumbswitch to control the discharge is mounted at the top of the grip. A defibrillator paddle and cable set using two of these electrodes is called an *anterior-anterior* set. To defibrillate, one electrode is placed on the chest directly over the heart, while the second electrode is placed on the left side of the patient's chest. A conductive paste is smeared on the electrodes to ensure an inefficient transfer of charge and reduce any burning of the patient's skin.

A *posterior* paddle is shown in Figure 9-47*b*. This electrode is constructed flat and is designed so that the patient can lie on it. Posterior paddles are always paired with one anterior paddle to form an *anterior-posterior* pair.

A more modern anterior paddle is the *D-ring* type shown in Figure 9-47*c*. This type of paddle is used on most current model defibrillators and has been popular on portable models for some time.

One final form of paddle set is the *internal* type shown in Figure 9-47*d*. Internal paddle sets use two of these electrodes, but one may not have the thumbswitch. These paddles are used during open-heart surgical procedures to apply the electrical shock directly to the myocardium.

In Figure 9-43, discharge switch S_1 is used to fire the defibrillator by energizing the charge transfer relay. In some models, S_1 will be mounted on the front panel, but in most models it will be on one of the patient electrode paddles. Some manufacturers actually use two switches in series for the sake of safety, one switch mounted on each of the paddles. Discharge of the defibrillator cannot occur unless *both* switches are closed. Some early models used a foot switch, but this proved to be too hazardous in the hectic and tense environment of a cardiac emergency.

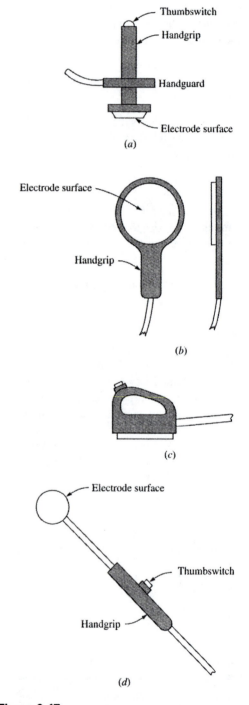

Figure 9-47
Defibrillator electrode handpieces. (*a*) Standard anterior. (*b*) Posterior. (*c*) D-ring anterior. (*d*) Internal.

It is absolutely essential that ventricular fibrillation is confirmed on an ECG machine, or monitor oscilloscope, before using a defibrillator. The nurse, physician, or other rescuer must first determine that fibrillation is in progress. Some defibrillator manufacturers have monitor oscilloscopes and ECG preamplifiers built into their products, but in others the user must provide an external ECG system. In some hospitals, an ECG or monitoring technician is responsible for bringing ECG equipment to the scene of a resuscitation attempt.

9-30 Defibrillator circuits

The circuit shown in Figure 9-43 is inadequate to describe modern defibrillators, although for certain older models it is nearly complete. Two approaches to the design of the *set level* control circuit are evident. One technique uses a *variac* (variable autotransformer) in the primary of the high-voltage transformer in the dc supply. The operator, then, is actually adjusting the high-voltage dc supply when setting the energy level. The dc output voltage of the power supply is a function of the variac setting. When the *charge* button is pressed, ac power is applied to the transformer through the variac. The capacitor will continue to

charge until its voltage is equal to the power supply voltage. When these two voltages are equal, the operator may discharge the defibrillator.

The other approach to control circuit design is shown in Figure 9-48. In this circuit, the dc output of the high-voltage power supply is fixed. A voltage comparator will turn the supply on and off, depending on the voltages applied to its inputs. One input of the comparator is connected to voltage divider R_1/R_2, which produces a low-voltage sample of the high voltage applied to capacitor C. The other input of the comparator is connected to a potentiometer designated as the *set level* control. When the operator selects an energy level, the voltage at the potentiometer wiper will represent the desired charge.

The operator initiates a *charge* cycle by pressing the *charge* button on the front panel. The voltage comparator sees the voltage from the *set level* control at one input and zero voltage at the other, so its output will snap high. When the comparator output is high, the relay or digital IC logic controlling the high-voltage supply latches *on*.

As the capacitor charges, however, the voltage at the comparator's inverting input rises. When the voltage rises to the point where it is equal to the voltage from the *set level* control, the comparator shuts off, stopping the charge cycle.

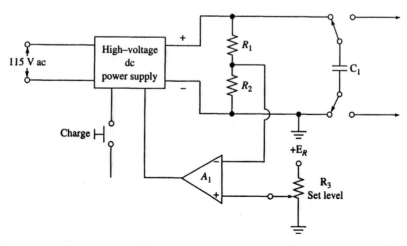

Figure 9-48
Electronic set charge circuit.

The *discharge* circuitry is very much like the previous design. A switch on the patient paddle set energizes the coil of a high-voltage vacuum relay, causing discharge of the capacitor's stored energy into the patient's body.

9-31 Cardioversion

In certain types of arrhythmia (e.g., atrial fibrillation), the patient's ventricles maintain their ability to pump blood, as evidenced by the existence of an *R* wave feature in the ECG waveform. These arrhythmias are also correctable by electrical shock to the heart, but it is necessary to avoid delivering the shock during the ventricles' refractory period (the *T* wave of the ECG waveform), or the shock intended to correct the problem will create a much more serious arrhythmia such as ventricular fibrillation. The shock is usually timed to occur approximately 30 μs after the *R* wave peak.

Human operators cannot be trusted to time the ECG waveform properly to avoid this problem, so an automatic electronic circuit is used. A machine equipped with the synchronizer circuit is called a *cardioverter.*

A switch on the machine allows the operator to select either *defibrillate* or *cardiovert* modes. In some machines, notably the Hewlett-Packard models, this control is labeled either *synchronized-instantaneous* or *sync-defib.*

Figure 9-49 shows a partial schematic of a synchronizer circuit. Relay K_1 and switch S_1 are the same as in the previous circuits. When switch S_2 is in the *defibrillate* position, the circuit operates in the manner of other circuits; depressing S_1 energizes the relay, discharging the capacitor.

But when switch S_2 is in the *cardiovert* position, the relay is not energized unless S_1 is closed and the silicon-controlled rectifier (SCR1) is turned on.

The SCR is turned on by an ECG *R* wave. The ECG preamplifier acquires the signal from the patient. This amplifier may be internal to the defibrillator or an external patient monitor. Many bedside monitors have an output jack labeled *defibrillator* to provide such a signal.

Regardless of the ECG amplifier configuration, it is necessary to also provide circuits that discriminate against any feature other than the *R* wave. In some early models, a simple threshold detector was used, depending on the fact that the *R* wave is

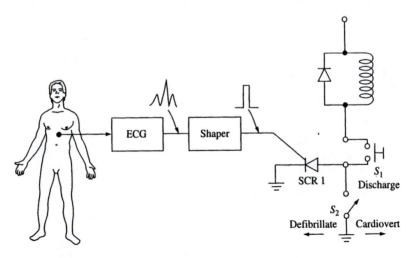

Figure 9-49
Block diagram for a cardioverter.

usually the highest amplitude feature of the ECG. But in some cases the *T*-wave amplitude would also exceed the threshold. To solve this problem, a *differentiator* circuit is used ahead of the threshold detector. The differentiator produces a much higher output on the *R* wave than on the *T* wave, because of the difference in their respective slopes (hence high-frequency content). The differentiator, therefore, ensures a greater difference in amplitude between the *R*-wave and the other major features. It is also necessary that a pacemaker rejection circuit be included, because the pacer spike will appear to the discriminator much the same as the *R*-wave.

Some manufacturers apply the output of the threshold detector directly to the SCR gate. But other manufacturers use the detector output to trigger a monostable multivibrator, whose output pulse then triggers the SCR gate. In some models the monostable pulse is also applied to an output jack.

Figure 9-50 shows a commercial defibrillator, the Hewlett-Packard Model 78620A installed on a Model 78630 resuscitation cart. An internal battery provides up to 100 discharges at the maximum 400 W-s level, or 7 hours of continuous monitoring. This instrument also includes a built-in patient monitor equipped with a nonfade oscilloscope.

9-32 Testing defibrillators

Defibrillators transfer large current charges at high electrical potentials. When trouble begins to develop, it develops rapidly. As a result, wisdom dictates frequent testing.

There are several defibrillator testers on the market. Most are basically integrating voltmeters that are calibrated in watt-seconds. An example of a defibrillator tester is shown in Figure 9-51. A 50-Ω dummy load is built into the tester and is connected between a pair of electrodes. The paddles are placed against the electrodes, and the capacitor is discharged into the load. The meter registers the delivered energy in watt-seconds.

It is preferable to specify a tester that has an oscilloscope output jack, so that the output

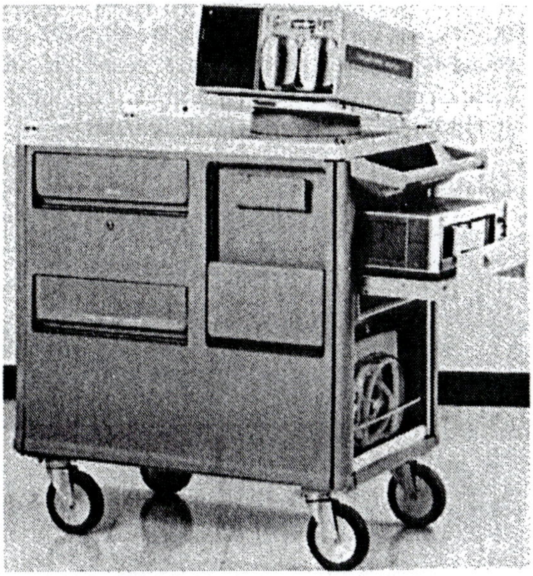

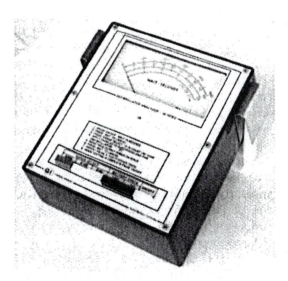

Figure 9-50
Typical defibrillator/crash cart. (Courtesy of Hewlett-Packard)

Figure 9-51
Defibrillator tester. (Photo courtesy of G.I. Medical Products, Inc., Santa Barbara, Calif.)

waveform may be viewed on an oscilloscope. Most authorities agree that a proper evaluation of defibrillator performance requires *both* determination of the delivered energy and examination of the waveform. An oscilloscope camera is usually preferred for making a permanent record of the waveform, although at least one tester uses special digital circuitry that allows recording of the defibrillator output waveform on a 25-mm/s strip-chart recorder.

9-33 Pacemakers

In previous sections we have discussed the electroconduction system of the heart. An electrical impulse is generated by the SA node, located in the vicinity of the right atrium. The pulse propagates down the electroconduction system, including the AV node (which acts as a delay line), to the ventricles. The system splits into left and right bundle branches in the ventricles.

If an interruption occurs in the electroconduction system, causing a condition called *heart block,* then the heart's ability to pump blood is disrupted or stopped. Physicians can maintain electrical stimulation of the heart using a *pacemaker*—an electrical generator that delivers the needed pulse at an appropriate time. Some pacemakers are external and are worn on the belt or placed at bedside. Others are surgically implanted inside the patient. It takes at least 10 μJ to pace the heart; more than 400 μJ is likely to cause ventricular fibrillation. Many commercial pacemakers deliver about 100 μJ and are thus safely within both limits.

External pacemakers are a temporary measure used following open-heart surgery for certain problems experienced by some myocardial infarction patients, and for patients who are to be evaluated as candidates for surgical implantation of a permanent model.

External models are usually adjustable from 50 to 150 BPM and produce fixed-duration, short-duty cycle pulses (i.e., 1.5 to 2.0 ms). The peak current amplitude is adjustable from 100 μA to 20 mA.

Permanent pacemakers (Figure 9-52) are built into molded epoxy-silicone rubber packages, although some recent models include an outer titanium shield that guards against interference from radio frequency fields. The device is implanted subcutaneously in either the abdomen or a region just below the collarbone.

Some implantable pacemakers have a single fixed rate, usually about 70 BPM, while others are dual-rate models. The latter type can be programmed from outside the patient's body using a magnet or induction coil. Still others are programmable from 30 to 150 BPM.

Two types of pacemaker lead wire are used: *endocardial* and *myocardial.* These categories are subdivided into *unipolar* and *bipolar.*

The endocardial lead is inserted through an opening in a vein and then threaded through the venous system and right atrium and into the right ventricle of the heart. On the other hand, the myocardial leads are connected directly to the heart muscle.

The pacemaker shown in Figure 9-52 uses a bipolar lead; both electrodes are inside a single catheter. The distal tip is one electrode, while the second is located a short distance behind the tip. These electrodes are made of platinum-iridium alloy to prevent interaction with body fluids.

The principal power source for *implantable* pacemakers is the *lithium iodine cell.* Mercury

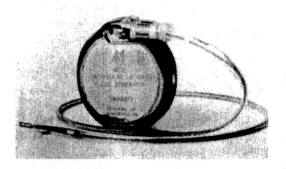

Figure 9-52
Internal pacemaker. (Courtesy of Medtronic, Inc., Minneapolis, Minn.)

pacemaker batteries are theoretically able to operate for as long as 4 to 5 years, but it is more usual to find service periods of 1.5 to 3 years. Pacemaker manufacturers go to great lengths to screen pacemaker batteries, even to the point of X-ray examination of the cell to spot assembly defects known to shorten life expectancy. The battery remains the weak point in the pacemaker, however. Some hospitals operate pacemaker surveillance clinics to spot premature battery failure. It is known that the pulse rate drops with decreased battery voltage. The heart rate of the patient, therefore, can sometimes serve as an early warning indicator of battery failure.

Some work has been done on a nuclear power source for the pacemaker. Early reports were optimistic about a 10-year life expectancy for a nuclear power pack. This type of power pack uses the heat generated by the natural decay of certain radionuclides to generate electricity in a thermocouple. At present, however, the mercury and lithium battery cells seem the most viable energy source for implantable pacemakers.

9-33-1 Pacemaker classifications

There are several ways to classify pacemakers besides the external versus internal scheme discussed in section 9-33. Pacemakers may also be classified by the type of output pulse that they produce. Some models produce a monopolar output pulse, while others produce a *biphasic* pulse (i.e., a high-amplitude pulse of one polarity followed by lower-amplitude pulse of the opposite polarity).

There are four general categories of pacemaker: *asynchronous, demand, R-wave inhibited,* and *AV synchronized.*

The asynchronous pacemaker produces pulses at a fixed rate in the 60- to 80-beats/min range. The standard rate is 70 beats/min, but rates within the specified range are obtainable on special order.

The demand pacemaker adjusts its firing rate to the patient's heart rate. It contains circuitry that senses the ECG *R* wave and measures the *R* to *R* interval. During the first quarter of this period, the

pacemaker is dormant to prevent response to the *T* wave feature of the ECG. But during the last three-quarters of the *R* to *R* interval, it is in a *sense* mode. If an *R* wave is not sensed within this period, then the pacemaker emits a pulse.

The *R*-wave inhibited pacemaker is similar to the demand type, except that it does not emit pulses during normal heart activity. The triggering circuits are inhibited for a period of time after each *R* wave. The pulse is enabled, however, if no *R* wave occurs for a preset period.

The AV synchronized pacemaker responds to the ECG *P* wave—the ECG feature created by contraction of the heart's atria. The atrial pacer circuitry contains a *P Q* delay circuit that simulates the propagation time in the heart's electroconduction system. Once the pacer senses a *P* wave, and the *P Q* delay of about 120 ms has elapsed, then the pacer will fire a pulse to stimulate the ventricles into conduction. The AV pacer has the advantage that it will follow the changing heart rate demands of the body. Pacers synchronized to the ventricles can result only in ventricular contractions independent of the atrial heart rate set by the SA node. The AV pacer will usually track heart rates in the 50- to 150-beats/min range but will revert to fixed rate if the atrial rate exceeds the 150-beats/min upper limit. This feature prevents atrial triggering if atrial flutter or atrial tachycardia occurs.

9-34 Heart-lung machines

The heart is unable to maintain circulation during surgery to either itself or the great vessels from the heart. During these types of surgical procedures, perfusion of the body tissues with blood is maintained by an *extracorporeal* (i.e., outside the body) pump called the *heart-lung machine.*

The heart-lung machine also oxygenates the blood. The lungs normally operate because of a partial vacuum inside of the thoracic cavity created when the diaphragm drops, thereby increasing the volume of the cavity. The pressure inside the lung is essentially atmospheric pressure, and the pressure in the interpleural space outside the

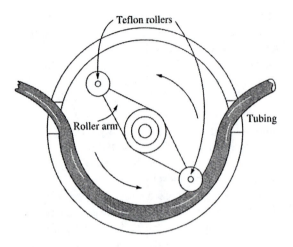

Figure 9-53
Peristaltic pump head.

lung is slightly less than atmospheric. This differential pressure is sufficient to cause the lungs to expand and fill with air. But during certain thoracic procedures, the chest is open, so *both* sides of the lung are at a pressure equal to atmospheric pressure.

Figure 9-53 is a diagram of a heart-lung machine *pump head*. This type of mechanism is called a *peristaltic pump*. The blood to and from the patient's body is carried in a length of sterile, clear plastic tubing called a *cannula*. Cannulas with appropriate fittings to accommodate the tubing are inserted into the vessels to take blood from and deliver blood to the patient. Pumping action occurs because the rollers on the rotating arm compress the tubing carrying the blood, forcing the blood ahead of the compressed section. This *peristaltic action* produces a wavelike, pulsatile flow of blood through the tubing.

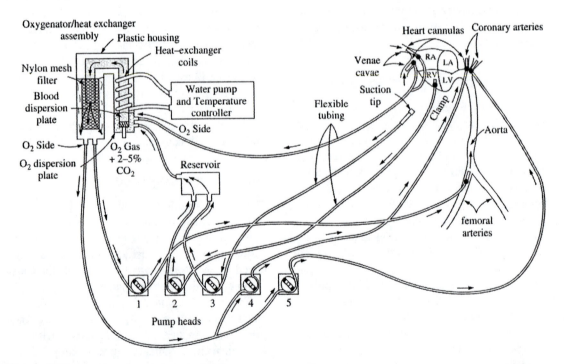

Figure 9-54
Schematic representation of the heart-lung machine.

The heart-lung machine diagrammed in Figure 9-54 uses five pump heads: one for perfusion of the body, two "suckers," and two for perfusion of the coronary arteries.

The main perfusion system includes pump head 1 and a combination *heat exchanger/oxygenator.* Some models separate these units, having separate oxygenator and heat exchanger devices. The heat exchanger consists of water coils isolated from, but thermally coupled to, the blood. A temperature controller permits the pump operator to keep the blood at a proper temperature and compensate for heat loss through radiation from the lines.

The input port of the oxygenator/exchanger assembly is called the O_2-minus side, while the output port is called the O_2-positive side.

Blood is taken from the patient's venae cavae. A cannula is placed into the superior vena cava and another into the inferior vena cava. These lines are joined into a single piece of tubing through a *Y-adapter.*

The blood flows from the venae cavae through the tubing to the O_2-minus side of the oxygenator/exchanger assembly. Another length of tubing carries blood from the O_2-positive side of the assembly, through the pump head, and back to the patient through a cannula inserted into the femoral artery.

Pump heads 2 and 3 are used as suckers. Pump head 2 has a *vent* function to perform in the heart, while head 3 is shown as a suction device. The surgeon can use the suction tip to collect blood that pools during surgery; this blood is ordinarily lost unless it is autotransfused back to the patient. Blood from the suckers is delivered to a reservoir tank and then transferred into the oxygen/exchanger assembly on the O_2-minus side.

The purpose of pump heads 4 and 5 is to perfuse the coronary arteries. A piece of tubing is routed from a port on the O_2-positive side of the oxygenator through the pump heads to the cannulas placed in the coronary arteries.

9-35 Summary

1. *Pressure* is measured in *force per unit of area.*

2. Human blood pressure is a *gauge pressure;* that is, it uses atmospheric pressure as the zero reference point.

3. An *indirect* method for measuring blood pressure called *auscultation* involves the use of a *sphygmomanometer* and a *stethoscope.* *Systolic* and *diastolic* pressures are indicated by the onset and disappearance, respectively, of characteristic *Korotkoff sounds.*

4. A *direct* method for measuring blood pressure involves the use of an *indwelling catheter,* a *transducer,* an *electronic amplifier,* and a *display.*

5. Proper reproduction of the waveform in an electronic arterial pressure monitor requires a plumbing system with a *high*-frequency response. *Clotting of blood* in the catheter, *air bubbles,* and *improper* or *overlong tubing* alter the *resonances* sufficiently to *distort* the waveform.

6. Three methods for determining cardiac output are the *Fick method* (using respiratory oxygen), *thermodilution,* and *dye dilution.* Radio-opaque, radioactive, or optical dyes might be used.

7. A *balloon-tipped* catheter is used to measure *right heart* and *pulmonary artery wedge pressures.*

8. *Plethysmography* measures blood flow volume by changes in the physical volume of a limb.

9. *Magnetic* transducers are most often used in *blood flow* measurements.

10. The graphical recording of heart sounds is called *phonocardiography.*

11. A *defibrillator* corrects certain cardiac arrhythmias by applying an electrical shock from a charge stored in a capacitor.

12. Four defibrillator waveshapes are *Lown*, *monopulse, tapered dc delay*, and *trapezoidal*.

13. *A cardioverter* is a defibrillator that is synchronized to discharge only on the patient's *R* wave.

14. A *pacemaker* is a device that supplies an electrical impulse to the heart to stimulate contraction.

15. A heart-lung machine maintains blood circulation and oxygenates the blood during heart surgery.

9-36 Recapitulation

Now return to the objectives and self-evaluation questions at the beginning of the chapter and see how well you can answer them. If you cannot answer certain questions, place a check mark next to each and review appropriate parts of the text. Next, try to answer the following questions using the same procedure. When you have answered all of the questions, solve the problems.

Questions

1. Human cardiac output is measured in units of _____ per _____.

2. The normal range of human cardiac output is _____ to _____.

3. Cardiac output can theoretically be measured by integrating _____ data.

4. Most clinical cardiac output computers use _____ techniques.

5. Define *pressure* (a) conceptually and (b) mathematically.

6. Define (a) *hydrodynamic* and (b) *hydrostatic* pressures.

7. Define Pascal's principle in your own words and give the limitations on it in *hydrodynamic* systems.

8. What are the (a) SI and (b) English engineering units for atmospheric pressure?

9. Give the *standard value* for a pressure of 1 atm in (a) SI, (b) English engineering, and (c) cgs units.

10. A pressure of 1 *atm* will support the weight of a column of mercury approximately _____ mm high.

11. One torr equals _____ mm Hg.

12. The *zero reference* pressure used for measuring a *gauge pressure* is _____.

13. Blood pressure measurements are referenced against _____. So are _____ pressures.

14. Stephen Hales's techniques for measuring arterial blood pressure are an example of a _____ technique.

15. Indirect methods for blood pressure measurement use an instrument called a _____.

16. The most common indirect method for measurement of arterial blood pressure is called _____.

17. Describe the apparatus and procedure for using *palpation* to measure arterial blood pressure.

18. The palpation method measures only the _____ value(s) of arterial blood pressure.

19. Describe the apparatus and procedure for using the *flush* method for determining arterial blood pressure.

20. The flush method obtains the _____ value(s).

21. Describe the apparatus and procedure for using *auscultation* to measure arterial blood pressure.

22. Auscultation determines the _____ value(s) of arterial blood pressure.

23. *Korotkoff sounds* occur in the _____ method of measuring arterial blood pressure at the instant when _____.

24. The _____ pressure is indicated by the *onset* of Korotkoff sounds.

25. The _____ pressure is indicated when the Korotkoff sounds _____.

26. Direct electronic measurement of arterial blood pressure uses a fluid column in an indwelling _____ between the patient and the transducer.

27. A _____ manometer is used to measure CVP.

28. Define in your own words (a) *mean arterial pressure* and (b) *functional mean pressure.* Use mathematical notation to describe and compare (a) and (b).

29. The two *basic* controls required on a clinical pressure monitor are _____ and _____.

30. Name four basic classes of pressure amplifier.

31. Describe in your own words the technique for calibrating a pressure amplifier using a mercury or aneroid manometer.

32. Describe in your own words how certain monitors use a *calibration factor* to calibrate the system. Is it permissible to use the *cal factor* for one transducer with another of the same model and similar serial number?

33. Draw the block diagram for an ac carrier amplifier.

34. Draw the block diagram for a pulsed-excitation pressure amplifier.

35. Draw the block diagram for an *auto-zero* circuit, and describe how it operates.

36. Describe how a blood pressure monitor could indicate a mean arterial pressure that is considerably different from the functional mean. Discuss cases in which (a) there is a fault on the system, (b) there is *no* fault on

the system, and (c) a method exists to tell you which is the case in any given situation.

37. The time constant of a pressure signal differentiator must be _____ compared with the rise time of the pressure signal waveform.

38. Describe the method used for calibrating a *dP/dT* output on a pressure amplifier.

39. Describe hydrostatic pressure as it affects the pressure monitoring system.

40. The technique using respiratory oxygen as a tracer is called the _____ method.

41. Iced or room-temperature IV solutions, such as saline or D_5W, are used in the _____ method of cardiac output measurement.

42. In optical dye dilution techniques for cardiac output measurement, a dye such as _____ is used.

43. Most thermodilution cardiac output computers use a thermistor-tipped catheter placed in the _____.

44. The input stage of most thermodilutioncardiac output computers is a _____ and an isolated differential amplifier.

45. The *recirculation artifact* can be ignored if the cardiac output computer uses _____ integration to approximate the exponential decay of the temperature signal.

46. A multilumen balloon-tipped catheter can be used to measure _____ and _____ pressures.

47. The catheter discussed in question 9-46 is introduced into the right side of the heart via the _____ venous system.

48. A plethysmograph measures _____ changes in a limb.

49. The _____ is a simple type of plethysmograph but is of limited usefulness because it cannot be calibrated accurately.

50. A true plethysmograph may be calibrated using a _____.

51. The blood pressure cuff used in plethysmography is inflated to a pressure greater than the _____ pressure but less than the _____ pressure.

52. Name two types of blood flowmeter.

53. Which type of blood flowmeter is most commonly used in clinical applications?

54. A _____ is a recording of heart sounds.

55. Name two types of microphones that are often used in the recording of heart sounds.

56. The *first* heart sound is correlated to _____.

57. The *second* heart sound is correlated to _____.

58. The *third* heart sound is correlated to _____.

59. The *fourth* heart sound is correlated to _____.

60. An _____-coupled microphone with a _____-s time constant is used to record the apical heart sounds.

61. _____ detection is sometimes used on phonocardiographs to allow recording on a low frequency strip-chart recorder.

62. A _____ records the ECG in the form of three loops on a CRT.

63. The instrument in question 9-62 uses the _____ lead system.

64. List three different catheterization techniques and describe each.

65. The heart's natural pacemaker is the _____.

66. The _____ system of the heart controls synchronization of the heart's pumping by controlling the distribution of the pacemaker impulse.

67. The _____ of the heart acts analogously to an electronic delay line.

68. List three cardiac arrhythmias that can be corrected by an electrical shock. Which of the arrhythmias cannot be corrected by an ac defibrillator? Which of the arrhythmias is corrected by using the *cardioversion* mode?

69. The purpose of using electrical shock to correct arrhythmias is to _____ the heart, so that all cells enter their refractory period together.

70. List four dc defibrillator waveforms.

71. A cardioverter is a dc defibrillator that is _____ to the _____ feature of the patient's ECG waveform.

72. A cardioverter contains three stages: _____, _____, and _____.

73. Testing a dc defibrillator requires both measurement of _____ and examination of the _____ _____.

74. What condition is the artificial pacemaker designed to correct?

75. What is the *minimum* energy required from a pacemaker?

76. Pacemaker output energy levels of _____ or more may cause ventricular fibrillation.

77. Most implantable pacemakers are packaged in molded _____, while some have an outer shield of _____ to guard against radio frequency interference.

78. Two types of pacemaker lead wire are _____ and _____.

79. Two batteries often used in pacemakers are _____ and _____.

80. Describe *biphasic* pacemaker pulses in your own words.

81. External pacemakers usually have a heart rate range of _____ to _____ BPM.

82. The output current of external pacemakers may be varied from _____ to _____ mA.

83. List four general types of pacemakers.

84. What is a principal advantage of the AV synchronized pacemaker? How is this advantage achieved?

85. The _____ _____ machine uses _____ circulation of the blood to bypass the heart and pulmonary arteries while maintaining perfusion of the body.

86. A _____ pump is used at each pump head on a heart-lung machine.

87. List the function of the five pump heads that might be used in a heart-lung machine.

88. List the major parts of the perfusion system in a heart-lung machine.

Problems

1. A coin has a mass of 1.8 g and a diameter of 14 mm. How much (a) force in millinewtons and (b) pressure in pascals is exerted when the coin is lying horizontally on a perfectly flat table top?

2. The bottom of a drinking glass has a diameter of 2 in. When empty, the glass weighs 4 oz. and when full, 16 oz. Calculate (a) the force in newtons and (b) the pressure in pascals exerted by the glass on a perfectly flat surface under *both* empty and full conditions.

3. A patient's arterial blood pressure is 130/85 mm Hg. Calculate the MAP.

4. A patient's arterial blood pressure is 140/85 mm Hg. Calculate the MAP.

5. A resistance Wheatstone bridge blood pressure transducer has a rated sensitivity of 50 μV/V/cm Hg. Calculate the *gain* required of the dc amplifier used with this transducer if the output scale factor is 10 mV/mm Hg and the full-scale pressure is 300 mm Hg.

6. Solve problem 9-5 with a maximum pressure of 100 mm Hg.

7. Solve Problem 9-5 with a sensitivity of 100 μV/V/mm Hg.

8. Calculate the stroke volume in milliliters if the CO is 3.75 L/m and the heart rate is 76 beats/min.

9. Calculate the blood flow if an injection rate of 3 mg/m results in a downstream concentration of 1 mg/L.

10. A cardiac output computer is tested by a thermistor simulator that uses a step-function change in resistance. Assuming that the correction factor for catheter temperature rise is 4.5, calculate the CO indicated if the integrator output rises 70°C-s. The computer controls are set as follows:

    Blood temperature: 37.6°C
    Injectate temperature: 23°C
    Injectate volume: 10 mL

11. Calculate the input voltage in microvolts to a magnetic blood flowmeter if the magnetic field is 325 G, the vessel diameter 0.65 cm, and the flow rate 200 cm^3/s.

12. Find the energy stored in a 16-μF capacitor that is charged to 6000 V dc.

13. Find the energy stored in a 16-μF capacitor that is charged to 2800 V dc.

14. Find the energy stored in a 25-μF capacitor that is charged to 2200 V dc.

15. Find the dc potential across a 16-μF capacitor that is charged to store an energy of 400 W-s.

16. Find the open-circuit (i.e., no-load) voltage across the patient paddle electrodes of a defibrillator using a 16-μF capacitor charged to 200 W-s (a) normally and (b) when the discharge button is pressed. Assume a patient resistance of 50 Ω and an internal resistance of 20 Ω.

17. Calculate the energy delivered to a 50-Ω noninductive load resistor by a Lown waveform defibrillator charged to 300 W-s. Assume an internal resistance of 25 Ω.

References

1. Carr, Joseph J., *Sensors and Circuits: Sensors, Transducers, and Supporting Circuits for Electronic Instrumentation, Measurement and*

Control, Prentice-Hall (Englewood Cliffs, N.J., 1993).

2. Cobbold, Richard S. C., *Transducers for Biomedical Measurements,* Wiley-Interscience (New York; 1974).

3. Edwards Laboratories, Inc., Instruction manual for model 9520 cardiac output computer, Edwards Laboratories, Inc. (Santa Ana, Calif., 1974).

4. Halliday, David and Robert Resnick, *Physics Parts I and II,* Wiley (New York, 1978).

5. Hewlett-Packard, *Guide to Physiological Pressure Monitoring. (a)* Applications Note AN-739, Hewlett-Packard (Waltham, Mass, 1977). *(b) Operating Notes Series 1280 Transducers,* Hewlett-Packard (Waltham, Mass., 1971).

6. Nara, Andrew et al, *Blood Pressure,* Spacelabs, Inc. (Redmond, Wash., 1989).

CHAPTER 10

The Human Respiratory System and Its Measurement

10-1 Objectives

1. Be able to introduce the biological principles underlying the respiratory system.
2. Be able to list and describe the gas laws.
3. Be able to describe internal (cellular) respiration.
4. Be able to describe external (pulmonary) respiration and pulmonary function (physical, chemical, and exchange of gases).
5. Be able to list the organs of respiration.
6. Be able to list and discuss mechanics of breathing and typical parameters of respiration (lung compliance, lung volumes/capacities, intraalveolar pressure, airway resistance, and intrathoracic pressure).
7. Be able to describe the regulation of respiration.

8. Be able to list and describe unbalanced and diseased states (hypoventilation, hyperventilation, dyspnea, hypercapnia, hypoxia, and apnea).
9. Be able to list the main threats of environmental pollution to the respiratory system.
10. Be able to list major measurements of pulmonary function.
11. Be able to list the principal pulmonary parameters measured.
12. Be able to describe the operation of various respiratory transducers.
13. Be able to list and describe the major instruments used in respiratory system measurement.

10-2 Self-evaluation questions

These questions test your prior knowledge of the material in this chapter. Look for the answers as you read the text. After you have finished studying the chapter, try answering these questions and

those at the end of the chapter.

1. List two purposes of the respiratory system.
2. State Boyle's, Charles's, Dalton's, and Henry's laws.

3. Describe internal respiration.

4. Which gas law describes gas exchange across cellular membranes?

5. Describe external respiration (inspiration and expiration) in terms of physical and chemical phenomena.

6. List and construct a block diagram of the organs of respiration and describe the function of each.

7. Describe the mechanics of breathing.

8. List and describe the major parameters of respiration.

9. Name and describe two control systems effecting the regulation of respiration.

10. State five unbalanced and diseased states of the respiratory system.

11. List and describe the major environmental threats to the respiratory system.

12. A *pneumotachometer* is used to measure _____.

13. Define *inspiratory reserve volume.*

14. Flow volume may be measured by using a _____.

15. Relationships between the various respiratory volumes are called _____.

16. What is an *apnea* alarm?

10-3 The human respiratory system

The *human respiratory system* is critical to immediate survival. The main organs affecting pulmonary function are the lungs, and these are surprisingly delicate, given that they interact with the external environment.

The respiratory system provides a means of acquiring oxygen (O_2) and eliminating carbon dioxide (CO_2).

Respiratory organs provide maximum *surface area* (alveolar spaces) for diffusion of O_2 and CO_2; the means of constantly renewing gases in contact with this surface (ventilation); the means of protecting surface membranes from harsh environmental factors, such as airborne toxic particles, microorganisms, drying, and extreme temperature; and a method of counteracting sudden shifts in pH of the body and body fluids.

10-4 Gas laws

The key to understanding of respiratory function lies in the laws of gases. These include *Boyle's law, Charles's law, Dalton's law,* and *Henry's law.*

Boyle's law states that the volume ofa gas varies inversely with the pressure if the temperature is held constant. The mathematical expression is:

$$\frac{V_2}{V_1} = \frac{P_1}{P_2} \tag{10-1}$$

where

V_1 = original volume

V_2 = final (new) volume

P_1 = original pressure

P_2 = final (new) pressure

Example 10-1 _____

A mass of oxygen gas occupies 6 L under a pressure of 720 mm Hg. Calculate the volume of the same mass of gas at a pressure of 760 mm Hg (standard). The temperature remains constant.

Solution

$$\frac{V_2}{V_1} = \frac{P_1}{P_2} \qquad V_1 = 6 \text{ L}$$

$$P_1 = 720 \text{ mm Hg}$$
$$P_2 = 760 \text{ mm Hg}$$
$$V_2 = \text{unknown}$$

$$V_2 = \frac{V_1 P_1}{P_2} = \frac{6 \text{ L} \times 720 \text{ mm Hg}}{760 \text{ mm Hg}}$$

$$V_2 = \textbf{5.681 L}$$

Charles's law states that the volume of a gas is directly proportional to its absolute temperature if the pressure is held constant. The mathematical expression is:

$$\frac{V_2}{V_1} = \frac{T_2}{T_1} \qquad (10\text{-}2)$$

where

V_1 = original volume

V_2 = final (new) volume

T_1 = original temperature

T_2 = final (new) temperature)

Example 10-2

Oxygen gas occupies 220 mL at 110°C. Calculate its volume at 0°C. The pressure remains constant.

Solution

$$\frac{V_2}{V_1} = \frac{T_2}{T_1} \qquad V_1 = 220 \text{ mL}$$

$$V_2 = \text{unknown}$$

$$T_1 = 100°C + 273 \text{ K} = 383 \text{ K}$$

$$T_2 = 0°C + 273 \text{ K} = 273 \text{ K}$$

$$V_2 = \frac{V_1 T_2}{T_1} = \frac{220 \text{ mL} \times 273 \text{ K}}{383 \text{ K}}$$

$$V_2 = 156.81 \text{ mL}$$

Dalton's law states that the total pressure exerted by a mixture of gases is equal to the sum of the partial pressures of the various gases. The partial pressure of a gas in a mixture is equal to the pressure of that gas if it were alone in the container. The mathematical expression is:

$$P_{total} = P_1 + P_2 + P_3 + \cdots + P_n \qquad (10\text{-}3)$$

where

P_{total} = combined pressure

P_1 = partial pressure of first gas

P_n = partial pressure of nth gas

Example 10-3

Atmospheric pressure at sea level is 760 mm Hg. Calculate the partial pressure of oxygen, nitrogen, and carbon dioxide.

Solution

$$P_{total} = P_{O_2} + P_{N_2} + P_{CO_2}$$

P_{O_2} by volume = 20.96% × 760 mm Hg

= 159.30 mm Hg

P_{N_2} = 79% × 760 mm Hg = **600.40 mm Hg**

P_{CO_2} = 0.04% × 760 mm Hg = **0.03 mm Hg**

P_{total} = 159.30 + 600.40 + 0.03

P_{total} = 760 mm Hg

Henry's law states that if the temperature is held constant, the quantity of a gas will go into solution proportional to the partial pressure of that gas. The gas with the greater partial pressure will have more mass in solution.

Example 10-4

Oxygen has a partial pressure of 120 mm Hg and carbon dioxide, 40 mm Hg, above a liquid with no initial dissolved gases. Which gas will have more mass in solution?

Solution

Oxygen will have more gas in solution due to its higher partial pressure.

10-5 Internal (cellular) respiration

Respiration is the interchange of gases between an organism and the medium in which it lives. *Internal respiration* is the exchange of gases between the bloodstream and nearby cells. Figure 10-1 shows a body cell exchanging gases with its environment (an adjacent capillary). During its passage through the body tissues, blood gives up approximately 5 to 7 *volume percent* (vol%) (number of cubic centimeters of a gas contained in 100 mL of blood) oxygen and absorbs 4 to 6 vol% carbon dioxide. When the temperature or acidity increases, more O_2 is released to the tissues. Most of the O_2

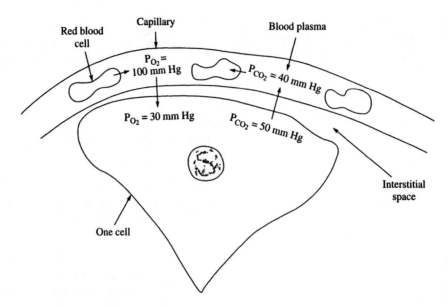

Figure 10-1
Internal respiration—exchange of O_2 and CO_2 between the capillary and the body cell.

(95%) is carried by the red blood cell (RBC) hemoglobin and, on release to tissues, the RBCs still remain 75% saturated. However, the RBCs carry only about 30% CO_2, and the remainder is carried in the plasma. The exchange of O_2 and CO_2 is dependent on *Dalton's law of partial pressures* (see section 10-4). For example, if the partial pressure of O_2 (PO_2) is 100 mm Hg in a capillary surrounding a cell and the internal cellular partial pressure is 30 mm Hg, O_2 moves into the cell. Similarly, CO_2 moves out of the cell into the capillary. It is the concentration of O_2 and CO_2 blood gases that is critical for sufficient gas exchange. The *oxygen dissociation curve* shows this condition in Figure 10-2. Notice that arterial blood is 100% oxygenated, containing oxyhemoglobin (oxygen chemically combined with hemoglobin within RBCs), and venous blood is normally 75% oxygenated.

10-6 External (lung) respiration

External respiration is the exchange of gases between the lungs and bloodstream. Most biomedical respiratory apparatus is concerned with measuring

or treating conditions of external respiration. Hence, the remainder of this chapter describes respiratory organs, physiology, and parameters.

Basically, external respiration includes *inspiration* (intake of air—79% nitrogen [N], 20.96% O, 0.04% CO_2) and *expiration (exhaust of waste gases—79% N, 17% O, 4% CO_2).* Pulmonary

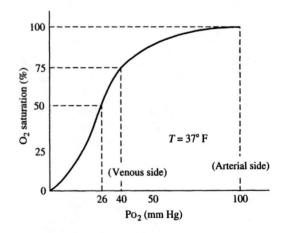

Figure 10-2
Oxygen dissociation curve.

function involves *physical* processes (mechanics of breathing) and *chemical* processes (reaction of gases with liquids or exchange of gases). All of these can be explained through the laws of physics and chemistry (gas laws).

10-7 Organs of respiration

The organs of respiration shown in Figure 10-3 are typically divided into the following:

1. Conducting division—containing thick walls (no gas exchange to capillaries) and including the nasal cavities, pharynx, larynx, trachea, bronchi, and bronchioles.

2. Respiratory division—containing thin walls (permitting gas exchange to blood capillaries) and including respiratory bronchioles, alveolar ducts, atria (space from which the alveoli of the sacs arise), and alveolar sacs.

Both divisions function through the muscles of respiration (diaphragm and intercostal or chest muscles), ribs, and sternum.

A block diagram of the passage of air from the nose to the capillaries is shown in Figure 10-4.

Specifically, the organs of respiration include the following:

1. *Nose and nasal cavities*—facial organ that serves for sense of olfaction (smell) and to warm, moisten, and filter air for respiratory tract.

2. *Pharynx (throat)*—there are three divisions:

   (a) *Nasopharynx* (near nose), including adenoids (mass of lymphatic tissue).
   (b) *Oropharynx,* including tonsils (mass of lymphatic tissue).
   (c) *Hypopharynx* or *laryngopharynx.*

3. *Larynx (voice box)*—houses the vocal cords that vibrate when air is forced upward.

4. *Trachea (windpipe)*—vertical tube kept open by rings of cartilage to allow passage of air to and from the lungs.

5. *Bronchi*—two branches of trachea that descend into each lung.

6. *Bronchioles*—smallest of the bronchial branches that form a network of tubes throughout the lungs.

7. *Alveoli (air sacs)*—air cavities (one cell thick) at the end of the bronchioles that trap air and allow exchange of gases to the blood capillaries.

8. *Lung capillaries*—thin tubes carrying blood that surround the alveoli and allow exchange of gases.

The *lungs* (Figure 10-5) consist of two cone-shaped spongy organs that contain the alveoli (air sacs) that trap air for gas exchange with the blood. Three lobes separated by fissures make up the right lung, and two make up the left. An indentation appears in the left lung (slightly larger than the right) to provide room for the heart. The *hilum,* through which the lymphatics, blood vessels, and bronchi enter and leave the lung, is located posteriorly. Both lungs lie within two lateral (side by side) *pleural cavities* of the thorax. A serous (moist) membrane, the *visceral pleura,* covers the lung surface, and the *parietal pleura* lines the thoracic cavity. These membranes contact one another and attach at the root of the lung. This fluid-lined potential space between two membranes accounts for easy slippage between lung and chest wall during breathing. The cohesive effect helps to keep the lung expanded.

Blood in need of oxygenation enters both lungs via the *pulmonary arteries* (from the heart's right ventricle). Oxygenated blood leaves the lungs through the *pulmonary veins* (to the heart's left atrium).

Air inspired through the nose, passed through the trachea, and branched to the bronchi eventually enters terminal bronchioles that separate into *respiratory bronchioles*. There, *alveoli,* or *air sacs,* each about 0.2 mm in diameter, are attached as shown in Figure 10-6. An estimated 300 million

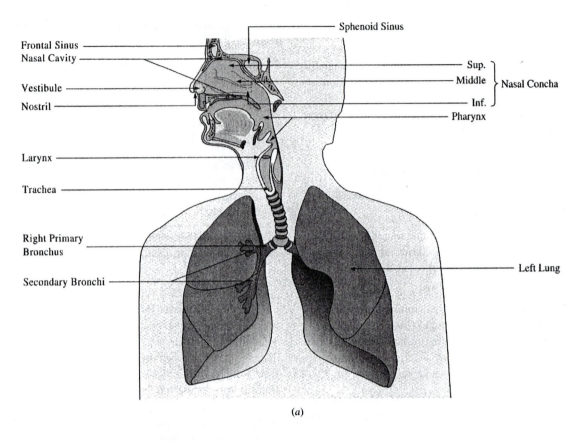

Frontal Sinus

Nasal Cavity

Vestibule

Nostril

Larynx

Trachea

Right Primary Bronchus

Secondary Bronchi

Sphenoid Sinus

Sup.

Middle ⎫ Nasal Concha

Inf. ⎭

Pharynx

Left Lung

(a)

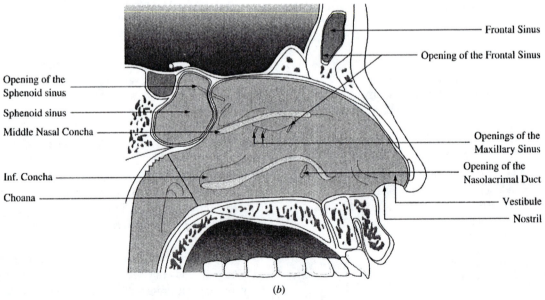

Opening of the Sphenoid sinus

Sphenoid sinus

Middle Nasal Concha

Inf. Concha

Choana

Frontal Sinus

Opening of the Frontal Sinus

Openings of the Maxillary Sinus

Opening of the Nasolacrimal Duct

Vestibule

Nostril

(b)

Figure 10-3
Organs of respiration. (a) Organs. (b) Left nasal cavity. (From *Human Anatomy and Physiology*, 2nd edition, by James E. Crouch, Ph.D. and J. Robert McClintic, Ph.D. John Wiley & Sons, New York, 1976. Used by permission.)

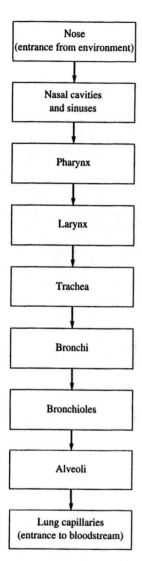

Figure 10-4
Block diagram of air pathway from nose to lung capillaries.

10-8 Mechanics of breathing

The *mechanics of breathing (respiration)* involve muscles that change the volume of the thoracic cavity to generate *inspiration* (intake) and *expiration* (exhaust).

The two sets of muscles involved are the *diaphragm*—the wall separating the abdomen from the thoracic (chest) cavity that moves up and down—and the *intercostal muscles*—muscles surrounding the thoracic cavity that move the rib cage in and out.

Inspiration (Figure 10-7) results from contraction of the diaphragm (downward movement) and intercostal muscles (rib cage swings up and outward). The enlarged cavity housing the lungs undergoes a pressure reduction (-3 mm Hg) with respect to the pressure outside the body. Since the lungs are passive (no muscle tissue), they expand because of the positive external pressure. If external environmental pressure is 760 mm Hg at sea level, the lung pressure is 757 mm Hg on inspiration. The closed nature of the thoracic chamber allows air to enter the lungs from one external opening.

Expiration (Figure 10-7) results from the relaxation of the diaphragm (upward movement) and intercostal muscles (inward and downward). The elastic recoil of the lungs creates a higher-than-atmospheric intrapulmonic pressure ($+3$ mm Hg) that forces air out of the lungs.

Mechanical and electrical analogies have been constructed to demonstrate and study respiratory function. One uses masses sliding along surfaces restrained by springs. The elasticity of the spring indicates lung compliance (ability to stretch). Another uses a volume-pressure piston pumping system. A bellows reflects compliance and bronchial airway resistance. A third is constructed of electrical components. A set of capacitors represents bronchial resistance and gas compressibility, while sets of resistors and capacitors give lung tissue elasticity. The muscles of respiration are simulated by ac generators.

alveoli are contained in the lung, generating about 70 m^3 of surface area (the size of the average tennis court). This gives rise to a total lung capacity of 3.6 to 9.4 L in adult men and 2.5 to 6.9 L in the adult women.

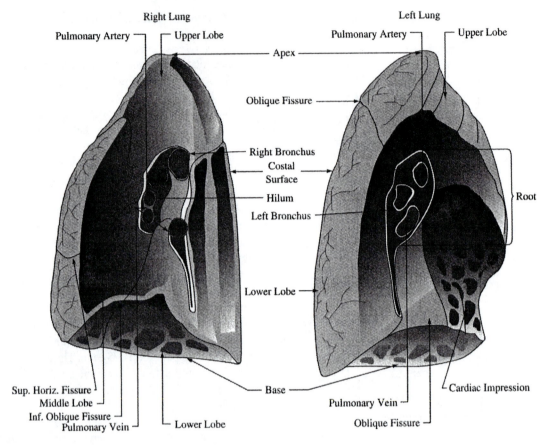

Figure 10-5
The lungs. (From *Human Anatomy and Physiology*, 2nd edition, by James E. Crouch, Ph.D.
and J. Robert McClintic, Ph.D. John Wiley & Sons, New York, 1976. Used by permission.)

10-9 Parameters of respiration

The parameters of respiration are measurements that indicate the state of respiratory function, including lung volumes and capacities, airway resistance, lung compliance and elasticity, and intrathoracic pressure.

Only a portion of the air entering the respiratory system actually reaches the alveoli. The volume of air that is not available for gas exchange with the blood resides in the conducting spaces. This is known as *dead air* and fills *dead space,* consisting of 150 mL. Because of uneven distribution of ventilation (exhaust) and perfusion (spread), *wasted ventilation* results in *wasted blood flow.* The total dead space is less than 30% of the total volume.

Important volumes to consider are shown in Figure 10-8. They are for a standard 70-kg male breathing at rest. The *tidal volume (TV)*—500 mL—is the depth of breathing or the volume of gas inspired or expired during each respiratory cycle. *Inspiratory reserve volume (IRV)*—3600 mL—is the maximal amount of gas that can be inspired from the end-inspiratory position (extra inspiration from the high peak tidal volume). *Expiratory*

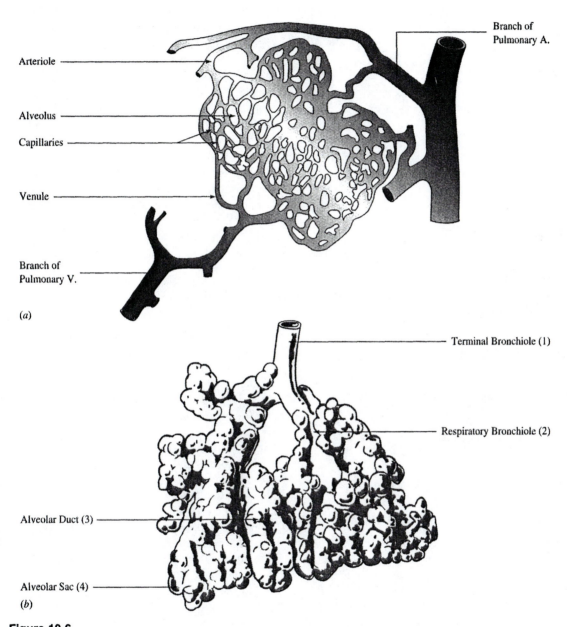

Arteriole

Alveolus

Capillaries

Venule

Branch of
Pulmonary V.

Branch of
Pulmonary A.

(a)

Terminal Bronchiole (1)

Respiratory Bronchiole (2)

Alveolar Duct (3)

Alveolar Sac (4)

(b)

Figure 10-6
Alveoli and blood circulation. (From *Human Anatomy and Physiology*, 2nd edition, by James
E. Crouch, Ph.D. and J. Robert McClintic, Ph.D. John Wiley & Sons, New York, 1976. Used by
permission.)

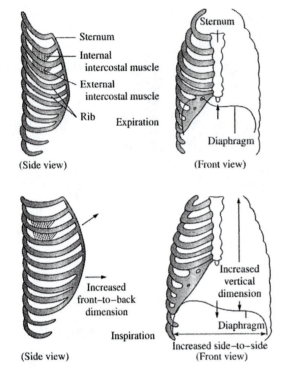

Figure 10-7
Expiration and inspiration (thoracic dimension changes.) (From *Human Anatomy and Physiology*, 2nd edition, by James E. Crouch, Ph.D. and J. Robert McClintic, Ph.D. John Wiley & Sons, New York, 1976. Used by permission.)

reserve volume *(ERV)*—1200 mL—is the maximal amount of gas that can be expired from end-expiratory level (extra expiration from the low peak tidal volume). *Residual volume (RV)*—1200 mL—is the amount of gas remaining in the lungs at the end of maximal expiration (amount that cannot be squeezed out of the lung). Even a collapsed lung contains 500 to 600 mL. *Minute volume* is the volume of air breathed normally for 1 minute.

Important capacities (addition of various volumes) to consider are shown in Figure 10-8. *Total lung capacity (TLC)*—6000 mL—is the amount of gas contained in the lungs at the end of maxi-

mal inspiration and is the sum of inspiratory capacity (IC) and functional residual capacity (FRC). *Vital capacity (VC)*—4800 mL—is the maximal amount of gas that can be expelled from the lungs by forceful effort from maximal inspiration. *IC*—3600 mL—is the maximal amount of gas that can be inspired from the resting expiratory level and is the sum of TV and IRV. *FRC*—2400 mL—is the amount of gas remaining in the lungs at the resting expiratory level (end-expiratory position is used as a base because it varies less than the end-inspiratory state). It is the sum of ERV and RV.

It is interesting to note the volume reserve available with respect to total lung volume. This equals:

$$\frac{RV}{TLC} \times 100 = 20\% \text{ in 25-year-old (70-kg) male}$$

$$= 40\% \text{ in 55-year-old (70-kg) male}$$

$$(10-4)$$

The *work of breathing* involves airway resistance, lung compliance, and lung elasticity.

Airway resistance relates to the ease with which air flows through tubular respiratory structures. Higher resistances occur in smaller tubes, such as the bronchioles and alveoli, that have not emptied properly.

Lung compliance is the ability of the alveoli and lung tissue to expand on inspiration. The lungs are passive, but they should stretch easily to ensure sufficient intake of air.

Lung elasticity is the ability of the lung's elastic tissues to recoil during expiration. The lungs should return to their rest (unstretched) state easily to ensure sufficient exhaust (ventilation) of gas.

Intrathoracic pressure is the positive and negative pressure occurring within the thoracic cavity. This is critical to proper inspiration (negative internal pressure) and expiration (positive internal pressure).

Intraalveolar pressure is important in maintaining proper respiration and gas exchange to and from the blood.

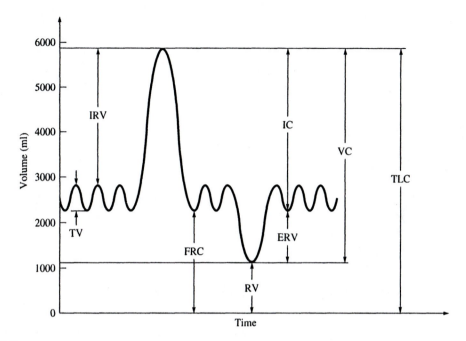

Figure 10-8
Lung volumes and capacities.

10-10 Regulation of respiration

Respiration rate and depth are controlled by (1) the nervous system and (2) the chemical concentration of CO_2 in the blood.

Respiration results from *involuntary neuronal activity* (see chapter 12, The Human Nervous System) modified by *chemical influences*. Voluntary control is also possible but is limited by internal body homeostasis. For example, voluntary deep breathing for a prolonged time may result in temporary unconsciousness to permit blood chemistry (pH level) to return to normal.

Respiratory centers in the brain are located within the *medulla* and *pons* of the brain stem. Nerve cells from the brain send out streams of impulses that stimulate the *diaphragm* and *intercostal muscles* to contract and effect *inspiration*. *Pneumotaxic centers* in the pons receive impulses that rise to a maximum at inspiration peak from *inspiratory centers* in the medulla. Messages relayed to the *expiratory centers* (located dorsally to inspi-

ratory centers in medulla) initiate expiration by sending out streams of pulses that inhibit inspiration. Muscles of inspiration relax, and *expiration* follows passively. This *feedback system* maintains *rhythmic breathing rate and depth (TV)*.

Respiratory activity is also affected by the chemistry and temperature of the blood passing through the brain. Changes in concentration of carbon dioxide in the blood changes the respiratory rate. The *acid base balance of the blood* (normally a pH of 7.4) arises from the following chemical reaction of carbon dioxide waste from cells with water in blood plasma.

$$CO_2 + H_2O \rightarrow H_2CO_3 \rightarrow H^+ + HCO_3^- \quad (10\text{-}5)$$

A *reflex mechanism* regulates breathing as shown in Figure 10-9. For example, if the accumulation of blood CO_2 from body cells should increase, more H;s+ and HCO_3^- ions will be

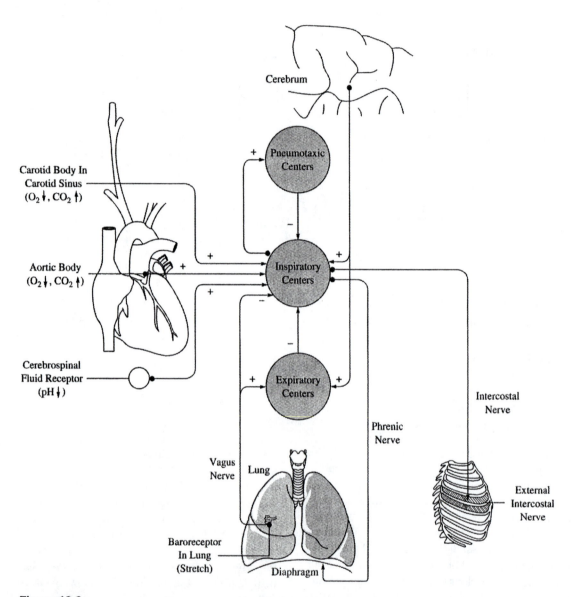

Figure 10-9
Breathing reflex mechanisms. (From *Human Anatomy and Physiology*, 2nd edition, by James E. Crouch, Ph.D. and J. Robert McClintic, Ph.D. John Wiley & Sons, New York, 1976. Used by permission.)

produced, leading to stimulation of the brain respiratory center. This increases the depth and, eventually, rate of breathing. The CO_2 level in the blood drops as a result of ventilation, and brain respiratory centers decrease breathing rate. The constitutes a *negative feedback loop,* and blood pH is maintained within normal limits (7.36 to 7.44). Stimulation and inhibition act through *baroreceptors* (stretch sensors in the lung), O_2 *chemoreceptors* (cells in the aorta), and *respiratory centers* (cells in the brain) to ensure the balance of the partial pressure of O_2 and CO_2 in the blood.

10-11 Unbalanced and diseased states

Unbalanced states of the respiratory system include the following: *Hyperventilation* is alveolar ventilation in excess of metabolic needs for CO_2 removal. Partial pressure of CO_2 in blood falls below 40 mm Hg. This results from voluntary or involuntary rapid or deep breathing, ridding the blood of excessive CO_2. *Hypoventilation* is alveolar ventilation inadequate for CO_2 removal. Partial pressure of CO_2 rises above 40 mm Hg. This results from voluntary or involuntary shallow breathing causing excessive buildup of CO_2 in the blood.

Diseased states of the respiratory system include the following: *Hypoxia* is low O_2 content in the blood, resulting in excessively reduced partial pressure of O_2 in the blood to the point of death. This results from damage to respiratory neurons, alveolar damage, respiratory tissue damage, or inadequate O_2 transport. *Apnea* is the cessation of breathing, usually temporary. This results from reduced stimulus to respiratory centers or brain center damage. *Hyperpnea* is the increased TV with or without increased breathing rate, which reduces alveolar and blood partial pressure of O_2. *Dyspnea* is labored breathing resulting from acidosis (low blood pH), pneumonia, cardiac failure, hemorrhage, or fever. *Polypnea* (tachypnea) is accelerated breathing rate without increase in breathing depth, resulting from fever or hypoxia. *Hypercapnia* is decreased ventilation (excessively low partial pressure of CO_2 in the blood) resulting from central nervous system disorders, disease of nerves or respiratory muscles, metabolic disorders, or respiratory obstruction.

10-12 Environmental threats to the respiratory system

The respiratory system, particularly the lungs, must withstand the insults of the external *environment*. Smoking cigarettes and inhaling gases, fibers, and liquids from occupational environments cause lung tissue damage. The National Institutes of Health has issued programs (since 1970) to manage the detection and prevention of respiratory disease resulting from environmental factors.

Mortality rates among cigarette smokers average about 70% greater than among nonsmokers. Breathing smog formed through chemical reactions of sulfur oxides and hydrocarbons with ozone in the atmosphere causes respiratory damage by means of acids that form deep within the lung alveoli destroying respiratory membranes and causing swelling. Particulate matter, such as smoke and dust, embeds within lung surfaces and causes insufficient oxygenation. Carbon monoxide (250 million metric tons annually) and other machine exhaust gases cause hypoxia and, ultimately, death.

Environmental impact assessment has become an essential part of industrial advance. Air quality took on a legal aspect with the introduction of the Clean Air Act in 1970. This act establishes air quality guidelines that all industry was required to meet by 1982. Part of assessing air quality deterioration includes *identifying* pollutants, describing existing air quality levels, summarizing meteorological data, gathering current air quality standard data, and determining whether air pollution is caused by new industrial construction.

Patients with disease resulting from organic or environmental factors often require *artificial respiratory ventilation*.

10-13 Major measurements of pulmonary function

Given all of the respiratory problems that can exist (organically and environmentally induced), *measurement of pulmonary function* is essential. This includes the following: *Maximum voluntary ventilation (MVV)* is the deep, rapid breathing measurement on a spirometer (respiratory volume measurement device). *Forced expiratory volume in 1 second (FEV_1)* is the rapid inhalation-exhalation as measured on a spirometer. *Maximum expiratory flow rate (MEFR)* is the forcible inhalation-exhalation measured on a pneumotachometer (flowmeter). *Intraalveolar pressure* is pressure in the alveolar sac as measured by a body plethysmograph (pressure-recording device). *Blood gas* *measurement* includes partial pressure of O_2 and CO_2 in the blood as measured by a blood gas analyzer. *Acid-base balance measurement* is the quantity of CO_2 in the blood as measured by a pH meter.

10-14 Respiratory system measurements

The respiratory system is responsible for bringing oxygen into the body and for discharging waste carbon dioxide from the body.

There are actually several different transducers used in respiratory measurements, although only a few different types of measurement are made. One class of instruments, known as *pneumographs,* is used to *detect* respiration, but these instruments do not deliver quantitative data about the system. These devices are, however, often paired with a *pneumotachometer* (i.e., respiration rate meter) to perform *monitoring* jobs in ICUs.

Instruments devised to quantitatively measure lung volumes are known as *spirometers;* both mechanical and electronic models are available. The measurements are as follows:

1. *Tidal volume* (TV)

2. *Inspiratory reserve volume* (IRV)

3. *Expiratory reserve volume* (ERV)

4. *Residual volume* (RV)

5. *Minute volume*

Relationships exist between the various volumes, and these are expressed as various *pulmonary capacities* and are calculated by the respiratory machine.

1. *Vital capacity* (VC)

2. *Functional residual capacity* (FRC)

3. *Inspiratory capacity* (IC)

4. *Total lung capacity* (TLC)

The amount of blood gases and CO_2 expired at the end of a normal TV respiration are also considered to be respiratory measurements.

10-15 Respiratory transducers and instruments

Respiratory instruments, like most other measurement instruments, tend to be little more than extensions of the transducers used to acquire the data from the subject. In some cases, no more than a simple dc amplifier is needed. It is, therefore, practically impossible to distinguish the transducers from the instruments. In this section, we discuss the transducers of respiratory instrumentation along with the instruments used to process the signals.

An *impedance pneumograph* is based on the fact that the ac impedance across the chest of a subject *changes* as respiration occurs. This technique is used in many neonatal *respiration monitors* and *apnea alarms.* Figure 10-10*a* shows the block diagram for an impedance pneumograph. A low-voltage, 50- to 500-kHz ac signal is applied to the chest of the patient through surface electrodes of the same type as used in ECG monitoring. In fact, many of these monitors are also ECG monitors, using a common set of electrodes and a single pair of lead wires. High-value fixed resistors connected in series with each electrode create a constant ac current source. The signal voltage applied to the differential ac amplifier is the voltage drop across the resistance, representing the patient's thoracic impedance (Figure 10-10*b*):

$$E_o = I(R \pm \Delta R) \qquad (10\text{-}6)$$

where

E_o is the output potential in *volts (V)*

I is the current through the chest in *amperes (A)**

R is the chest impedance, *without* respiration, in ohms (Ω)

ΔR is the change of chest impedance caused by respiration, in ohms ($\Delta\Omega$)

---

*Although the ampere unit is used in Equation 10-6, the current would be inthe microampere range.

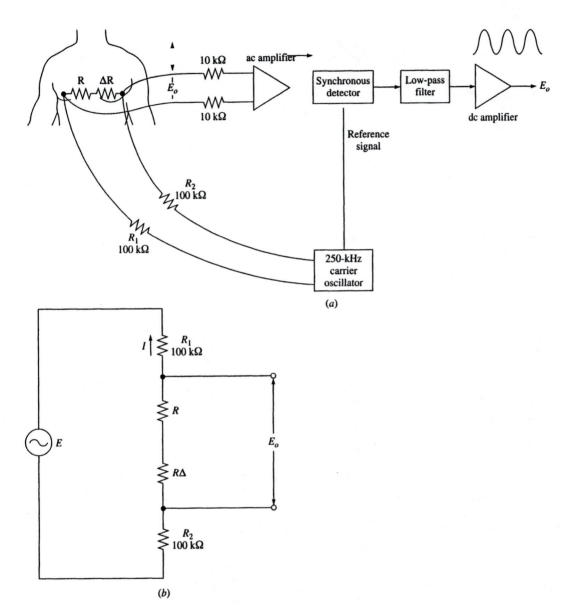

Figure 10-10
Impedance pneumograph. *(a)* Block diagram. *(b)* Equivalent circuit.

The current passed through the patient's chest is very small and is nearly constant without respiration because the source voltage E is constant and the term ΔR is very small with respect to the sum $R_1 + R_2 + R_3$.

The signal E_o is amplified and then applied to a synchronous amplitude modulation (AM) detector; the respiration waveform is contained within amplitude variations in E_o caused ΔR. A low-pass filter following the detector removes residual carrier signal, and a dc amplifier scales the output waveform to the level required by the display device or pneumotachometer following this circuit.

The output of the impedance pneumograph contains only *rate* data and the *existence* of respiration, hence its use in monitoring and apnea alarm devices.

These are two types of pneumograph that use piezoresistive strain gauge transducers to detect respiration. One type, now largely obsolete, is the *mercury strain gauge*. In this instrument, a very thin elastic tube filled with mercury is stretched across the patient's chest. The tube is typically of 0.5 mm inside diameter and perhaps 2 mm outside diameter. Most are about 3 cm long. The ends of the tube are typically plugged with amalgamated copper, silver, or platinum. Modern versions of this elastic strain gauge use copper sulfate or an electrolytic paste instead of mercury. These materials have a higher resting resistance, therefore reducing the electrical current needed to create a usable output voltage.

The other type of piezoresistive strain gauge transducer uses the same wire, foil, or semiconductor piezoresistive devices. In pneumograph applications, however, the strain gauge element is attached between two elastic bands. When this assembly is stretched across the patient's chest, the strain gauge element will change resistance with movement of the patient's chest. As the chest rises and falls with respiration, therefore, a ΔR component is created that is translatable into a changing voltage signal. Again, no flow volume data is obtained; only rate and existence information is contained within the output signal.

Both of these strain gauges, as well as the thermistor transducers to follow, may be used in either a half or a full Wheatstone bridge (Figures 10-11 and 10-12).

In Figure 10-11, the resistive strain gauge element is in series with constant current I. Output voltage E_o represents the respiration signal and is also given by Equation 10-6 (used previously in the discussion on the impedance pneumograph, section 10-15). But this circuit has one serious drawback: Voltage E_o is *not* zero when there is no respiration but is equal to $I \times R$. Pneumographs that use this circuit, therefore, are either ac-

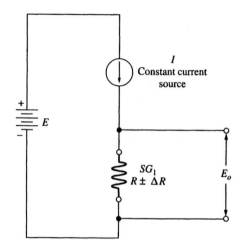

Figure 10-11
Half-bridge circuit.

coupled (the lower -3 dB frequency is 0.05 Hz) or have an *offset control* to compensate for the static value of E_o.

The full Wheatstone bridge circuit in Figure 10-12 eliminates the offset problem; the static value of E_o in this circuit is zero volts. In some cases R_2 will also be a transducer element connected in opposition to SG_1; that is, it changes to $+\Delta R$ when SG_1 becomes $-\Delta R$, and vice versa.

Thermistors are also used as flow detectors in some pneumographs. One type of transducer con-

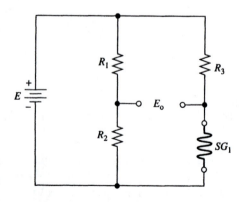

Figure 10-12
Full-bridge circuit.

sists of a bead thermistor placed just inside the patient's nostril. A constant current is passed through the thermistor (i.e., Figure 10-11), but its value is limited to the current required to barely allow self-heating of the thermistor. This level will be 5 to 10 mA in most thermistors. The power dissipation is usually limited to less than 40 mW in order to avoid injury or discomfort to the patient. The thermistor changes resistance because of the temperature difference between inspired and expired air.

A thermistor transducer that can be used on a patient who is fitted with an endotracheal tube or is on a respirator or ventilator is shown in Figure 10-13. Two thermistors are mounted inside of a *tee piece* (a standard piece of apparatus used in respiratory therapy). Thermistor R_1 is in the flow of in-

haled and exhaled gases, while thermistor R_2 forms a reference point by being placed in nonturbulent gas dead space. External resistors R_3 and R_4 form the other half of a Wheatstone bridge. Again, the current flowing through the thermistors is limited to the point of self-heating.

Output voltage E_o is normally zero when there is no gas flow but takes on a nonzero value when gas flows through the tube. A voltage waveform representing respiration is created because thermistor R_1 responds to the difference in temperature between inhaled and exhaled air.

In some transducers, the thermistor is replaced with a thin platinum wire (Figure 10-14) stretched taut across a short section of tubing. As in the previous cases, the wire is treated as a resistor at the point of self-heating. Also, as in thermistor types,

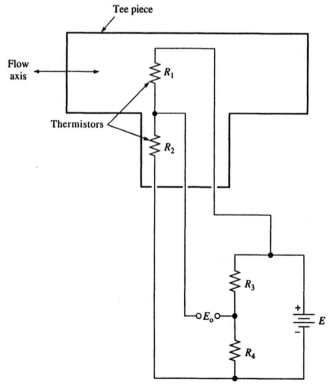

Figure 10-13
Thermistor airway flow detector.

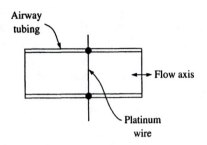

Figure 10-14
Platinum wire flow detector.

the platinum wire does not yield numerical flow data, only respiration rate and existence.

Figure 10-15 shows a flow volume transducer that is capable of quantitative measurement. The flow volume is measured in liters per minute.

The transducer assembly consists of a differential pressure transducer (see chapter 6) and an *airway* containing a *wire mesh* obstruction.

When a wire mesh is placed in an airway, it causes a *pressure drop* that is measured as a differential pressure across the mesh. The pressure transducer is connected so that this difference can be measured.

It is necessary to keep the pressure drop to less than 1 cm H_2O, or normal breathing will be affected. The standard transducer, therefore, offers a 50-mm diameter mesh that has a grid density of 158 wires per centimeter (i.e., 400 per inch). This mesh offers a pressure difference of approximately 0.09 cm H_2O per 10 L/min gas flow (i.e., 9×10^{-3} cm H_2O/L).

The manufacturers of respiratory instruments using the mesh transducer calibrate the instrument to the transducer, but the calibration may be checked in the field by using a precision pneumatic flowmeter to create a known flow volume.

Air flow rate is flow volume per unit of time and may be obtained by integrating the volume-time signal for a known time period. One version of this measurement frequently seen in medical equipment is the *minute volume* measurement, in which the inspiratory volume is measured only for a period of one minute. This is usually obtained by integrating the volume signal for a 1-min period.

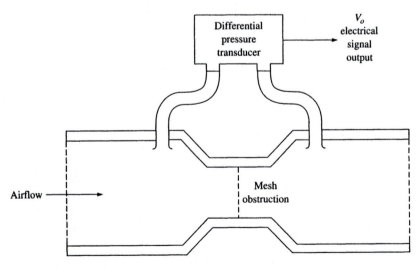

Figure 10-15
A common form of flow rate transducer.

10-16 Spirometers

A conventional spirometer is shown in Figure 10-16. This instrument uses a bell jar, suspended from above, in a tank of water. An air hose leads from a mouthpiece to the space inside of the bell above the water level. A weight is suspended from the string that holds the bell in such a way that it places a tension force on the string that exactly balances the weight of the bell at atmospheric pressure. When no one is breathing into the mouthpiece, therefore, the bell will be at rest with a fixed volume above the water level. But when the subject *exhales,* the pressure inside the bell *increases* above atmospheric pressure, causing the bell to rise. Similarly, when the patient *inhales,* the pressure inside the bell *decreases.* The bell will *rise* when the pressure increases and *drop* when the pressure decreases.

The change in bell pressure changes the volume inside the bell, which also causes the position of the counterweight to change. We may record the volume changes on a piece of graph paper by at-taching a pen to the counterweight or tension string.

The chart recorder is a rotary drum model called a *kymograph.* It rotates slowly at speeds between 30 and 2000 mm/min.

Some spirometers also offer an electrical output that is the electrical analog of the respiration waveform. Most frequently the electrical output is generated by connecting the pen and weight assembly to a linear potentiometer. If precise positive and negative potentials are connected to the ends of the potentiometer, then the electrical signal will represent the same data as the pen. When no one is breathing into the mouthpiece, E_o will be zero. But when a patient is breathing into the tube, E_o will take a value proportional to the volume and a polarity that indicates inspiration or expiration.

There have also been some ultrasonic flowmeters on the market. These instruments work on the Doppler shift difference noted on ultrasonic waves traveling with and against the direction of flow. The principles of operation for this instrument are covered in chapter 17.

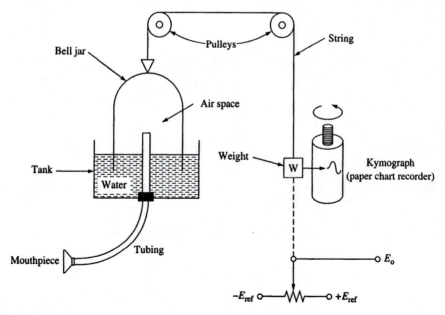

Figure 10-16
Bell-jar mechanical spirometer.

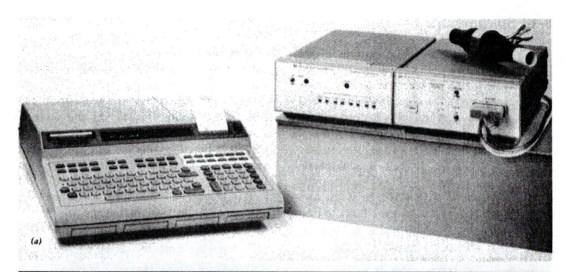

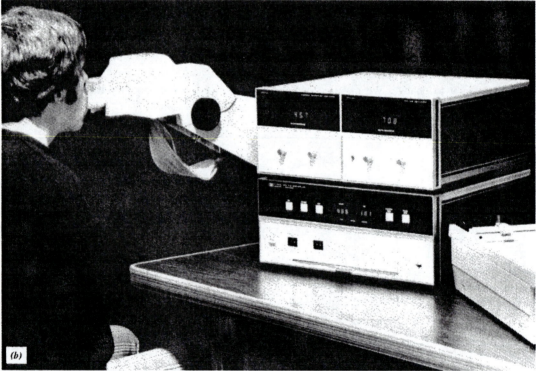

Figure 10-17
Pulmonary function analyzers. (*a*) H-P Model 47804A Pulmonary Data Acquisition System.
(*b*) H-P Model 47404A Single-Breath Diffusion System. (Photo courtesy of Hewlett-Packard)

A few instruments use a pinwheel transducer. A pinwheel is either connected to an alternator or interrupts a photocell light path to produce an output frequency that is proportional to the gas flow rate.

10-17 Pulmonary measurement systems and instruments

For many years, pulmonary instrumentation was limited to the bell spirometer and a few other pieces of equipment. This was not because of a lack of importance, only a certain difficulty in making the measurements. Cardiovascular measurements (i.e., ECG tracings and pressures) are easier to make and so were developed first. Today, however, the range of pulmonary instrumentation available to hospital pulmonary function laboratories; ICU, CCU, and OR staffs; researchers; and even physicians in private practice has increased dramatically.

Figure 10-17 shows two pulmonary measurement systems that are used in pulmonary function laboratories in hospitals and medical centers. The instrument in Figure 10-17a is the Hewlett-Packard (H-P) Model 47804A Pulmonary Data Acquisition System, while that in Figure 10-17b is the H-P Model 47404A Single-Breath Diffusion System. The 47804A uses a microcomputer terminal (at left) to process the data.

The various volumes and capacities are often regarded as the only pulmonary measurements. But also considered in this class are PO_2 and PCO_2, which are measurements of arterial and venous blood and of the exhaled gases. Blood gas analyzers are discussed in Chapter 16 and are not covered here. We will, however, discuss a gaseous CO_2 analyzer.

Figure 10-18 shows an instrument that measures the percentage of carbon dioxide in a sample of gas. When the sensor is placed in the exhalation

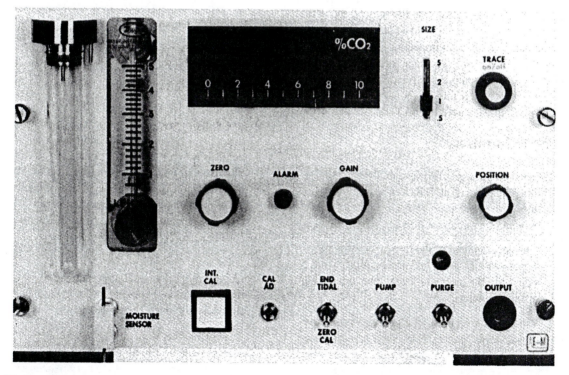

Figure 10-18
CO_2 analyzer.

line of a respirator or anesthesia machine, it will measure the *end tidal volume CO₂* content.

The device on the left of the CO_2 analyzer is a cold trap that reduces the moisture content of the incoming gas. The device immediately to the right of the cold trap is a flowmeter. An internal pump creates a reduced pressure so that a sample of the exhaled gases is drawn into the instrument. The flowmeter allows the operator to determine whether the flow rate is sufficient to permit an accurate measurement.

Function of the typical clinical CO_2 analyzer is based on the fact that CO_2 will absorb infrared energy, while O_2 and N will not. The gas sample is made to pass through a transparent cell that is in the light path between an infrared source and a photocell or phototransistor that is a filter for, or sensitive only to, infrared energy.

Calibration is performed by adjusting the *zero* control for a zero reading on the %CO_2 meter when ordinary room air, or some other gas free of CO_2, is being drawn into the instrument. Once the zero is obtained, the gain can be adjusted by drawing a sample from a calibrated gas cylinder into the machine. A relatively common standard gas available from most compressed gas distributors is 95% O_2 and 5% CO_2. If this gas is used, then the *gain* control is adjusted until the %CO_2 meter reads 5%.

10-18 Summary

1. The human respiratory system is critical to immediate survival. This system provides a means of *acquisition of oxygen* and *elimination of carbon dioxide*.

2. The development of the respiratory system begins with the nose and nasal passages and ends with the laryngotracheal tube and alveoli within the lungs.

3. *Major gas laws* in the study of respiration are *Boyle's law, Charles's law, Dalton's law,* and *Henry's law.* Dalton's law of partial pressures explains gas exchange between lungs and blood and blood and body cells.

4. *Internal respiration* is the exchange of gases between the bloodstream and nearby cells.

5. *External respiration* is the exchange of gases between the lungs and bloodstream. This involves the process of *inspiration* (intake of air) and *expiration* (exhaust of gases). Physical (mechanics of breathing) and chemical (gas exchange) phenomena underlie respiration.

6. The system of respiration is separated into *conducting* and *respiratory* divisions and include the nose, nasal cavities, pharynx (throat), larynx (voice box), trachea (windpipe), lungs, bronchi, bronchioles, alveoli, and lung capillaries.

7. The *mechanics of breathing* involve the diaphragm and intercostal (rib cage) muscles. Through these, the thoracic cavity (chest) enlarges (negative internal pressure generated on inspiration) and relaxes (positive internal pressure generated on expiration).

8. *Parameters of respiration* include lung volume and capacities, compliance and elasticity, airway resistance, and intrathoracic pressure.

9. *Regulation of respiration* rate and depth depends on *nervous system* and *chemical* controls. CO_2 concentration in the bloodstream indicates ventilation level to brain respiratory centers. Negative feedback loops exist among lungs, heart, and brain centers to maintain constant blood pH (acid-base balance).

10. *Unbalanced and diseased states* of the respiratory system are hyperventilation, hypoventilation, hypoxia, apnea, hyperpnea, dyspnea, polypnea, and hypercapnia.

11. *Environmental threats* to the respiratory system include smoking cigarettes and inhaling liquids, vapors, fumes, smoke, and dust from occupational environments.

12. *Major measurements* of pulmonary function are MVV, FEV_1, MEFR, intraalveolar pressure, blood and gas measurement, and pH.

13. Nonquantitative volume transducers may use transthoracic impedance changes, an elastic strain gauge, or a thermistor to acquire a respiration signal. Only the existence of respiration and respiration rate, however, can be determined with these transducers.

14. Two common transducers that are capable of yielding quantitative data are the *wire mesh* and *pinwheel* transducers.

15. Most end-tidal CO_2 analyzers used in clinical work use infrared absorption, but a few research instruments use mass spectometry.

16. A mechanical device called a bell-jar spirometer is used to record respiration volumes. This instrument will record the volumes on a chart recorder called a kymograph.

10-19 Recapitulation

Now return to the objectives and self-evaluation questions at the beginning of the chapter and see how well you can answer them. If you cannot answer certain questions, place a check mark next to each and review appropriate parts of the text. Next, try to answer the following questions using the same procedure. When you have answered all of the questions, solve the problems.

Questions

1. Two purposes of the respiratory system are _____ and _____ of _____.

2. The respiratory system counteracts sudden changes in blood _____.

3. *Boyle's law* states that the volume of a gas varies inversely with the _____.

4. *Charles's law* states that the volume of a gas is directly proportional to its absolute _____ if the _____ is _____.

5. *Dalton's law* states that the total pressure exerted by a gas mixture equals the sum of the _____ _____.

6. *Henry's law* states that if the _____ remains constant, a quantity of gas that goes into solution is proportional to its _____.

7. Internal respiration is the _____ of _____ between the _____ and nearby _____.

8. Blood is _____% oxygenated in the _____ vein and _____% oxygenated in the _____ artery.

9. The term *oxyhemoglobin* refers to oxygenated _____.

10. What is the percentage of oxygen, nitrogen, and carbon dioxide in inspired and expired air?

11. List eight major organs of respiration.

12. What is the approximate surface area of the internal lung alveoli?

13. Mechanical motion of breathing occurs through which two sets of muscles?

14. State the following approximate volumes of these lung parameters: tidal volume, residual volume, total lung capacity, and vital capacity.

15. Define *lung compliance*.

16. What two major factors control the rate and depth of respiration?

17. Do positive or negative feedback systems control respiration?

18. State the normal regulated pH range of the blood.

19. Define unbalanced states of hyperventilation and hypoventilation.

20. Describe the respiratory diseases of hypoxia, apnea, and hypercapnia.

21. How does environmental pollution affect respiratory function?

22. State four major measurements of pulmonary function.

23. What are the functions of the human respiratory system?

24. A _____ can be used to detect the presence of respiration but is not able to make quantitative volume measurements.

25. Respiration rate can be determined from the instrument in question 10-24 if the output signal is applied to a _____.

26. What general class of respiration instruments is used in ICU and CCU monitoring applications?

27. A _____ is capable of making quantitative lung volume measurements.

28. Define *tidal volume*.

29. Define *inspiratory reserve volume*.

30. Define *expiratory reserve volume*.

31. Define *residual volume*.

32. Define *minimal volume*.

33. Define *minute volume*.

34. Define *vital capacity*.

35. Define *functional residual capacity*.

36. Define *total lung capacity*.

37. List three different types of transducers that might be used with a simple pneumograph.

38. List materials other than mercury that might be used in an elastic strain gauge.

39. Elastic strain gauges operate on the principle of _____.

40. An impedance pneumograph measures the change in _____ _____ as the patient breathes.

41. When thermistors and platinum wires are used to detect respiration, they are energized with just enough current to cause _____ _____.

42. The wire-mesh transducer produces a signal proportional to flow _____ in liters per minute.

43. The wire mesh transducer depends on the _____ across the mesh when gas flows through the mesh.

44. The approximate density of a typical wire mesh used in the transducer of question 10-42 is _____ per centimeter.

45. The _____ volume can be measured by integrating a flow signal for a period of 60 s.

46. Describe in your own words (a) a bell-jar spirometer and (b) the operation of the bell-jar spirometer.

47. The chart recorder that is used with a mechanical bell-jar spirometer is called a _____.

48. The bell-jar spirometer will produce an analog electrical output representing flow volume if a _____ is mechanically connected to the weight or pen of the spirometer.

49. Most clinical end-tidal CO_2 analyzers, especially those intended for bedside use, operate on the principle of _____ absorption.

Problems

1. Given a 4-L container of oxygen gas under a pressure of 780 mm Hg, calculate the volume of the same mass of gas at a pressure of 760 mm Hg.

2. Given 200 mL of oxygen gas at 100°C, calculate the volume at 0°C if the pressure remains constant.

3. Given expiratory gas (79% N, 17% O, and 4% CO_2) at 40 mm Hg, calculate the partial pressure of oxygen, nitrogen, and carbon dioxide.

4. Calculate the IRV of a patient in whom the VC is 4130 mL, TV is 480 mL, and the ERV is 1156 mL.

5. Find the TV of a patient in whom the IRV is 2100 mL and the IC is 2580 mL.

6. Find the *total lung capacity* for a patient in whom the TV is 500 mL, IRV is 2300 mL, ERV is 1050 mL, and RV is 1200 mL.

7. Calculate the current required in an impedance pneumograph if the output potential is to be 1 mV when the patient's chest resistance varies $\pm 20\ \Omega$ with respiration from a resting resistance of 15 kΩ.

8. Find the output potential of a half-bridge circuit energized by a 500-nA constant current source if the resting resistance is 30 kΩ.

9. Calculate the amplitude of the respiration signal in Problem 10-8 if the resistance changes $\pm 90\ \Omega$ as the patient breathes.

Suggested readings

1. Carola, Robert, John P. Harley, Charles R. Noback, *Human Anatomy and Physiology,* 2nd Edition, McGraw-Hill (New York, 1992).

2. Crouch, James E. and Robert J. McClintic, *Human Anatomy and Physiology,* Wiley (New York, 1976).

3. Guyton, Arthur C., *Textbook of Medical Physiology,* W. B. Saunders (Philadelphia, 1976).

4. McNaught, Ann B. and Robin Challander, *Illustrated Physiology,* Churchill Livingstone (New York, 1975).

5. Koa, Frederick F., *An Introduction to Respiratory Physiology,* American Elsevier Publishing (New York, 1972).

6. Peters, Richard M., *The Mechanical Basis of Respiration,* Little, Brown (Boston, Mass., 1969).

CHAPTER 11
Respiratory Therapy Equipment

11-1 Objectives

1. Be able to describe the physiological basis (diseased states) for requiring artificial respiratory therapy.
2. Be able to describe medical gases and safety systems (cylinders, high-pressure control).
3. Be able to describe the procedure and equipment used in oxygen therapy (regulators, flowmeters, humidifiers/nebulizers, cannulas, oxygen masks, and oxygen tents).
4. Be able to describe the procedure and equipment used in intermittent positive pressure breathing (IPPB) therapy.

5. Be able to describe the procedure and equipment used in artificial mechanical ventilation.
6. Know how to describe accessory devices used in respiratory therapy apparatus (respiratory monitors and alarms, oxygen analyzer).
7. Know how to describe sterilization and isolation procedures used in respiratory therapy units.
8. Be able to list typical faults and maintenance procedures for artificialrespiratory ventilators.

11-2 Self-evaluation questions

These questions test your prior knowledge of the material in this chapter. Look for the answers as you read the text. After you have finished studying the chapter, try answering these questions and those at the end of the chapter.

1. List two general respiratory diseases that may require artificial respiratory therapy.

2. What is the goal of artificial ventilatory control mechanisms?

3. What is the difference between controlled artificial ventilation and mechanically assisted ventilation?

4. List six regulating agencies involved in compressed gas cylinder safety during manufacture, transportation, storage, and usage.

5. What safety systems are used throughout the hospital for oxygen, carbon dioxide, helium, and nitrous oxide?

6. Define *oxygen therapy*.

7. Name four specific diseases requiring oxygen therapy.

8. How should respiratory therapists and physicians orient patients to respiratory therapy?

9. Describe gas regulators, flowmeters, humidifiers, nebulizers, and oxygen masks and tents.

10. Define IPPB therapy and list its objectives.

11. Describe the hardware and operation of an IPPB unit (include block diagram of Bennett valve and accessories).

12. Describe the operation of two major types of artificial respiratory ventilators (include block diagram and external controls).

13. Describe respiratory therapy equipment sterilization and isolation procedures, including special sterilization equipment.

14. List typical faults and maintenance procedures for artificial respiratory ventilators.

11-3 Disease states requiring artificial respiratory therapy

Four basic *pulmonary abnormalities* (see Chapter 10) that require *artificial respiratory ventilation* are abnormalities of ventilation (hypoventilation), ventilation/perfusion problems, membrane permeability defects (diffusion impairment), and arteriovenous shunts (abnormal bypassing of blood).

Essentially, two respiratory diseases cause respiratory (ventilation) failure:

1. *Hypoxia*—low oxygen level in the blood resulting from improper ventilation. This is caused by pulmonary emphysema (stretched alveoli lead to loss of lung elasticity), chronic bronchitis, pulmonary tumors, aspiration pneumonia, interstitial fibrosis, or pulmonary infarction (tissue death resulting from lack of blood supply).

2. *Hypercapnia*—poor alveolar ventilation causing an accumulation of carbon dioxide in the blood. This results from central nervous system disorders, diseases of nerves and muscle weakness, metabolic diseases, pulmonary emphysema, chronic bronchitis, or lung obstruction.

The goal of an *artificial ventilatory control mechanism* (correction of pulmonary abnormalities) is to adjust alveolar ventilation to changing body needs of oxygen intake and carbon dioxide removal. Alveolar ventilation depends on the relationship between respiratory rate, tidal volume (TV), and dead space.

In addition, *tracheostomy* (surgical technique to overcome obstructions of the upper respiratory tract) may be performed to permit prolonged artificial ventilation.

11-4 Overview and terminology of ventilation

Various types of mechanical devices can assist the patient in the ventilation process. However, when *lung damage* or *blood perfusion* (saturation of lung tissue with blood) occurs, cures for ventilation problems cannot always be complete. Essentially, the following ventilating processes are common:

1. *Mechanically assisted ventilation*—all ventilation by mechanical means.

2. *Controlled artificial ventilation*—process in which the patient plays no role in initiating the respiratory cycle.

3. *Patient-cycled artificial ventilation*—process in which the patient initiates the inspiratory cycle.

4. *Volume-cycled ventilation*—process by which inspiration is terminated after a preset volume is delivered.

5. *Pressure-cycled ventilation*—process by which inspiration is terminated when a preset pressure is reached.

Ventilation *terms* relate to the parameters of pulmonary function (see chapter 10), including the following:

1. *Peak pressure*—maximum airway pressure reached in distending the lungs during artificial ventilation.

2. *Respiratory failure*—failure of the respiratory system to meet body needs for O_2 uptake and CO_2 removal.

3. *Ventilatory failure*—failure of the respiratory system to meetthe body needs for CO_2 removal.

4. *Venous return*—minute volume of blood flow into right atrium. Normal minute volume is the tidal volume (500 mL) times the breaths per minute (about 16), which is 8000 mL. *Respiratory minute volume* is known as *pulmonary ventilation*.

5. *Lung volumes*—TLC, VC, RV, IC, IRV, ERV, FRC (see chapter 10).

11-5 Historical perspective of artificial respiratory ventilation

The understanding of pulmonary physiology followed the discovery of oxygen by Joseph Priestley (1733-1804) and Joseph Black (1728-1799).

In 1790, Thomas Beddoes (1760-1808) founded the Pneumatic Institute for the treatment of diseases by inhalation of gases. The era of inhalation therapy took form when Sir Arbuthnot Lane invented the nasal catheter in 1907 and John Haldane (1860-1936) introduced the oxygen mask (for World War I poison-gas victims with pulmonary edema). The oxygen tent constructed by

Sir Leonard Hill in 1920 also showed promise. Later, the foot bellows, *Fell-O'Dwyer respiration apparatus,* and *compressed air techniques* paved the way for invention of the modern artificial respiratory ventilator.

11-6 Medical gases and safety systems

A variety of *medical gases, cylinders,* and *regulating equipment* is used by the respiratory therapist. The following *regulating agencies* and *acts* are important to the therapist:

1. *National Fire Protection Agency* (NFPA)— voluntary agency (National Consensus Standards) that promotes prevention and detection of fire hazards.

2. *U.S. Department of Transportation* (DOT)— regulates gas cylinder construction, testing, and maintenance.

3. *Compressed Gas Association* (CGA)— develops safest methods for handling compressed gases.

4. *Federal Food, Drug, and Cosmetic Act*— regulates shipment of medical gases in interstate commerce and provides standards through the Pharmacopeia of the United States (USP).

5. *Federal Occupational Safety and Health Act of 1970* (OSHA)—provides for federal inspections of facilities used for storage of flammable gases.

6. *Local and state agencies*—providing safeguards for their communities from hazards of storage, transportation, and use of compressed gases.

Gas cylinders are made from seamless tubing (brazed or welded) or from flat sheets of drawn steel shaped into a cylinder. Some common types are the ICC-3A (seamless high pressure, 150 to 15,000 psig), ICC-3AA (seamless high pressure above 3A rating), ICC-3B (seamless, 150 to 500 psig), ICC-3E (seamless, 2 in. maximum diameter, 24 in. maximum length, 1800 psig), and ICC-8 (seamless low pressure, 250 psig, for acetylene service). *Gas cylinders are dangerous* and if mishandled may result in fire and explosion.

Markings on gas cylinders are required. For example, first line: ICC spec 3AA, 2015 psig; second line: H 396042; third line: BAP (manufacture marking); and fourth line: 8-70 (month and year of qualification test).

Piping systems, as shown in Figure 11-1, are used throughout the hospital. Central oxygen cylinders supply oxygen to specific hospital areas through a pressure regulating valve, which maintains a pressure between 50 and 100 psi at the service outlet. The main supply must have a shutoff valve and an alarm system. Separate station manual or automatic shutoff valves are also required. All personnel must be educated as to the placement and use of these valves.

Therapeutic gases include: oxygen—essential to life (normally 21% of room air); carbon dioxide—important to the control of respiration and circulation (normally 0.025% of room air); helium—lightweight inert gas used in cases of respiratory obstruction; nitrous oxide—inorganic gas used as an anesthetic agent; helium-oxygen mixtures—low-density gas used on asthmatic patients; and oxygen-carbon dioxide mixtures—used to stimulate deep breathing and to relieve cerebral vascular spasm.

Safety systems for compressed gases in hospitals are essential. The Diameter-Index Safety System (DISS) was developed by the CGA to provide interchangeable threaded connections. Each connection of DISS (make-and-break threaded connections) consists of a body, nipple, and nut. The Pin-Index Safety System (two-pin approach) prevents incorrect interchange of medical gas cylinders with flush-type valves. Ten combinations are possible, of which eight are in current use. With the two-pin approach, no two incompatible cylinders can be attached together.

11-7 Oxygen therapy

Oxygen therapy is the administration of oxygen for the treatment of conditions resulting from oxygen deficiency. These conditions result from pneumonia, pulmonary edema (swelling), obstruction to breathing, congestive heart failure, coronary thrombosis (blood blockage), and complications following surgery. Oxygen is administered through nasal catheters, masks (nasal or oronasal), funnels or cones, tents, or special chambers. A typical oxygen mixture is 70% to 100% by volume. Oxygen is usually introduced together with medicines, water vapor, other gases (carbon dioxide or helium), and anesthetics.

Oxygen therapy is accomplished through the use of special procedures and equipment, such as

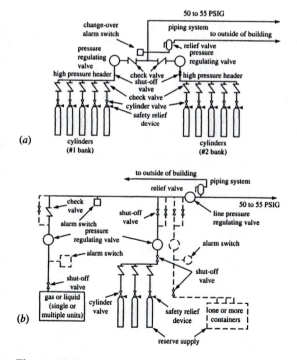

Figure 11-1
Oxygen supply systems. (*a*) Oxygen cylinder system. (*b*) Oxygen bulk system. (Dotted lines are alternates.) (Reprinted with permission of Prentice Hall)

gas regulator or flowmeter control devices, humidifier or nebulizer conditioning units, and oxygen mask or tent administering systems.

Gas regulators are used to reduce cylinder pressure to a safer level, such as 50 psig. A flowmeter adjusts the gas flow in liters per minute. Cylinder regulators are typed as *preset* (reduction to working pressure of 50 psig through one chamber and one safety valve), *adjustable* (reduction to 50 to 100 psig through one chamber and one safety valve), and *multiple stage* (reduction to 50 psig through two or three chambers and the same number of safety valves). Figure 11-2 shows a cylinder regulator, with a flowmeter attached, and a flow-adjusting valve.

A *flowmeter* is a device that contains a calibrated tube to indicate oxygen flow in liters per minute and a valve to control the rate of flow. It must be in the upright position to obtain an accurate reading. Becauseof the back pressure generated in the flow line by these devices, back pressure compensated flowmeters must be used to give correct indications. Figure 11-3 shows the uncompensated Thorpe flowmeter (needle valve control), Bourdon flow gauge (needle-valve, fixed-size orifice control), and pressure-compensated flowmeter (rising ball that partially drops from back pressure in the line-variable area flowmeter).

Wall outlets and adapters are extensive in number. Some standard ones appear in Figure 11-4.

Humidifiers add water vapor to medical gases administered to a patient. This is necessary because alveolar-capillary gas transfer membranes require high humidity to be effective. This is accomplished by passing the gas through sterile water, which creates tiny bubbles. Two types are the Ohio Medical *jet humidifier* and Puritan-Bennett *bubble-jet humidifier,* shown in Figure 11-5. Some have temperature regulation units, such as the Bennett cascade humidifiers. All must be sterilized after each use.

Nebulizers are aerosol therapy units in which suspended fine particles or droplets appear in the administered gas. This is accomplished by the *Bernoulli principle,* which is that greater fluid velocity through a restriction causes a reduction in its pressure. Nebulizers of this type are all-purpose and rely on the restriction to convert liquid to vapor. Others are *ultrasonic nebulizers.* These operate on the principle of breaking the water into uniform particles by passing high-frequency (1.35 MHz) sound waves through the liquid. This type of aerosol can penetrate deeper into the bronchial tree. The De-Vilbiss *ultrasonic nebulizer* is a mobile unit that can be cleaned easily.

Oxygen therapy is primarily administered through oxygen masks or tents. *Oxygen masks* are devices that fit over the patient's face and allow oxygen to pass to the nose and mouth. They are dangerous because suffocation will result if oxygen is cut off and the patient cannot remove the mask. Nevertheless, they are more effective than the *nasal cannulas* (simple inexpensive flexible tubes at each nostril opening for 22% to 30% oxygen delivery) or *nasal catheters* (plastic tube placed into a nostril for 30% to 35% oxygen delivery). *Oxygen tents,* such as the *Bunn tent,* provide the patient with a regulated temperature humidity, oxygen concentration and environment. A canopy surrounds the patient, gas is pumped in,

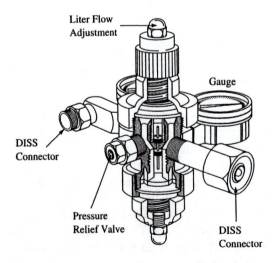

Figure 11-2
Cylinder regulator. (Reprinted with permission of Prentice Hall)

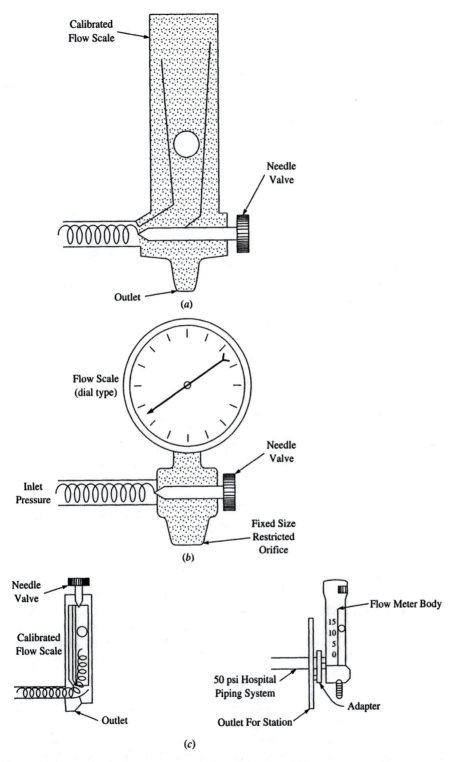

Figure 11-3

Flow gages. (*a*) Thorpe uncompensated flowmeter. (*b*) Bourdon uncompensated flow gage.
(*c*) Pressure-compensated flowmeter.

335

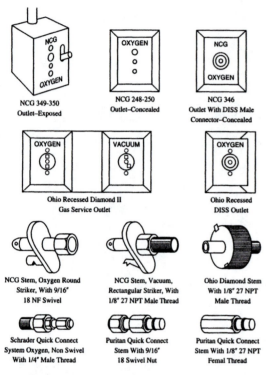

Figure 11-4
Wall outlets and adapters. (Reprinted with permission of Prentice Hall)

and waste gases are removed. *Oxygen hoods,* such as the Olympic Oxyhood, deliver high concentrations of oxygen to infants. Special *infant incubators,* such as the Ohio-Armstrong *isolation incubator,* supply heated, filtered, humidified air for newborns.

It is important to remember that technology and machines are only aids. *Respiratory therapists* and the *respiratory therapy department* treat patients. Recordkeeping provides physicians, nurses, therapists, and other allied health personnel with a valuable guide for treating the patient.

Since city and industrial area air is polluted, respiratory irritation frequently occurs. Increasing numbers of people will require artificial ventilatory machines as our modern growth expands.

11-8 Intermittent positive pressure breathing therapy

Intermittent positive pressure breathing (IPPB) therapy involves special procedures and equipment. IPPB is a type of assisted breathing pattern in which the lungs are inflated by positive pressure during *inspiration* and, on release of the pressure, *expiration* occurs passively.

IPPB is indicated for patients with the following problems: chest disorders, such as bronchitis, bronchiectasis, asthma, pulmonary emphysema, and edema; central nervous system disorders (e.g., drug overdose); chronic bronchopulmonary diseases (e.g., bronchial infections, respiratory acidosis); and postoperative conditions (to prevent pneumonia).

The *objectives* of IPPB are to assist and promote more uniform ventilation, facilitate better O_2 and CO_2 exchange and aspiration of antibiotic drugs, relieve bronchospasm, assist in removal of bronchopulmonary secretions (drainage), and exercise respiratory muscles. Medical gases commonly used are oxygen, compressed air, and oxygen-helium mixtures.

Under emergency circumstances in which IPPB respirators are not available, *cardiopulmonary resuscitation* (CPR) may save the patient's life. This is a technique used to maintain blood flow and oxygenation when heart attack (fibrillation) or respiratory arrest is present. In simple terms, it consists of pumping rhythmically on the patient's chest with the palm of one hand while periodically blowing air into the patient's mouth. For long-term respiratory treatment, respiratory therapy devices must be used. All patient care personnel should be familiar with CPR.

Patient orientation is extremely important for IPPB therapy success. Respiratory therapists should greet and treat patients with a cheerful attitude, explaining that this treatment is easy but requires the patient's cooperation. Should the patient fight the machine, total success is uncertain. The therapist should also explain the procedure of treatment and entertain any questions from the patient.

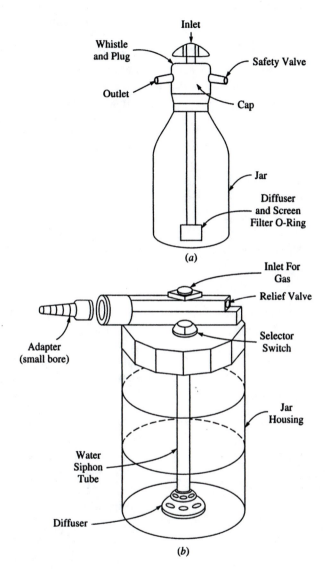

Figure 11-5
Humidifiers. (*a*) Ohio Medical jet. (*b*) Puritan-Bennett bubble-jet.

IPPB unit hardware includes a special device known as the *Bennett valve*. This valve controls an intermittent positive inspiration pressure that assists in inflating the lungs. The patient's respiratory effort (rate and rhythm) controls valve cycling. Connection between the patient and gas reservoir through the valve is such that, in the automatic mode, the patient can take over both inspiration and expiration.

Figure 11-6 shows a Bennett respiration unit that operates from a standard 50-psi pressure source. Supply can be through a standard hospital

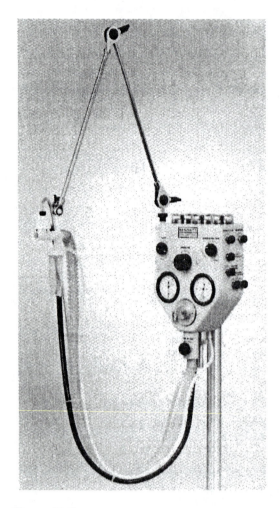

Figure 11-6
Bennett respirator. (Photo courtesy of Puritan-
Bennett)

nett valve for manually adjusted control. Terminal and negative pressures are also controlled from the main line. The *Bennett valve rotating internal ball* closes during patient expiration, and the exhalation diaphragm opens to release exhaust gases. Upon inspiration, the diaphragm closes, and the Bennett valve opens to deliver oxygen and water vapor (from the nebulizer) to the patient.

Accessories can be used with this unit, as shown in Figure 11-6. These include a *monitoring spirometer,* which indicates each expiration volume; an *alarm* set to sound below a preset tidal volume; a *humidifier* cascade type for counteracting drying effects of anhydrous gas; an *oxygen adder,* which mixes oxygen from a metered supply with air from the main line; *bacterial filters,* which reduce infection between patients; and *volumetric ventilation control,* which delivers a preset tidal volume to the patient, independent of lung compliance.

The assembly and operation procedures for the Bennett IPPB unit are important. During the performance of these procedures, problems that can cause serious injury to the patient are uncovered.

An *assembly procedure* consists of the following steps:

1. Blow out the dust particles from the cylinder valve and connect it to the compressed gas cylinder (tighten with a wrench and avoid stripping the threads).

2. Screw the support arm into the threaded hole on the unit head (tighten using wing nuts, and avoid forcing any section into place).

3. Attach the manifold, including exhalation valve, to the end of the support arm (exhalation port should face the patient).

4. Attach one end of the large main air tube to the port beneath the Bennett valve.

5. Attach the remaining end of the main air tube to the bottom manifold port for horizontal nebulizer use and attach to the back of the manifold for vertical nebulizer use.

piped system of 40 to 70 psi or from a separate gas cylinder of 50 psi regulated.

Figure 11-7 shows a block diagram of the functional features of the Bennett-type IPPB unit. Air pressure at 50 psi is fed to the Bennett valve through an adjustable-diluter regulator. The control and system pressure are recorded on front panel gauges. From the main input gas line, a low-pressure regulator supplies the input for sensitivity, rate, and expiration control. These lead to the Ben-

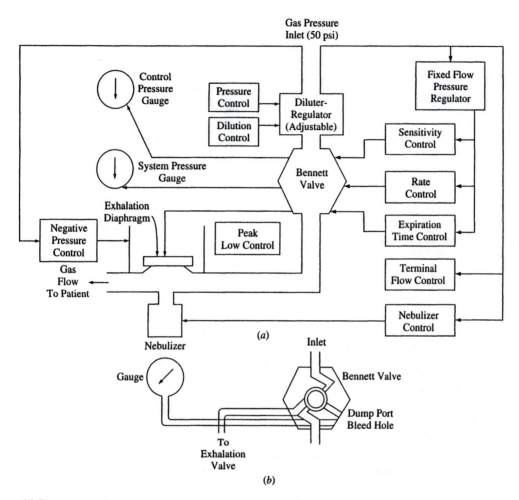

Figure 11-7
IPPB respirator. (*a*) Functional block diagram. (*b*) Internal structure of the Bennett valve.

6. Connect the smaller diameter tubing to the exhalation port on the manifold and the other end below the Bennett valve.

7. Connect the larger diameter tubing to the nebulizer tailpiece and the remaining end to the nebulizer control (top of unit head).

8. Secure the flex tube and mouthpiece (or mask) to the manifold end nearest the exhalation valve.

It is important to remember that other assembly techniques yield a system that appears to be functional but may be erratic or marginal for patient therapy success.

The *operation procedure* is as follows:

1. With both hands, open the cylinder valve fully (stand in back of the unit for safety; a burst of gas may dislodge any unit member).

2. Move the shutoff lever on the unit head downward to the vertical position ("on" position).

3. Turn the pressure control clockwise until the gage registers the amount prescribed by the physician (typically 10 to 20 cm H_2O).

4. Set the dilution control prescribed by the physician to either the 100% oxygen setting or the room-air oxygen setting.

5. Place the nebulizer medication in the canister (always have medication, distilled water, or physiological saline present, as dry gas will harm the patient).

6. Open the nebulizer control and observe a slight mist or fog.

The foregoing procedure involves an *operating sequence* that involves setting inspiratory flow start (patient cycled or automatic time cycling), expiratory start (inspiratory end), system cycling (rate control), inspiration/expiration ratio, nebulizer flow, and breathing system (lung flow resistance and lung and thoracic compliance and leaks).

The biomedical equipment technician *should not* set up or administer respiratory treatment. This operation is the responsibility of a trained respiratory therapist or physician.

Automatic electronically controlled IPPB therapy units are also on the market (e.g., the Bennett AP-5). These use a motorand pump assembly that drives filtered air through a Bennett valve to the patient. Most often these are used in the patient's home, physician's office, or outpatient clinic, because they do not require a tank air pressure cylinder supply. They can also be fitted with accessories, such as cascaded humidifiers, nebulizers, and bacteria filters.

Some *manual IPPB units* operate by compressing room air and are equipped to provide additional oxygen, if required (e.g., the Bennett Model TA-1, shown in Figure 11-8).

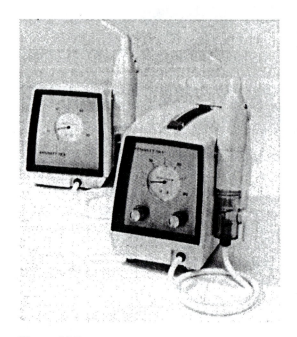

Figure 11-8
Bennett TA-1 manual IPPB unit model. (Photo courtesy of Puritan-Bennett)

11-9 Artificial mechanical ventilation

Artificial lung ventilators are devices that connect to the patient's airway and are designed to augment or replace the patient's ventilation automatically. They are used with a mask, endotracheal tube (within the trachea), or tracheostomy tube (through an artificial opening in the trachea via the throat). These ventilators consist of a controller, which operates independently of the patient's inspiratory effort; an assistor, which augments or assists inspiration of the spontaneously breathing patient; and an assist-controller, which assists and/or controls. Some lung ventilators are *pressure preset* and others are *volume preset* (tidal or minute volume). Some *cycle inspiratory to expiratory* (volume, pressure, time, or a combination). Others *cycle expiratory to inspiratory* (pressure, time, and combined; patient-controlled or manual override). Safety limits are *volume pressure* or *time set*. Pressure patterns are positive atmospheric, positive-negative, or positive-positive. Most operate pneumatically; others are electrically powered.

Essentially, ventilators are classified into two types:

1. *Pressure-cycled (pressure-limited)*—those that continue to inflate the patient's lungs until a preset pressure is reached, at which time expiration stops and inspiration starts. These units maintain ventilation with small system leaks but compensate poorly for obstruction.

2. *Volume-controlled (volume-limited)*—those that permit maintenance of constant minute and tidal ventilation even though changes in pulmonary compliance and airway resistance occur. Safety valves for maximum preset pressure should be included. These units maintain steady tidal volume, but with partial obstruction they compensate poorly for system leaks.

Pressure-cycled, assistor-controlled pneumatic ventilators (Bird Mark-8, shown in Figure 11-9) are used for patients with apnea, for assisted ventilation, and for patients with airway resistance. This system pressure is adjusted by the operator, and the patient-delivered volume is variable, depending on lung compliance. The Bird Mark-14, shown in Figure 11-10, has all the capabilities of the Bird Mark-8 and also has leak-compensated, positive-phase operation, automatic flow accelerator, and provisions for handling airway pressures of up to 140 mm Hg and flow rate up to 160 L/min.

Volume-limited ventilators (Bennett Respiration Unit Model MA-1, shown in Figure 11-11) are used for patients who can initiate their own inspiration. The MA-1 is an electrically powered device that uses *ambient air* as the principal gas, with provisions for oxygen enrichment up to 100%. It can initiate inspiration by a *timing mechanism*. Inspiration may also be initiated by the patient, and under this condition, the unit becomes an assistor. Adjustments are also available

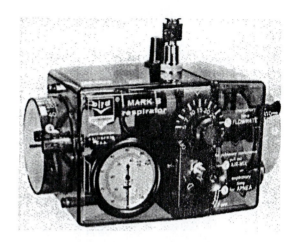

Figure 11-9
Bird Mark-8 ventilator. (Photo courtesy of the Bird Corporation)

to permit the ventilator to take over respiratory control should the patient become apneic (cease to breathe). *Adjustable volume and pressure limits* set the end of the inspiration. Essentially, these controls are positioned to deliver a fixed volume at each inspiration that is below the selected maximum safety pressure. The *breaths per minute* setting is set on the timer dial. This is chosen based on the volume or pressure limits and calibrated

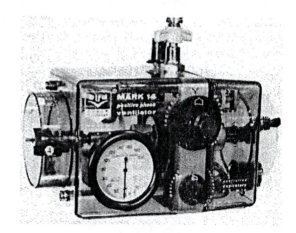

Figure 11-10
Bird Mark-14 ventilator. (Photo courtesy of the Bird Corporation)

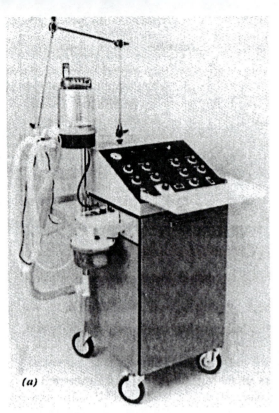

(a)

Figure 11-11

(a) Bennett respirator unit Model MA-1 solid-state IPPB unit. (Photo courtesy of Puritan-Bennett) (b) Flow block diagram.

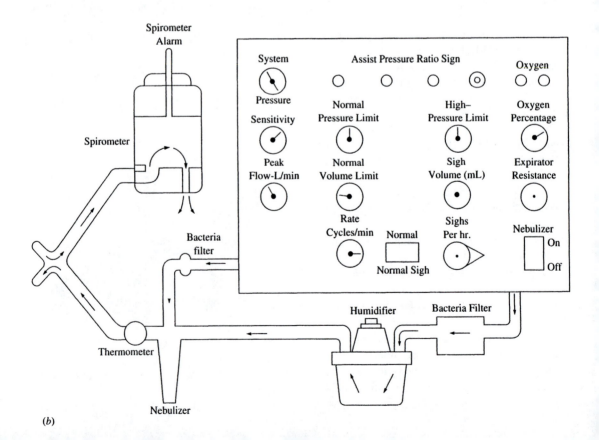

(b)

maximum flow rate. Periodic deep breaths (sighs), volume and pressure limits, oxygen percentage, and nebulizer controls are also on the front panel. There are nine *output displays:*

1. System pressure gauge.

2. Spirometer below volume and spirometer audible alarm.

3. Adverse ratio.

4. Warning light.

5. Oxygen-deficiency audible alarm.

6. Sigh inspiration warning light.

7. Pressure warning limit light or audible alarm.

8. Thermometer.

9. Elapsed-time indicator.

The MA-1 unit operates from a 115-V, 60-Hz power line with chassis grounding for electrical safety (low-leakage current). As shown in Figure 11-11, the *external controls* are as follows:

1. Adjustable calibrated normal volume (0 to 2200 mL)

2. Adjustable calibrated normal rate (6 to 60 cpm).

3. Adjustable calibrated normal pressure limit (20 to 80 cm H_2O).

4. Manual normal inspiration start control.

5. Adjustable calibrated sigh volume (0 to 2200 mL).

6. Adjustable calibrated sigh intervals (4, 6, 8, 10, or 15 times, or number of deep breaths per hour to remove blockages).

7. Adjustable calibrated multiples (1, 2, 3 sighs per interval).

8. Adjustable calibrated sigh pressure limit (28 to 80 cm H_2O).

9. Controlled expiration after sigh inspiration.

10. Manual sigh inspiration start control.

11. Adjustable calibrated O_2 percentage (21% to 100%).

12. Adjustable assist sensitivity control with lockout position.

13. Adjustable calibrated maximum flow (15 to 100 L/min).

14. Adjustable inspiratory plateau and expiratory flow resistance.

15. Nebulizer on-off control.

16. Adjustable heated humidifier.

17. Power on-off switch.

11-10 Accessory devices used in respiratory therapy apparatus

Accessory devices used with respiratory therapy apparatus enhance the possibilities for quality patient treatment.

Respiratory monitors (see chapter 9) typically have meter displays for tidal volume, minute volume, and respiratory rate, or low and high pressure alarm settings and audible tones. These monitors are portable and operate from 60-Hz power lines or internal rechargeable batteries. Output signals are usually provided for oscilloscopes or strip-chart recorders. Respiration transducers are thermistor probes that change temperature as the patient breathes air across the probe's surface. *Pneumographs* plot physical respiratory excursions.

Portable oxygen analyzers are also used to give oxygen concentrations in controlled environments (refer to chapter 9), such as tents, incubators, oxygen hoods, and ventilators.

Ventilation failure devices attach to the patient's gas delivery line and give audible warning for respiratory malfunction, supply gas loss, massive leaks, compliance-obstruction changes, and loose tracheostomy fittings.

11-11 Sterilization and isolation procedures in respiratory therapy units

Sterilization of respiratory therapy equipment results in the destruction of all microorganisms and their spores. This is necessary because gases carrying bacteria into the lungs can cause severe lung damage due to infection. The effect of respiratory treatment is then reduced, and, in the extreme case, the patient may die.

Sterilization processing of contaminated equipment should be done in an area separate from clean storage. All equipment should be dismantled as completely as possible and washed with a brush in a detergent. Thorough rinsing and draining is then required. Equipment should be packaged or arranged for sterilization by one of the following methods:

1. *Autoclave*—steam treatment at temperatures higher than 212°F (100°C) for 20 minutes or longer.

2. *Ethylene oxide gas*—microbicidal and sporicidal agent in contact with equipment parts for at least 5 minutes (45 minutes or longer is also common).

3. *Cold sterilization using glutaraldehyde (Cidex)*—2% aqueous activated dialdehyde used as a bactericidal, tuberculocidal, virucidal, and sporicidal agent poured over equipment for 10 minutes to 10 hours.

4. *Automatic decontamination system (Cidematic)*—device that cleans, disinfects, and dries equipment automatically.

5. *Sonacide (potentiated acid glutaraldehyde)*—lemon-scented sterilizing and disinfecting solution.

These techniques are selectively designed to kill *fungi, bacteria,* and most *viruses.* However, regardless of the method used, *periodic bacteriological cultures* should be taken to evaluate sterilization effectiveness.

In addition to sterilization, *isolation* should be required for certain patients to prevent the transmission of infection. Infection may be caused by direct or indirect contact, through a *vehicle route* (blood, water, drugs, food), *vector route* (insects), or *airborne route* (droplet and dust). *Frequent hand washing* is always a good practice. *Wearing gloves, gowns, and masks* is an added precaution near infected patients. Isolation is required for patients with the following *infections: Staphylococcus aureus, Streptococcus species,* diphtheria, herpes simplex, plague, rubella, smallpox, rubella (congenital syndrome), meningitis, mumps, tuberculosis, and any aspergillosis, *Pseudomonas species,* bacillus, or coccidioidomycosis (pneumonia) conditions.

11-12 Typical faults and maintenance procedures for ventilators

In general, *air tubes and their connections* cause considerable difficulty. This can be minimized by frequent inspections, especially before patient use. *Worn clamps and tubing* should be replaced immediately. Humidifiers and nebulizers frequently become *clogged,* but constant cleaning reduces this occurrence. Occasionally, someone will accidently *spill some fluid* (e.g., blood, urine, saline, antiseptic, Betadine, or water) into the machine. Extensive disassembly and parts replacement (e.g., switches, relays, motors, and air filters) often become necessary.

Leaks in compressed gas (oxygenated helium) cylinders and ventilator systems occur despite attentive inspections. These are tracked down by rating differential pressures in various parts of the system. Obviously, leaks reduce gas pressure and volume delivered to the patient.

Routine preventive maintenance consists of periodic inspections of system connections and functional operation. Electrical leakage current (less than 10 μA) checks should be done monthly. *Calibration* is usually performed every 6 months. The applicable operation and maintenance manual should always be consulted for calibration procedures.

Intake and patient line *air filters* must be cleaned or replaced periodically (every few weeks depending on use and patient infection). This ensures proper air flow to the patient.

Electrical components that require routine replacement include lamps, switches, actuating devices, motors, and heaters. *Electronic problems* (faulty capacitors, diodes, transistors, and integrated circuits) are relatively rare.

11-13 Summary

1. Two general *respiratory diseases* that may require artificial respiratory therapy are *hypoxia* (low blood oxygen content) and *hypercapnia* (poor alveolar ventilation).

2. The *goal* of an *artificial ventilatory* control mechanism is to adjust alveolar ventilation to changing body needs for oxygen intake and carbon dioxide removal.

3. *Medical gas safety* is regulated by the NFPA, DOT, FDA, OSHA, and state and local agencies. Gas cylinders are dangerous since compressed air, oxygen, helium, and nitrous oxide gas may cause fire, explosion, or direct physical injury. Interchangeable threaded piping is controlled by specific systems, e.g., DISS.

4. *Oxygen therapy* is the administration (treatment) of oxygen for treatment of conditions (e.g., pneumonia, edema, obstruction, heart failure, and thrombosis) resulting in patient oxygen deficiency. Devices such as gas regulators, flowmeters, humidifiers, nebulizers, masks, tents, and incubators are commonly used.

5. *IPPB* therapy is a type of assisted breathing pattern in which the lungs are inflated with air, O_2, or O_2-helium by a positive pressure during inspiration. Upon release of the pressure, expiration occurs passively. IPPB

therapy promotes more uniform breathing, facilitates better O_2 and CO_2 gas exchange, and removes secretions. Patient orientation is extremely important. Assembly and operating procedures should be followed carefully. Most IPPBs use a Bennett valve to control inspiration and expiration. Spirometer, alarms, humidifiers, and filters are common accessories used.

6. *CPR* is a mechanical manual method for maintaining respiration under emergency conditions.

7. *Artificial mechanical ventilators* are devices that connect to the patient's airway and are designed to augment or replace the patient's ventilation. They work automatically and are either *pressure-cycled* (pressure-limited) or *volume-controlled* (volume-limited). The applicable *operation and maintenance manual* should always be consulted for instructions (guessing can be dangerous to the patient).

8. Respiratory therapy apparatus *accessories* include respiratory monitors, pneumographs, O_2 analyzers, and alarms.

9. *Sterilization* of respiratory therapy equipment is a process of cleaning deposits and destroying bacteria and viruses. This is accomplished by using an autoclave, ethylene oxide gas, cold liquid (dialdehyde), and automatic decontamination chambers.

10. Typical *faults* in artificial respiratory ventilators include broken or leaky air tubes or clamps, clogged devices or filters, leaks, burned-out lamps, broken switches, and rare electronic failures (e.g., capacitors, diodes, transistors, and integrated circuits).

11-14 Recapitulation

Now return to the objectives and self-evaluation questions at the beginning of the chapter and see how well you can answer them. If you cannot answer certain questions, place a check mark next to each and review appropriate parts of the text. Next, try to answer the following questions using the same procedure. When you have answered all of the questions, solve the problems.

Questions

1. Two general respiratory therapy diseases, _____ and _____, cause patient ventilation difficulties.

2. The goal of an artificial ventilatory control mechanism is to adjust _____ ventilation to body needs of _____ intake and _____ _____ removal.

3. The following six regulatory agencies are involved in compressed gas safety: _____, _____, _____, _____, _____, _____.

4. Compressed gas in an ICC-3B seamless tank at 150 psig is considered *high* or *low* pressure by industrial standards.

5. For hospital piping system safety, automatic _____ valves as well as separate station manual _____ valves are required.

6. Therapeutic gases include _____, _____, _____, _____-_____ mixture, and _____-_____ _____ mixture.

7. Interchangeable threaded connections on gas cylinders are provided by the _____-_____ _____ System developed by the _____ _____ Association.

8. The _____-_____ _____ System provides the two-pin approach, which prevents incorrect _____ of medical gas cylinders with flush-type valves.

9. Oxygen therapy is the _____ of _____ gas for treatment of conditions resulting from _____ deficiency.

10. Oxygen can be introduced through nasal _____, _____, or _____.

11. Gas regulators are used to _____ cylinder _____ to a safer level, such as _____ psig.

12. A flowmeter is a device that controls and _____ gas flow in units of _____ _____ _____.

13. Aerosol therapy units are known as _____ and may operate on the _____ principle or from _____ energy.

14. Infant incubators are a type of _____ therapy apparatus.

15. IPPB represents _____ _____ _____ _____ and is defined as a type of assisted _____ pattern in which the _____ are inflated by a _____ pressure during inspiration.

16. The objectives of IPPB therapy are to promote more _____ ventilation, facilitate better _____ and _____ _____ exchange, relieve _____, assist in removal of _____, and _____ respiratory muscles.

17. Medical gases commonly used are _____, _____, _____, and _____.

18. IPPB units commonly use a _____ valve, which contains a rotating internal ball. This controls an intermittent _____ _____ pressure that assists in inflating the patient's _____.

19. CPR refers to what procedure?

20. How much pressure is usually fed to a Bennett valve?

21. Can the Bennett valve be adjusted to respond to the patient's inspiratory initiation?

22. What accessories can be used with IPPB units?

23. Why are the assembly and operating procedures for IPPB units important?

24. Artificial mechanical ventilators are generally cycled by which two methods?

25. The Bennett MA-1 ventilator cycles by what method?

26. What are the maximum oxygen concentration, breaths per minute, and flow rate on the Bennett MA-1 ventilator?

27. Why are pressure limit settings available on the Bennett MA-1 ventilator?

28. The sigh control on the Bennett MA-1 ventilator serves what long-term purpose?

29. Name four types of accessory devices used with artificial respiratory ventilators.

30. What is the purpose of sterilization for respiratory therapy equipment?

31. How would one proceed to sterilize respiratory apparatus using available sterilizing equipment?

32. Should gloves, gown, and mask be worn to repair disease-contaminated respiratory therapy equipment?

33. Name five of the most common faults with artificial respiratory ventilators and list their solutions.

Problems

1. A respiratory therapist reports that a mechanical ventilator does not turn on when the power switch is toggled. What checkout procedure would you use and which system components would be suspected first?

2. A nurse reports that an artificial respiratory ventilator appears to be delivering insufficient gas flow to the patient with proper flow, pressure, and gas-mixture front-panel settings (based on the nurse's experience). What checkout procedure would you use and which system components would be suspected first?

Suggested reading

1. Hunsinger, Doris L., Karl Lisnerski, Jerome J. Maurizi, and Mary Phillips, *Respiratory Technology—A Procedure Manual,* Reston Publishing Co., Inc. (Reston, Va., 1976).

2. Moore, Francis D., John H. Lyons, Jr., Ellison C. Pierce, Jr., Alfred P. Morgan, Jr., Philip A. Drinker, John D. MacArthur, and Gustave J. Kammin, *Post-Traumatic Pulmonary Insufficiency,* W. B. Saunders Co. (Philadelphia, 1969).

3. Petty, Thomas L., *Intensive and Rehabilitative Respiratory Care—A Practical Approach to the Management of Acute and Chronic Respiratory Failure,* Lea and Febiger (Philadelphia, 1971).

4. Beall, Cheryl E., Harold A. Brown, and Frederick W. Cheney, Jr., *Physiological Basis for Respiratory Care,* Mountain Press Publishing Co. (1974).

5. "A Comprehensive Volume-Cycled Ventilator Embodying Feedback Control." *Medical and Biological Engineering, 12* (2): 160-169 (1974).

6. Pace, William R., Jr., *Pulmonary Physiology in Clinical Practice,* F. A. Davis Company (Philadelphia, 1970).

7. *Operation and Service Manual* for Bennett TV-2P IPPB Pressure Breathing Therapy Unit, Puritan-Bennett Corp. (Kansas City, Mo., 1969).

8. *Operation and Service Manuals* for Bird Mark 1,7,8,10,14 Intermittent Positive Pressure Ventilator, Bird Corp. (Palm Springs, Calif., 1974).

9. Kurtzweil, Paula, *"When Machines Do The Breathing,"* FDA Consumer, September-October, 1999, Vol. 33, No. 5.) Describes portable ventilator at the base of actor

Christopher Reeve's wheelchair that allows this paralyzed person to breath assisted by a tube in his throat.

10. Cornwell, Anne Christake, *"Apnea Monitors," Medical Electronics and Equipment Manufacturing,* Measurement and Data Corp., 2994 W. Liberty Ave., Pittsburg, PA 15216, June, 1999 Phone: 412-343-9685. Describes devices to measure cessation of breathing syndrome (SIDS) in the home setting as part of screening for prolonged apnea and bradycardia.

CHAPTER 12

The Human Nervous System

12-1 Objectives

1. Be able to introduce the biological principles underlying the human central nervous system (CNS), the peripheral nervous system (PNS), and the autonomic nervous system (ANS).
2. Be able to describe the structure and function of the *neuron* (single nerve cell), *CNS* (brain and spinal cord), *PNS* (nerve pairs), and *ANS* (sympathetic and parasympathetic systems).
3. Be able to identify specific areas of the brain concerned with bodily sensory and motor functions.

12-2 Self-evaluation questions

These questions test your prior knowledge of the material in this chapter. Look for the answers as you read the text. After you have finished studying the chapter, try answering these questions and those at the end of the chapter.

1. List the major divisions of the nervous system.

2. Draw a diagram and define various portions of a *neuron* (single nerve cell).

3. Describe *nerve impulse conduction* through one neuron and several neurons connected together.

4. Describe the basic structure and function of the *CNS, PNS,* and *ANS.*

5. Name the four lobes of the cerebrum.

6. Identify the areas of the brain responsible for the senses of sight, sound, touch, smell, and taste.

7. Identify the areas of the brain responsible for the function of muscle movement, memory, intelligence, judgment, imagination, creativity, and conscious thought.

8. How does blood circulate through the brain?

9. What is the purpose of the three membranes (meninges) covering the brain?

10. Does human behavior control brain function, or does brain function control human behavior?

12-3 Organization of the nervous system

The nervous system is a complex interconnection of nervous tissue that is concerned with the *integration* and *control* of all bodily functions. We know that this system allows an individual to *detect* internal and external environmental *changes* (stimuli) and to *interpret* (analyze) the resulting nerve impulses.

Homeostasis (constancy or stability in internal body states) is achieved through a network of *negative feedback loops* involving nervous (electrochemical) and humoral (biochemical) components. For example, blood carbonate is detected in the brain. If it is too high (indicating too much carbon dioxide in the blood), the brain initiates movement of breathing muscles. This, in turn, increases breathing rate and rids (ventilates) the body of carbon dioxide gas through the lungs.

The nervous system is generally considered the most complex bodily system. It is divided into several major divisions distinguished by *anatomy* (structure and location) and *physiology* (function), including the following:

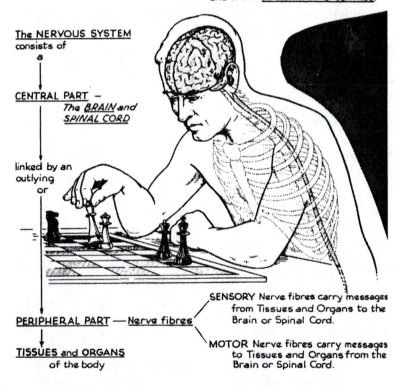

NERVOUS SYSTEM

The Nervous System is concerned with the INTEGRATION and CONTROL of all bodily functions.
It has specialized in IRRITABILITY— *the ability to receive and respond to messages from the external and internal environments* and also in CONDUCTION ~ *the ability to transmit messages to and from CO-ORDINATING CENTRES.*

The NERVOUS SYSTEM consists of a

CENTRAL PART —
The *BRAIN* and *SPINAL CORD*

linked by an outlying or

PERIPHERAL PART —Nerve fibres

TISSUES and ORGANS of the body

SENSORY Nerve fibres carry messages from Tissues and Organs to the Brain or Spinal Cord.

MOTOR Nerve fibres carry messages to Tissues and Organs from the Brain or Spinal Cord.

Figure 12-1
The nervous system. (McNaught, Ann B. and Robin Callander, *Illustrated Physiology,* Churchill Livingstone, New York, 1976. Used by permission.)

1. *Central nervous system (CNS)*, which is enclosed within the skull and vertebral column—*brain and spinal cord*.

2. *Peripheral nervous system (PNS)*, which consists of nervous tissue outside the skull and vertebral column—periphery (extremity) of the body. Subdivisions of the PNS include:

a. *Somatic system*, which supplies sensory motor and sensory fibers to the skin and skeletal muscles.

b. *Autonomic nervous system (ANS)*, which supplies smooth muscle, cardiac muscle, and glands in the body viscera. The *sympathetic* (stimulatory) *system* causes organ changes that help the body resist stress. The *parasympathetic* (inhibitory) *system* maintains normal function and conserves body resources.

Figure 12-1 shows an overview of the nervous system.

Humans have the ability to perceive their environment as well as to receive it. *Reception*

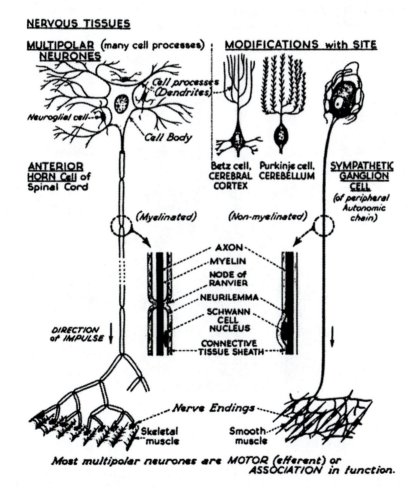

Figure 12-2
Nervous tissue. (From McNaught & Callander, *Illustrated Physiology*. Used by permission of Churchill Livingstone.)

involves response to environmental stimuli, while *perception* relates to the recognition of symbolic patterns. These patterns are abstract (not physical) and are composed of linguistic symbols. The ability of the human to think of the physical world in abstract terms accounts for the extraordinary talent to manipulate objects, construct houses, and control his or her environment.

12-4 The neuron (single nerve cell)

The *neuron* is the fundamental unit of the nervous system. It is a single cell composed of a *cell body (soma),* several short *input projections (dendrites),* and a *long propagation channel (axon).* The axon together with its sheath (covering) forms the nerve

fiber. Figure 12-2 shows a nerve cell connected to *skeletal muscle* and to *smooth muscle.* Notice that the nerve impulse travels in one direction only from dendrites to nerve endings. The *axon* extends the entire length of the nerve cell, and some are surrounded by a *myelin sheath* (segmented insulating covering). The *neurilemma* encompasses this sheath and is composed of *Schwann cells. Nodes of Ranvier* act to speed up the nerve impulse transmission.

The *transmission of the nerve impulse* is actually a result of biochemicals that travel across the *synapse* (space between nerve cells). The change in membrane permeability is the chief reason for nerve pulse transfer across the synaptic junction. Figure 12-3 shows the synaptic ultrastructure. Observe the

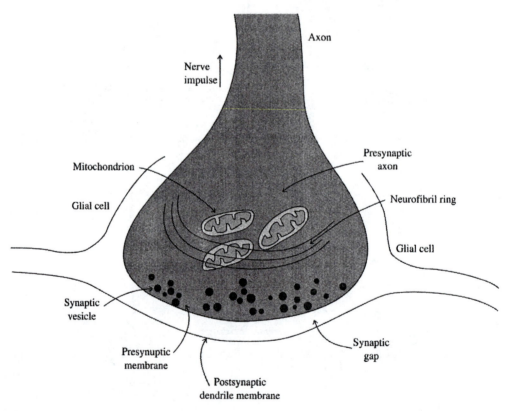

Figure 12-3
Synaptic ultrastructure.

presynaptic and postsynaptic membranes and synaptic gap. The excitatory postsynaptic potential (EPSP) results in *higher* levels of conduction, and the inhibitory postsynaptic potential (IPSP) results in *decreased,* or inhibited, conduction.

The conduction pulse results in a wave of depolarization (action potential) similar to that presented for heart muscle in chapter 2, particularly Figures 2-3 and 2-4. *Nerve conduction* is in one direction only (constant speed) from dendrites through axon to nerve endings. Neurons can con-

nect to each other in the following arrangements: one to one, one to many, many to one, or many to many. Figure 12-4 shows these possibilities.

The axons and dendrites (nerve fibers) bundle together to form a *nerve.* The sensory nerves carried to the brain are known as *afferent nerves,* and the ones carried away from the brain are called *efferent nerves.* Nerves switch on and off in such a manner as to cause abrupt changes in cell voltages. In effect, this nerve impulse switching is similar to electronic digital circuit logic. Several nerve cells

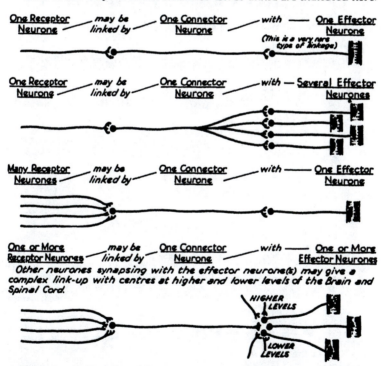

Figure 12-4

Arrangements of neurons (neurones). (From McNaught & Callander, *Illustrated Physiology.* Used by permission of Churchill Livingstone.)

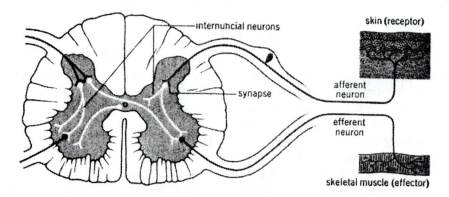

Figure 12-5
Components of reflex arc. (From *Human Anatomy and Physiology,* 2nd edition, by James E. Crouch, Ph.D. and J. Robert McClintic, Ph.D. John Wiley & Sons, New York, 1976. Used by permission.)

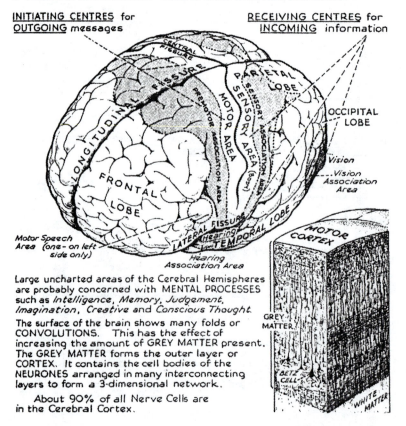

Figure 12-6
The cerebrum. (From McNaught & Callander, *Illustrated Physiology.* Used by permission of Churchill Livingstone.)

354

may be required to conduct before a triggering threshold is reached. The *AND* and *OR* functions performed by nerve cells act to control bodily coordination and reflexes.

Reflex action in the human involves many reflex arcs. A nervous reflex is an *involuntary* action response caused by stimulation of an afferent nerve ending or receptor. The knee jerk in response to the tap of a hammer is one example of a reflex arc, the components of which are shown in Figure 12-5. The components of the arc are:

1. A *receptor*, which detects change.

2. An *afferent neuron*, which conducts the nerve impulse from the sensory area to the CNS.

3. A *center or synapse*, which connects neurons together.

4. A brain processing area.

5. An *efferent neuron*, which conducts nerve impulses from the CNS to an organ for appropriate response.

6. An *effector or organ*, which responds to maintain homeostasis.

12-5 Structure and function of the central nervous system*

The brain is defined as "a large soft mass of nerve tissue contained within the cranium, the *encephalon*."[†] Three major structures compose the brain (Figures 12-6 through 12-9): the *brain stem*—automatic vital system control, the *cerebellum*—involuntary muscle control and coordina-

tion, and the *cerebrum*—voluntary movement, sensation, and intelligence.

12-5-1 Brain stem

The *brain stem* consists of the *medulla* (oblongata), *pons, midbrain,* and *diencephalon.*

The *medulla* automatically controls heart rate and breathing. (Actually, most essential life systems are controlled here.) Reflex functions such as coughing, sneezing, and vomiting are associated with the medulla. Indeed, one modern definition of clinical death is the absence of lower brain EEG activity.

The *pons* is about 2.5 cm long and forms a noticeable bulge on the anterior surface of the brain stem. It *functions* as a relay station for motor respiratory and auditory fibers from the cerebrum and cerebellum. Other impulses from eye movement, head muscles, and taste sensors also pass through here.

The *midbrain* is a wedge-shaped portion of the stem. Midbrain tissues function as a motor relay station for fibers passing from the cerebrum to the cord and cerebellum. Integration of visual and auditory reflexes, including those concerned with avoiding objects, also occur here.

The *diencephalon* forms the superior (top) part of the brain stem. As part of the original forebrain, it develops into the *thalamus* and *hypothalamus.*

The *thalamus* receives fibers from the hearing structures of the inner ear and visual system. It also provides pathways for somatic sensory systems. All this sensory information eventually reaches the *cerebrum,* where it is processed.

The *hypothalamus* responds to the properties of blood passing through nerve connections. The *endocrine system* is controlled through nerve responses, affecting emotional behavior patterns. Other functions controlled via chemical interaction with the *pituitary gland* are temperature regulation, water balance, food intake, gastric secretion, sexual behavior, and sleeping patterns.

As a general arousal mechanism, the *reticular activation system (RAS)* functions with the thalamus to prepare the cerebral cortex (higher parts of

---

*The central nervous system is composed of the brain and spinal cord. Many excellent drawings and photographs have been presented by anatomists. *Yokochi* has excellent pictures of actual brain tissue. Frank H. Netter, *Ciba Pharmaceutical Products, Inc.,* has a superb 13-minute motion picture presentation from the Department of Anatomy, U.C.L.A. Medical School (Teaching Films, Houston, Texas, Clemintine and Hardwick) entitled *Guides to Dissection, The Cranial Cavity—Removal of the Brain.*

[†]*Taber's Cyclopedic Medical Dictionary,* F.A. Davis Co. (Philadelphia, 1973).

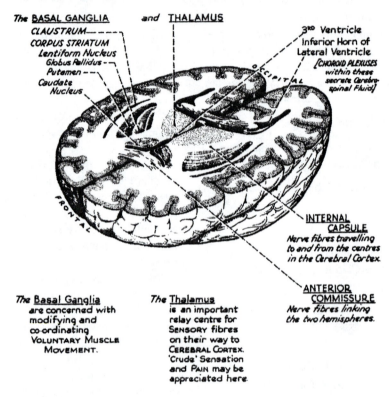

HORIZONTAL SECTION through BRAIN

This view shows surface GREY MATTER containing Nerve Cells and inner WHITE MATTER made up of Nerve Fibres.

Deep in the substance of the Cerebral Hemispheres there are additional masses of GREY MATTER:-

The BASAL GANGLIA   *and* THALAMUS

CLAUSTRUM
CORPUS STRIATUM
Lentiform Nucleus
Globus Pallidus
Putamen
Caudate
Nucleus

3ᴿᴰ Ventricle
Inferior Horn of
Lateral Ventricle
[CHOROID PLEXUSES
within these
secrete Cerebro-
spinal Fluid]

OCCIPITAL

FRONTAL

INTERNAL
CAPSULE
Nerve fibres travelling
to and from the centres
in the Cerebral Cortex.

ANTERIOR
COMMISSURE
Nerve fibres linking
the two hemispheres.

The Basal Ganglia
are concerned with
modifying and
co-ordinating
VOLUNTARY MUSCLE
MOVEMENT.

The Thalamus
is an important
relay centre for
SENSORY fibres
on their way to
CEREBRAL CORTEX.
'Crude' Sensation
and PAIN may be
appreciated here.

Figure 12-7
Horizontal brain section. (From McNaught & Callander, *Illustrated Physiology.* Used by permission of Churchill Livingstone.)

the brain) for incoming sensory stimulation data. This system is a network of gray matter placed centrally in the brain stem.

12-5-2 Cerebellum

The *cerebellum* (Figures 12-8 and 12-9) is the second largest portion of the brain (the cerebrum is the largest) and, essentially, integrates incoming sensory messages to provide smooth body *muscle movements, balance,* and *equilibrium.* This portion of the brain has an outer *cortex* of gray matter and

an inner *medulla* composed of white matter. The cerebellum acts at the subconscious level in coordinating reflexes that automatically establish an upright posture. Thus, *proprioception* (information on position of limbs and movements of muscles) is established through general and special body proprioceptors. Some consider the cerebellum to be a part of the "old" brain, involving basic locomotion but not intellectual thought.

As an example, consider yourself driving a bicycle or car down a road that has frequent turns. When you begin drifting to the right (1/4 ft), you

This is a Vertical Section through the LONGITUDINAL FISSURE— a deep cleft which separates the two Cerebral Hemispheres. At the bottom of this cleft are tracts of nerve fibres which link up the different LOBES of each hemisphere and also link the two hemispheres with each other — the CORPUS CALLOSUM.

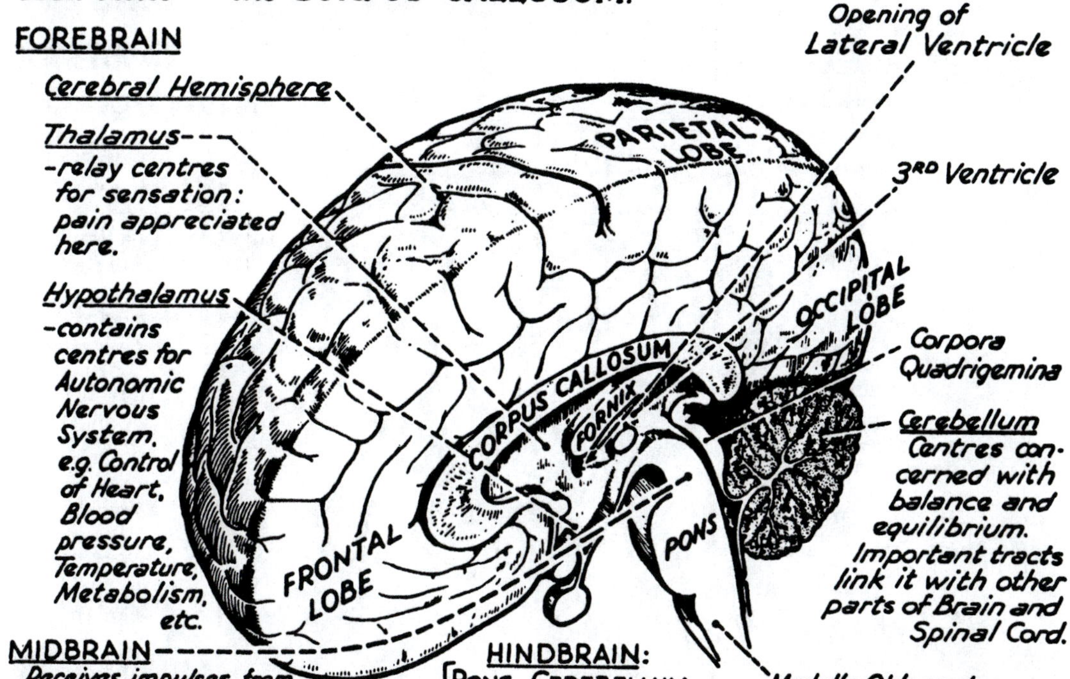

FOREBRAIN

Cerebral Hemisphere

Thalamus—
-relay centres for sensation: pain appreciated here.

Hypothalamus
-contains centres for Autonomic Nervous System, e.g. Control of Heart, Blood pressure, Temperature, Metabolism, etc.

Opening of Lateral Ventricle

3RD Ventricle

PARIETAL LOBE

OCCIPITAL LOBE

CORPUS CALLOSUM

FORNIX

FRONTAL LOBE

PONS

Corpora Quadrigemina

Cerebellum
Centres concerned with balance and equilibrium. Important tracts link it with other parts of Brain and Spinal Cord.

MIDBRAIN
Receives impulses from Retina and Ear. Serves as a centre for Visual and Auditory Reflexes. In the Grey Matter are nerve cell bodies of III, IV Cranial nerves and the Red Nucleus which helps to control skilled muscular movements. The White Matter carries nerve fibres linking Red Nucleus with Cerebral Cortex, Thalamus, Cerebellum, Corpus Striatum and Spinal Cord. It also carries Ascending Sensory fibres in Lateral and Medial Lemnisci, and Descending Motor fibres on their way to Pons and Spinal Cord.

HINDBRAIN:
[PONS, CEREBELLUM, MEDULLA OBLONGATA]

Pons: Groups of Neurones form sensory nucleus of V and also nuclei of VI and VII Cranial nerves. Other nerve cells here relay impulses along their axons to Cerebellum and Cerebrum. Rubrospinal tract, Lateral and Medial Lemnisci pass through Pons and nerve fibres linking Cerebral Cortex with Medulla Oblongata and Spinal Cord.

Medulla Oblongata:
Groups of Neurones form Nuclei of VIII, IX, X, XI, XII Cranial nerves. Gracile and Cuneate Nuclei -second sensory neurones in cutaneous pathways. Tracts of Sensory fibres decussate and ascend to other side of Cerebral Cortex. Some fibres remain uncrossed. The larger part of each Motor pyramidal tract crosses and descends in other side of Spinal Cord.

Figure 12-8
Vertical brain section. (From McNaught & Callander, *Illustrated Physiology*. Used by permission of Churchill Livingstone.)

CORONAL SECTION through BRAIN

This is a section through the TRANSVERSE (CENTRAL) FISSURE.
It shows each of the major developments of the BRAIN –

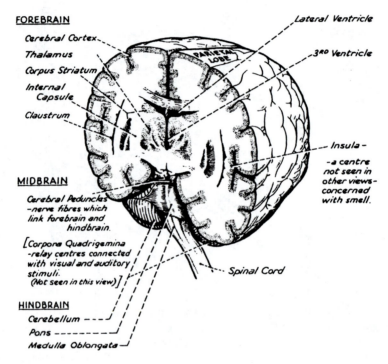

Figure 12-9
Coronal brain section. (From McNaught & Callander, *Illustrated Physiology.* Used by permission
of Churchill Livingstone.)

take no action to correct your position until the drift becomes appreciable (2 ft). You then apply a force opposite in direction to that which caused the drift until a center of the lane position is obtained. This constitutes *negative feedback* from a macroscopic point of view and allows you to maintain a relatively smooth path down a winding road. Of course, each person has a different perception threshold (ability to sense appreciable drift), but we do manage (most of the time) to speed smoothly past each other at speeds of 10 to 70 mph. If this integrated brain-muscle action were

not present, you would travel down the road in short, jerky paths, using much more muscle energy.

12-5-3 Cerebrum

The *cerebrum* (Figure 12-6) is the largest part of the brain in humans and acts as a nerve impulse processor as well as a memory bank and controller of voluntary motor actions. A *longitudinal fissure* (a groove or natural division) divides the cerebrum into lateral halves or *hemispheres.* Each hemisphere is further subdivided by other fissures. The surface area of the brain is large because of the many folds of the cerebrum.

The outer layer of the cerebrum forms the *cerebral cortex* and is composed of gray matter. Approximately 90% of all nerve cells are in this cortex. Inner portions of the brain are comprised of white matter.

John Von Neumann[‡] (mid–twentieth-century mathematician—Von Neumann Computer Architecture) had calculated that in a 60-year lifetime a human would store about 2.8×10^{20} bits of information in the nearly 10 billion neurons found in the cerebrum. The conclusion of this grand computer-type model of the brain reveals that every neuron must have a memory capacity equivalent to 30 billion off-on switches. This seems inconsistent with the (early) idea that one neuron stores only one bit of data. But recent evidence indicates that neuronal activity does increase the amount of ribonucleic acid. Although a firm conclusion is not yet available, Von Neumann might have been correct in his estimation of the mechanism of human memory, and this is only a fraction (one-third) of the total brain capability. Humans do seem, however, to be more than just learning machines or computers.

The structure of the cerebrum is typically divided into the following two *lobes* (two each, one on each side) that are named for the bones they lie beneath: frontal, temporal, parietal, and occipital. These areas of the brain are, in part, concerned with the sensation of sight, sound, smell, taste, and touch.

Frontal lobes contain motor neurons that control certain body muscles. Within the lobe on the left side, speech action is initiated. Figure 12-10 shows the *motor homunculus* (little man), which indicates the proportions of the brain designated to

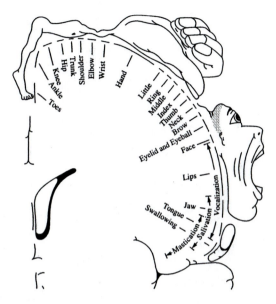

Figure 12-10
Motor locations in the cortex. (From *Human Anatomy and Physiology*, 2nd edition, by James E. Crouch, Ph.D. and J. Robert McClintic, Ph.D. John Wiley & Sons, New York, 1976. Used by permission.)

control various motor actions. Notice that a large portion of the frontal lobe is dedicated to the face, especially the lips and tongue. This accounts for human speech development. The speech center is much less predominant in most animals. Figure 12-11 shows the *sensory homunculus.*

The *prefrontal lobes* are most likely related to mental processes, such as intelligence, memory, judgment, imagination, and creative and conscious thought. Disease of these areas, such as anoxia (lack of oxygen) at birth, can lead to mental retardation or even behavioral disorders.

Temporal lobes house the auditory sensory areas above the ears. High-frequency auditory sensation seems to occur in the temporal areas closest to the frontal lobes. These lobes are also concerned with learning and memory of visual and auditory images. Damage to these areas can result in epilepsy, with severe behavioral disorders and aggressive outbursts. Even the loud, excitable, noisy child (*hyperkinetic syndrome*) may have brain

---

[‡]Before the age of 25, Von Neumann wrote *The Theory of Games and Economic Behavior,* which characterized the theoretical precise steps and outcomes of games such as poker. He also wrote *The Computer and the Brain* (1956), in which he described the brain as having a language that involves specific activities that are related.

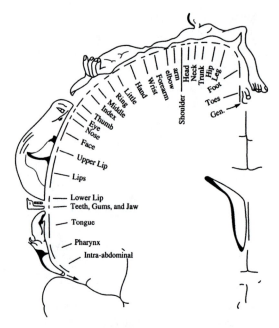

Figure 12-11
Sensory locations in the cortex. (From *Human Anatomy and Physiology*, 2nd edition, by James E. Crouch, Ph.D. and J. Robert McClintic, Ph.D. John Wiley & Sons, New York, 1976. Used by permission.)

damage. Although brain and nervous tissue will not regenerate once damaged, other nearby portions may take over the intended functions.

Minimal cerebral dysfunction (minimal brain dysfunction) has been recognized in recent years as a very subtle cerebral palsy. Mild frontal and temporal lobe damage might be more widespread than previously anticipated.

The *parietal lobes* facilitate the interpretation of size, shape, texture, and other qualities of touch. As seen in Figure 12-11, large sensory areas are devoted to the head, especially the lips, face, and tongue. Greater motor brain area is devoted to thumb movement than to thumb sensation.

The *occipital lobes* at the back of the head contain the visual cortex. This region of the brain receives impulses from the eyes by way of optic nerves. The left eye is controlled by the right occipital cortex and the right eye by the left. The

nerve impulses cross over in the brain through the *optic chiasma* (common crossing point). In fact, much of the left half of the body is controlled by the right brain, and vice versa.

The senses of *smell* and *taste* do not have specific cerebral areas associated with them, although the *olfactory bulb* (smell) is near the center of the brain.

Association areas are those areas of the cerebrum from which specific motor responses or sensations cannot be elicited when stimulated (link of many sensations). Internal brain communication occurs across bands of tissues (corpus collosum, fornix, and commissures seen in Figures 12-7 and 12-8).

The cerebrum also contains four major ventricles, through which *cerebrospinal fluid* (CSF) circulates, which is similar to blood plasma but contains no clotting agents. Three major functions for this fluid are known: protective covering against physical shock, constant cranial fluid volume regulation, and exchange of metabolic substances to nerve cells. CSF circulation occurs because of the forces of *hydrostatic pressure*. Internal hemorrhaging (bleeding) near the brain or nervous system can be detected by withdrawing a sample of CSF from the vertebral column (called a *spinal tap*). No red blood cells should appear in the CSF.

Blood circulation is another circulatory system in the brain. Arterial blood is pumped to the head and brain via the *common carotid artery*. Venous blood is returned to the superior vena cava of the heart through the *jugular vein*.

The brain is covered by three major *membranes (meninges)*. The meninges protect and transfer CSF. The common term for inflammation of these membranes is *meningitis*.

Cranial nerves supply the head, neck, and most of the viscera. The 12 pairs of nerves arise directly from the undersurface of the brain, as shown in Figure 12-12. *Sensory* and *motor* nerves are evident.

The *spinal cord* can be described as a long column of nervous tissue. The cord is protected within the bony *spinal column*. All nerves to the trunk and limbs arise from the spinal cord, which

Twelve pairs of nerves arise directly from the undersurface of the Brain to supply Head and Neck and most of the viscera.

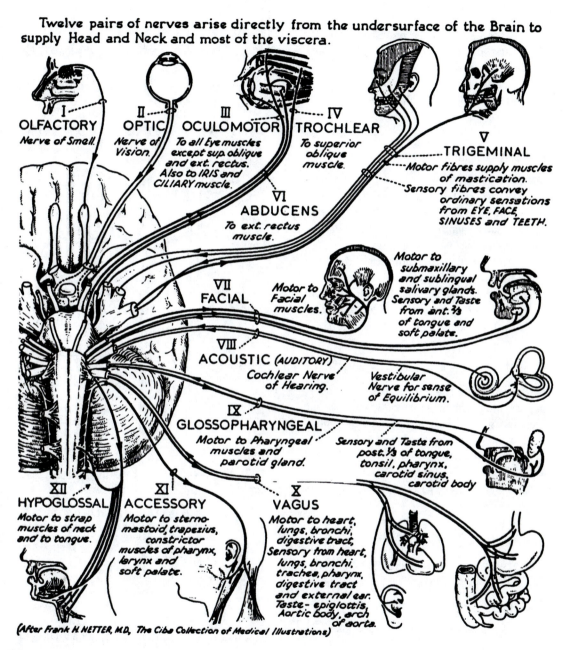

I OLFACTORY
Nerve of Smell.

II OPTIC
Nerve of Vision.

III OCULOMOTOR
To all Eye muscles except sup. oblique and ext. rectus. Also to IRIS and CILIARY muscle.

IV TROCHLEAR
To superior oblique muscle.

V TRIGEMINAL
Motor fibres supply muscles of mastication.
Sensory fibres convey ordinary sensations from EYE, FACE, SINUSES and TEETH.

VI ABDUCENS
To ext. rectus muscle.

VII FACIAL
Motor to Facial muscles.
Motor to submaxillary and sublingual salivary glands. Sensory and Taste from ant. ⅓ of tongue and soft palate.

VIII ACOUSTIC (AUDITORY)
Cochlear Nerve of Hearing.
Vestibular Nerve for sense of Equilibrium.

IX GLOSSOPHARYNGEAL
Motor to Pharyngeal muscles and parotid gland.
Sensory and Taste from post. ⅓ of tongue, tonsil, pharynx, carotid sinus, carotid body

XII HYPOGLOSSAL
Motor to strap muscles of neck and to tongue.

XI ACCESSORY
Motor to sterno-mastoid, trapezius, constrictor muscles of pharynx, larynx and soft palate.

X VAGUS
Motor to heart, lungs, bronchi, digestive tract, Sensory from heart, lungs, bronchi, trachea, pharynx, digestive tract and external ear. Taste- epiglottis, Aortic body, arch of aorta.

(After Frank H. NETTER, M.D., The Ciba Collection of Medical Illustrations)

Figure 12-12
Cranial nerves. (From McNaught & Callander, *Illustrated Physiology.* Used by permission of Churchill Livingstone.)

is the center of reflex action containing the conductive paths to and from the brain. It is bathed in CSF, which also circulates through the brain. Figure 12-13 shows the spinal cord and vertebral canal. Notice the five general divisions with 31 pairs of spinal nerves (cervical, thoracic, lumbar, sacral, and coccygeal).

12-6 Peripheral nervous system

The PNS (which functions away from the brain) includes the *craniosacral nerves* or *spinal nerves;* the organs of special sense, or body, skin, and muscle receptors; and the sympathetic nervous system or stimulatory nerve responses.

This system acts on the extremities of the body to control muscles that permit mobility.

All of the nerves that branch from the CNS and link to the body are either *motor* (efferent) or *sensory* (afferent), or a combination of the two.

12-7 Autonomic nervous system

The ANS is typically classified as part of the PNS. It supplies motor fibers to smooth and cardiac muscles and glands, functioning "automatically" at the reflex and subconscious levels to keep basic body systems operating (e.g., heart rate and breathing). Figure 12-14 shows the ANS, including *sympathetic* (stimulatory) and *parasympathetic* (inhibitory) areas.

12-7-1 Dynamic equilibrium

Equilibrium of the following bodily functions is obtained through the ANS:

1. Heart function—rate and volume output.

2. Blood pressure—arteriovenous vessel size.

3. Blood sugar—regulation of liver action.

4. Digestion—regulation of gastric secretions.

5. Growth—hormone secretion through the endocrine system.

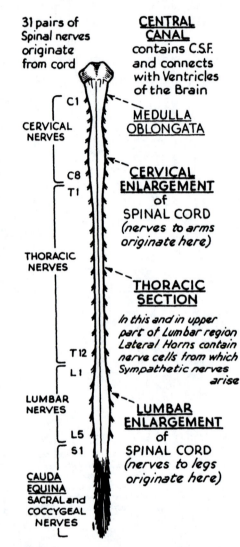

The SPINAL CORD lies within the Vertebral Canal. It is continuous above with the Medulla Oblongata.

31 pairs of Spinal nerves originate from cord

CENTRAL CANAL contains C.S.F. and connects with Ventricles of the Brain

C1

CERVICAL NERVES

MEDULLA OBLONGATA

C8

T1

CERVICAL ENLARGEMENT of SPINAL CORD (*nerves to arms originate here*)

THORACIC NERVES

THORACIC SECTION

In this and in upper part of Lumbar region Lateral Horns contain nerve cells from which Sympathetic nerves arise

T12

L1

LUMBAR NERVES

L5

S1

LUMBAR ENLARGEMENT of SPINAL CORD (*nerves to legs originate here*)

CAUDA EQUINA SACRAL and COCCYGEAL NERVES

The spinal nerves travel to all parts of the trunk and limbs.

Figure 12-13
Spinal cord. (From McNaught & Callander, *Illustrated Physiology.* Used by permission of Churchill Livingstone.)

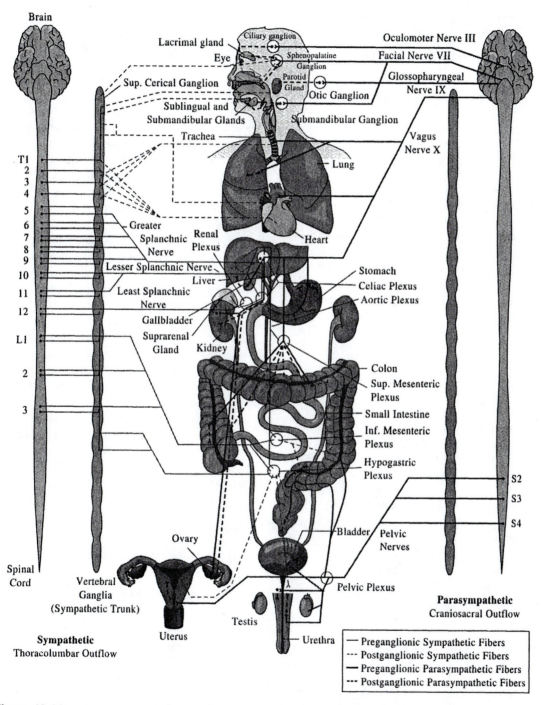

Figure 12-14
Autonomic nervous system. (From *Dorland's Illustrated Medical Dictionary*, 25th edition, W.B. Saunders Co., Philadelphia, 1974.)

363

6. Body temperature—sweat glands.

7. Body fluid balance—sweat and kidney functions.

8. Emotional reactions—endocrine system and the brain.

12-7-2 Sympathetic nervous system

This system is formed by thoracic and lumbar nerve outflows. Body resources are made more available through stimulation by this system. Visceral functions are involved. For example, a massive sympathetic discharge is associated with the liberation of *epinephrine (adrenalin)* from the adrenal glands (on top of the renal glands or kidneys). This increases heart rate and skeletal muscle movements that characterize the "fight-or-flight" state.

12-7-3 Parasympathetic nervous system

This system arises from cranial motor nerve outflows from the brain stem and spinal nerves. During sleep, this system acts to slow the heart rate down to conserve energy.

The *master tissues* (nervous system) control the *vegetative systems* (e.g., respiration, digestion, growth, repair, reproduction, and others). Essentially, body control mechanisms originate and are communicated through *nerve impulse* transmission and reception or through *hormonal secretions.* Thus, the body is a conglomerate of *electrochemical* and *biochemical* activity.

12-8 Behavior and the nervous system

The most sophisticated computer system or machine that humans have ever built has but a fraction of the complexity of the human brain. The hereditary carrier, *deoxyribonucleic acid (DNA),*

within a cell's nucleus, stores an extensive amount of information concerning structure and function. The most complex organ in the body, the brain, is still greatly uncharted in terms of function, although its structure has been identified.

Linking human brain activity and behavior is uncertain. We do know, however, that human behavior is *adaptive,* and this trait seems to be controlled by the *prefrontal lobes.* The electrical activity of the brain (recorded as EEG tracings) changes during sleep and other forms of behavior but is difficult to relate to specific patterns of behavior.

The process of *memory* appears to involve three mechanisms: (1) *momentary retention* (recall of a phone number long enough to dial it), (2) *short-term memory* of events occurring minutes to hours before (classroom lecture), and (3) *long-term memory* of events occurring in the past (e.g., childhood joys, successes, sorrows, failures, and horrors). Most of our memory bank is hidden from us in the *subconscious.* Nevertheless, stimulation of areas within the *temporal lobes* evokes recall of long-past experiences.

As we will see in chapter 13, EEG waveforms can easily be obtained from the EEG machine. The biomedical equipment technology is well developed, even if the interpretation of the recording is not.

12-9 Summary

1. The nervous system is the *most complex* system in the body.

2. The major divisions of the nervous system distinguished by *anatomy* (structure and location) and *physiology* (function) are the *central nervous system* (brain and spinal cord), *peripheral nervous system* (periphery or extremities), *somatic system* (body sensory and motor areas), and *autonomic nervous system* (sympathetic stimulatory), and *parasympathetic* (inhibitory nervous systems).

3. The *neuron* (a single nerve cell) is the fundamental unit of the nervous system. It consists of a cell body *(soma),* several short "input" projections *(dendrites),* and a long propagation "output" channel *(axon).*

4. Neurons may be connected one to one, one to many, many to one, or many to many. These combinations may form *afferent nerves* (sensory, toward the brain) and *efferent nerves* (motor, away from the brain). The multiconnection off/on action is similar to that of digital logic circuits (AND/OR).

5. *Reflex arc action* is an involuntary response caused by stimulation of an afferent nerve ending or receptor. The knee jerk in response to the tap of a hammer is one example.

6. The *central nervous system* is composed of the *brain* (soft mass of nerve tissue within the skull) and *brain stem* (long column of nervous tissue).

7. The *cerebellum* is the second largest part of the brain and integrates incoming sensory messages to provide smooth body muscle movements, balance, and equilibrium *(proprioception).* It acts below the level of consciousness to control such functions as *breathing* through *negative feedback loops.*

8. The *cerebrum* is the largest part of the brain and acts as a nerve impulse processor as well as a memory bank and controller of voluntary motor actions. The *longitudinal fissure* separates the cerebrum into two hemispheres. The *cerebral cortex* is composed of *gray matter.* Inner portions consist of *white matter.* Four pairs of lobes are noticeable in the cerebrum:
   a. *Frontal lobes* (voluntary movements, intelligence, memory, thought).
   b. *Temporal lobes* (auditory and visual sensation, learning, memory).
   c. *Parietal lobes* (touch; object size, shape, and texture sensation; thumb).

d. *Occipital lobes* (visual sensation, crossover in optic chiasma).

9. The CSF circulatory system operates on hydrostatic pressure, and the CSF circulates between the cerebrum and spinal cord (vertebral column).

10. Blood circulates to the brain via the *common carotid artery* (arterial flow) and from the brain via the *jugular vein* (venous flow).

11. The *peripheral nervous system* includes nerves that supply the extremities of the body.

12. The *autonomic nervous system* includes nerves that supply motor fibers, smooth and cardiac muscles, and glands. It functions automatically at the reflex and subconscious levels to keep basic body systems operating. The *sympathetic* (stimulatory) and *parasympathetic* (inhibitory) nervous systems function as antagonists to regulate these body systems.

13. The body is composed of *master tissues* (nervous system) and *vegetative systems* (respiration, digestion, growth, repair, reproduction, and others).

14. *Human behavior* and *brain activity* are difficult to relate.

15. Electrical activity of the brain can be measured and recorded on EEG machines. The biomedical equipment technology for EEG measurement is well developed.

12-10 Recapitulation

Now return to the objectives and self-evaluation questions at the beginning of the chapter and see how well you can answer them. If you cannot answer certain questions, place a check next to each and review appropriate parts of the text. Next, try to answer the following questions using the same procedure. When you have answered all of the questions, solve the problems.

Questions

1. The most complex system in the body is the _____ _____.

2. The major divisions of the nervous system are the central nervous system, the _____ _____ _____, and the _____ _____ _____.

3. The CNS consists of _____ and _____ _____.

4. The neuron is composed of a soma, many _____, and an _____, and has a nerve impulse traveling in _____ direction.

5. A synapse is a _____ between neurons across which electrochemical substances pass.

6. Afferent nerves carry nerve impulses *to* or *away from* the brain.

7. Efferent nerves carry nerve impulses *to* or *away from* the brain.

8. A reflex arc is an _____ action caused by stimulation of an afferent nerve ending.

9. The CNS is composed of the _____ and _____.

10. The medulla acts to _____ control basic physiological systems such as _____ _____ and _____.

11. The cerebellum (cortex and medulla) provides the body with smooth _____ _____ and balance or _____.

12. Biological and physiological negative feedback loops act to *increase* or *decrease* the output when an *increase* or *decrease* in the input occurs.

13. Four lobes make up the _____ according to the _____ structures they lie beneath.

14. Frontal lobes control voluntary _____, _____, and _____.

15. Temporal lobes control _____ sensation and _____.

16. Parietal lobes control the qualities of _____.

17. Occipital lobes control _____ sensation.

18. CSF circulates through _____ in the brain and functions to provide the brain with _____, constant _____ _____ _____, and exchange of _____.

19. Blood circulates through the brain via the _____ _____ artery and returns through the _____ vein.

20. Meningitis refers to _____ of brain membranes.

21. The PNS consists partly of _____ nerves.

22. The ANS consists of the _____ or stimulatory and _____ or inhibitory nervous systems.

23. Dynamic body function equilibrium control through the ANS involves _____ rate, _____ pressure, _____ sugar, _____ temperature, and _____ reactions, among others.

24. Modern understanding of the brain *does* or *does not* include knowledge of which brain areas control which body sensory and motor functions.

25. Electroencephalography refers to _____ activity of the brain.

26. EEG patterns change with the behavior of _____.

27. Visual or auditory sensory stimulation *does* or *does not* change the EEG pattern.

Problems

The human nervous system is more complex than any invented device.

1. **a.** Some scientists, including John Von Neumann, have estimated that the human brain has *10 billion neurons,* each capable of storing 30 billion bits of data (one bit equals one

off-on switch) over a *60-year lifetime.* From this postulated information, *how many total bits* of data can the human store in an average lifetime?

b. Given a large modern electronic computer with 12 computer memory banks (internal and external) each capable of storing *200 million bits* of data, *how many total bits* can the computer store?

c. Approximately (because numbers on the brain are difficult to prove exactly) *how many times more data* can the brain store than the electronic computer?

d. What can you say about the relative physical size of the biological versus the electronic device?

2. **a.** The *human eye* passes nerve impulses to the brain through the optic nerve and cranial nerve II. The band of frequencies passed by the eye range from *red* (0.7 μm wavelength, 4.3×10^{14} Hz) to *violet* (0.4 μm wavelength, 7.5×10^{14} Hz). *What is the approximate bandwidth* of the *human visual system?*

b. Commercial VHF and UHF electronic television operates on frequencies (granted by the Federal Communications Commission [FCC] that range from *channel 2* (54 MHz) to *channel 83* (890 MHz), neglecting the break in the band between channels 6 and 7 and channels 13 and 14. *What is the approximate bandwidth* of the *television system?*

c. Approximately *how many times wider* is the bandwidth of the *human visual system* than that of the television system?

d. What can you say about the *relative physical* size of the biological versus the electronic device?

Suggested reading

1. Crouch, James E. and Robert J. McClintic, *Human Anatomy and Physiology,* Wiley (New York, 1976).

2. Guyton, Arthur C., *Textbook of Medical Physiology,* W. B. Saunders Co. (Philadelphia, 1976).

3. McNaught, Ann B. and Robin Callander, *Illustrated Physiology,* Churchill Livingstone (Edinburgh/London/New York, 1975).

4. Yokochi, Chihiro, *Photographic Anatomy of the Human Body,* University Park Press (Baltimore/London, 1971).

5. Smith, C. U. M., *The Brain—Towards Understanding,* G. P. Putnam's Sons (New York, 1970).

6. Chusid, Joseph G. and Joseph J. McDonald, *Correlative Neuroanatomy and Functional Neurology,* Lange Medical Publications (Los Altos, Calif., 1967).

7. Karczmar, A. G. and J. C. Eccles, *Brain and Human Behavior,* Springer-Verlag (New York, 1972).

8. Bruch, Neil and H. I. Altshuler, *Behavior and Brain Electrical Activity,* Plenum Press (New York, 1973).

9. Eccles, John, *The Understanding of the Brain,* McGraw-Hill (New York, 1973).

10. Khanna, J. L., *Brain Damage and Mental Retardation—A Psychological Evaluation,* Charles C. Thomas (Springfield, Ill., 1973).

11. Walton, John N. and Lord Brain, *Brain's Diseases of the Nervous System* (1933-1977), Oxford University Press (New York, 1977).

12. Avers, Charlotte, *Evolution,* Douglass College, Rutgers University, Harper and Row (New York, 1974).

13. Saparina, Y., *Cybernetics Within Us,* Wilshire Book Co. (Calif., 1967). Foreword by Maxwell Maltz, author of *Psycho-Cybernetics).*

14. Bronowski, Jacob, *The Ascent of Man,* Little, Brown (Boston, 1973).

15. Cooper, R. J. W. Osselton, and J. C. Shaw, *EEG Technology,* Butterworth (London, England, 1974).

16. Strong, Peter, *Biophysical Measurements,* Tektronix, Inc. (Beaverton, Ore., 1970/1973).

17. Bachrach, Henry and Jim Mixtz, "The Wechsler Scale as a Tool for the Detection of Mild Cerebral Dysfunction," *J. Clinical Psychology, 30* (1):58-61 (January 1974).

18. Kaufman, Nadeen L. and Alan S. Kaufman, "Comparison of Normal and Minimally Brain Dysfunctioned Children on the McCarthy Scales of Children's Abilities (MSCA)," *J. Clinical Psychology, 30* (1):69-72 (January 1974).

CHAPTER 13
Instrumentation for Measuring Brain Function

13-1 Objectives

1. Be able to describe biomedical instrumentation for measuring anatomical and physiological parameters of the brain.
2. Be able to describe the procedure and equipment used in cerebral angiography, cranial X-rays, and brain scans.
3. Be able to describe the procedure and equipment used in echoencephalography.
4. Be able to describe the procedures and equipment used in electroencephalography (EEG).
5. Be able to describe the origin, cranial location, amplitude, and frequency bands of EEG signals.
6. Be able to describe EEG electrodes and the 10-20 electrode placement system.
7. Be able to describe diagnostic uses of EEG patterns (waking, sleeping, and diseased states).
8. Be able to describe multichannel EEG recording systems, including a simplified block diagram.
9. Be able to list typical external controls on EEG machines.
10. Be able to list typical characteristics of EEG preamplifiers and machine specifications.
11. Be able to describe the setup and equipment used to obtain visual and auditory evoked potential recordings.
12. Be able to describe the setup and equipment used for EEG telemetry.
13. Be able to list typical EEG system artifacts, faults, troubleshooting techniques, and maintenance.

13-2 Self-evaluation questions

These questions test your prior knowledge of the material in this chapter. Look for the answers as you read the text. After you have finished studying the chapter, try answering these questions and those at the end of the chapter.

1. What is the origin of the physiological parameter (EEG signal) measured by the EEG machine?

2. Give the frequency bands usually specified for EEG signals.

3. What is meant by the 10-20 EEG electrode placement system? Describe it.

4. Name five common EEG machine malfunctions.

13-3 Instrumentation for measuring anatomical and physiological parameters of the brain

Instrumentation used to measure *anatomical* (structure) and *physiological* (function) parameters of the brain includes X-ray equipment, ultrasonic equipment, and electrophysiological equipment.

X-ray equipment transmits high-energy electromagnetic (light) waves (0.05-100 Å) that pass through the body and indicate relative tissue density on a photographic plate. X-ray brain measurements include cerebral angiography, cranial X-rays, and brain scans.

Ultrasonic equipment transmits high-frequency sound waves (1-ms bursts at 2.5 MHz) that pass into the body and indicate tissue location by reflecting waves. This measurement is made by means of *echoencephalography* (echo ranging from the brain).

Electrophysiological equipment detects low-voltage (1 to 100 μV) and low-frequency (0.1 to 100 Hz) bioelectric signals that are *picked up* by electrodes, signal *conditioned* by amplifiers or filters, and *displayed* on graphic recorders or cathode-ray tubes (CRTs). This measurement involves electrical activity produced in the brain measured by means of EEG.

13-4 Cerebral angiography

Cerebral angiography is an X-ray technique used to display brain structures and blood vessels with the aid of a contrast medium. Radiopaque dyes

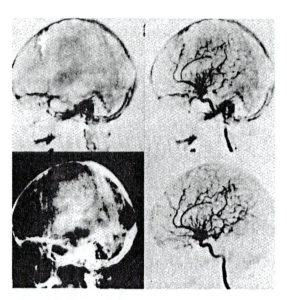

Figure 13-1
Cerebral angiography.

that block X-rays are injected in an artery (e.g., common carotid) and disperse throughout the cerebrovascular tree. X-ray images are taken at 1-s intervals and can reveal blockages or tumors, as shown in Figure 13-1.

Recent techniques in *nuclear medicine* are somewhat different from angiography and considerably safer. Small amounts of short-lived *radioactive isotopes* (e.g., iodine 131 taken up by the thyroid gland) are introduced into the cardiovascular system, accumulating in various organs throughout the body. The concentrated radioactivity is measured with a *scintillation counter* that responds to impinging alpha, beta, or gamma rays, depending on and given off by the radioactive material used. The amount of substance taken up by a specific gland indicates the physiological function of the gland. Since very little radioactive substance is required and its emission life is very short, the danger is minimal.

13-5 Cranial X-rays

Cranial X-ray pictures are simply two-dimensional X-ray exposures taken of the cranium. They may be used to indicate fractures in cranial bones and,

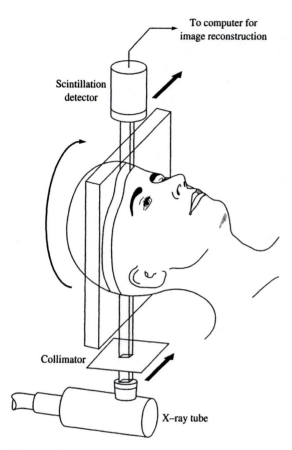

Figure 13-2
Pencil beam multiprojection cerebral scanning. (From *Medicine and Clinical Engineering,* by Bertil Jacobson and John Webster, Prentice Hall, Englewood Cliffs, N.J. 1977. Used by permission.)

on occasion, blood clots or tumors. The problem in cranial diagnosis, as in chest X-ray exposures, is the difficulty in reading (evaluating) the exposure. Only when the contrast is high, indicating relatively large tissue density differences, can positive diagnoses be made. Therefore, in the early 1970s, the practice of X-ray scans became more popular.

13-6 Brain scans

Brain scans are radiographs that are taken through successive scanning by highly collimated X-ray beams. Small-contrast differences in selected planes can be seen on the picture and thus provide considerably more information than simple cranial X-ray exposures.

13-6-1 Computed tomography (CT)

CT scanning is a technique of recording and processing a set of image projections that represent a reconstruction of the object scanned. A *thin layer* of the object is *tomographically* (sectioned) scanned with a pencil beam. The X-ray attenuation is then recorded with a *scintillation counter* in groups of parallel scans. Many-angle X-ray exposures are obtained every degree for 180°, as shown in Figure 13-2. Many projection scans (three-dimensional) are stored in a computer, and, through a complex program, the original object is redrawn (two-dimensional) on a CRT screen by the computer. The CT scanner is, then, capable of producing a tomogram of the skull and brain (Figure 13-3) that shows the ventricles of the brain.

13-6-2 Whole-body scanners

These scanners present views of whole body areas. Such tomographic X-ray results are more costly than regular X-ray patterns. However, they show more detail and resolution and have much higher diagnostic quality. This is especially true for color presentations, in which different colors represent fine differences in tissue density. One such device is the *ACTA* (automatic computerized transaxial) X-ray tomographic scanner developed by Robert

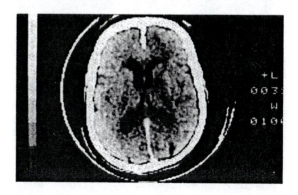

Figure 13-3
Data tomogram of normal skull.

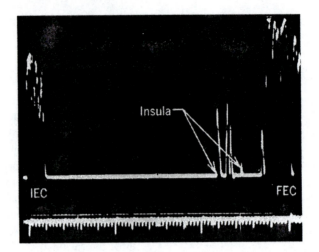

Figure 13-4
Cerebral sonogram reflection from sylvian fissure. IEC, initial echo complex; FEC, far echo complex. (From M. S. Tenner and G. M. Wodraska, *Diagnostic Ultrasound in Neurology: Methods and Techniques,* John Wiley & Sons, New York, 1975. Used by permission.)

S. Ledley and his colleagues at Georgetown University in Washington, D.C.

13-7 Ultrasonic equipment

Diagnostic ultrasonography may prove to be as great a medical discovery as the X-ray and diagnostic radiology. Diagnostic ultrasound is described in detail in chapter 17.

In this chapter, we are concerned with some diagnostic qualities of *echoencephalography* (echo ranging from the brain to reveal abnormal brain structures, such as tumors and dilated brain ventricles). Diagnostic success in such ultrasound neurological examinations depends as much on the operator as the equipment. The principle that underlies diagnostic ultrasound is similar to that of radar and sonar. All ultrasonic equipment emits short bursts of sound at pulse frequencies at or near 2.5 MHz. The sound energy is formed into a beam by a transducer (usually piezoelectric) and directed into the body. The echo received back indicates the distance of the reflecting tissues. The *reflections* are displayed as *peaks versus distance* and show symmetry of brain structures. Asymmetrical peaks may indicate tumors or swellings in the

brain. Figure 13-4 shows a *normal* sonogram with reflected echo from the sylvian fissure (see chapter 12 for brain anatomy). Figure 13-5 shows an abnormal echo resulting from a subarachnoid (second of threebrain meninges) hemorrhage.

13-8 Electroencephalography

EEG is a representation (writing on paper or display on CRT) of the electrical activity of the brain. The technique involves the following:

1. Biopotential pickup—cranial or cerebral surface transducer electrodes.

2. EEG signal conditioning—transducer output amplification and filtering (0.1 to 100 Hz).

3. EEG signal recording—signal displayed on graphic recorder or CRT.

4. EEG signal analysis—visual or computer interpretation of resulting EEG.

The record obtained is called the electroencephalogram.

The *EEG record* obtained in item 3 in the preceding list is used primarily for diagnosis, including the following:

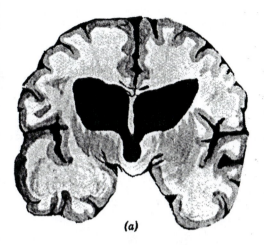

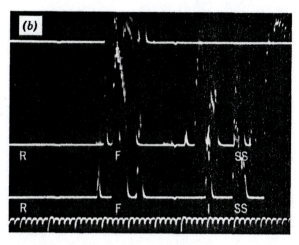

Figure 13-5
Subarachnoid hemorrhage. *(a)* Brain structure. *(b)* Prominent echoes and hemisphere symmetrical reflections indicate an enlarged subarachnoid space (SS). (From M. S. Tenner and G. M. Wodraska, *Diagnostic Ultrasound in Neurology: Methods and Techniques,* John Wiley & Sons, New York, 1975. Used by permission.)

1. Help detect and localize cerebral brain lesions (asymmetry/irregularity in EEG tracings).

2. Aid in studying epilepsy (recurrent, transient attacks of disturbed brain function with irregular sensory and motor activity such as convulsions).

3. Assist in diagnosing mental disorders.

4. Assist in studying sleep patterns.

5. Allow observation and analysis of brain responses to sensory stimuli.

Notice the words *help, aid,* and *assist* in the preceding list. They indicate that the EEG is a *collaborative tool* in diagnosing brain function and disease. Many physicians and neurologists view EEG signals as interesting artifacts but confess that they are not certain of the signal origins. In fact, until recently, EEG waveforms were originally thought to be a summation of action potentials of neurons as they made their way to the cranial surface. Later ideas reflect stimulation associated by diverse neurons.

Modern interpretation of EEG origin rests with knowledge of basic *neuronal electrochemical processes.* The *action potential* (AP) from neurons has been recorded with microelectrodes at the cellular level. Essentially, the synaptic fibers, terminal boutons, neuronal membrane, and axon contribute the distinguishable response characteristics. Electrical reaction of neurons includes the following potentials:

1. *Presynaptic spike potential* (rapid 1-ms positive event resulting from presynaptic depolarization).

2. *Excitatory postsynaptic potential (EPSP)* (prolonged 2-ms graded *positive* potential).

3. *Spike potential* (high-voltage, sudden 2-ms *positive* discharge of 10 to 30 mV).

4. *After hyperpolarization* (prolonged *positive* potential).

5. *Inhibitory postsynaptic potential (IPSP)* (*negative* potential associated with neuronal inhibition).

Figure 13-6 shows the various neuron membrane potentials. Because of the short durations, a high-frequency oscilloscope (500-Hz bandwidth) and

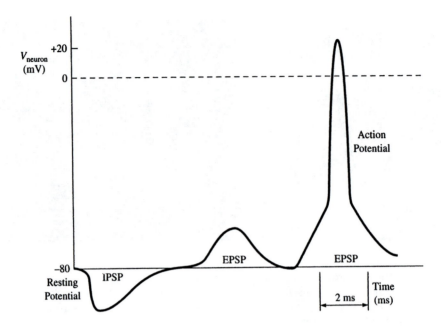

Figure 13-6
Neuron membrane potentials.

Polaroid camera are used in place of chart recorders (150-Hz bandwidth) to display the neuron potentials.

The EEG is composed of *electrical rhythms* and transient discharges which are distinguished by *location, frequency, amplitude, form, periodicity,* and *functional properties. Synchronization* appears in the EEG, and the resulting slow activity is evident. In fact, some EEG investigators have discovered an "EEG pacemaker" located just above the brain stem. Cats have displayed this synchronism from their unanesthetized cerebrum.

EEG measurements from the cranial surface can be considered by the following analogy. Imagine a Martian who visits Earth and lands on the Astrodome during a football game. If this being places a microphone on the Astrodome surface (similar to cranial surface), many sounds are heard (similar to EEG patterns). The complex sound patterns are difficult to interpret on a gross scale. The Martian may hear loud sounds from one side of the dome (cheering) but cannot distinguish their origin. The Martian may also lower a microphone and listen to one person (similar to one neuron), who is selling "hot dogs." Again, this one set of sounds is hardly representative of the entire situation and what is happening in the stadium. EEG signals are, in many respects, just as foreign to us as diverse football game noises might be to an extraterrestrial visitor.

13-9 EEG electrodes and the 10-20 system

EEG electrodes transform ionic currents from cerebral tissue into electrical currents used in EEG preamplifiers. The electrical characteristics are determined primarily by the type of metal used. Silver-silver chloride (Ag-Ag Cl)lis commonly found in electrode discs.

Essentially, five types of electrodes are typically used:

1. *Scalp*—silver pads, discs, or cups; stainless steel rods; and chlorided silver wires.

2. *Sphenoidal*—alternating insulated silver and bare wire and chlorided tip inserted through muscle tissue by a needle.

3. *Nasopharyngeal*—silver rod with silver ball at the tip inserted through the nostrils.

4. *Electrocorticographic*—cotton wicks soaked in saline solution that rests on the brain surface (removes artifacts generated in the cerebrum by each heartbeat).

5. *Intracerebral*—sheaves of Teflon-coated gold or platinum wires cut at various distances from the sheaf tip and used to electrically stimulate the brain.

Reusable scalp disc or cup electrodes (most common in the clinic) are placed on the head using a *conductive cream* (similar consistency to body fluids or electrolytes). The area is first *cleaned* with *alcohol* or *acetone* to remove skin oils. It is good practice (using conductive paste) to lower this contact resistance *below* 10 kΩ to ensure good EEG signal recording. A test of this resistance can be made with a dc ohmmeter, but electrode polarization results after a few seconds. A better approach is to use an *ac ohmmeter*, which applies an ac signal between two electrodes, avoiding polarization.

The amplitude, phase, and frequency of EEG signals depend on electrode *placement*. This placement is based on the frontal, parietal, temporal, and occipital cranial areas described in Section 12-5-3. One of the most popular schemes is the *10-20 EEG electrode placement system* (Figure 13-7) established by the International Federation of EEG Societies. In this setup, the head is mapped by four standard points: the *nasion* (nose), the *inion* (external occipital protuberance or projection), and the *left* and *right* preauricular points (ears). Lead

F_{p1}, for example, is in the frontal area and lies on a circle with other leads. Nineteen electrodes, plus one for grounding the subject, are used. Electrodes are placed (using a flexible tape measure) by measuring the nasion-inion distance and marking points on the (shaved) head *10%, 20%, 20%, 20%,* and *10%* of this length. The *vertex, C_2* electrode is the midpoint. Figure 13-7 shows the complete 10-20 electrode placement system. Here, 19 electrodes are used on the scalp, plus one for grounding the subject.

Electrode arrangements may be either *unipolar* or *bipolar,* as shown in Figure 13-8. A *unipolar arrangement* (Figure 13-8a) is composed of a number of scalp leads connected to a *common indifference point* such as an earlobe. Hence, one electrode is common to all channels. For example, F_{p2} may be measured with respect to two ear electrodes connected together (Figure 13-8a) or summation of scalp electrodes (Figure 13-8b). A *bipolar arrangement* (Figure 13-8c) is achieved by the interconnection of scalp electrodes. The difference of voltage between F_{p2} and F_{p8} may also be measured (Figure 13-8c). *Montages* are patterns of connections between electrodes and recording channels. All of these combinations have inputs to a three-lead differential amplifier and use a third connection for the reference (two ears, forehead, or nose).

13-10 EEG amplitude and frequency bands

EEG signal voltage amplitudes range from about 1 to 100 μV peak-to-peak at low frequencies (0.5 to 100 Hz) at the *cranial* surface. At the surface of the *cerebrum,* signals may be 10 times stronger. Also, brain-stem signals measured at the cranial surface are often no larger than 0.25 μV peak-to-peak (100 to 3000 Hz). In contrast, ECG chest-to-surface signals are about 500 to 100,000 μV peak-to-peak. Weak EEG signals require input preamplifiers (differential type) that have high gain

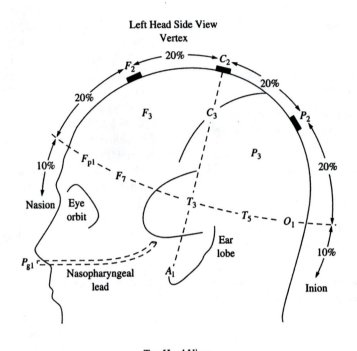

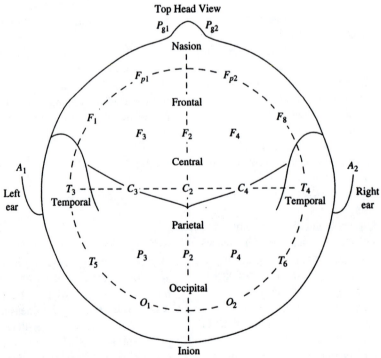

Figure 13-7
The 10-20 EEG electrode placement system.

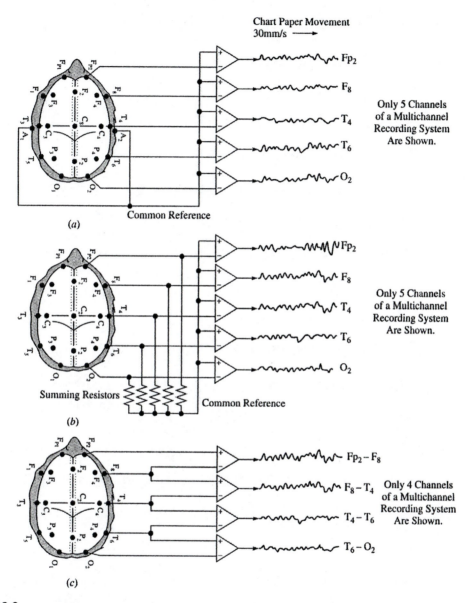

Figure 13-8

EEG recording modes. *(a)* Unipolar. *(b)* Average. *(c)* Bipolar. (Courtesy of Tektronix, Inc. Copyright 1970. All rights reserved.)

and internal or external noise rejection. Typical EEG signals for *wakefulness* and *sleep* in a normal adult are shown in Figure 13-9.

EEG *frequency* bands are normally classified into five categories:

Delta (δ)	0.5-4 Hz
Theta (θ)	4-8 Hz
Alpha (α)	8-13 Hz
Beta (β)	13-22 Hz
Gamma (γ)	22-30 Hz and higher

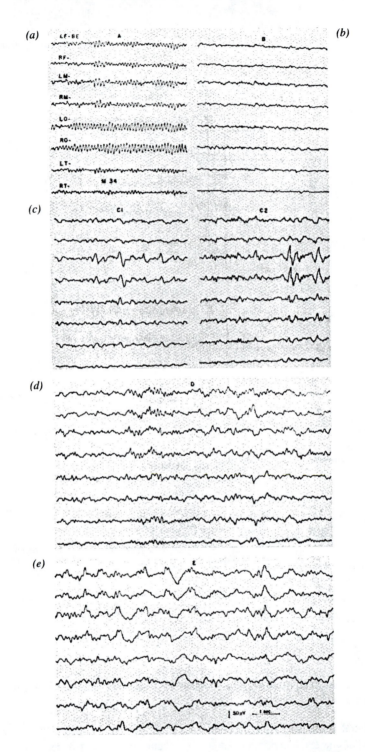

Figure 13-9

EEG patterns. *(a)* Alert state. *(b)* Drowsiness. *(c)* Theta and beta waves. *(d)* Moderately deep sleep. *(e)* Deep sleep. (From *Fundamentals of Electroencephalography,* by Kenneth A. Kooi, M.D., Harper & Row, New York, 1971. Used by permission.)

The meaning of these different frequencies is not completely known. However, *alpha activity* is less than 10 μV peak-to-peak and reasonably stable (deviating less than 0.5 Hz). These signals arise from the posterior brain in the waking person with eyes closed. Opening the eyes and focusing attention greatly reduces alpha waves.

Beta activity is less than 20 μV peak-to-peak over the entire brain but is most predominant over the central region at rest. High states of wakefulness and desynchronized alpha patterns produce beta waves.

Gamma activity is less than 2 μV peak-to-peak and consists of low-amplitude, high-frequency waves that result from attention or sensory stimulation.

Theta and *delta activity* (less than 100 μV peak-to-peak) are strongest over the central region and are indications of sleep. The waveforms in Figure 13-9 represent *adult* EEG patterns; those of infants are almost nonexistent (lack of brain development). Children show increasingly stronger signals as their brain matures (a 12-year-old child has an EEG pattern similar to an adult).

The *frequency spectrum* of the EEG is shown for the normal adult in Figure 13-10. This reveals alpha (10-Hz) and beta (18-Hz) peaks with eyes opened and closed. The usable bandwidth is not much beyond 50 Hz.

13-11 EEG diagnostic uses and sleep patterns

EEG waveforms show remarkable changes just before an *epileptic seizure. Grand mal* seizures are associated with wild, uncontrollable muscle contractions (convulsions) and may be accompanied by coma (unconscious state in which the patient cannot be aroused by external stimuli). Changes in EEG patterns are predominant and usually reflect a large-amplitude, random, low- to high-frequency EEG oscillation, especially near brain motor areas. *Petite mal* seizures are associated with small muscle movements and, occasion-

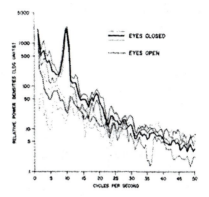

Figure 13-10
EEG frequency spectrum of normal adult. (From *Fundamentals of Electroencephalography,* by Kenneth A. Kooi, M.D., Harper & Row, New York, 1971. Used by permission.)

ally, temporary loss of consciousness. Some symptoms in young children involve simply a few moments staring into space (hardly noticeable). Evoked cerebral potentials to visual or auditory stimuli are also useful in diagnosing brain disorders (section 13-15).

EEG sleep patterns show dramatic changes to the five *stages of sleep,* as shown in Figure 13-9. These are *drowsiness, light sleep, moderately deep sleep, deep sleep,* and *rapid eye movement (REM)* sleep, which usually follows deep sleep. Notice the progressively higher amplitude and lower frequency as sleep occurs. EEG changes are also apparent in patients with sleep disorders, such as *insomnia* (most prevalent complaint: lack of adequate sleep), *narcolepsy* (recurring, uncontrollable sleep episodes), *chronic hypersomnia* (excessive sleep or sleepiness), *sleep paralysis* (characterized by an inability to move during apparent full consciousness), and *nightmares* (night terrors revealed by sudden scream and arousal).

EEG pattern changes are also present with changes in behavior. Examples are relative depressions of EEG peaks in *alcoholics,* sporadic runs of slow waves in *drug addicts,* and depth EEG abnormalities in those who display *violence and aggression* (more conclusive studies are under investigation).

13-12 Multichannel EEG recording systems and typical external controls

Clinical EEG machines typically consist of 8, 16, or 32 channels, as shown in Figures 13-11 and 13-12. *Eight-channel* devices are most common and record eight switch-selectable signals from the 20 cranial electrodes (10-20 system). The older EEG machine (Figure 13-11) is rather large but tends to be very reliable. Newer solid-state EEG devices have very stable circuitry; their weakest section is often the ink-pen graphic display.

A large selector-switch box usually accompanies the EEG machine proper. These switches allow the selection of particular *montages* (specific electrodes connected to EEG input amplifiers for eventual graphic display). The International Federation of EEG Societies suggests the following guidelines for setting up montages:

1. Recording channels should be connected, in sequence, to rows of electrodes along the anteroposterior or traverse lines of the head.

2. The sequences should run from the front to the back of the head and from right to left.

3. For bipolar recordings, channels should be connected so that the black lead of an amplifier (grid 1—right side of head near nose) is anterior to or to the right of the white lead (grid 2—right side of head near ear).

The *EEG technician,* psychologist, physiologist, researcher, or physician selects these montages to obtain desired recordings. The biomedical equipment technician (BMET) sometimes encounters

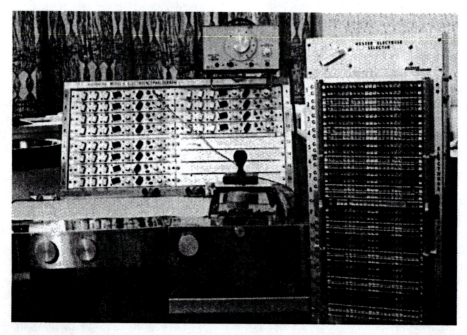

Figure 13-11
EEG machine (vacuum-tube type).

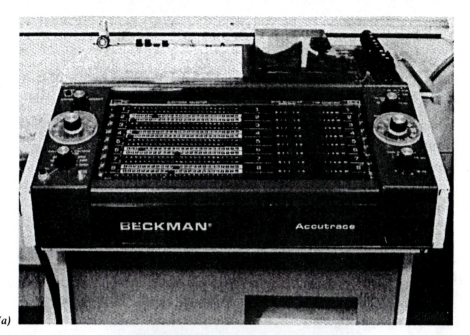

(a)

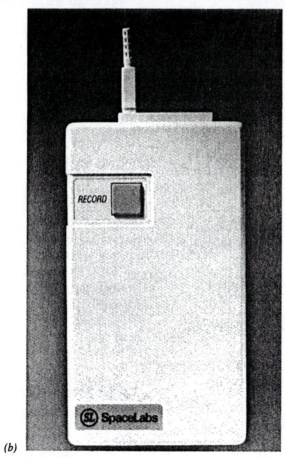

(b)

Figure 13-12
EEG machine (solid-state type).

381

switch problems, which can be solved using an ohmmeter or by viewing problems in the EEG recording.

External controls on EEG machines usually include the following (Figures 13-11 and 13-12):

1. Gain or sensitivity multiplier switch—selects sensitivity ranges, usually ×20, ×4, ×1, ×500, and ×250.

2. Gain control or sensitivity potentiometer—sets the overall system gain (must be high enough to give good pen deflection but not high enough to clip EEG peaks). It is useful to plot gain in μV/cm for specific machines, because most EEGs have all-channel master control and individual channel control.

3. Low-frequency (time constant) filter attenuator or high-pass filter switch—selects low-frequency cutoff, usually 0.16, 0.53, 1.0, and 5.3 Hz.

4. High-frequency filter attenuator or low-pass filter switch—selects high-frequency cutoff, usually 15, 35, 50, 70, and 100 Hz.

5. Sixty-hertz notch filter switch—connects or removes 60-Hz filtering (reduces 60 ± 0.5 Hz by -60 dB typically but does cause some signal phase distortion).

6. Calibration push button—sets 5 to 1000 μV peak-to-peak for rectangular-wave calibration pen deflection.

7. Baseline (position) potentiometer—sets graphic display baseline.

8. Individual electrode selection switches—selects specific electrodes.

9. Event marker push button—places a graphic display mark to identify desired events.

10. Chart speed switch—selects speed of graphic display chart paper, usually 10, 15, 30, and 60 mm/s.

13-13 The EEG system: Simplified block diagram

System operation can be understood by studying a *simplified block diagram*. For specific EEGs, detailed manufacturer's block diagrams and schematics must be consulted. If a block is not available, an industrious investigator could draw one from observation of the schematics. Figure 13-13 shows a simplified block diagram for an EEG. Twenty electrodes are placed on the patient's scalp, and these are switch-selected to the input of eight differential preamplifiers (differential input, single-ended output). The eight outputs are further amplified and presented to eight driver or power amplifiers that supply sufficient current to drive the pen deflectors. A calibration signal, usually in the form of a pulse, is generated by a separate circuit and applied to the *diff-amp inputs*. It is advantageous to connect the calibration signal to the electrode switch selector box to check the system operation. *Calibration signal amplitude* gives an indication of correct sensitivity settings. If the reading is not within specifications, the amplifier system must be adjusted. *Calibration signal waveform* gives an indication of frequency response. As with the ECG machine, *pulse ringing* will occur when underdamping exists, and *rounded pulse corners* will be evident when overdamping occurs.

The low-voltage power supply (Figure 13-13) design and operation is very important in EEG systems because the low-level input signals (as small as 5 μV peak-to-peak), can easily pick up extraneous 60-Hz internal as well as external noise.

EEG output signals can be digitized in an analog-to-digital converter and then analyzed in a digital analyzer (computer) or stored on digital magnetic tape.

13-14 Preamplifiers and EEG system specifications

EEG preamplifiers are perhaps the most important link in the EEG system. They are usually differ-

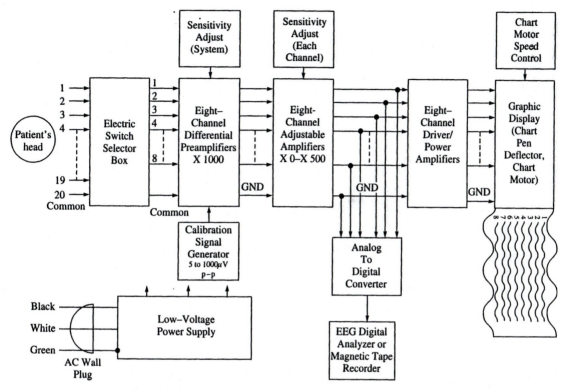

Figure 13-13
Simplified block diagram of an eight-channel EEG system.

ential amplifiers and have the following characteristics: low internal noise, high gain (X 5k-X 10k), high common-mode rejection ratio (CMRR of 100 dB), low-frequency ac-coupled operation (1 Hz and below), low dc drift, and high input impedance (10 mΩ and above). Figure 13-14*a* shows single-ended input and differential input amplifier diagrams. The single-ended amplifier simply provides a ground for one scalp electrode and uses the other as an active site. The current resulting from the "cranial voltage source" is as follows:

$$i = \frac{e}{r + R_1 + R_2 + R_{in}}$$ (13-3)

where

- *e* is the cranial voltage source acting through cranial impedance, *r*

- R_1 and R_2 represent equivalent electrode scalp resistance

- R_{in} is the input impedance of the electronic amplifier

Example 13-2

Given the cranial generator voltage (*e*) to be 100 μV_{p-p}, impedance (*r*) to be 10 kΩ, the equivalent electrode-scalp resistances (R_1 and R_2) to be 10 kΩ each, and the amplifier input impedance (R_{in}) to be 10 MΩ, calculate the amplifier input voltage ($e_{amp_{in}}$) (refer to Figure 13-14*a*).

384   CHAPTER 13

Solution

$$i = \frac{e}{r + R_1 + R_2 + R_{in}}$$

$$= \frac{100\ \mu V_{p-p}}{10\ k\Omega + 10\ k\Omega + 10\ k\Omega + 10\ M\Omega}$$

$$i = \frac{100\ \mu V_{p-p}}{10.03\ M\Omega} = 10 \times 10^{-12} a_{p-p}$$

$$e_{amp_{in}} = iR_{in} = 10 \times 10^{-12} a_{p-p} \times 10\ M\Omega$$

$$e_{amp_{in}} = \mathbf{100\ \mu V_{p-p}}$$

The amplifier input voltage is calculated as:

$$e_{amp_{in}} = iR_{in} = \frac{eR_{in}}{r + R_1 + R_2 + R_{in}}$$

$$= \frac{e}{1 + (r + R_1 + R_2)/R_{in}} \quad (13\text{-}4)$$

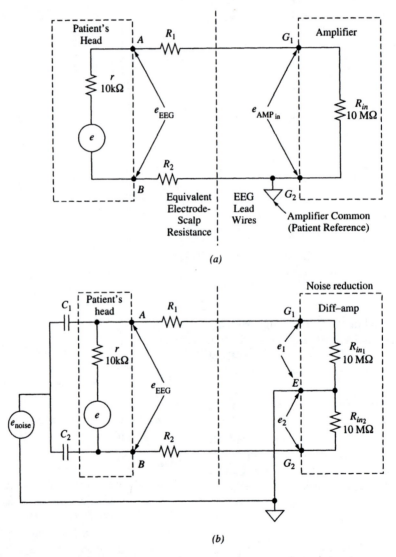

(a)

(b)

Figure 13-14
EEG amplifiers. *(a)* EEG input circuit—single-ended. *(b)* EEG input circuit—differential amplifier.

When $(r + R_1 + R_2)/R_{in}$ in Example 13-2 is small, $e_{amp_{in}}$ nearly equals e_{EEG}. That is, when R_{in} is large compared to $(r + R_1 + R_2)$, say 100 times greater, the amplifier receives the *cranial-generated* EEG signal. That is one reason EEG preamplifiers have such high input impedance: to avoid signal attenuation (and also reduce possible shock hazard). Fig-

ure 13-15a shows one such amplifier. This circuit (single-ended input operational amplifier) has one serious disadvantage. It will amplify noise voltages induced from lights or power equipment by the same amount as the signal. If the noise amplitude is larger than the EEG signal, the EEG recordings will be obscured.

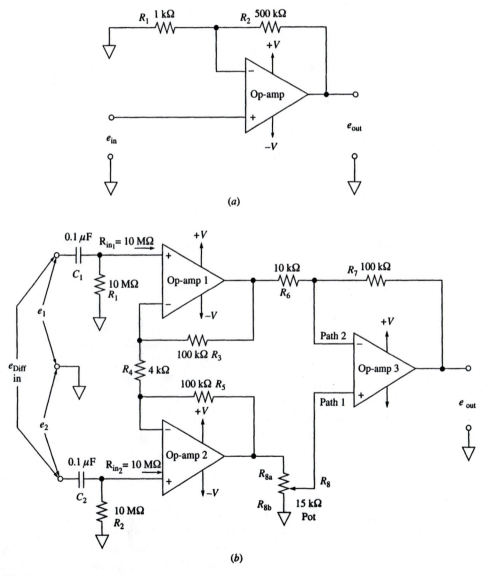

(a)

(b)

Figure 13-15
Preamplifiers. (a) Single-ended. (b) Differential.

The balance or *differential input amplifier,* shown in Figures 13-14*b* and 13-15*b,* cures most of the noise pickup problem. Noise is usually capacitively coupled (C_1 and C_2) into *both* inputs. If the gain of path 1 (G_1) equals the gain of path 2 (G_2), then equal noise signals will be cancelled (ideally). This results because amplifier gain equals $G_1 - G_2$ and amplified noise equals ($e_{1\ noise} - e_{2\ noise}$)$G$. G equals total gain, and $e_{1\ noise} - e_{2\ noise}$ equals zero. Since $e_{1\ EEG}$ is not equal to $e_{2\ EEG}$, the difference is not zero. The differential amplifier then subtracts the two unequal input EEG signals to produce an amplified EEG output. But it also subtracts the *equal* noise signals to produce zero (or a very small) noise output.

Example 13-3

Given $R_1 = 1\ k\Omega$ and $R_2 = 500\ k\Omega$ in Figure 13-15*a,* calculate the gain of the op-amp (see chapter 7 for op-amp details).

Solution

$$A_v = 1 + \frac{R_2}{R_1} = 1 + \frac{500\ k\Omega}{1\ k\Omega}$$

$$A_v = 501 \tag{13-5}$$

The input impedance is on the order of 10 MΩ (typical for a noninverting op-amp). This circuit arrangement is *not* particularly suitable for EEG preamplifiers.

Example 13-4

Given $R_3 = R_4 = 100\ k\Omega$, $R_4 = 4\ k\Omega$, $R_6 = 10\ k\Omega$, and $R_7 = 100\ k\Omega$ in Figure 13-15*b,* calculate the output voltage for the *differential EEG input signal.*

Solution

$$e_{o\ EEG} = e_{in\ EEG}\ A_v$$

$$= (e_{2\ EEG} - e_{1\ EEG})\left(\frac{1 + 2R_3}{R_4}\right)\left(\frac{R_7}{R_6}\right)$$

$$= e_{in\ EEG}^{diff}\left(1 + 2\frac{100\ k\Omega}{4\ k\Omega}\right)\left(\frac{100\ k\Omega}{10\ k\Omega}\right)$$

$$e_{o\ EEG} = e_{in\ EEG}^{diff}\ 510 \tag{13-6}$$

If $e_{in\ EEG}^{diff} = 100\ \mu V_{p-p}$, then $e_{o\ EEG} = 51\ mV_{p-p}$

Example 13-5

Given the same values in Example 13-4, calculate the output voltage for the noise input.

Solution

$$e_{o\ noise} = e_{in\ noise}\ A_v$$

$$= (e_{2\ noise} - e_{1\ noise})\left(1 + 2\frac{R_3}{R_4}\right)\left(\frac{R_7}{R_6}\right)$$

$$= e_{in\ EEG}^{diff}\left(1 + 2\frac{100\ k\Omega}{4\ k\Omega}\right)\left(\frac{100\ k\Omega}{10\ k\Omega}\right)$$

$$e_{o\ noise} = e_{in\ noise}^{diff}\ 510 \tag{13-7}$$

If $e_{in\ noise}^{diff} = 0$, that is, input noise signals on two EEG leads are equal, then $e_{o\ noise} = 0\ V_{p-p}$ ideally.

R_8 is adjusted to give equal gain in both paths 1 and 2 (balancing the diff-amp). Even with careful adjustment, some gain differences are present; thus, some residue noise voltage is present in the output.

Example 13-6

Given that the EEG output is 51 mV$_{p-p}$ (to a 100 μV$_{p-p}$ differential EEG input) and the noise output is 0.005mV$_{p-p}$ (to a 100 μV$_{p-p}$ common-mode noise input), calculate the CMRR. Refer to Figure 13-15*b.*

Solution

$$CMRR_{ratio} = \frac{e_{o\ EEG}}{e_{o\ noise}} = \frac{51\ mV_{p-p}}{0.005\ mV_{p-p}} = 10,200$$

$$CMRR_{dB} = 20\ log_{10}CMRR_{ratio}$$

$$= 20\ log_{10}\ 10,200 = 80\ dB \tag{13-8}$$

The CMRR is a number that indicates, in this case, that the *differential input gain* is 10,200 times the *single-ended input gain.* Most EEG machines have 60 to 120 dB of CMRR.

Example 13-7 _____

Given the preamplifiers shown in Figure 13-15*b*, which is also ac-coupled to reduce slow baseline drift, calculate the *low-cutoff frequency (half power* or -3 dB down frequency).

Solution

$$f_{low} = \frac{1}{2\pi(R_1 \| R_{in1})(C_1)}$$

$$= \frac{1}{2\pi(5 \text{ M}\Omega)(0.1 \text{ }\mu\text{F})}$$

$$= \textbf{0.318 Hz} \qquad (13\text{-}9)$$

The *single-ended input impedance* in Figure 13-15*b* is approximately 5 MΩ.

EEG preamplifiers are the predominant stage that influences EEG machine specifications.

EEG machine specifications typically include:

1. Input impedance: 12 MΩ minimum at 10 Hz.

2. Sensitivity: 0.5 μV/mm maximum.

3. Sensitivity controls: 10-position master (2 to 75 μV/mm), six-position individual channel (X 20 to X 0.25), and individual-channel gain equalizer.

4. Calibration voltages: 5 to 1000 μV.

5. CMRR: 2000 or 66 dB minimum at 60 Hz and 10,000 or 80 dB minimum at 10 Hz.

6. Noise: 1 μV$_{rms}$ (equivalent referred to input) with input shorted.

7. Low frequency (time constant): 30% attenuation—0.16 through 5.3 Hz, at time constants of one through 0.03 s, respectively.

8. High-frequency response: 30% attenuation at 1 to 1000 Hz.

9. 60-Hz filter: 50 dB down at 60 Hz.

10. Chart speeds: 10 to 60 mm/s.

13-15 Visual and auditory evoked potential recordings

Early EEG investigators discovered that *cortical potentials* could be evoked from sensory stimuli. EEG changes were noted when loud sounds were present. Although wave and spike resources, as well as K-complexes, are evident in the primary record (real time), most evoked responses on the scalp are too small to be recorded by typical EEG machines.

The technique of *averaging repetitive EEG signals* allows the tiny evoked potential to be separated from the background EEG. Each EEG response (5 μV$_{p-p}$) to a sensory stimulus is added to produce a readable signal. Along with this evoked signal enhancement, the ongoing EEG signal (100 μV$_{p-p}$) is reduced (averaged out due to its random nature). Some information is lost in this process; therefore, the number of stimulations should be kept to a minimum. Unfortunately, each response is unique, and the result can only represent the addition of all 100 different potentials.

The *block diagram* in Figure 13-16 shows a *visual and auditory evoked potential system*. Three electrodes pick up a one-channel EEG signal. This signal is then filtered through a 60-Hz notch filter and presented to the *evoked potential averaging computer*. The raw or ongoing EEG signal is available at the 60-Hz filter output. The computer can be set, for example, to give 100 trigger pulses to the visual or auditory stimulator. Each brain response is added synchronously with each trigger in the computer. The computer output is then the *summed response potentials* divided by the number of responses (an *average* of 100 signals). This information can be on magnetic tape or hard-copied onto a strip-chart recorder. A 5 μV$_{p-p}$ *calibration signal* can be used to test the averaging process accuracy.

Figure 13-17 shows an *auditory (tone burst) evoked potential* from a 22-year-old male. Notice the positive response at 5 ms and the negative peak at 15 ms. Early responses probably indicate lower-level brain reactions and later ones, higher-level (cerebral cortex) reactions. Waveform origin is still

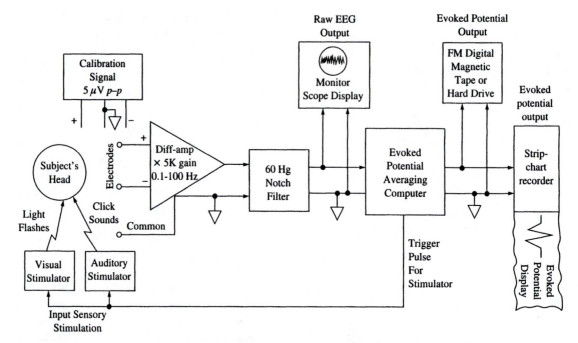

Figure 13-16
Block diagram of a visual and auditory evoked potential system.

being investigated. Evoked potentials can be used to evaluate sensory action and impairment.

13-16 EEG telemetry system

EEG telemetry systems are used to transfer the EEG from the patient's cranium to a remote site without encumbering wires. This technique is useful for children or mentally disturbed persons who may be uncooperative in the data-gathering process. Young children can be monitored while they play; epileptic patients can be monitored while active or just before an attack.

Figure 13-18 shows a block diagram for a two-way telemetry system. From this system, evoked responses can be studied in free-roaming patients. The EEG is amplified and then modulated—amplitude-modulated (AM), frequency-modulated (FM), or pulse-modulated (PM)—and transmitted to a remote site. There, the EEG is demodulated and presented to an EEG machine and evoked-response computer. Tone bursts or clicks can also

be transmitted via radio. Radio transmission is, however, plagued with noise interference. Control of the frequency band and power output is required by the Federal Communications Commission (FCC) in the United States. Furthermore, it is difficult to transmit multichannel because bandwidth problems become important. Transmission media other than radio may prove more suitable for line-of-sight EEG telemetry.

13-17 Typical EEG system artifacts, faults, troubleshooting, and maintenance

EEG recording systems suffer from artifacts that can obscure the signals of interest and render diagnosis impossible. Figure 13-19 shows typical artifacts. Aside from 60-Hz interference and *eye blinks* that result in spikes, *muscle activity* from the scalp causes significant interference (Figure 13-19a). This can be reduced by adjusting external EEG

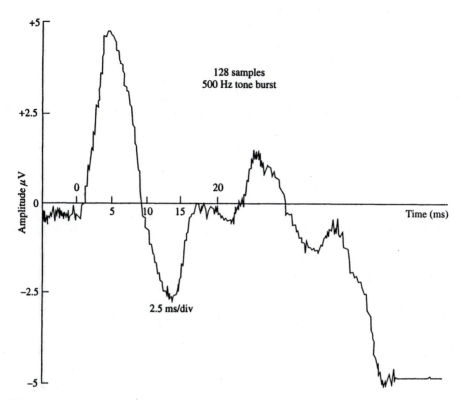

Figure 13-17
Auditory (tone burst) evoked potential from a 22-year-old male.

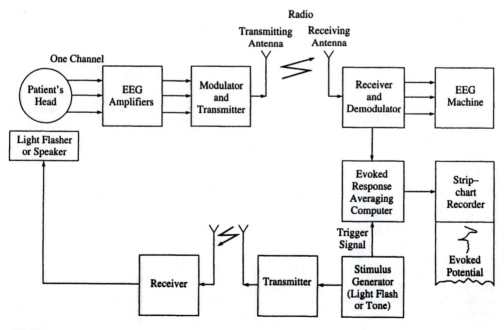

Figure 13-18
EEG telemetry system block diagram.

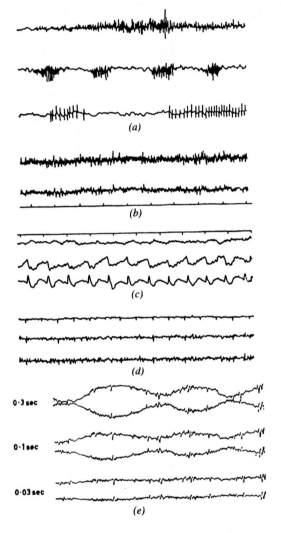

Figure 13-19
Typical EEG recording artifacts. *(a)* Examples of muscle activity recorded from scalp electrodes. *(b)* The effect of high-frequency attenuation (30% cut at 25 Hz) on the muscle activity shown in the upper trace. Artifacts caused by cardiac activity. *(c)* Pulse artifacts from the same subject. *(d)* ECG artifacts from the same subject. *(e)* Effects of progressively reducing the time constant in a pair of channels affected by perspiration under the common electrode. (From *Fundamentals of Electroencephalography,* by Kenneth A. Kooi, M.D. Harper & Row, New York, 1971. Used by permission.)

machine control to give 30% high-frequency attenuation at 25 Hz (higher frequencies are effectively removed in Figure 13-19*b*). *Cardiac activity* may be evident as arterial pulse (Figure 13-19*c*) or *R*-wave peaks (Figure 13-19*d*). *Perspiration* under the common electrode, for example, can cause a progressive reduction in time constant (Figure 13-19*e*).

Typical faults fall into the following categories:

1. Patient electrode connection problems—high-impedance connections to the scalp or broken electrode wires.

2. Cable connection problems—broken wires and bent connector pins.

3. Incorrect switch position—operator error or broken knob indicators.

4. Broken switches—faulty switch contacts.

5. Graphic recorder malfunctions—drive roller slipping or ink pens clogged or unseated.

6. Electronic malfunctions—circuit faults in individual channels, system control, or power supply.

Troubleshooting, maintenance, and *repair* of EEG machines is similar to that of ECG machines (see chapter 5, sections 5-9 and 5-10, particularly examples 5-1, 5-2, and 5-3). EEG machines are typically less rugged than clinical ECG machines but need not be inspected by the BMET on a daily basis. However, the EEG technician should perform a routine inspection procedure before daily use, as follows:

1. Machine turned on to warm up.

2. Calibration set, usually at 100 μV, and rectangular pulse observed on all channels (pen recorder).

3. Sensitivity set (system and individual channel) for proper deflection corresponding to 100 μV.

4. Pressing and holding calibration switch set to observe time constant decay.

5. All inputs grounded to observe zero signal on all channels.

Individual manufacturer's *operation and maintenance manuals* give specific calibration and maintenance procedures.

Electrical or electronic and mechanical faults rarely occur in clinical EEG machines. EEG machine faults occur much more frequently as a result of heavy use, but even these are relatively few. Manufacturer's troubleshooting trees (charts) are often helpful. The following examples are representative of typical problems.

Example 13-10

Symptom: Machine runs, but the tracing on one or more channels is missing.
Possible Causes:

1. Ink reservoirs for pens are dry [on missing channel(s)].

2. Ink tubes are clogged.

3. Pen is not touching.

Troubleshooting (machine off):

1. Check ink reservoirs.

2. Check ink tube for clogging.

3. Check for upwardly bent pens—gently push pen onto paper with finger or pencil to observe any tracing.

Solutions

1. For dry ink reservoirs, fill to level suggested by manufacturer (usually just below top rim). To overfill causes messy operation and can damage circuitry and mechanisms if allowed to drip into the machine.

2. For clogged ink tubes, remove the tube and pen and soak in warm water. Use a fine wire to gently push the clog through. Be certain not to punch a hole in the tube.

3. For bent pens, remove the pen in question and gently bend the pen downward. Be careful not to bend at right angles, as these pens are delicate and will crack.

Example 13-11

Symptoms: Spotty recordings (light or dark).
Possible Causes: Worn pens or incorrectly loaded paper.
Troubleshooting: Check paper loading, and if proper, then check pen for worn tip (ink not feeding properly).

Solutions

1. For paper loading, perform manufacturer's procedure.

2. For worn pen tip, replace with manufacturer's part or equivalent.

Example 13-12

Symptoms: Noisy or poor recording.
Possible Causes: Lead connection or electronic or mechanical problems.
Troubleshooting:

1. Place selector switches to standard calibration position and check for noise and improper operation.

2. If calibration operation is normal, the problem is probably the patient connection.

3. Ground all EEG leads and check for straight line tracing (noiseless) and, if good, connect an EEG simulator, if available. Check for good tracings. If noise appears on the trace, the problem is probably inside the machine. Refer to the service manual for troubleshooting.

Solutions

1. For patient connection, physically inspect all electrodes and connectors to the machine.

2. For machine problem, internal repair will be necessary.

Interference (60 Hz) in EEG machines is the most common problem next to chart-recorder difficulties. Since EEG signals are very low amplitude (5-100 μV_{p-p}), great care must be taken to shield and connect the patient leads. Open power supply filter capacitors and shorted voltage regulators cause symptoms that often appear to be similar to lead problems.

Muscle jitter (Figure 13-19*a*) is different in both *amplitude* and *frequency* from 60-Hz interference. *Filtering* may be used, but it is almost imperative that the patient be helped to relax.

Erratic or *wandering baseline* can be caused by poor electrode connections or long-term patient connection (Figure 13-19*e*). Clean, well-secured electrodes (low electrode resistance below 10 kΩ) are the only sure cure for this phenomenon. Also, junction box leads may have intermittent connections. Occasionally, amplifiers may have excessive dc drift.

13-18 Summary

1. Instrumentation for measuring anatomical and physiological parameters of the brain include *X-ray equipment* (cerebral angiography, cranial X-rays, and brain scans), *ultrasonic equipment* (echo encephalography), and *electrophysiological equipment* (electroencephalography and brain stimulators).

2. X-rays pass more readily through soft tissue than bone and reveal *differences in tissue density.* They are dangerous and can cause mutations, physical illness, and death.

3. *Cerebral angiography* is an X-ray technique used to display brain structures (tumors) and blood vessels (blockages) by circulating a radiopaque dye contrast medium.

4. *Cranial X-rays* are two-dimensional exposures taken of the cranium and can reveal cranial fractures and tumors.

5. *Brain scans* (computed tomography) are radiographs that are taken through successive scanning by highly collimated X-ray beams. They show small differences in tissue densities and reveal obscure tumors and swellings.

6. *Echoencephalography* is an ultrasound pulsing Doppler-shift technique that shows differences in acoustic properties of various tissues. It shows brain structures and blood flow.

7. *EEG* is a representation (writing on paper or display on CRT) of the electrical activity of the brain. It is used to help detect and localize cerebral brain lesions and to study epilepsy, mental disorders, sleep patterns, and brain responses to sensory stimuli.

8. *Neuronal electrochemical processes* form the basis for EEG activity.

9. The *10-20 EEG electrode placement system* establishes 10% to 20% distances across the cranium *(naision to inion)* for electrode positions. Nineteen electrodes are used with one as a reference. EEG patterns are distinguished by location, frequency, amplitude, form, periodicity, and functional properties. A common, or indifference, point (earlobe) is used to supply the differential amplifier input with an inactive reference. *Unipolar* recordings indicate the difference between an active and inactive site, while *bipolar* recordings are between two active sites.

10. *EEG amplitude* ranges from 1 μV to 100 μV_{p-p} at 0.5 to 100 Hz. The following signal waves are defined: delta (0.5 to 4 Hz), theta (4 to 8 Hz), alpha (8 to 13 Hz), beta (13 to 22 Hz),and gamma (22 to 30 Hz and above).

    Alpha activity (the most predominant) occurs when the subject is awake with eyes closed. *Beta waves* begin with eyes open. *Delta* and *theta waves* appear at various stages of drowsiness and sleep.

11. *Clinical EEG machines* typically consist of 8 (most common), 16, or 32 channels. Switch-selectable electrode signals make up the montage.

12. External EEG machine *controls* consist of gain or sensitivity control (system and individual channel), low- and high-frequency attenuation filter adjusts, 60-Hz notch filter switch, calibration push button, baseline (position) potentiometer, electrode selection switch box, event marker push button, and chart speed switch.

13. The *basic EEG block diagram* consists of electrode switch-selector box, differential amplifiers (system), adjustable gain amplifier (individual channel), driver amplifiers, graphic display, and power supply.

14. *EEG preamplifiers* (differential amplifiers) compose the most important section of the EEG machine. Their characteristics are low internal noise, high gain (X 5k to X 10k), high external noise rejection (CMRR of 100 dB), low-frequency ac-coupled operation (1 Hz), low dc drift, and high input impedance.

15. EEG machine *specifications* typically include 12 MΩ input impedance, 0.5 μV/mm sensitivity, 5 to 1000 μV calibration voltages, CMRR of 60 to 120 dB, low-frequency attenuation (30% cutoff) at 0.16 through 5.3 Hz, high-frequency attenuation at 1 to 100 Hz, 60-Hz notch filtering (50 dB down), and chart speeds of 10 to 60 mm/s.

16. Sensory (visual and auditory) *evoked potential* recordings are obtained by repetitive sensory stimulation and synchronous computer averaging of the low-amplitude evoked signal ($5 \ \mu V_{p-p}$).

17. *EEG telemetry systems* are used to transmit and receive EEG signals via radio (AM, FM, PM) and other media for mobile or uncooperative patients.

18. EEG recording systems are susceptible to *artifacts* (60-Hz noise, eye blinks, muscle tremor or activity, cardiac activity, and perspiration). These may obscure the recording but can be corrected by good electrode technique, high-quality preamplifiers, and filtering.

19. *Typical EEG machine faults* are poor patient-electrode connection, broken cable wires, bent connector pins, broken switches, problems with graphic recorder paper drive and ink, electronic or mechanical malfunction, and operator error.

20. *Troubleshooting and maintenance* takes the form of an inspection procedure (calibration, control check, tracing evaluation). Individual equipment manufacturer's operation and maintenance manuals must be consulted for proper maintenance. Typical trouble symptoms include missing trace; spotty, noisy, or poor recordings; 60-Hz noise interference; muscle jitter; and erratic or wandering baseline.

13-19 Recapitulation

Now return to the objectives and self-evaluation questions at the beginning of the chapter and see how well you can answer them. If you cannot answer certain questions, place a check mark next to each and review appropriate parts of the text. Next, try to answer the following questions using the same procedure. When you have answered all the questions, solve the problems.

Questions

1. Three classes of instrumentation used to measure anatomical and physiological parameters of the brain are _____, _____, and _____.

2. Cerebral angiography and brain scans both use _____.

3. Mutations, physical illness, and death are hazards that can result from overexposure to _____.

4. During cerebral angiography, _____ or contrast media are injected into the circulatory system of the brain.

5. In brain scans, CT refers to _____ _____.

6. The ACTA scanner uses a _____ counter to record X-ray beam attenuation.

7. Diagnostic ultrasonic brain instrumentation is known as _____ and uses frequencies of _____ MHz.

8. Brain *symmetry* or *asymmetry*, indicated by ultrasonic reflections in the cranium, shows normal conditions.

9. EEG results from _____ activity of the _____.

10. EEG systems include _____ pickup, signal _____, signal _____, and signal _____.

11. EEG recordings are used to detect cerebral _____, study convulsive problems of patients with _____, assist in diagnosing mental _____, study _____ patterns, and observe _____ brain responses to _____ stimuli.

12. Neuronal action potentials can be measured with _____ electrodes.

13. EEG patterns are distinguished by _____, _____, _____, and _____.

14. The 10-20 EEG electrode placement system derives its name from what measurements?

15. How many EEG electrodes are typically used?

16. The EEG vertex electrode is half of what distance?

17. Why is a common, or indifference, point used for EEG recordings?

18. What is the difference between unipolar and biopolar recordings?

19. EEG electrode resistance should be below what level?

20. State the typical amplitude range for EEG signals.

21. List the names and frequency bands of EEG waveforms.

22. EEG multichannel recording systems typically use how many channels?

23. Montage refers to the selection of what connections?

24. List 10 typical EEG machine external controls and describe each.

25. List the main sections of a typical EEG machine block diagram and describe the flow of signals.

26. List six characteristics typical of EEG preamplifiers (differential amplifiers).

27. List 10 typical EEG machine specifications.

28. In sensory evoked potential systems, the averaging computer performs what two functions?

29. List two uses for evoked potential studies.

30. EEG telemetry systems transmit signals (wireless) and are used for which type of patients?

31. List four types of EEG artifacts.

32. List six typical EEG machine or system faults.

33. Troubleshooting and maintenance of EEG machines includes a routine inspection procedure typically consisting of which steps?

34. Describe two EEG machine problems (symptoms, causes, troubleshooting, and solutions).

Problems

1. What peak-to-peak output voltage level will be present from an EEG input level of 50 μV_{p-p} and EEG system gain of 5000?

2. From Figure 13-15*b*, what voltage gain will result if $R_3 = R_5 = 150$ kΩ, $R_4 = 10$ kΩ,

$R_6 = 5$ kΩ, $R_7 = 100$ kΩ, and R_8 is set to balance the diff-amp?

3. From Figure 13-15b, will the low-frequency response be satisfactory if capacitor C_1 leaks and becomes 0.005 μF?

4. What CMRR (number ratio and dB) exists if the EEG output is 1 V_{p-p} (to a 100-μV_{p-p} EEG input) and the noise output is 0.01 mV_{p-p} (to a 100 μV_{p-p} noise input)?

Suggested readings

1. Scott, Donald, *Understanding the EEG, An Introduction to Electroencephalography,* J. B. Lippincott Co. (Philadelphia, 1975).

2. Kooi, Kenneth A., *Fundamentals of Electroencephalography,* Medical Department, Harper and Row Publishers, (New York, 1971).

3. Kiloh, L. G., A. J. McComas, and J. W. Osselton, *Clinical Electroencephalography,* Appleton-Century-Crofts Educational Division/Meredith Corp. (New York, 1972).

4. Cooper, R., J. W. Osselton, and J. C. Shaw, *EEG Technology,* Butterworths (London, 1974).

5. Strong, Peter, *Biophysical Measurements,* Tektronix, Inc., Measurement Series (Beaverton, Ore., 1970).

6. Williams, Robert L. and Carolyn J. Hursch, *Electroencephalography (EEG) of Human Sleep: Clinical Applications.* Wiley (New York, 1974).

7. Burch, Neil and H. I. Altshuler, *Behavior and Brain Electrical Activity,* Plenum Press (New York, 1975).

8. Mishkin, Fred S. and John Mealey, Jr., *Use and Interpretation of the Brain Scan,* Charles C Thomas (Springfield, Ill., 1969).

9. Tenner, Michael S. and Georgina M. Wodraska, *Diagnostic Ultrasound in Neurology,* Wiley (New York, 1975).

10. Jacobson, Bertil and John Webster, *Medicine and Clinical Engineering,* Prentice Hall, Inc. (Englewood Cliffs, N.J., 1977).

11. Geddes, L. A. and L. E. Baker, *Principles of Applied Biomedical Instrumentation,* Wiley (New York, 1975).

12. Ledley, Robert S., "Computerized Transaxial X-Ray Tomography of the Human Body," *Science, 186:*207-212 (1974).

CHAPTER 14

Intensive and Coronary Care Units

14-1 Objectives

1. Be able to describe the functions and purpose of special care units in the hospital.
2. Be able to list the types of instrumentation systems used in the ICU/CCU.

3. Be able to identify and troubleshoot common ICU/CCU instruments.

14-2 Self-evaluation questions

These questions test your prior knowledge of the material in this chapter. Look for the answers as you read the text. After you have finished studying the chapter, try answering these questions and those at the end of the chapter.

1. List the types of monitoring equipment normally found in the ICU/CCU of a hospital.

2. What is the function of a *cardiac memory unit?*

3. What is an *arrhythmia monitor?*

4. Describe the principal functions of a *bedside monitor.*

14-3 Special care units

Special care units go by a variety of names, some of which are descriptive of function, such as intensive care unit (ICU) and critical or coronary care unit (CCU). But all of these units are designed to offer the advantages of a low nurse-patient ratio and concentration of the equipment and resources needed to take care of critically ill or seriously injured patients.

The situation "on the floor"—on the regular medical and surgical wards of the hospitals—is quite different. It is not unusual in some hospitals on the night shift to find one or two nurses caring for 50 to 80 patients, with the ratios as high as 50 patients per nurse when crowded. In the not-too-distant past a critically ill patient would be as-signed to such a ward, possibly with a one-on-one private duty nurse. But in the event of a crisis, few resources were available soon enough to do any good. Even today in some rural hospitals, there might not be a physician in the building at odd hours, especially from midnight to morning.

But in the ICU/CCUs of modern hospitals, physicians are available, and nurses are specially trained to recognize and deal with signs of im-pending disaster. Rapid action can be taken to counter the event. The critical care nurse is spe-cially trained to do this job. In medical and surgi-cal ICUs, there are usually one or two patients per nurse, and in many cases the ratio is one to one. Additionally, the staff has the physical resources, supplementing their skills and abilities, necessary to handle emergencies.

Most hospitals have medical-surgical emer-gency teams that rush to the scene of a situation that could be life threatening. Most hospitals call the team by radio pager (beeper) and by voice page over the public address system. It is common to find the team called using a cryptic phrase, such as "code 2 MICU," which might be inter-preted by appropriate personnel as "respond im-mediately to an emergency in the medical ICU." The use of a cryptic code for an emergency may stem from a desire to avoid alarming the visitors to the hospital but also serves a communications role in that it provides an unmistakable command to the team. Since emergencies rarely follow a schedule, it is not likely that team members will be expecting trouble. The use of a code allows them to be trained to respond immediately even though they were otherwise engaged at the mo-ment. The emergency team will respond to emer-gency situations anywhere in the hospital, includ-ing the ICU/CCU areas that will need additional help in such cases.

A key factor in the success of the ICU/CCU is the information that is available to the staff. Pro-viding that information is the role of the technol-ogy and equipment.

14-4 ICU/CCU equipment

The information used by physicians and nurses in the ICU/CCU comes from several sources, includ-ing their own skilled observations, the laboratory, and an array of electronic monitoring equipment at each bedside. The particular parameters mea-sured on any given patient vary from one hospital to another and from one physician to another. There is some disagreement over certain types of monitoring, but in all cases the ECG waveform is monitored.

Arterial blood pressures are routinely moni-tored in some units. Less often, but becoming more popular, we find monitors for temperature, respiration rate/apnea, venous pressure, right arte-rial pressure, cardiac output, and EEG. Almost all monitors include a heart rate meter that is trig-gered from the ECG waveform and, in some cases, the arterial pressure waveform.

Additionally, other equipment may be present for use as required. Examples are respirators and ventilators, hypothermia and hyperthermia ma-chines, defibrillators, rotating tourniquets, and aor-tic balloon pumps.

Most ICU/CCU facilities provide a bedside monitor near the patient, complete with an oscillo-scope and sometimes with its own dedicated strip-chart recorders. The bedside monitor will have auxiliary outputs that are connected by wire to re-mote readouts at a central console (Figure 14-1). On computer-based systems, which are common today, a *local area network* (LAN) may be used for intercommunications.

The console will display physiological wave-forms and numerical data on one or more patients; a popular unit size seems to be eight patients, al-though that is not a general rule.

Several philosophies regarding ICU/CCU lay-out seem to be prevalent. In some, all of the beds can be monitored from a single console. In some cases, the console is at the nurses' station, al-though in others it is at a nearby location. Monitor watching may be the responsibility of a designated

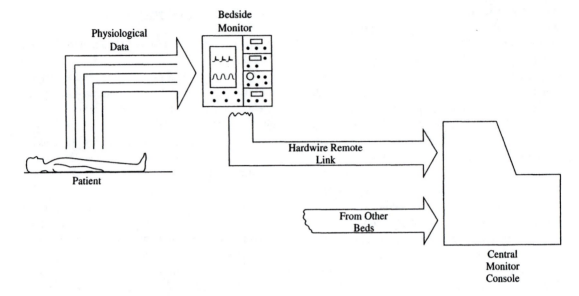

Figure 14-1
ICU/CCU central monitoring system.

person (e.g., a nurse or a specially trained "monitoring technician"), or it may be a general responsibility shared by everyone on duty at the time. A variation is to have several consoles, each carrying part of the load, no more than a few patients. This design concept minimizes the possibility that a single equipment failure will cost the unit all of its monitoring capability.

14-5 Bedside monitors

The bedside monitor in the ICU/CCU may consist of a simple ECG amplifier, oscilloscope, and heart rate meter package or a complex array of physiological instruments. Despite differences in features, however, all bedside monitors will be equipped with alarms, at least for heart rate, so that the staff is warned if the patient gets into trouble. Alarm circuitry will be discussed more fully in a later section.

Figure 14-2 shows several types of bedside monitoring equipment. The instrument shown in Figure 14-2*a* is an older style self-contained basic

monitor, the Hewlett-Packard Model 78330A. The oscilloscope in this model is nonfade; that is, the waveform is stored on the CRT screen until it is erased by an updated waveform on the next sweep. The oscilloscope sweep rate is selectable between 25 and 50 mm/s.

The ECG waveform displayed may be any of the standard leads. Additionally, the monitor can be used to display EEG or the output of a photoplethysmograph. The display selector in the upper left-hand corner shows both ECG-DIAG and ECG-MON positions, which refer to *diagnostic* and *monitoring* grade displays, respectively. These switch positions select different amplifier bandwidths in the ECG channel (i.e., 0.05 to 100 Hz in diagnostic mode, and 0.05 to 45 Hz in monitoring mode). The ECG-MON mode provides for reducing the muscle artifact and gross patient movement artifact, without sacrificing the ability to display and recognize life-threatening cardiac arrhythmias.

The alarms are set by front panel controls. A switch allows them to be turned on and off and to be reset once the condition that caused the alarm

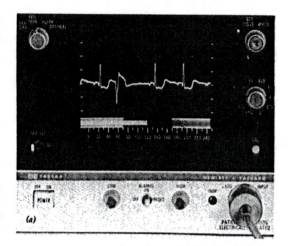

(a)

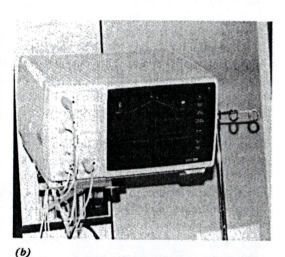

(b)

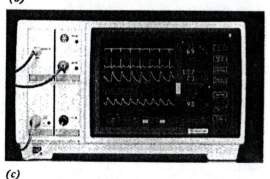

(c)

Figure 14-2

Bedside monitors. *(a)* H-P Model 78330A. (Photo courtesy of Hewlett-Packard) *(b)* and *(c)* Integrated bedside monitors. (Photos courtesy of Spacelabs)

ceases to exist. The alarm limits are displayed on the CRT screen along with the heart rate. The display is in the form of a band of light at the bottom of the screen. The low limit is indicated by the end of the thick band from the left side of the screen, in this case 70 BPM. The *high* alarm limit is indicated by the end of the band coming from the right side of the CRT, in this example 170 BPM. The patient's actual heart rate is determined by the narrow band of light from the left side of the CRT, in this case 120 BPM.

The patient monitor unit depicted in Figure 14-2*b* represents a trend away from rigidly defined "black-box" models that offered only what the manufacturer thought was needed. While that type of design is still common among portable monitors, it has long since departed from the formal bedside monitor scene. The modular design still survives because it allows the manufacturer, the hospital, and the nursing and physician staffs to custom configure a monitor for a patient's needs. In one unit, for example, it may be policy to provide continuous arterial pressure and ECG monitoring for all patients. All of the bedside monitors in that unit would be equipped with these modules. Other measurements, such as venous pressure or continuous rectal temperature or EEG, on the other hand, would typically be ordered for fewer patients. The physician could order these services, and they could then be provided by a monitoring technician or biomedical equipment technician. The hospital would thus be spared the cost of completely equipping each bed with all functions, while still providing the functions whenever needed. A related bedside monitor unit is shown in Figure 14-2*c*. This model shows the various physiological traces that can be displayed.

These monitors have a built-in self-test mode. Modern microprocessor electronic monitors can conduct self-tests and display the results. Thus, the unit will self-test whenever it is first turned on and whenever a self-test is initiated by the medical, nursing, or biomedical equipment staff. With proper design, self-test results can be reported over the data lines to the central computer and be used there for recordkeeping purposes. Some self-tests can locate the problems in the system to the printed circuit board level and therefore tell the repair technician which subassembly to replace.

The Hewlett-Packard instrument in Figure 14-2c is an integrated bedside monitor that makes extensive use of digital electronic circuitry. The unit contains ECG, heart rate, two pressure channels, respiration, temperature, and (optionally) a second temperature channel with ΔT capability. An internal character display generator, such as those used in computer video terminals, displays the numerical data along the right-hand vertical edge of the CRT.

14-6 Bedside monitor circuits

Most of the circuits in the bedside monitor are ordinary ECG or pressure amplifiers, covered in detail elsewhere in this text. In this section, we will discuss those circuits that are unique to, or commonly employed in, bedside monitors.

14-6-1 Cardiotachometers

The *cardiotachometer* is a heart rate meter. It provides an analog or digital display of the heart rate, usually developed from the patient's ECG signal but sometimes derived from the arterial pressure waveform.

The vast majority of all cardiotachometers are analog circuits that produce a *dc voltage* proportional to the patient's heart rate. This dc voltage will be displayed on an analog or digital voltmeter. The block diagram of an analog cardiotachometer is shown in Figure 14-3a and consists of four sections: *R-wave discriminator, monostable multivibrator* (i.e., *one-shot*), *integrator,* and *readout.*

The R-wave discriminator is necessary so that the circuit will count only once for each heart beat, and the R-wave is the most easily identified feature of the ECG waveform. All R-wave discriminators use a *level detector* (i.e., a circuit that will produce an output change only when the predetermined input voltage level is exceeded). A simple voltage comparator will perform this function.

But a simple voltage comparison circuit is not sufficient to prevent false counting. Equipment that uses only level detection often suffers from double counting because, in some patients, the T-wave amplitude also exceeds the level detector threshold.

A *differentiator* stage *(dE/dt)* preceding the level detector is used by some manufacturers to reduce the double counting artifact. This circuit is called a *high-pass filter* in some service manuals, but it is the same circuit under a different name. The high-pass filter produces an output voltage that is proportional to the *slope* (i.e., *rate of change* of the input signal). The fast-changing R-wave, therefore, will produce a much larger output voltage than will the slow-rising, low-frequency T-wave and P-wave features.

The output of the R-wave discriminator triggers a monostable multivibrator. This one-shot stage will generate one output pulse for each R-wave. These pulses have *constant duration* and *amplitude;* only the pulse repetition rate varies with the patient's heart rate.

The one-shot stage is required because the dc output voltage, which must be proportional to the heart rate, is obtained from an *integrator* (called a *low-pass filter* in some service manuals) stage. The integrator *averages* the pulses applied to its input and produces an output voltage proportional to the total area under the pulses. This area is determined by the number of pulses received and the area of each pulse (i.e., *duration × height*). The one-shot stage, however, produces constant-area pulses, and only one output pulse is generated for each R-wave. The dc output of the integrator, therefore, is proportional only to the time average of the heart rate (i.e., number of R-waves per unit of time).

The readout device will be a simple voltmeter. Even many digital heart rate meters use analog circuitry and then display the result on a digital voltmeter.

A *systole lamp* and a *systole beeper* may also be driven by the output of the one-shot stage. The systole lamp or light-emitting diode (LED) is turned on by a drive transistor that becomes forward

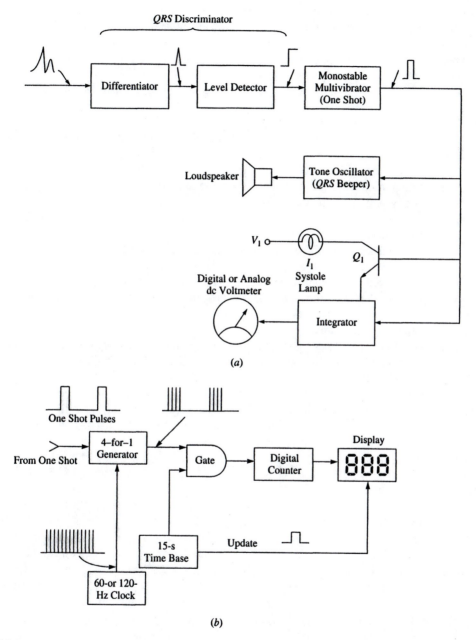

Figure 14-3
Cardiotachometer circuits. *(a)* Integrating analog type. *(b)* Digital type.

biased only when the output of the one-shot is high. The systole beeper is a tone oscillator that is turned on by the output pulse from the one-shot stage. The beeper is especially useful when transporting the patient on a stretcher and in other cases when the oscilloscope screen is not always in view, or the alarms are inoperative. At most other times the beeper is an annoyance and so will remain turned off.

Figure 14-3*b* shows a digital cardiotachometer. This circuit, or a similar one, is found only in a few instruments. The input section of the circuit is the same as the analog type, until the output of the one-shot stage.

The one-shot pulses occur at the same rate as the patient's *R* waves and are used to trigger a *four-for-one* circuit, which outputs four clock pulses for each pulse received at the input. In most cases, the clock signal is derived from either a free-running *R-C* oscillator or a 120-Hz wave train from the full wave rectified power supply.

The digital counter circuit, then, sees four input pulses for each *R* wave and is gated on for 15 s. After the 15-s count period, the accumulated data is equal to the patient's heart rate in BPM, so the time base issues an *update* command to the display and then initiates a new count cycle. This allows the digital counter to measure the averaged heart rate in 15 s (i.e., one-fourth of a minute).

Computer-based bedside monitors have cardiotachometer functions that are similar to the digital type but with the functionality implemented in software instead of hardware. It is relatively easy to get a computer to count (indeed, some have onboard counter chips), so it is easy to measure the beat-to-beat interval and then take the reciprocal and convert to BPM. The software can provide the instantaneous heart rate (one beat to the next) or a sliding window average of the past several heart beat rates (the integrated or average value).

These cardiotachometer circuits are basically averaging types. It is not generally deemed prudent to use a short time constant in these circuits because many patients' heart rates may normally change slightly from beat to beat (i.e., the *period*

of R-R interval changes). This is one reason that few instruments use the period to derive heart rate.

14-6-2 Alarms

Alarm circuits are provided on bedside monitors to warn the staff of an emergency condition. On heart rate, for example, it is normal practice to bracket the patient's indicated heart rate with high and low alarm limits. If the patient's rate either speeds up or slows down significantly, then an alarm sounds.

Two common approaches are taken in the design of alarm circuits, as shown in Figures 14-4 and 14-5. The photocell type of alarm circuit in Figure 14-4 is used in analog readout meters. Inside the meter housing are two lamp-photocell assemblies (Figure 14-4*a*), one each for high and low alarms. These assemblies are positioned by the *alarm set* tabs on the front of the meter housing. A metal vane attached to the rear of the meter pointer is used to trigger the alarm condition. The photocell assembly is built such that the light will shine on the photocell element, keeping its resistance low all the time unless the limit is exceeded. If that situation should occur, then the vane of the meter pointer will blind the photocell assembly, causing its resistance to increase substantially. In one model, the dark resistance is over 1 MΩ, while lighted resistance is under 20 kΩ.

The alarm circuit is shown in Figure 14-4*b*. Only one is shown here, but two will be in each monitor; one each for high and low.

Alarm driver transistor Q_1 is normally reverse biased by the potential across capacitor C_1. This voltage is the sum of two sources, $V-$ and $V+$. Under normal conditions the resistance of the photocell is low, so the voltage across C_1 is negative, thereby reverse biasing Q_1. If the photocell is *blinded* when an alarm situation occurs, then its resistance goes very high, and the voltage across C_1 goes positive to forward bias Q_1 and turns on the alarm circuit.

Figure 14-5 shows two alarm circuits that use voltage comparators to detect the alarm condition.

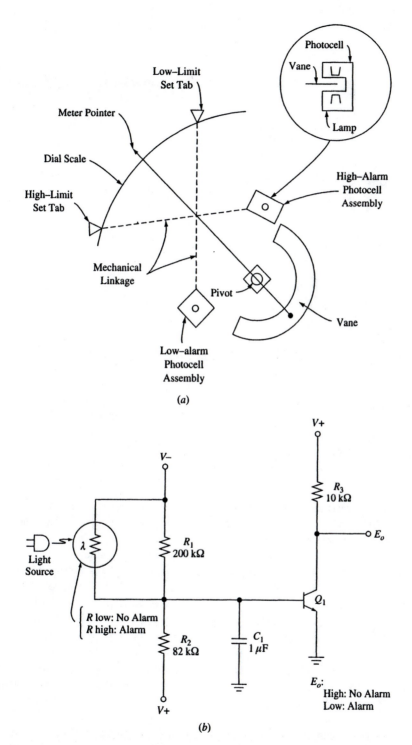

Figure 14-4
Photocell alarm. *(a)* Mechanical arrangement (top view). *(b)* Circuit.

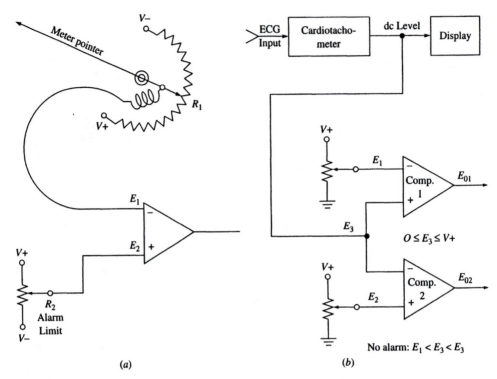

Figure 14-5
Alarm circuits. *(a)* Comparator alarm with special meter movement. *(b)* Alarm circuit using cardiotachometer output.

In Figure 14-5a there is a resistance element inside the analog meter movement. The output voltage, E_1, indicates the heart rate, while the alarm limit voltage E_2 is produced by a front panel potentiometer. As long as the set limit is not exceeded by E_1, no alarm occurs. But if the limit is exceeded, then the alarm triggers.

A similar, and more popular, circuit is shown in Figure 14-5b. In this case the cardiotachometer output voltage, a dc level, is fed to the input of a standard dual-limit window comparator. No alarm occurs if E_3 remains between E_1 and E_2.

14-6-3 Lead fault indicator

When a monitor electrode or its lead wire comes loose, the appearance of the display will be either 60-Hz interference or a flat baseline (i.e., no signal at all). In the latter case, the flat baseline may be mistaken for asystole and emergency resuscitation procedures initiated inappropriately. A *lead fault indicator* will help prevent this occurrence.

A simplified version of the lead fault circuit used in the Tektronix Model 414 monitor is shown in Figure 14-6a. Two very high-value resistors (R_1 and R_2) place a 10-nA current on each lead from the patient. Voltages E_1 and E_2 are formed by voltage divider action of the patient-electrode resistance and resistors R_1/R_2, respectively. Ordinarily, E_1 and E_2 are very low and nearly equal to each other and so do not affect the ECG preamplifier output. For example, E_1 is

$$E_1 = \frac{ER}{R + R_1} \qquad (14\text{-}1)$$

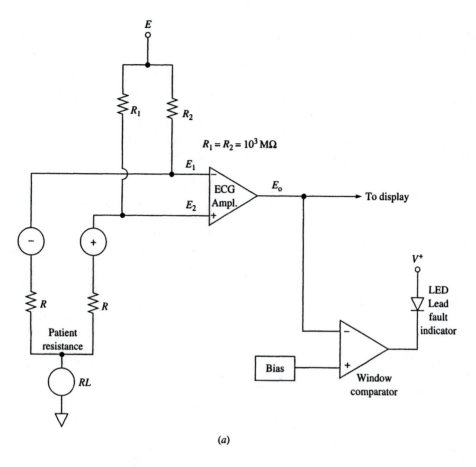

$R_1 = R_2 = 10^3 \, \text{M}\Omega$

(a)

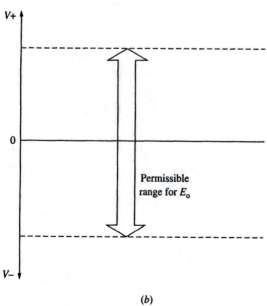

(b)

Figure 14-6

Lead fault indicator. (a) Circuit. (b) Range of E_o.

where

E_1 is the dc voltage at the inverting input of the ECG preamplifier

E is the reference voltage

R is the patient resistance in ohms (Ω)

R_1 is the value of resistor R_1 (10^9 Ω)

Example 14-1

Calculate the value of E_1 in Figure 14-6a if $E = +10$ V dc, and R is 10 Ω.

Solution

$$E_1 = ER/(R + R_1) \qquad (14-1)$$
$$E_1 = (10\ V)(10^4\ \Omega/10^4 + 10^9)\Omega$$
$$E_1 = (10^5\ V)/(10^4 + 10^9) \approx \textbf{100 } \boldsymbol{\mu}\textbf{V}$$

If a lead should come off the patient's body, however, the voltage at the input of the ECG preamplifier rises to almost $+10$ V, saturating the output. A level detector turns on the *lead fault* lamp if E_o exceeds the limits due to the offset caused by the loss of R, the patient resistance. Figure 14-6b shows the permissible limits of E_o.

14-7 Central monitoring consoles

The central monitoring console is credited with allowing each critical care nurse to attend more patients. Without central monitoring, critical care would be more one to one, and the total number of nursing personnel would be greater. But life-threatening events do not usually occur for all patients in the unit at the same time, so such a costly nurse-patient ratio would not be cost-effective.

The central station serves several functions in the intensive care environment. One, which is immediately apparent, is that it amplifies the abilities of the staff to keep track of the situation and so reduces the number of nurses and doctors needed to staff a unit. All of the analog signals, plus numerical data and the alarm status signals, are routed from each bedside monitor to the central nurses' station unit. The console will provide an array of multichannel oscilloscopes, heart rate meters (plus

occasionally blood pressure meters), a computer terminal, an alarm status annunciator panel, and a communications system. On modern systems, the entire information display may be part of a video terminal controlled by a personal computer, with a strip-chart recorder for hard-copy readout (Figure 14-7). With this information a single operator can keep track of the condition of several patients at once, relieving the need to station a nurse in each patient room all of the time.

Figure 14-8 shows the block diagram of a typical central monitoring system. Electrodes and transducers (sensors) attached to the patient provide signals through an array of input amplifiers to the local bedside monitor. These signals are locally displayed on a monitor oscilloscope, various numerical (digital) readouts, and sometimes a local strip-chart (paper) recorder. Local alarms are also provided to alert the staff if any parameter (e.g., heart rate) goes outside of set limits.

There will be a transmission path between the bedside monitors and the central station. The

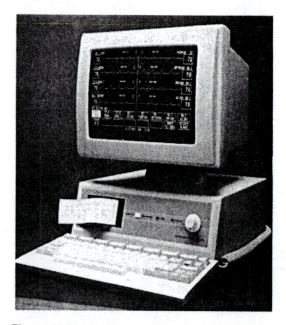

Figure 14-7
Modern centralmonitoring system.

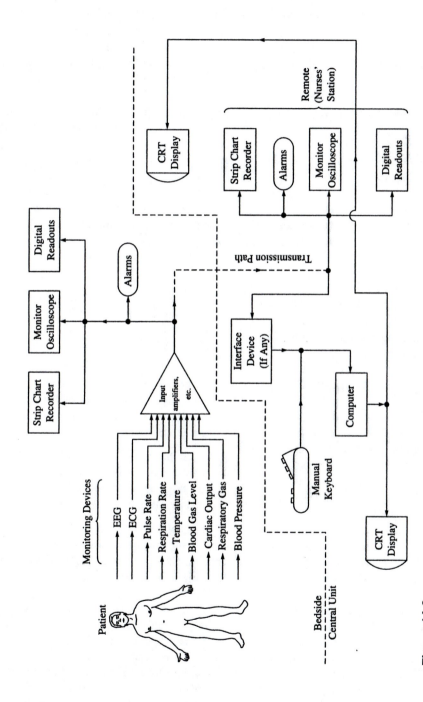

Figure 14-8
Block diagram of a typical central monitoring system.

transmission path might be analog or digital, or a combination of both. We will discuss these options later.

The signals from the bedside units are routed to the central nurses' station console, where they are displayed on slave units of the bedside monitors. Shown in the system in Figure 14-8 are the following units: oscilloscope (usually multichannel), digital readouts for numerical data, alarms, and a strip-chart recorder. In many modern designs, the numerical data and analog data are both displayed simultaneously on the screen of a video terminal.

Although older central station units (some of which are still in use) were simple analog instruments that were slaved to the bedside monitors, modern design uses a microcomputer to monitor patient status and record data. The typical system contains a computer (often an IBM XT or AT machine), a manual data entry keyboard, a video CRT display, and an interface device (not always used). The *architecture* of the central monitoring system determines how the various units relate to one another and how the system is interconnected. Figure 14-8 shows one example of system architecture.

Older systems were strictly analog and so used the type of system shown in Figure 14-9. The bedside monitor is equipped with an output interface that consists of a large multiconductor cable that carries two types of signal: analog waveforms and alarm or control *discretes*. A "discrete" is a single wire or wire pair that is either open-circuited or closed-circuited when a certain condition exists. The ECG alarm "discrete," for example, is "open" when no alarm is present and is shorted to ground when the alarm occurs. These conditions signal the central station circuits as to the alarm condition. This type of architecture requires a large number of wires to implement. A 24-bed ICU system, for example, has as many as 20 discrete and analog signal lines per bed, for a total of 480 analog lines.

Note in Figure 14-9 that the output of the ECG amplifier (labeled "analog ECG signal") is not fed directly to the multiconductor cable, but rather is directed to a buffer amplifier. This stage is used to isolate the bedside monitor from faults in either the multiconductor cable, the interconnections, or the central station itself. If, for example, a short circuit occurs in the transmission path, the output of the buffer will be shorted to ground. But, because of the buffer amplifier stage, the local oscilloscope and alarm system remains working—protecting the patient. If the external fault does not affect the alarm "discrete," then even the central station alarm function will remain (even though the analog signal disappears).

Buffering in analog signals has its parallel in digital systems and represents a feature that should be required in specifying any new systems or modifications to existing systems. Some items to include in the purchase order or request for quotation are as follows:

1. No single-point fault will remove more than one single patient unit from service (i.e., a fault on, say, bedside monitor 2 only affects that unit and does not affect all other units).

2. No single-point fault, such as an output short, on a bedside monitor unit shall remove all functions of that unit either locally or at the nurses' station.

3. It shall be possible to disconnect any bedside monitor unit from the system without adversely affecting any other unit or function either in the local rooms or at the central station.

Most modern bedside monitor (BSM) units are digitized to allow their use with a computer. Early computerized monitoring systems were configured like any analog system, except that *digitization* took place at the central nurses' station computer. In modern systems, however, the BSM itself may include a microprocessor to perform many of the chores once performed elsewhere (in addition to chores not offered before).

Figure 14-10 shows the block diagram for a simple digitized ECG monitor or BSM. The ECG amplifier, local alarm, and local oscilloscope are

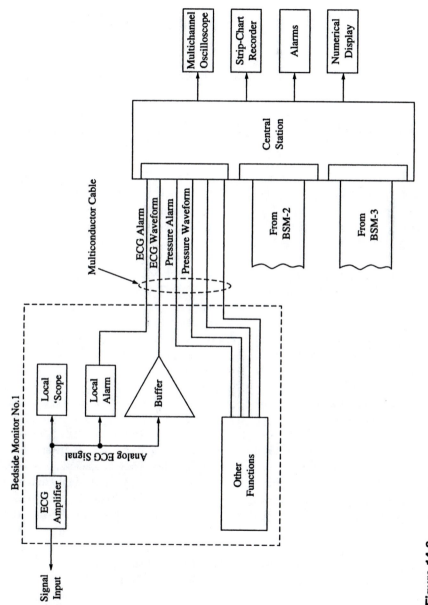

Figure 14-9
Older analog monitoring system.

409

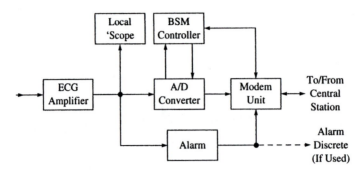

Figure 14-10
Digitized ECG bedside monitor system.

similar (often identical) to those of the strictly analog system. The difference is that no analog signals are passed to the central station. An *analog-to-digital* (A/D) *converter* is used to convert the analog voltage that represents the ECG signal into binary "words" that are transmitted to the central computer over a data bus. Because the voltage levels of the binary word do not transmit well over distances greater thanabout 20 yards, it is often the practice to use a modulator/demodulator (MODEM) unit to convert the binary signals to a series of audio tones. These tones are transmitted to the central station computer, where another MODEM unit reconverts them to data words.

The alarms can be sent along the bus as a tone by way of the modem or via a separate discrete line. Both systems are known. In some cases, both MODEM and discrete alarms might be used as a safety feature.

The BSM controller module usually contains a microprocessor or simple digital computer to control the operation of the bedside monitor, run self-tests, and perform the alarm functions. It can communicate with the main computer unit to synchronize operations. In some systems "handshaking" between the central computer and BSMs indicates when data is ready or may be transmitted.

A function of the controller is to respond to the central computer when it is being polled for data. Each BSM is given a unique *address*. The BSM will not respond to traffic on the bus unless it

"hears" either its own address or an "all units listen" broadcast address.

Although there are many variations on the following themes, and variations also exist in the specifics of implementation, the systems shown in Figure 14-11 represent a large number of data connection schemes between BSMs and central stations. Figure 14-11*a* shows the system in which a local area controller receives the data lines from each BSM, prioritizes the signals, and then transmits the data to the central station computer. In some implementations this system is called a *star* connection.

A parallel connection is shown in Figure 14-11*b*. In this case, a common main data bus connects all of the BSMs and the central stationcomputer. The controller is located inside the computer. Be sure to avoid connections that are truly *daisy chained*. These modules should be paralleled (and isolated to prevent a single failure from taking out the whole system). In a daisy chain system, data is passed from BSM-1 to BSM-2 to BSM-3 to BSM-4 and then to the computer. In that type of system, which is analogous to a series of strung Christmas tree lights, a single failure in BSM-4 blocks all data from the other three units. In other words, the entire ICU monitoring system goes down because of a single failure.

The actual data bus between the bedside units might be any one of the following: twisted pair wires, multiconductor wires, coaxial cables (like

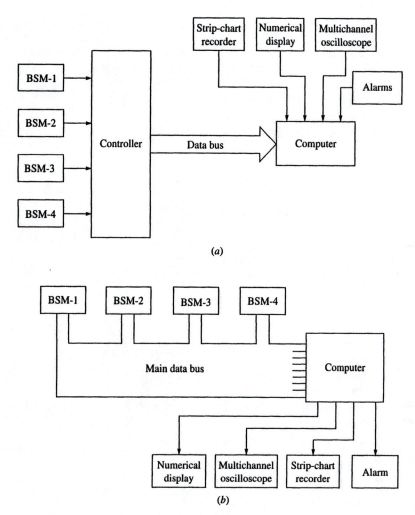

Figure 14-11
Data connection schemes, BSM to central station. *(a)* Local area controller configuration.
(b) Parallel connection configuration.

television antenna cables) for a computer LAN, or special wires.

14-8 ECG and physiological telemetry

Telemetry systems are special CCU patient monitoring systems in which the monitoring function is performed from a remote location. There are two basic forms of telemetry systems: *radio telemetry* and *landline telemetry*. The radio form, which is used in CCU *step-down* units, uses a small radio transmitter attached to the patient that picks up the electrocardiograph (ECG)—or other physiological data—waveform and transmits it via radio waves to a receiver at a central monitoring station. The landline form of telemetry uses an audio tone, or computer-like modem, to represent the analog ECG signal and then transmit it over telephone lines to a central office. We will discuss both forms.

14-8-1 Radio telemetry systems

Many hospitals use radio telemetry systems to monitor certain patients. The most common use of radio telemetry is to keep track of improving cardiac patients and at the same time keep them ambulatory. These units are sometimes called *post-coronary care units* (PCCUs), or *step-down CCUs,* or some other name that indicates a less rigorous monitoring regimen than the full CCU, where new heart patients are treated. The telemetry unit is sort of a "halfway house" between the CCU and either the general medical floor patient population or home care.

The telemetry unit uses a tiny VHF or UHF radio transmitter (Figure 14-12) that is attached to the patient by either a belt clip or a small sack hung around the patient's neck. Most transmitters contain an analog ECG section that acquires the signal and uses it to modulate the frequency of the radio transmitter. The nurses' station is equipped with a bank of radio receivers tuned to the same frequencies as the transmitters. The receiver demodulates the frequency modulation (FM) signal to recover ECG waveform. The waveform is then displayed on an oscilloscope or strip-chart recorder, as in any other patient monitoring system. The signal may also be input to a computerized monitoring system.

It is common practice to use either specialized radio frequencies set aside by the FCC for medical telemetry or unused television channel frequencies. It is not unusual for a telemetry transmitter to operate in the quieted "guard band" between the sound and video carrier of a television signal. These VHF and UHF frequency allocations allow the telemetry system designer to use hardware that was originally designed for the master antenna television (MATV) or cable TV markets to process signals for medical systems.

Figure 14-13 shows the block diagram of a typical analog ECG telemetry system. Several patients (*A, B,* and *C*) are wearing the miniature transmitters that pick up and then transmit the ECG waveform over a VHF or UHF radio fre-

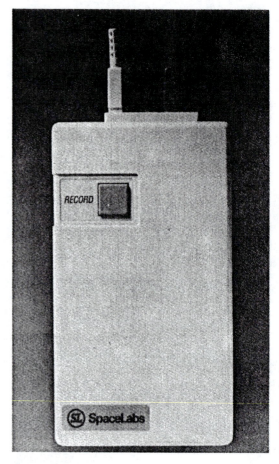

Figure 14-12
UHF ECG telemetry unit.

quency. In each case, a radio receiver picks up and demodulates the signal, recovering the analog waveform. This waveform is output to an oscilloscope display and a pulse rate meter. The pulse rate meter also has a high-rate (tachycardia) alarm and a low-rate (bradycardia) alarm built in. The analog signal is also sent through a patient selection switch to a strip-chart recorder that can provide a hard copy of the waveform for the nurses and doctors who care for the patient.

Some telemetry systems now use an A/D converter inside the transmitter to digitize the analog waveform before transmission. The transmitter

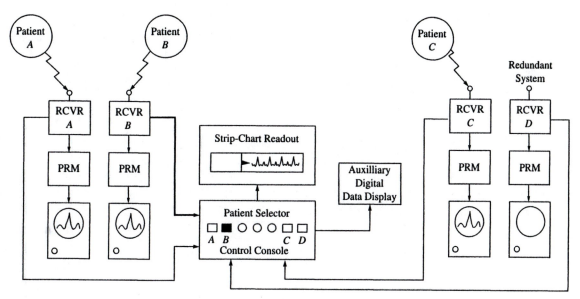

Figure 14-13
Block diagram for an analog ECG telemetry system. PRM = Pulse rate monitor (beats per minute).

then sends a series of tones that represent the ones and zeros of the binary numbers recognized by the computer attached to the receivers.

A practical analog telemetry system is shown in Figure 14-14a. The corridors around the nurses' station are set aside for use by ambulatory patients. However, there are defined limits to the patients' permitted zone of travel. Some hospitals paint the walls of the permitted zone of travel. Some hospitals paint the walls of the permitted area a different color from the rest of the building or use a color-coded stripe on the walls. Other hospitals make no modifications of the paint scheme but rather depend on telling the patient where to stop walking, or rely on a prominent landmark such as a fire door or elevator lobby to limit the zone. The nurses' station is usually located to permit surveillance of all the permitted area in case a patient has problems.

The transmitters carried by the patient are very low-power units, on the order of a few milliwatts at best. Therefore, it is possible for the signal levels to be too low for the receiver, even at a short distance, even though the area permitted for travel is not extensive. As a result, a series of small whip antennas are placed at strategic locations throughout the unit. These antennas usually hang from the false ceilings (Figure 14-14b) in a manner that does not interfere with pedestrian traffic in the corridor.

Even with several antennas in place, however, the losses in the system added to the low power of the original signal conspire to prevent adequate reception. As a result, booster amplifiers (labeled "Amp" in Figure 14-14a) are placed at each antenna site. Gains up to 60 dB are required. These amplifiers are usually selected from MATV and cable TV equipment.

The outputs of the various amplifiers are mixed together in standard VHF/UHF two-set TV couplers ("Coup" in Figure 14-14a). It is common to find ordinary TV receiver couplers in this application. These devices are passive and so will offer losses of −2 to −9 dB.

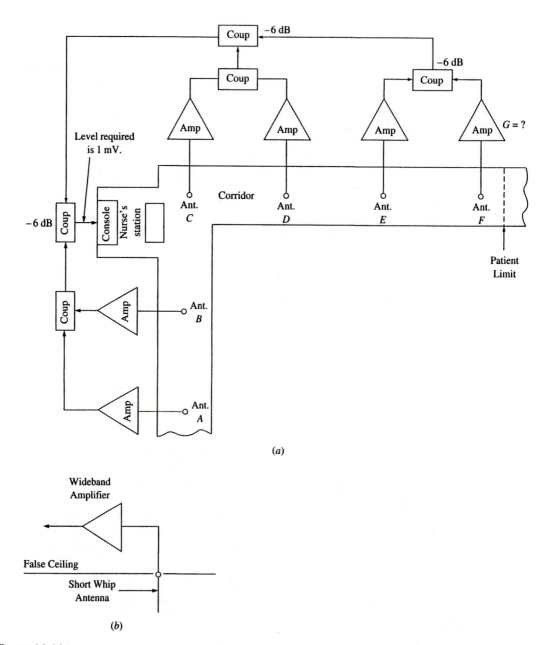

(a)

Wideband
Amplifier

False Ceiling

Short Whip
Antenna

(b)

Figure 14-14
Analog telemetry connection. *(a)* Practical analog telemetry system. *(b)* Antenna installation in
false ceiling.

Some modern ECG telemetry systems are classified as *digital telemetry*. These systems are more sophisticated than analog systems and are freer of fading and signal artifacts than analog systems. Digital technology allows the use of frequency synthesis for the transmitter and receiver, which means that the frequency can be entered for each unit (making them more interchangeable). In addition, complex error correction and checking schemes can be incorporated to ensure proper transmission of the waveform and other data. Some systems incorporate a zone pattern scheme like that of cellular radio (i.e., a unit alters its operation as it travels from one antenna cell to another), a scheme that reduces—some claim eliminates—fading or mutual interference.

14-8-2 Troubleshooting telemetry systems

ECG telemetry systems are like all other hardware systems, so from time to time they malfunction. Some of the faults can be handled directly by the user, while others must be referred to various grades or levels of service shop.

Nurses, emergency medical technicians (EMTs), and other medical personnel can perform several minor troubleshooting tests. First, the patient electrodes and the wires that connect them to the transmitter are usually replaceable by the user, so they can be checked before taking a unit out of service. Second, the battery (which isa common fault) can be replaced on most units by the user (alternatively, a battery charger is used). Finally, it is permissible for users to swap telemetry transmitters and receivers on most systems and therefore restore operation (if on a different channel) by the simple process of elimination. The problem on single-channel systems is that this process does not reveal whether the receiver or the transmitter is at fault.

For routine troubleshooting of the telemetry system by a service technician, much can be said for owning either a TV field strength meter (FSM),

which can also be used for making site surveys before installation or ordering, or a continuously tunable VHF/UHF receiver that covers all of the operating frequencies that might normally be expected to be covered (Figure 14-15). The receiver or FSM can be used to monitor the output of the transmitter to determine whether the transmitter is putting out a signal.

Perhaps the most useful form of service instrument for telemetry equipment is the *spectrum analyzer.* This device is a swept frequency receiver in which the signals received are displayed in the form of amplitude versus frequency. The spectrum analyzer can show output signal strength, its harmonic content, and interactions between two units or a unit and some external signal source. Spectrum analyzers are now less expensive.

Receiver troubleshooting requires a signal generator that covers the frequency of operation. The

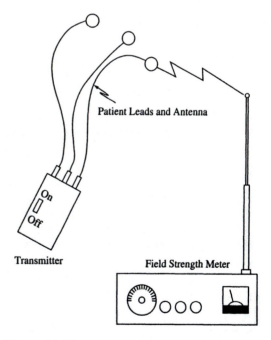

Patient Leads and Antenna

On
Off

Transmitter

Field Strength Meter

Figure 14-15
Using a field strength meter to check ECG telemetry transmitter.

selected instrument should be an FM signal generator that is capable of external modulation so that a low-frequency square wave, simulated ECG from a "chicken heart" generator, or other signal source can be used to modulate the FM output of the generator. The FM signal generator should be capable of deviating at least 25 kHz and preferably the entire range of the deviation expected in the system.

If no FM generator is available, then a common continuous wave (CW) generator can be used by an experienced, knowledgeable technician. The telemetry transmitter can also be used as a signal source, but this approach is fraught with difficulty when it is uncertain whether the receiver or transmitter is at fault.

Also useful for troubleshooting telemetry systems is the usual collection of dc multimeters and oscilloscopes that are needed for all forms of complex electronic service work. However, be aware that most of the faults are "trauma" items, such as broken battery connectors, open switches, and other components that are subject to abuse in normal service.

14-8-3 Portable telemetry units

The increase in emergency medical technicians (EMTs) in the rescue services of local communities gives us an immensely useful tool in dealing with trauma and coronary victims outside the hospital. Although very highly trained, the EMT is not a physician, so some means is often required to communicate physiological data to the local hospital emergency department to be interpreted by a trained physician. In addition, two-way voice communications must be established for the EMT team to converse with and receive instructions from the physician at the hospital. Specialized communications equipment is needed for this.

Figure 14-16 shows a portable telemetry system that has the range and power needed for the EMT or ambulance crew to establish a data link to the hospital. The transmitter might be a special unit, or a modified version of the standard handheld transceivers normally used by fire, police, and other services. The modulating signal, however, is either the analog or digitized ECG. The signal is transmitted over the airwaves to a base station transceiver at the hospital. From there, the demodulation and display is similar to that of other telemetry systems.

Because the size of handheld radio transceivers used for telemetry and voice communications is necessarily very small, the available radio frequency (RF) power is low. As a result, the range is short for these units. When the required range is greater, however, a *repeater* system can be used. At critical locations around the city, receiver sites can pick up a small signal from handheld units. This scheme is commonly used in police and fire communications systems, so it is no great leap in technology to extend it to EMT communications. Another method, shown in Figure 14-17, is to install the repeater on the ambulance or rescue vehicle itself. The handheld unit only has to transmit on frequency F_1 as far as the vehicle, where the signal is picked up and retransmitted at a higher power level on frequency F_2 to the hospital site.

14-8-4 Landline telemetry

It is possible to transmit ECG signals over the telephone lines (called *landlines* in the trade). Both analog and digitized ECG signals can be transmitted. This form of telemetry is used for several purposes. For example, the converted ECG waveforms can be transmitted to a distant location for interpretation by either a computer or a specialist physician.

In other cases, some patients are asked to send in their ECG waveforms on a periodic basis. For example, some cardiac pacemaker clinics ask the patient to start sending in the waveform after so many months, because it is known that an imminent failure of the battery is usually preceded by a sudden shift of heart rate. Because the approximate life expectancy of the battery is known statistically, the monitoring can commence when the

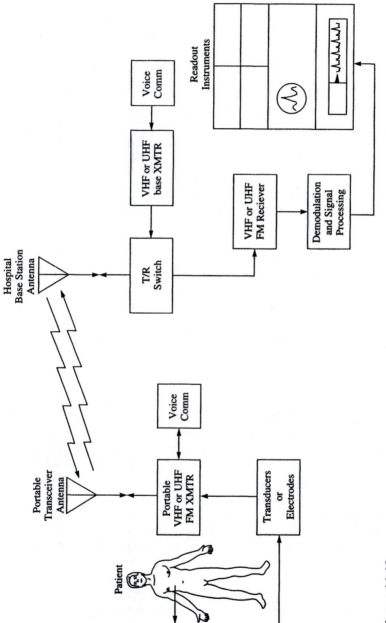

Figure 14-16
Portable telemetry system.

417

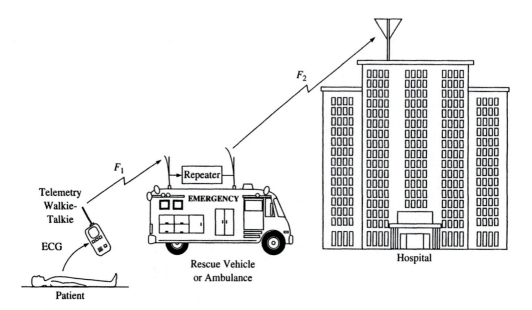

Figure 14-17
Repeater ECG telemetry system.

patient is in the dangerous period between the onset of permanent failure and the routine replacement cycle.

Figure 14-18 shows the block diagram for a typical landline telemetry unit. The basis for this system is a voltage-controlled oscillator (VCO), or digital MODEM, as is used in radio telemetry. The signal will be acquired from ECG electrodes or a photoplethysmograph (PPG) sensor. The waveform is applied to the input of a signal processor (which includes filtering) and the modulator, where it is converted to the audio FM or digital signal. This signal can be recorded on an ordinary audiotape recorder or a digital recorder, or it can be transmitted over telephone lines to the central station.

A digital landline telemetry system is shown in Figure 14-19. This system is similar to those that transmit the ECG waveform from doctors' offices or hospital rooms to a central computer for reading and diagnosis. The analog waveform from the patient is amplified and then digitized in an A/D con-

verter. Also generated is any patient data needed (e.g., name, identification number, social security number, age, physician's name).

The data can be entered in a number of ways, including a standard keyboard. At least one system uses a bar-code scanner that is used to pick up and decode the bar codes on a hospital patient's ID bracelet. The patient data is alphanumeric and thus may be in ASCII format, while the ECG data is binary. The alphanumeric and binary data are combined in a processor, which today usually means a microcomputer. The data is then transmitted to the telephone lines by a MODEM. The MODEM converts the binary bits to corresponding audio tones that will pass through the telephone system.

Another MODEM at the computer end of the landline receives the audio tones and converts them back into binary signals that the computer can read. Software in the computer strips the ECG waveform and various alphanumeric characters and sends them to their respective functions.

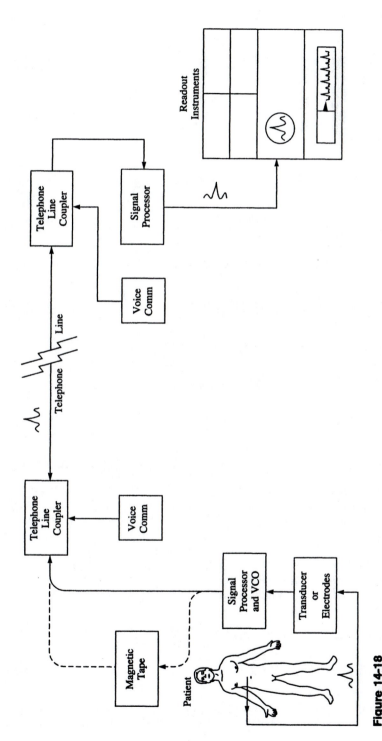

Figure 14-18
Block diagram of an analog landline telemetry system.

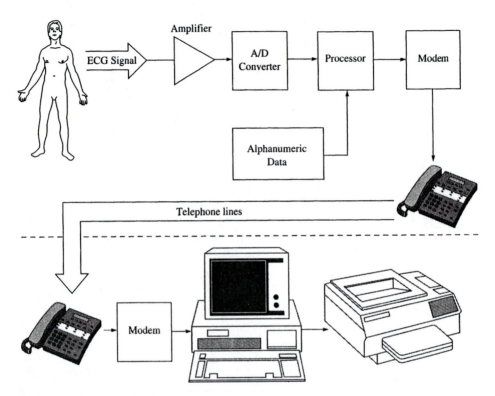

Figure 14-19
Digital landline telemetry system.

14-9 Summary

1. In the ICU and CCU, patients are continuously monitored. All units monitor ECG, and some also monitor pressures, temperatures, and other body functions.

2. The principal instrument is a bedside monitor (BSM), which may be able to monitor the ECG only, or a combination of several physiological parameters.

3. In many units, the ECG and other waveforms, in addition to certain physiological data, are remotely displayed at a central console.

4. Computerized monitoring systems are used to automatically classify and record heart rate, life-threatening or premonitory arrhythmias, and alarm conditions.

14-10 Recapitulation

Now return to the objectives and self-evaluation questions at the beginning of the chapter and see how well you can answer them. If you cannot answer certain questions, place a check mark next to each and review appropriate parts of the text. Next, try to answer the following questions using the same procedure.

Questions

1. Discuss in your own words the purpose and function of an ICU.

2. Each patient's ECG is continuously monitored for _____ and _____ cardiac arrhythmias.

3. List five physiological parameters, other than ECG and heart rate, that might be measured in an ICU or CCU.

4. List four pieces of nonmonitoring equipment often found in the ICU or CCU.

5. Describe a typical bedside monitor.

6. What is the principal difference between *monitoring* and *diagnostic* ECG modes in a bedside monitor?

7. Why are two ECG monitoring modes needed?

8. What is the frequency range of a typical ECG radio telemetry transmitter?

9. List two different types of ECG telemetry transmitter.

10. What is the function of a *cardiotachometer?*

11. Draw a block diagram for, and discuss the operation of, an integrating cardiotachometer.

12. What is a *systole* lamp? What does it indicate?

13. Describe the operation of a digital cardiotachometer.

14. List two types of alarm circuit used in bedside monitors.

15. What is the function of a cardiac memory unit?

16. List two types of cardiac memory unit.

17. Describe in your own words, using diagrams if needed, the operation of a low-frequency tape recorder using FM. Why is it necessary to use an FM recording system?

18. Describe the operation of a lead fault indicator circuit.

19. Draw the block diagram for a digital landline telemetry system.

CHAPTER 15
Operating Rooms

15-1 Objectives

1. Be able to describe the protocols for working in the operating room (OR) suite.
2. Be able to list sterilization techniques.
3. Be able to describe the different types of personnel employed in the OR.
4. Be able to list the different types of surgical specialties.
5. Be able to list and describe special equipment used in the OR.

15-2 Self-evaluation questions

These questions test your prior knowledge of the material in this chapter. Look for the answers as you read the text. After you have finished studying the chapter, try answering these questions and those at the end of the chapter.

1. Why are aseptic working procedures and techniques required in surgery?

2. List four methods for sterilizing surgical instruments.

3. List four types of workers employed in the OR, other than the surgeon.

4. Anesthesia is used to manage _____ in surgical procedures.

5. True or false? You may enter the OR suite (for brief periods only) wearing street clothes.

15-3 Surgery

Three challenges of surgery are *pain* associated with cutting into the body, the tendency to *bleed,* and the problem of *infection.*

Pain is managed by the use of anesthesia agents that put the patient to sleep or, alternatively, deaden sensation in the region where the surgeon is working.

The bleeding is managed mainly by the practices of the surgeon, who must continually stop bleeding as it occurs during the procedure. The surgeon will tie off cut blood vessels with su-

422

ture or cauterize them with an electrical device called an *electrosurgery machine* (discussed in chapter 18).

Infection is caused by microorganisms that exist almost everywhere on earth. In past centuries, before the role of these microorganisms in infection was discovered and before the introduction of drugs that fight infection, surgery was considerably more dangerous than it is now. Many patients survived an operation only to succumb to an infection a little later. Today, however, the threat of infection is reduced by the use of antibiotic drugs and aseptic techniques in the OR.

Aseptic technique requires that a zone be created surrounding the operation site that is essentially free of microorganisms. The surgeon and any assistants wash their hands extensively and then are dressed in a sterile gown and wear sterile gloves. All instruments used during the procedure have been sterilized. Those instruments capable of withstanding high temperatures and humidity are steam-sterilized in an *autoclave,* and more sensitive devices are gas-sterilized in an ethylene oxide atmosphere (see section 15-6).

All personnel in the OR must wear special clothing provided by the hospital (i.e., scrub suits). These garments are not sterile but are well laundered. Their use is to limit the introduction of microorganisms from outside. Although the specific dress codes vary slightly from one hospital to another, it is never proper to wear street clothes in an OR suite, even for a few seconds. Before you enter the OR suite, you must go to an appropriate locker room and change clothes. If you are not sure of the dress code in any particular hospital, then ask somebody to explain it to you.

15-4 Types of surgery

The use of surgical techniques is found in general surgery, several surgical specialties, and other areas of medicine in which surgery is but one of several different treatment options. Dentists also perform *oral surgery* in hospital operating rooms. Several specialty areas are as follows:

1. *Ophthalmology*—treats diseases of the eye by various methods, including surgery.

2. *Otolaryngology*—treats diseases of the ear, nose, and throat using various techniques, including surgery.

3. *Orthopedics*—treats diseases of the bones, joints, and other locomotor organs and structures, often surgically.

4. *Neurosurgery*—treats certain diseases of the brain and nervous system using surgical techniques.

5. *Thoracic surgery*—surgical specialty that performs operations to treat diseases of the organs in the chest cavity.

6. *Urology*—treats diseases of the urinary system using various techniques, including surgery.

7. *Obstetrics*—manages pregnancy and delivers babies.

8. *Gynecology*—treats diseases of the female reproductive system using various techniques, including surgery. Many physicians in this specialty area are also obstetricians.

15-5 OR personnel

The *surgeon* is a physician who has been trained beyond medical school in the art of performing operations and the postsurgical management of the patient's recovery. In many, perhaps most, states any licensed physician may legally perform surgery. But most large hospitals require additional training in a residency program, if not board certification of the physician as a surgeon. There may also be another physician assisting the surgeon, very often a resident or an intern.

The anesthesia agent is administered and managed either by a specially trained physician called an *anesthesiologist,* or a nurse trained in anesthesia called a *nurse anesthetist* or, simply, *anesthetist.* Some nurse anesthetists who pass a certification procedure are called *certified registered nurse anesthetists* (CRNA).

At least two other persons are assigned to each case. A *circulating nurse* (usually an RN) is outside of the sterile zone and performs various services, including (but certainly not limited to) keeping records, obtaining supplies, and preparing drugs. Because of the drugs and certain medical-legal problems, most hospitals require an RN in the circulator's position.

The *scrub nurse* may be an RN, a licensed practical nurse (LPN), or an OR technician. This person works in the sterile zone and must follow the same antiseptic rules as the surgeon. The scrub nurse or technician is responsible for keeping the instruments, tools, and supplies straight. This job is not similar to that of the so-called mechanic's helper, who merely hands tools to the mechanic, but is a skilled job in its own right and is often done by registered nurses.

Anesthesia technicians assist the anesthesiologists and anesthetists by bringing supplies, running errands during the procedure, and cleaning or maintaining the anesthesia machines and related equipment after the day's case load is finished.

Monitoring technicians operate the physiological monitoring equipment, such as pressure monitors and ECG machines. These people may have a minimal skill level or may be indistinguishable from cardiovascular technicians.

The *cardiovascular technician* is trained to operate and perform elementary maintenance on a wide variety of physiological monitoring and measurement equipment, intraaortic balloon pumps, heart-lung machines, blood gas machines, and so forth. Cardiovascular technicians who mainly operate the heart-lung machine are sometimes called *perfusionists* or *perfusion technicians*.

Orderlies and *nursing assistants* perform menial to semiskilled work in the OR, usually under the direct supervision of an RN or other personnel.

15-6 Sterilization

Sterilization is the process of killing microorganisms on tools, instruments, and other objects used in surgery. It is also applied to linen and clothing,

and in some cases, to objects and tools that are not normally used in surgery or other sterile fields to prevent the spread of disease from one patient to another as the tool is used. Blood pressure transducers (those not using sterile disposable domes) and certain equipment in respiratory therapy, for example, are not used in a sterile environment but could possibly spread pathogenic (disease-causing) microorganisms among patients.

Several different methods are used for sterilization: *steam heat, dry heat, gas, liquid,* and *radiation.*

Steam sterilization is done in a device called a *steam autoclave,* which is a pressure lock chamber of rather substantial construction. Temperatures inside of an autoclave are in excess of 100°C (212°F), so the pressure must also be elevated. Never attempt to operate or service a steam autoclave without first receiving instructions for that particular model. In some localities, a steam "engineer's" license is required of anyone who services the autoclave.

The objects being sterilized are wrapped in a double thickness of linen or other suitable material that is porous to pressurized steam. They are then loosely packed with other such bundles inside the autoclave chamber. There are three periods of the steam sterilization cycle:

1. *Vacuum period*—The air is withdrawn from the sealed autoclave chamber, producing a vacuum.

2. *Sterilization period*—Superheated (over 100°C) steam is introduced into the chamber. The temperature will be either 120°C for 15 min or 144°C for 2 min. These temperatures correspond to pressures of 10^5 Pa (1 atm) and 3×10^5 Pa (3 atm), respectively.

3. *Poststerilization period*—The steam is withdrawn, allowing the wrapped packs to dry before readmitting room air and unlocking the door.

A special tape is applied to the wrapped packs, and special indicator strips are placed inside the pack to give the user an indication of whether the sterilization process was completed. There are marks on these indicators that become visible or change color when sterilized. Most autoclaved bundles can be stored for a considerable length of time provided that they are not opened or become damp. The efficacy of the autoclave is checked periodically by sterilizing a *spore strip*. After the process, the strip is sent to the laboratory in a sterile container. It is placed in an incubator that allows any live spores (those not killed in the autoclave) to grow and reproduce.

The use of dry heat allows sterilization in room air, at room pressures. The dry heat process requires that objects or bundles be in an environment with temperatures of 160°C for 120 min, 170°C for 60 min, or 180°C for 30 min. Dry heat is considered to be less effective than steam sterilization.

Gas sterilization uses *formalin* gas, or more commonly, *ethylene oxide* gas. The wrapped bundles are exposed to the gas for 10 to 12 hours and then must be allowed to vent for 24 hours or more to get rid of gas residue. Gas sterilizers are typically more difficult to use than are steam or dry heat models. As a result, many hospitals place steam and dry heat sterilizers in the OR suite and send objects requiring gas sterilization to a central supply department.

Gas methods are used to sterilize objects that cannot withstand the high temperatures of the steam and dry heat methods but can tolerate the 30 to 60°C temperatures used in the gas autoclave. Typically, plastics, rubbers, synthetics, fabrics, and certain sharp-edged metal objects that become dull in high-temperature environments are candidates for gas sterilization. Occasionally, a question arises as to whether certain objects are immune to reaction with the gas used in the process because they seem to deteriorate rapidly under gas sterilization.

Several antiseptic liquids can be used to sterilize objects. The object is left immersed in the liquid for periods ranging from 30 min to several hours, depending upon the type of solution and the nature of the object being sterilized.

Ionizing radiation (gamma and X-rays from a cobalt-60 source) can also be used for sterilizing objects. The object must be exposed to the radiation for as long as 24 hours, so the process is used primarily in industrial situations in which the high degree of sterilization of medical products being manufactured requires and justifies the radiation equipment.

15-7 OR equipment

The range of medical equipment found in various ORs depends on several factors, such as the types of surgery performed, the physician's preferences, and the level of activity. There are, however, certain items that are found in all ORs.

Electrosurgery (ES) *machines* (see chapter 18) are radio frequency ac generators that produce currents of the intensity needed to cut tissue and cauterize bleeding blood vessels. These machines are commonly, if erroneously, called *Bovies* after the inventor. But the word *Bovie* is the brand name of one of the oldest producers of ES equipment, Liebel-Flarshiem. The word has become, however, a generic term in jargon.

Light sources are used with fiber-optic endoscopes to view inside the patient's body through certain openings or surgical incisions. They are also used to illuminate the surgeon's head lamp. Most light sources are quartz-halogen lamps, either 110 or 21 V.

Suction apparatus is used to remove blood, mucus, and other material from the patient's body and mouth or the surgical wound. The suction device usually has a bottle to hold the material that is removed but may be powered by either its own compressor or a vacuum port in the OR wall.

Anesthesia machines are used to control and deliver oxygen and the anesthesia gas to the patient. It is not wise to attempt to work on these machines without training in that area. While they are not terribly complicated, they can be an issue in a malpractice case.

Most hospitals now routinely use ECG and blood pressure monitors during surgical procedures. These instruments are essentially the same as those devices discussed in chapters 3 through 8.

15-8 Summary

1. Three problems in all surgery are *pain, bleeding,* and *infection.*

2. *Aseptic* techniques and working practices are designed to reduce the incidence of infection.

3. The most commonly used forms of sterilization are *steam heat, dry heat, gas, liquid,* and *radiation.*

4. Anesthesia agents are administered by either a physician (called an *anesthesiologist*) or a *nurse anesthetist.*

15-9 Recapitulation

Now return to the objectives and self-evaluation questions at the beginning of the chapter and see how well you can answer them. If you cannot answer certain questions, place a check mark next to each and review appropriate parts of the text. Next, try to answer the following questions, using the same procedure.

Questions

1. Three problems common to all surgery are _____, _____, and _____.

2. Pain is managed by _____ agents administered by an _____ (MD) or _____ (nurse).

3. List two practices used to control bleeding during surgery.

4. Infection is controlled through the use of _____ drugs and _____ techniques.

5. List five medical or surgical specialties that use surgical treatment as all or part of their repertoire.

6. The _____ nurse works in the sterile zone, while the _____ nurse works outside of the zone.

7. List four types of sterilization for objects used in the OR.

8. In a steam autoclave, the temperature is raised to _____ °C for 15 min or _____ °C for 2 min.

9. In a dry heat autoclave, the temperature is maintained at _____ °C for 2 hours, _____ °C for 1 hour, or _____ °C for 30 min.

10. Ethylene oxide autoclaves operate at a temperature between _____ °C and _____ °C.

CHAPTER 16
Medical Laboratory Instrumentation

16-1 Objectives

1. Be able to state the purpose of blood.
2. Be able to list the components and describe the composition of blood.
3. Be able to list and describe blood tests (cells and chemistry).
4. Be able to state the purpose, uses, principle of operation, and maintenance of the following equipment: colorimeter, densitometer, flame photometer, spectrophotometer, blood cell counter, blood gas analyzers (pH, Po_2, and Pco_2), chromatograph, and autoanalyzers.
5. Be able to describe renal physiology, including types of renal failure and the hemodialysis machine operation, safety, and maintenance.

16-2 Self-evaluation questions

These questions test your prior knowledge of the material in this chapter. Look for the answers as you read the text. After you have finished studying the chapter, try answering these questions and those at the end of the chapter.

1. Define *blood* and state its purposes.

2. Name the components of blood (cells and plasma).

3. What is the difference between blood cell tests and blood chemistry analysis?

4. Why is the medical laboratory department of critical importance in diagnosing the disease and treating the patient?

5. Describe the principle of operation and maintenance of the colorimeter, flame photometer, spectrophotometer, blood cell analyzer, blood gas analyzer (pH, Po_2, and Pco_2), chromatograph, autoanalyzer, and hemodialysis machine.

16-3 Blood (purpose and components)

Blood is the fluid that circulates through the heart, arteries, veins, and capillaries, carrying nourishment, electrolytes, hormones, vitamins, antibodies, heat, and oxygen to body tissues and taking away waste matter and carbon dioxide.

Whole blood, as shown in Figure 16-1, is composed of *cells* and *plasma* (fluid containing dissolved and suspended substances). The *blood cell portion* consists of the following elements:

1. *Red blood cells* (RBCs) or *erythrocytes*—these are concave, disc-shaped cells (8 μ long, 3 μ wide) that contain no nucleus and live about 120 days before being replaced by the bone marrow. Their number is 4.5 to 5.5×10^6 cells/mm^3. Internally, each RBC contains four iron atoms in a structure known as the

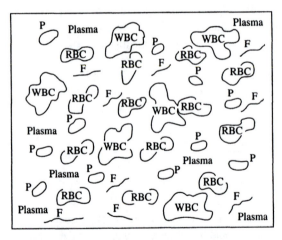

Figure 16-1
Whole blood composed of cells and plasma. RBC—red blood cell. 4.5–5.5 × 10^6 cells/mm^3, 8 × 3 μ, no nucleus, 120-day life. WBC—white blood cell. 6–10 × 10^3 cells/mm^3, 10 μ diam., nucleus, 15-day life. P—platelet cell. 200–800 × 10^3 cells/mm^3, μ diam., no nucleus. F—fibrinogen protein. Plasma—fluid portion. Inorganic and organic substances dissolved in H$_2$O. Whole blood = RBC + WBC + P + F + plasma. Plasma = whole blood − (RBC + WBC + P). Serum = plasma − fibrinogen.

hemoglobin molecule. Oxygen from the lung alveoli enters the bloodstream and chemically combines with hemoglobin to form *oxyhemoglobin.* RBCs transport oxygen to the tissues and pick up carbon dioxide to form *carbaminohemoglobin.*

2. *White blood cells (WBCs) or leukocytes*—these are amoebalike cells (10 μ in diameter) that contain a nucleus and live from 13 to 20 days. Their number is 6 to 10×10^3 cells/mm^3. They are also present in the lymph fluid and engulf invading bacteria and foreign substances to destroy the invaders' effect. For example, bacteria invading the leg are encapsulated by WBCs in the lymph fluid, transported to the inferior vena cava, circulated through the right atrium/ventricle, through the lungs to the left atrium/ventricle, and pumped to the kidneys, where they are extracted in the urine. They are then excreted from the body as harmless cell fragments. Specific *antibodies* are also produced to kill the invaders' *antigen* (toxin).

3. *Platelets*—these are cell fragments (3 μ in diameter) that contain no nucleus. Their number is 200 to 800×10^3 cells/mm^3. These form a repair substance that initiates blood coagulation and clotting. A protein, *thrombin,* also acts on *fibrinogen* (soluble protein formed in the liver) to generate insoluble *fibrin.* Fibrin deposits as fine threads to form the framework of the blood clot. *Platelets* cling to intersections of fibrin threads. As fibrinogen is used up, serum is secreted. *Serum* will not clot, as it contains no fibrinogen.

Blood plasma consists of the following elements:

1. *Plasma proteins*—organic *repair* substances. These are *albumins* (synthesized in the liver) that help regulate plasma/tissue cell osmotic pressure. *Fibrinogen* and *prothrombin* are used in the clotting process. *Globulin* substances (alpha, beta, and gamma) are catalysts and aid in the immunizing (disease protection) process.

2. *Plasma nutrients—energy-storing* substances. These are *glucose* (blood sugar), *lipids* (fats), and *amino acids* (proteins for tissue growth).

3. *Regulatory and protective substances—* these are *enzymes* (catalysts for digestion and cell metabolism), *hormones* (stimulatory/ inhibitory function to target organs), and *antibodies* (providing immunity against infection).

4. *Plasma electrolytes—*acid-base and *nerve-impulse* transmission substances. These are inorganic salts (metal and nonmetal combination) and pure chemical substances (Na^+, K^+, Cl^-).

5. *Metabolic waste substances—these include* urea and *uric acid* waste from the kidneys and carbon dioxide waste from cellular metabolism.

Figure 16-2 shows blood that has been spun in a centrifuge (motor-driven mechanical device that generates a circular motion). A centrifuge is shown in Figure 16-3. Since the RBCs are the heaviest, they sink to the bottom and form 45% of the total by volume. Plasma occupies 55%. Blood plasma does contain some dissolved oxygen, but 97% of the transported oxygen is carried in the RBC hemoglobin molecules. During its passage through the body, blood hemoglobin still remains 70% oxygen-saturated per the oxygen dissociation curve. The total carbon dioxide carried by the blood is 30% in the RBCs and 60% in the blood plasma.

The body functions as a biological machine that receives life-giving input substances of oxygen and food nutrients and gives off waste substances. All living creatures typically display the characteristics of *organization* (life process control),

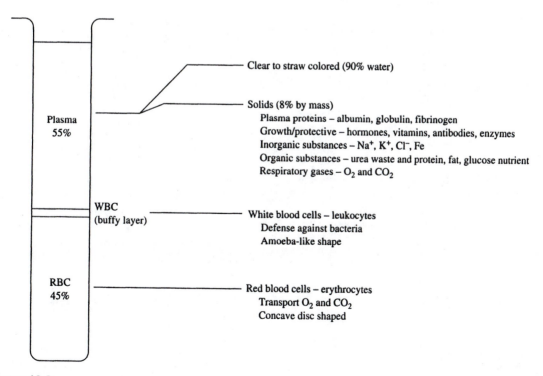

Clear to straw colored (90% water)

Solids (8% by mass)
Plasma proteins – albumin, globulin, fibrinogen
Growth/protective – hormones, vitamins, antibodies, enzymes
Inorganic substances – Na^+, K^+, Cl^-, Fe
Organic substances – urea waste and protein, fat, glucose nutrient
Respiratory gases – O_2 and CO_2

White blood cells – leukocytes
Defense against bacteria
Amoeba-like shape

Red blood cells – erythrocytes
Transport O_2 and CO_2
Concave disc shaped

Plasma 55%

WBC (buffy layer)

RBC 45%

Figure 16-2
Blood that has been spun in a centrifuge.

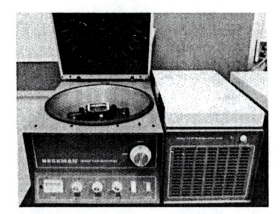

Figure 16-3
Refrigerated centrifuge.

irritability (response to change), *contractility* (movement), *nutrition* (ingestion and digestion of food), *metabolism* and *growth* (liberation of stored chemical energy), *respiration* (intake of O_2 and ventilation of CO_2), *excretion* (elimination of waste), and *reproduction* (generation of a new structure).

Metabolism is the sum total of all chemical and biochemical processes in the body. It involves *catabolism* (breaking down of complex protein and sugar substances to simpler ones) and *anabolism* (building up of complex substances for body use). Waste products from the digestive process are eliminated in the feces. Toxic substances that result from metabolic processes are removed from the blood by the kidneys and excreted in the urine.

The purpose of *medical laboratory instrumentation* is to provide a means of measuring required substances and metabolic waste products in urine and blood.

16-4 Blood tests (cells and chemistry)

Blood cell tests include the following elements:

1. *RBC count*—accomplished manually (diluting a blood sample 100:1 and counting the cells per cubic millimeter by use of a microscope) or automatically (blood cell counting analyzers).

2. *WBC count*—accomplished manually (10:1 dilution) or automatically (blood cell analyzer).

3. *Platelet count*—accomplished automatically by a blood cell analyzer.

4. *Hematocrit (Hct)*—percentage of total blood volume that is solid (WBC volume is negligible). This is measured by spinning a blood sample in a test tube and optically observing the percentage of packed RBCs (Figure 16-2). It normally ranges from 45% to 55%.

5. *Mean cell (corpuscular) volume (MCV)—average volume* of an RBC measured by a value based on the RBC count (number per mm^3). This volume is measured in femtoliters $(10^{-15}$ L).

$$MCV = \frac{Hct}{RBC} \qquad (16\text{-}1)$$

6. *Mean cell hemoglobin (MCH)*—the *proportional mass* of RBC/100 mL to the total number of RBCs is expressed as:

$$MCHC = \frac{\text{hemoglobin in grams/100 mL}}{Hct} \qquad (16\text{-}2)$$

This value is indicated in picograms $(10^{-12}$ g).

7. *Mean cell hemoglobin concentration (MCHC)*—hemoglobin *color concentration* measured by lysing RBCs (breaking their membranes) to release hemoglobin. Acid hematin or cyanmethemoglobin can be generated by hemoglobin chemical reaction. The resultant value is measured by a colorimeter and normally indicates 32% to 36% color index.

$$MCHC = \frac{\text{hemoglobin in grams/100 mL}}{Hct} \qquad (16\text{-}3)$$

Blood chemical tests check for amounts of *acidity*—pH normally 7.36 to 7.44 (blood is normally slightly alkaline); *glucose*—lactic acid, lactose sugar; *nonprotein nitrogen substances*—

amino acids, peptides, urea waste, and uric acid; *lipids*—fatty acids of cholesterol and triglycerides; *proteins*—plasma albumin, globulins, and fibrinogen; and *enzymes and steroids,* among other elements.

Blood serological tests involve testing for agglutination (clumping) of cells due to the addition of *antigens* (bacterial toxins) to blood serum. This occurs following thethe reaction of a specific *antibody* produced by WBCs in response to the specific invader.

Blood bacteriological tests include growth of blood bacteria in a petri dish with appropriate nutrients.

Historical tests are studies of small, thin tissue samples under the microscope. Specimens are obtained by cutting tissues with a precision slicer known as a *microtome.*

16-5 Medical laboratory department

The *medical laboratory department* includes facilities, personnel, and equipment within the hospital or public or private location. The facilities must include a clean, safe surrounding with a special area for sterilization of contaminated blood urine samples and equipment. Since high-volume blood testing occurs in this department, sufficient storage and cleaning areas must be designated. In such a situation, the chance of error (misreading or a patient record mixup) is high.

Medical laboratory *personnel* include equipment operators (medical technologists), supervisors, and physicians. The director of these facilities is usually a physician.

Equipment contained in the laboratory includes glassware, centrifuges, suction devices, and sophisticated instrumentation, such as colorimeters, spectrophotometers, blood cell and gas analyzers, chromatographs, autoanalyzers, and computer-based record and operation systems.

Recordkeeping is extremely important. This information is used by physicians as an aid in diagnosing disease and imbalanced physiological

states. Standard cards with printouts of RBC or WBC counts, Hct, MCV, MCHC, and blood chemistry are presented by most clinical instrumentation.

16-6 Overview of clinical instrumentation

Clinical instrumentation in the early 1900s was almost nonexistent. Since the 1950s, sophisticated apparatus has been developed to measure blood parameters, as described in section 16-4. The complex substances appearing in blood serum can be evaluated for concentration based on chemical color reactions. Blood cells can be counted by electrical conductivity changes as they pass through a fixed diameter aperture. The following types of instrumentation are used to analyze blood:

1. *Colorimeter* or *filter photometer* is an optical electronic device that measures the color concentration of a substance in solution (following the reaction between the original substance and a reagent). The results are displayed in percentage of optical color transmittance or absorbance to indicate hemoglobin concentration, for example. The *densitometer* is a device similar to the colorimeter and measures optical transmittance (density) of particles in fluid suspension.

2. *Flame photometer* is an optical electronic device that measures the color intensity of substances (i.e., sodium or potassium) that have been aspirated into a flame.

3. *Spectrophotometer* is an optical electronic device that measures light absorption at various wavelengths for a given liquid sample. This is a type of sophisticated colorimeter.

4. *Blood cell analyzer* is a device that measures the number of red and white blood cells per scaled volume. This is accomplished in either of two ways. The *aperture impedance* method looks at the change in electrical impedance as

cells pass through a fixed diameter opening, while the *flow cytometry* method uses the scattering of light from a laser source.

5. *pH* and *blood gas analyzer* is a device which measures blood pH (acid-base balance), P_{O_2} (partial pressure of blood oxygen), and P_{CO_2} (partialoxygen), and $P;I_{CO_2}$ (partical pressure of blood carbon dioxide). This is accomplished through use of glass electrode transducers.

6. *Chromatograph* is an electromechanical device used to separate, identify, and measure the concentration of substances in a liquid medium. Results are displayed as colored bands in a liquid column or as colored strips on paper.

7. *Autoanalyzer* is an electromechanical-electronic device that sequentially measures and displays blood chemistry analysis. This is accomplished by use of mixing tubes and colorimeters arranged in a serial system connection.

16-7 Colorimeter

The *colorimeter,* shown in Figure 16-4, is a filter photometer that measures the color concentration of a substance in solution. This is accomplished electronically by detecting the color light intensity passing through a sample containing the reaction products of the original substance and a reagent. A yellow urine sample, for example, passes yellow

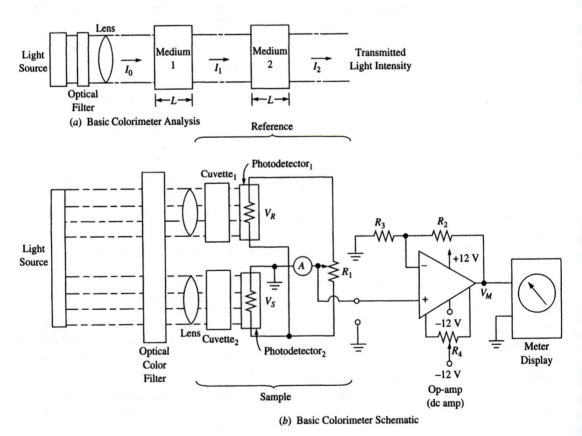

(*a*) Basic Colorimeter Analysis

(*b*) Basic Colorimeter Schematic

Figure 16-4
Colorimeter—filter photometer. (*a*) Basic colorimeter analysis. (*b*) Basic colorimeter schematic.

light and absorbs blue and green. For this reason, and to obtain purity in measurement, optical color filters are used to select a narrow wavelength spread (bandwidth) of light that shines on the photodetectors. Laser light-emitting diodes are also used and are preferred if the wavelength is suitable because of the inherent monochromaticity of light emitted.

Basic colorimeter analysis (Figure 16-4a) involves the precise measurement of light intensity. Transmittance is defined as:

$$T = \frac{I_1}{I_0} \times 100\% \qquad (16\text{-}4a)$$

also
$$I_2 = TI_1 \qquad (16\text{-}4b)$$

then
$$I_2 = T^2I_0 \qquad (16\text{-}4c)$$

I_0 is initial light intensity

I_1 is first attenuated light intensity

I_2 is second attenuated light intensity

T is transmittance in percent

Absorbance (optical density) is defined as:

$$A = \log\frac{I_0}{I_1} = \log\frac{1}{T} \qquad (16\text{-}5)$$

where

A is absorbance

I_1 and I_2 are as before

If the path length or concentration increases, the transmittance decreases and the absorbance increases. Essentially, this phenomenon can be expressed by *Beer's law:*

$$A = aCL \qquad (16\text{-}6)$$

where

A is absorbance

L is cuvette path length

C is concentration of absorbing substance

a is absorbtivity related to the nature of the absorbing substance and optical wavelength (known for a standard solution concentration)

Therefore, the concentration of the unknown solution can be found from the following relationship:

$$C\mu = Cs\,\frac{A_\mu}{A_s} \qquad (16\text{-}7)$$

where

C_μ is unknown concentration

C_s standard concentration (for calibration)

A_μ is unknown absorbance

A_s is standard absorbance

A *basic colorimeter schematic* is shown in Figure 16-4b. Observe that light passes through an optical color filter, is focused by lenses on the reference and sample cuvettes, and falls on the reference and sample photodetectors. The difference in voltage between the two detectors is increased by a dc amplifier and applied to a meter. A *calibration procedure* is as follows:

1. Ground the amplifier input (V_1) and adjust potentiometer (R_4) and adjust potentiometer (R_4) for 0 V $\pm$ 5 mV at the amplifier output.

2. Remove the ground and place reference concentrations in cuvettes 1 and 2 (empty cuvettes or open spaces may also be used).

3. Adjust potentiometer (R_1) for 0 V $\pm$ 10 mV at the amplifier output.

4. Leave the reference concentration in cuvette 1 and replace cuvette 2 with a cuvette containing the sample.

5. Read the unbalanced voltage on the meter in percentage of transmittance or absorbance units.

A photo of a colorimeter is shown in Figure 16-5.

Example 16-1

(Refer to Figure 16-4b)

Given $V_1 = +1$ mV with reference cuvettes (step 3 in calibration procedure), $V_1 = +25$ mV with

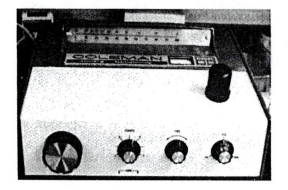

Figure 16-5
Colorimeter.

reference and sample cuvettes (step 5 in calibra-tion procedure), $R_2 = 2k\Omega$, $R_3 = 1$ kΩ, *calculate* the voltage read on the meter display for both con-ditions of V_1. (Noninverting op-amp voltage gain.)

$$A_r = 1 + \frac{R_2}{R_3}$$

$$A_v = 3 = 1 + \frac{2\text{ k}\Omega}{1\text{ k}\Omega} = 3 \qquad (16\text{-}8)$$

Condition 1:

$$V_1 = +1\text{ mV} \qquad (16\text{-}9)$$

$$A_v = \frac{V_m}{V_1} \qquad (16\text{-}10)$$

$$V_m = A_v V_1 = 3\,(+1\text{ mV})$$
$$V_m = \textbf{+3 mV}$$

Condition 2:

$$V_1 = +25\text{ mV} = A_v V_1$$
$$V_m = 3(+25\text{ mV})$$
$$V_m = \textbf{+75 mV}$$

Note that the sample measurement (balanced) volt-age is 25 times larger than the reference measure-ment (unbalanced) voltage. This is a desirable low-error situation.

Precipitating reagents are usually mixed with samples to remove substances from the sample.

TABLE 16-1   COMMON CHEMICAL BLOOD TESTS AND NORMAL RANGES

Test	Normal range	Units
Sodium	135–145	mEq/L*
Potassium	3.5–5	"
Chloride	95–105	"
Total CO_2	24–32	"
Blood urea nitrogen	8–16	mg/100 mL
Glucose	70–90	mg/100 mL
Inorganic phosphate	3–4.5	"
Calcium	9–11.5	"
Creatine	0.6–1.1	"
Uric acid	3–6	"
Total protein	6–8	g/100 mL
Albumin	4–6	"
Cholesterol	160–200	mg/100 mL
Bilirubin	0.2–1	"
SGOT	20–50	mU/mL

$$*\ \frac{1\text{ mEq}}{\text{L}} = \frac{\text{concentration}\left(\frac{\text{mg}}{\text{L}}\right)}{\text{molecular weight}}$$

Table 16-1 shows common chemical tests and their normal ranges.

Maintenance includes calibration adjustment and replacement of burned-out lamps and photode-tectors. Colorimeters are very reliable and usually do not often have electronic problems.

16-8 Flame photometer

The *flame photometer,* shown in Figure 16-6, measures the color intensity of a flame that is supported by oxygen and a specific substance. The basic schematic shows that a reference gas containing a *lithium salt* causes a *red light* to shine on the *reference photodetector* through the reference optical filter. A yellow or violet light from sample sodium or potassium falls on the *sample photodetector.* Basically, the flame pho-tometer is *calibrated* in a manner similar to that of the colorimeter. However, continuous calibration can be accomplished by inspiration of air (oxygen

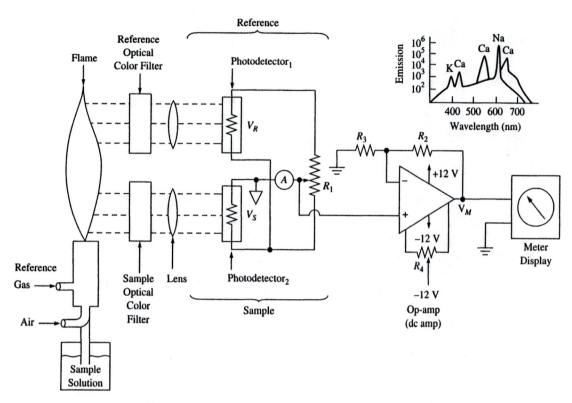

Figure 16-6
Flame photometer—simplified schematic.

to support combustion) and lithium. The output is read in units of sodium or potassium concentration. A photo of a flame photometer is shown in Figure 16-7.

   Maintenance includes calibration adjustment and replacement of bulbs and photodetectors. Aspiration devices and flame chambers occasionally require cleaning. Electronic failures are usually infrequent.

16-9 Spectrophotometer

The *spectrophotometer,* as shown in Figure 16-8, measures light absorption by a liquid substance at various wavelengths. Form this, the components of an unknown material can be determined, or the concentration of a number of known substances can be measured. A *monochromator* uses a diffrac-

tion grating or prism to disperse the light from the lamp (slit S_1). The light is broken into its spectral components as it arises from slit S_2 and falls on the sample in the cuvette. Narrower slits give rise to shorter wavelengths. The angle of the diffraction grating determines light wavelength if all other parameters are fixed and the mirror reduces equipment size. Light output, photodetector sensitivity, and sample substance absorption change with wavelength, and this necessitates zero calibration for each wavelength measurement. The *double-bean* spectrophotometer accomplishes this automatically by beam path switching (sample to reference) via a mechanical shutter or rotating mirror. The ratio of path absorbances can then be computed. Figure 16-9 shows a photograph of a spectrophotometer with input sample to the left and output graph to the right.

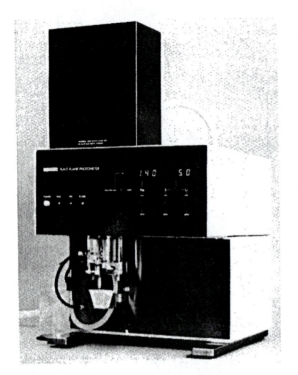

Figure 16-7
Flame photometer. (Courtesy of The London Co.)

Maintenance includes calibration adjustment and replacement of light source bulbs and photodetectors. Also, mechanically rotating assemblies (mirrors, diffraction grating) occasionally malfunction. The electronics, however, are very reliable.

16-10 Blood cell counters

The blood cell counters count the number of RBCs or WBCs per unit of volume of blood using either of two methods: an electrical method called *aperture impedance change* and an optical method called *flow cytometry*.

16-10-1 Aperture impedance change (ΔR_A) counters

The *aperture impedance* method of counting blood cells depends on the fact that, when blood is diluted in the proper type of solution, the electrical

resistivity of blood cells (ρ_c) is higher than the resistivity of the surrounding fluid (ρ_f). By contriving a situation in which these resistivities can be differentiated from each other, we can count cells.

Figure 16-10 shows the basic sensing cell that allows us to make use of that fact. The original impedance aperture cell counter was in an instrument called the Coulter counter, after its inventor and the company that produced it. The sensor consists of a two-chamber vessel in which the dilute incoming blood is on one side of a barrier, and the waste blood to be discarded is on the other. A hole with a small diameter (50 μm) is placed in the partition between the two halves of the cell. A pair of electrodes from an ohmmeter are placed, one in each chamber, so that the resistance of the path through the hole is measured. When no blood cell is in the aperture (Figure 16-10a), this resistance is:

$$R = \frac{\rho_f L}{A} \qquad (16\text{-}11)$$

where

R is the resistance in ohms (Ω)

ρ_f is the resistivity of the fluid (Ω-cm)

L is the length of the path (cm)

A is the cross-sectional area of the aperture (cm)

Under the condition in which no blood cell is in the aperture, the resistance of the path is low, and is so indicated on the ohmmeter. But when the aperture is filled with a blood cell, which has a significantly higher resistivity, the resistance of the path rises sharply (Figure 16-10b). The change of resistance (R) is described by:

$$\Delta R = Kv\left[1 + \frac{4X}{5} + \frac{843\,X^2}{1120} + \cdots \right] \qquad (16\text{-}11a)$$

where

K is the ratio of the aperture resistance to its volume

v is the volume of the sphere (e.g., blood cell) being measured

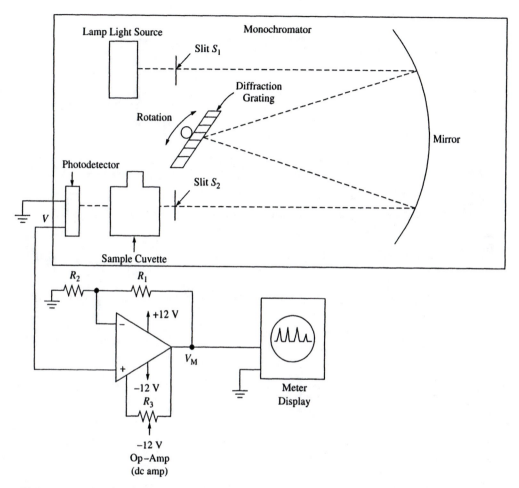

Figure 16-8
Spectrophotometer—simplified schematic.

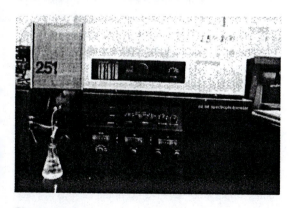

Figure 16-9
Spectrophotometer.

X is the ratio of the cross-section of the sphere to the cross-section of the aperture

In an actual counter, a *constant current source* (CCS) and voltage amplifier replaces the ohmmeter of Figure 16-10. A suitable front-end configuration is shown in Figure 16-11. The CCS is connected to a voltage source, V. Because the CCS has high resistance, circuit variations in the voltage (within reason) do not show up as changes of current (I) level. The resistance R_A is the resistance of the aperture-electrode path and will be either high or low, depending on whether or not the blood cell is inside the aperture. Because I is a

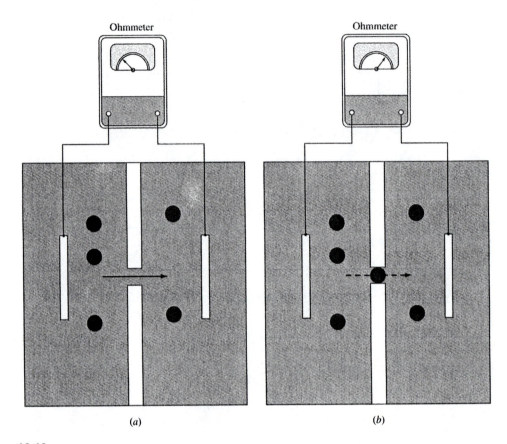

Figure 16-10
Blood sensing cell.

constant current, the voltage drop across the aperture-path resistance will be solely a function of the resistance value.

Although the sensor cell produces current pulse changes, the use of a differential amplifier (A1) to measure the voltage drop across R_A converts the current pulses into voltage pulses. These voltage pulses can be further processed in the circuit that follows the amplifier.

The block diagram to an impedance aperture cell counter is shown in Figure 16-12. The sensor and differential amplifier (A1) are as described above. There are two outputs from amplifier A1. One goes directly to the vertical input of the oscilloscope, while the other goes to a threshold detector circuit. The threshold detector is a circuit (dis-

cussed later) that discriminates against pulses that are too high or too low. Because the signal from the sensor is quite weak compared with ordinary Johnson (1/F) noise, it is necessary to provide such discrimination. The output of the threshold detector is supplied to a digital counter and to the oscilloscope Z-axis (i.e., brightness modulation) input.

A control section of the circuit provides gating to the counter, triggering to the oscilloscope time base, and blood sample acquisition commands to the pump used to move the fluid.

Threshold Detection. The threshold detector is a circuit that passes only those pulses that fit within an amplitude window (Figure 16-13). It establishes upper and lower amplitude bounds for acceptance, and issues an output only if the received

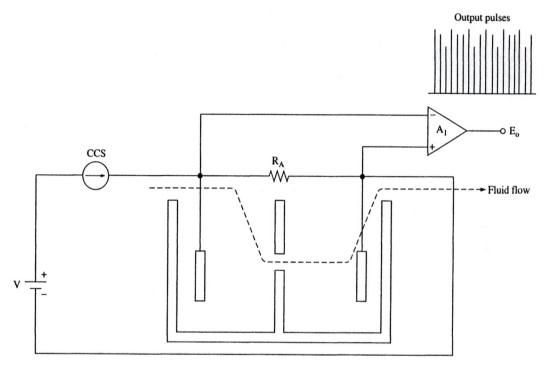

Figure 16-11
Blood cell counters. *(a)* Coulter model F. *(b)* Coulter model senior.

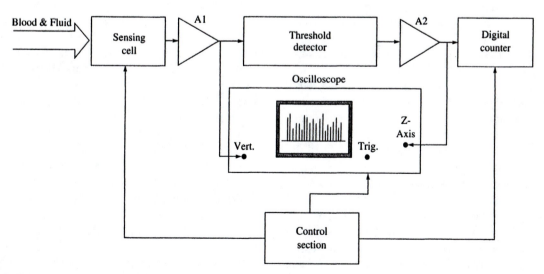

Figure 16-12
Impedance aperture cell counter.

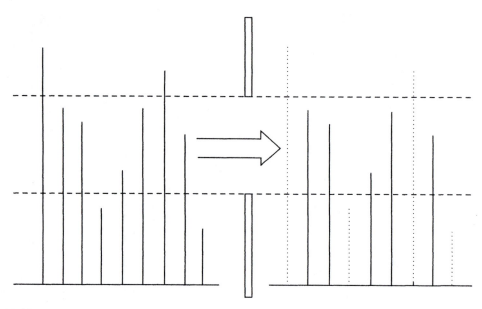

Figure 16-13
Threshold detector.

pulse is higher than the minimum and lower than the maximum. By this means, the threshold detector screens out noise artifacts. Regardless of whether the counting is done by a digital counter or microcomputer, this stage will clean up the analog input signal before applying it to the counter stage.

An example of a threshold detector is shown in Figure 16-14. It consists of two sections: a *window comparator* (A1 and A2) and a *coincidence detector* (AND gate).

A window comparator is a circuit based on operational amplifier voltage comparators. It uses two such circuits, one for the lower limit and the other for the upper limit. A comparator is made by connecting an operational amplifier with no negative feedback, so the gain is the open-loop gain of the device; in other words, it is very high. The high gain means that only a very small differential voltage between the inverting (−IN) and noninverting (+IN) inputs will cause the output to snap back and forth between the V− and V+ supply. Only when the voltages applied to both inputs are equal

(i.e., there is a zero differential voltage) will the output of the operational amplifier be zero. By the correct choice of reference voltage to bias one input, one can select whether or not the output will occur when a pulse is received.

A coincidence detector is nothing more than a digital AND gate. It will produce a HIGH output only if both inputs are HIGH. If either input is LOW, indicating a lack of coincidence between the two comparators (A1 and A2), then the output will be LOW also.

Aperture Impedance Counters. Some instruments based on the aperture impedance method uses both direct current (dc) excitation, as in the discussion above, and radio frequency (RF) excitation. The RF excitation allows the instrument to discriminate between various types of cells.

16-10-2 Flow cytometry cell counters

The optical flow cytometry sensor is shown in Figure 16-15. It consists of a quartz sensing sheath designed with a hydrodynamic focusing region

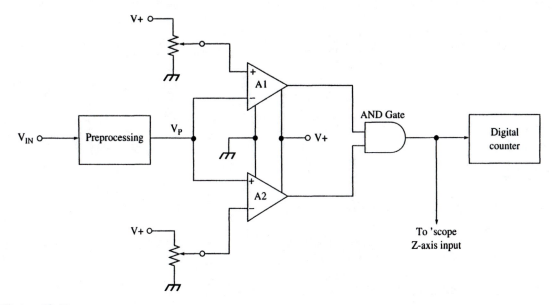

Figure 16-14
Threshold detector.

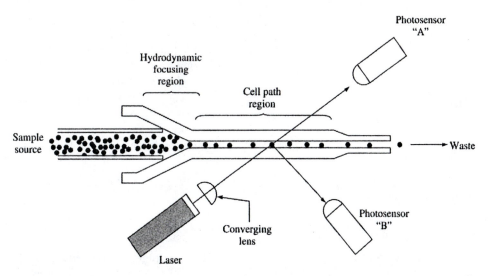

Figure 16-15
Optical flow cytometry sensor.

and a cell path region that passes only a single cell at a time. The focusing is done by decreasing the diameter of the aperture until it reaches the cell path region. A small section (about 18 to 20 μm) of the cell path region is illuminated by light from a helium-neon (He-Ne) laser (see chapter 21). When a cell enters this sensing region, it scatters light. From the scatter data one can drive the cell volume, its time of flight (TOF) through the sensing region, and the refractive index of the cell.

Two photosensors are used to detect the scattered light. Photosensor A detects forward scattered light, while photosensor B detects light scattered orthogonal to the path of the cells.

The flow in the cell path region of the sensor is interesting. The blood is mixed with a diluting solution as it enters the sensor. Because the hydrodynamic focusing and cell path regions do not allow the rise of turbulence, the fluid in the cell path exhibits laminar flow. The blood forms into a thin line about 20 μm in diameter within a "sheath" of the other fluid. The laser is designed to focus onto a segment of that small cell column flowing within the sheath.

When the blood sample enters the analyzer, it is split into two paths. One path goes through an optical counter (as above) to count the WBCs. The second path is split into two additional paths. One path measures the hemoglobin by passing the diluted sample through a colorimeter that uses a 539-nm light-emitting diode as the light source. The remaining stream is mixed with an isotonic diluting fluid and passed through an optical flow sensor to count the red cells.

The flow rate of the sample is:

$$r = kXe^{KX} \qquad (16\text{-}12)$$

where

r is the rate of output pulses

K is the flow in meters per second

K is volume of the sensing section

X is the cell concentration

The term KX is the probability of coincidence, and the term e^{KX} is $1 + KX + (KX)^2$. For small values of KX, the expression e^{KX} evaluates to $r \propto KX$.

The count can be in error because of noise pulses and coincidence of two cells in the sensing volume. The time required for the cell to clear the sensing volume sets the width of the pulse (τ) from the photosensors. The probability of coincidence is the product of the cell rate and pulse width τ. The count can be corrected by:

$$r_C = \frac{r}{1 - \tau} \qquad (16\text{-}13)$$

where

r_C is the corrected rate

r is the observed rate

τ is the pulse width

The two methods of cell counting are sometimes combined in one instrument. Certain instruments use both the aperture impedance and flow cytometry methods.

16-11 pH and blood gas analyzers

Acid-base balance of the blood is generated by body electrolytes and measured by a pH meter. The *respiratory system* provides an immediate buffer to sudden blood pH changes, and the *renal system* provides a slower, longer-range balance adjustment protection.

The *glass pH electrode* is the heart of the pH meter. Acidity or alkalinity is indicated by the concentration of hydronium ions (H_3O^+) in solution. This gives rise to hydrogen ions (H^+). PH is a measure of this ion concentration and is defined as:

$$pH = \log_{10}\frac{1}{(H^+)} = \log_{10}(H^+) \qquad (16\text{-}14)$$

where

pH is acidity

H^+ is hydrogen ion concentration

Pure water has a pH of 7 (neutral, $H^+ = 10^{-7}$). *Stomach acid* has a pH of 1.5 (greatly acid,

$H^+ = 10^{-1.5}$). *Blood* has a pH of 7.36 to 7.44 (slightly alkaline, $H^+ = 10^{-7.4}$ average).

The glass electrode, shown in Figure 16-16, consists of a platinum wire immersed in a highly acidic buffer solution contained within a thin *glass bulb*. This bulb wall is 0.1 mm thick and has an electrical resistance of *1000 MΩ*. It passes hydrogen ions only and thus acts as a *membrane* for separating out these ions. Also immersed in the test solution is a *calomel reference cell* (mercurous chloride). The platinum-wire electrode generates a *half-cell* electrical potential that acts in combination with the stable reference calomel half-cell. The test solution is in common with both half-cells. The resultant voltage is amplified by a high-input impedance amplifier, such as a MOSFET input op-amp (10^{12} Ω differential input impedance). Op-amp baseline drift (dc voltage stability) is important since the glass electrode signal is low level dc (50 mV). These amplifiers are often chopper stabilized, which returns the amplifier to ground potential at a relatively high rate (1 kHz).

Blood gas analyzers measure the P_{O_2} and P_{CO_2} in solution. This gives an indication of respiratory function. The *carbon dioxide electrode* is known as the *Severinghaus* electrode. It has a thin Teflon CO_2-permeable membrane over the glass bulb of the pH electrode. Final readings are reached

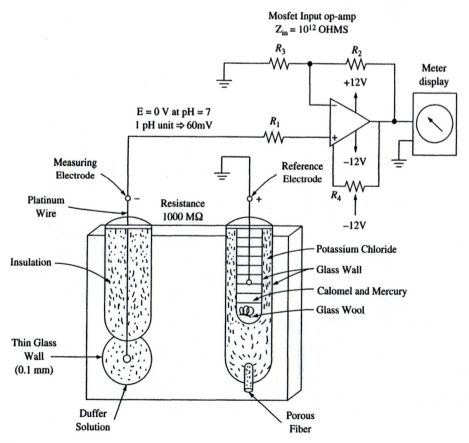

Figure 16-16
Basic pH glass electrode.

quickly. PH values are measured and compared to pH values of standard calibration solutions with partial pressures of 60 and 30 torr (mm Hg). This is done on a *nomograph* and is called the *Astrup method*. Essentially, partial pressures correspond to specific pH values, and thus P_{CO_2} electrodes are actually modified pH electrodes.

The *oxygen electrode* is composed of a thin platinum wire and a reference silver-silver chloride (Ag-Ag Cl) electrode. The magnitude of a small current generated by a battery connected across the electrodes is proportional to the oxygen concentration of the solution. Modern measurement techniques use the *Clark P_{O_2} electrode*. This consists of a platinum wire and Ag-Ag Cl electrode mounted inside a glass housing containing a saturated potassium-chloride (KCl) solution. A polythene membrane, semipermeable to oxygen molecules, covers an opening at the bottom. A current driven by a battery indicates P_{O_2}.

A combination electrode that measures blood pH and gases can also be designed. This is known as the *Clark-Severinghaus* electrode assembly.

Modern blood gas analyzers are precision devices that typically measure blood *pH*, P_{CO_2}, and P_{O_2} (Figure 16-17). The blood micro system is a thermostated unit incorporating a micro pH electrode (40-μL sample), a microtonometer for four disposable equilibrium tubes, and a high-value suction pump. The glass electrode is seen at the middle and the suction nozzle at the upper left. The *pH/blood gas monitor* gives accurate pH, P_{CO_2}, and P_{O_2} determinations on the blood sample or other body fluids. It is designed so that less frequently used controls are covered by a hinged front panel. Essentially, the blood sample can be measured for a preset (delay function) time following the push of the measure button. The unit will measure pH (15 s typically), P_{CO_2} (30 s typically), and P_{O_2} (50 s typically) and then display the values. The values shown in the photograph are within normal ranges. Calibration can be accomplished easily. This unit contains a combination of

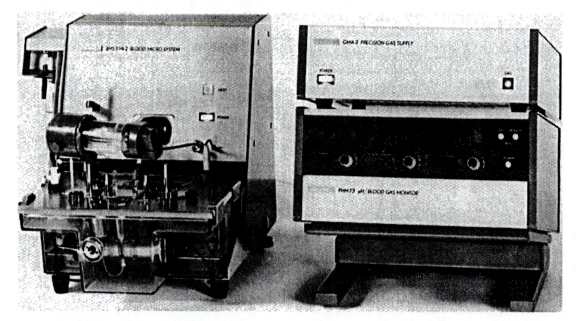

Figure 16-17
Blood gases/blood pH analysis system. (Photo courtesy of The London Co. [Radiometer]).

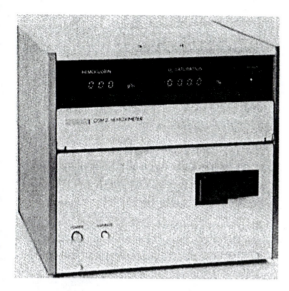

Figure 16-18
Hemoximeter photometric analyzer. (Photo courtesy of The London Co. [Radiometer])

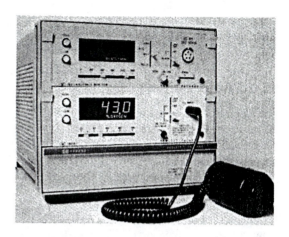

Figure 16-19
Gaseous oxygen analyzer. (Photo courtesy of Hewlett-Packard)

stable analog amplifiers and many digital control and storage circuits.

A *fully automated photometric analyzer* is shown in Figure 16-18. This unit measures hemoglobin concentration and oxygen saturation. Whole blood or erythrocyte concentrate is aspirated into the system, where hemolysis (breaking open of RBCs by 40-kHz ultrasonic energy), measurement, calculation, and rinsing are performed automatically. A precision colorimeter is used to measure hemoglobin concentration.

Neonatal oxygen monitors are commonly found in nurseries to continuously monitor environmental oxygen concentration inside the incubator. The one shown in Figure 16-19 monitors infant ECG, heart rate, and incubator Po_2. A transducer is placed next to the child, and a manually selected alarm setting permits warning of low or high Po_2.

Maintenance of pH meters and blood gas analyzers includes frequent adjustment of calibration and replacement of glass electrodes. These electrodes age and require increasing times to produce accurate readings. For continuous Po_2 monitors, electrodes must be periodically cleaned and occasionally replaced. Electronic failures are relatively few.

16-12 Chromatograph

The *chromatograph* provides a means for separation and assay of complex substances. Material identification and concentration can be determined by any one of the following methods.

1. *Liquid column chromatography*—Liquid is percolated down a tube, and the bands formed along the tube (as well as the time to travel through) indicate the type of substance present.

2. *Paper partition chromatography*—Solid and liquid phases are separated out on strips or hollow cylinders of filter paper. The solvent movement is timed.

3. *Gas chromatography*—Movement of gas instead of liquid is used to separate out samples. Gas passing through a solid is known as *gas solid (adsorption) chromatography (GSC)* and gas through liquid as *gas liquid chromatography (GLC)*.

Figure 16-20 shows a gas chromatograph with input to the left and graph output to the upper right.

16-13 Autoanalyzer

The *autoanalyzer* sequentially measures blood chemistry and displays this on a graphic readout. As shown in Figure 16-21, this is accomplished by *mixing, reagent reaction,* and *colorimetric measurement* in a continuous stream. The system includes the following elements.

1. *Sampler*—aspirates samples, standards, and wash solutions to the autoanalyzer system.

2. *Proportioning pump and manifold*—introduces (mixes) samples with reagents to effect the proper chemical color reaction to be read by the colorimeter. It also pumps fluids at precise flow rates to other modules, as proper color development depends on reaction time and temperature.

3. *Dialyzer*—separates interfacing substances from the sample material by permitting selective passage of sample components through a semipermeable membrane.

4. *Heating bath*—heats fluids continuously to exact temperature (typically 37°C incubation, equivalent to body temperature). Temperature is critical to color development.

5. *Colorimeter*—monitors the changes in optical density of the fluid stream flowing through a tubular flow cell. Color intensities (optical densities) proportional to substance concentrations are converted to equivalent electrical voltages.

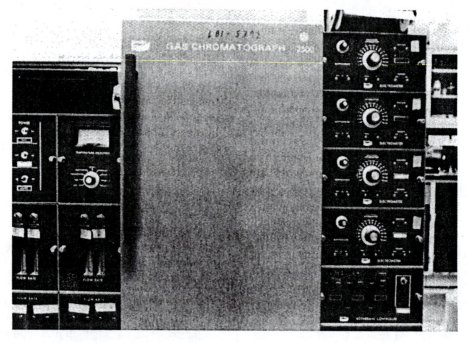

Figure 16-20
Gas chromatograph.

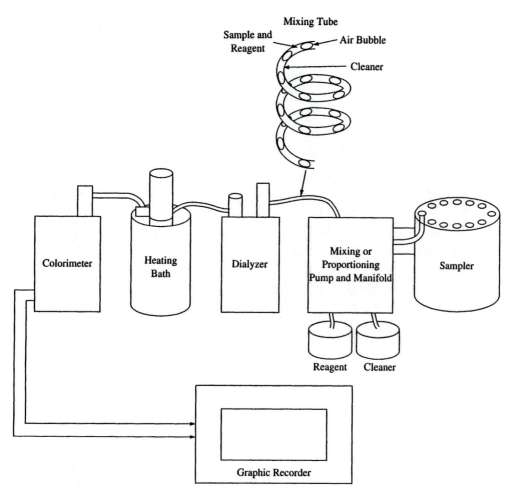

Figure 16-21
Autoanalyzer system.

6. *Recorder*—converts optical density electrical signal from the colorimeter into a graphic display on a moving chart.

The heart of the autoanalyzer system is the *proportioning pump*. This consists of a *peristaltic* (occluding or roller) *pump*. Air segmentation in the *mixing tube* separates the sample/reagent mixture from the cleaning fluid and other samples. As these air-separated fluids traverse the coil of the mixing tube, effective mixing action is achieved.

The Technicon SMA 12/60, shown in Figure 16-22, is a sequential multiple analyzer that performs 12 different tests on 60 samples per hour. It is a continuous flow process that produces a chemical profile read on a graphic chart. Tests accomplished include most of those shown in Table 16-1.

A later computerized version is shown in Figure 16-23. This is the Technicon SMAC. Up to 40 different tests can be performed on an individual serum sample.

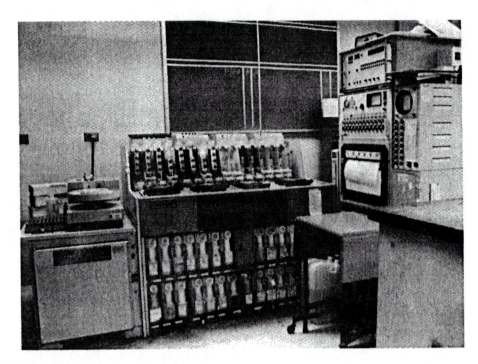

Figure 16-22
Technicon SMA 12/60.

One problem with automatic analyzers is certain identification of samples. Patient data can be intermixed with that of other patients if care is not taken.

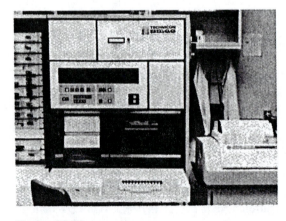

Figure 16-23
Computerized autoanalyzer.

Sterilization is also needed for samples, glassware, and equipment parts that are contaminated with disease. Diseases such as hepatitis or other communicable infections can be spread to equipment operators. Figure 16-24 shows an *autoclave* unit used to sterilize small and large items. It operates at saturated steam pressures and temperatures of 120°C for 20 minutes to 1 hour.

Maintenance on autoanalyzers includes frequent calibration adjustment. Most problems are mechanical (tubes, moving pump parts) and electrical (switches, motors). Electronic failures are few. Sophisticated autoanalyzer system maintenance and repair requires the biomedical equipment technician to complete the manufacturers' schools. Operation and service manuals must always be consulted. A patient's life may hinge on accurate measurement obtained by clinical instrumentation.

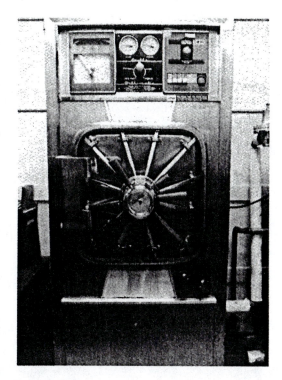

Figure 16-24
Autoclave sterilizer.

16-14 Basic Renal Physiology

The main *excretory systems* of the body are the gastrointestinal system (digestive-mouth, stomach, intestine, bowels), respiratory system (lungs), skin (sweat glands), and renal system (kidneys).

The *renal system* is composed of the *kidneys.* As shown in Figure 16-25, these are organs that perform the following functions:

1. Excretion of waste products from metabolic processes.

2. Regulation of constancy of body fluids (water and electrolytes).

3. Regulation (assist) of constant blood pH (acid-base balance).

4. Maintenance (assist) of constant blood pressure.

5. Regulation (assist) of blood sodium, potassium, calcium, magnesium, chlorides, phosphates, sulfates, carbonates, and proteins.

6. Control (assist) of erythrocyte discharge.

The kidneys remove toxic substances and salts from the blood through a process involving *filtration, reabsorption,* and *excretion.* This is accomplished within each kidney (input blood through renal artery, output blood through renal vein, and output urine to the bladder through the ureter). Approximately 25% of systemic blood flow occurs in the kidneys, and urine is formed in the loop of Henle. Each kidney supplies 100% of body requirements (2 to 1 reserve).

16-15 Renal Failure

Renal disease is classified as *primary* (internal to kidneys) and *secondary* (external to kidneys, such as urinary blockage). Renal failure results in little or no urine formation. Hence, toxic substances accumulate in the body, causing symptoms such as headaches, dry blotches on the skin, dizziness, and eventual death. Kidney stones (calcium deposits) may cause kidney blockage.

Renal disease can be detected by the following methods.

1. Clinical examination of the abdomen (kidney region).

2. Two-dimensional X-ray of the abdomen (kidney region).

3. Intravenous pyelography (IVP)–X-ray exposures taken of a radiopaque substance (i.e., sodium diatrizoate) injected into a vein and filtered through the kidneys.

4. Renal tomograms–X-ray scans.

5. Renal angiography–motion picture X-rays of radiopaque dye circulation through the kidney.

6. Examination of the urine.

KIDNEY

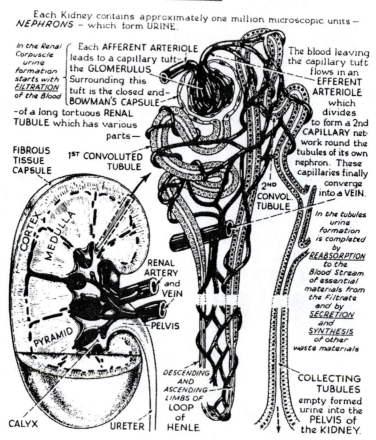

Each Kidney contains approximately one million microscopic units — NEPHRONS - which form URINE.

In the Renal Corpuscle urine formation starts with FILTRATION of the Blood

Each AFFERENT ARTERIOLE leads to a capillary tuft — the GLOMERULUS Surrounding this tuft is the closed end — BOWMAN'S CAPSULE —

-of a long tortuous RENAL TUBULE which has various parts —

The blood leaving the capillary tuft flows in an EFFERENT ARTERIOLE which divides to form a 2nd CAPILLARY network round the tubules of its own nephron. These capillaries finally converge into a VEIN.

FIBROUS TISSUE CAPSULE

1ST CONVOLUTED TUBULE

2ND CONVOL TUBULE

In the tubules urine formation is completed by REABSORPTION to the Blood Stream of essential materials from the Filtrate and by SECRETION and SYNTHESIS of other waste materials

CORTEX
MEDULLA
PYRAMID

RENAL ARTERY and VEIN

PELVIS

COLLECTING TUBULES empty formed urine into the PELVIS of the KIDNEY.

DESCENDING AND ASCENDING LIMBS OF LOOP of HENLE

CALYX   URETER

Figure 16-25
Human kidney. (From McNaught & Callander, *Illustrated Physiology.* Used by permission of Churchill Livingstone.)

When *kidney failure* occurs, *kidney transplantation* may be undertaken. This procedure, if successful, results in the most comprehensive cure. However, transplants last only a few years due to complications and tissue rejection.

Peritoneal dialysis or hemodialysis is recommended for those who are not candidates for transplantation.

16-16 Peritoneal Dialysis

Peritoneal dialysis is accomplished by puncturing two needles through the abdominal wall (peri-

toneum) and washing out the peritoneal cavity with a saline solution. This solution flows through a semipermeable membrane outside the body. Toxic substances are, thus, removed. This type of dialysis is performed under emergency conditions.

16-17 Hemodialysis

Hemodialysis is a process that involves the removal of chemical substances from the blood by passing it through tubes surrounded by semipermeable membranes. It is accomplished by puncturing two needles through an artery and vein and circulating the patient's blood through a coiled plastic tube. This coiled tube is bathed in a *dialysate solution* (dextrose and salts of Ca, Mg, K, and Na). Osmotic pressures are balanced in such a way that toxins (urea, creatinine, and uric acid) gradually pass through the plastic tube and cellophane wrapping (membrane) into the dialysate solution. The *semipermeable membrane* passes salts and small molecules but not blood cells and large protein molecules.

16-18 The Hemodialysis Machine

Hemodialysis can be administered by registered nurses with particular familiarity with the he-

modialysis process and the machine used to administer it. Even patients with special training can use machines at home. This machine must replace vital kidney functions. Unfortunately, this artificial kidney, as it is often called, cannot replace total kidney operation. Patients may live 6 years or more, depending on kidney disease and complications.

The *hemodialysis machine,* whose block diagram appears in Figure 16-26 consists of the following systems.

1. A *power system* composed of 120-V input power plug, off/on switch, time-delay fuse or circuit breaker, and wiring distribution to lights, controls, heaters, and pumps.

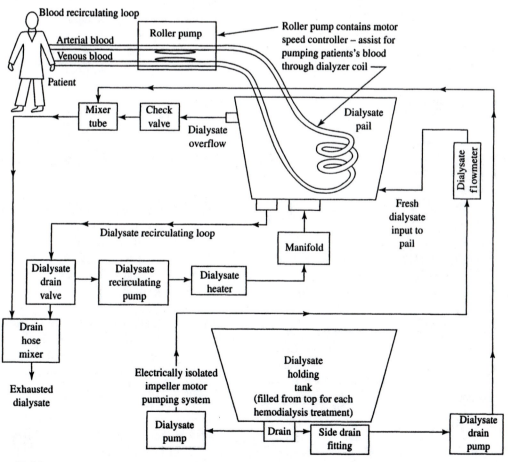

Figure 16-26
Block diagram of hemodialysis machine (blood and dialysate recirculating loops).

2. A *control panel light system* consisting of terminal boards, printed circuit boards, lamps, and transformer.

3. A *dialysate recirculating system* consisting of a recirculating pump and switch, seals, housing, and plastic tubes.

4. A *dialysate drain system* consisting of an electromechanical compartment drain switch and valve, drain pump, seals, housing, and plastic drain tubing.

5. A *dialysis bath delivery system* consisting of a dialysate pump and switch, seals, housing, flowmeter, 120-L dialysate holding tank, plastic tubing, and *dialyzer coil* (blood input/output and surrounding dialyzer bath).

6. A *temperature system* consisting of a heater element and switch, seals, housing temperature gage, and control. Usual temperature range is 25°C to 50°C (37°C is body temperature). Overtemperature shutoff and audible alarm are also included.

7 A *blood pump* consisting of a roller (peristaltic) pump and switch, time delay fuse, motor clutch, electronic motor speed control circuit, potentiometer speed control on front panel, plastic tubing for blood passage, and venous bubble trap.

8. A *positive/negative pressure monitor* consisting of a dialysis bath overtemperature shut off and audible alarm, blood leak detector, and pressure monitor microswitch in the venous line (return to the patient).

In essence, the hemodialysis machine is much like a washing machine with dialysate recirculating pumps and blood pumps. The functional heart of the system is the dialyzer coil through which chemicals pass into the dialysate solution.

The *patient-hemodialysis setup procedure* consists of the following steps.

1. Preparation of hemodialysis machine (makeup of dialysate solution and machine control pumping action and dialysate temperature checkout).

2. Preparation of the patient (blood test, physical condition).

3. Connection of the patient to the machine.
   a. *Internal arterial and venous puncture* with special needles into a subcutaneous artery and vein or plastic shunt (a tube below the skin that connects an artery to a vein—also called a fistula). This must be preceded by sterile preparation and sometimes local anesthetic. *External arterial and venous* blood shunt tubing connection is also used.
   b. Blood circulation connection to the dialyzing coil through plastic tubing.
   c. Dialysis liquid recirculating pump turn-on.
   d. Roller pump turn-on and speed adjustment.
   e. Bubble trap connection on venous side.
   f. Low-pressure alarm setting on venous side.

16-19 High-Flux and High-Efficiency Dialysis

The cost of dialysis in the United States is now more than $1 billion, because of the growing number of elderly and diabetic patients.

With the advent of modern medical equipment, based on progressive research, new therapy strategies have become available for the dialysis patient.

Problems in new technology have emerged in the areas of dialyzer reuse, high-flux/high-efficiency procedures, and infection, such as hepatitis and HIV.

Great advances in two areas have occurred from 1985 to 1992. High-flux and high-efficiency dialysis offers patients faster treatment (about 3 hours versus double that with older machines) and more effective results. Today about 60% of total dialysis units use some form of the advanced technique.

The two therapies are essentially the same, but high-flux dialyzers have larger pore sizes, which provides better clearance of large-molecular-weight solutes, and higher ultrafiltration rates. The higher solute removal efficiency is a clear benefit, a result of in part the cellulosic-based membranes, including cuprophane, hemophan, cellulose acetate, and cuproammonium. High-efficiency types typically have ultrafiltration coefficients of less than 15 mL/hr per millimeter of mercury (mm Hg). These dialyzers have large surface areas of 1.7 to 2.0 m^2. High-flux dialyzers have lower coefficients and are made of the synthetic, polysulfone.

Accompanying the advantages of these treatments are the dangers of hypotension (low pressure) if the membrane pressure is not carefully controlled. Therefore, considerable technical requirements are placed on the equipment and operators.

Further improvements in ultrafiltration control systems have relied on microprocessor-based electronic measurement and processing techniques. Electromagnetic flow sensors measure dialysate inflow and outflow with servo-control systems in place to regulate transmembrane pressure. This multisensor and feedback approach is similar to modern aircraft, which would not operate properly without the computer. Although it is easier to lose control with these new hemodialysis systems, they are increasingly helping patients live better lives.

16-20 Electrical Safety Precautions

Electrical safety on hemodialysis machines is very important because the entire system involves wet components, direct patient bloodstream connection (leading to the heart), and electrically operated devices.

Leakage current is difficult to minimize. Leakages of less than 10 μA under normal clinical operating conditions may never be achieved on some units. Patient protection is enhanced by doing the following:

1. Using a special *magnetically coupled* motor shaft dialysate impeller system. In this scheme there is no direct electrical connection between the dialysate pump motor and dialysate solution.

2. Using carefully secured separate machine ground wire.

3. Checking frequently for electrical safety leakage current.

4. Avoiding fluid (blood and dialysate) leaks by frequent tubing and pump inspections.

Ground fault interruptors (GFI) are sometimes used in these wet areas.

16-21 Typical Faults, Troubleshooting, and Maintenance

Typical faults (system symptom) and troubleshooting points (possible cause) on hemodialysis machines include the following:

1. All lights are out when power switch is turned on: AC fuse is blown due to loose ac wire connections or component/wiring short due to leaking dialysate.

2. Individual or all light bulbs on the control panel are out: Blown light bulb or damaged circuit board.

3. Dialysis bath solution does not flow through the dialyzer: Open or damaged switch or foreign object is stuck in recirculating pump housing (hum sound) or there is a damaged pump.

4. Recirculating pump or pumping system leaks: Pump fitting or seals are worn, hose clamps are loose, or hoses have holes.

5. Dialyzing compartment overflows: Check whether valve ball is stuck, foreign object is blocking the drain hose, or the drain hose is kinked.

6. Dialyzing compartment does not drain: There is a faulty drain switch or sticking or inoperative electromechanical drain valve.

7. One hundred twenty-liter dialysate tank leaks: Drain cap is not in place, seals are worn, or tank is cracked.

8. Dialysate bath does not heat or wrong temperature is indicated: There is a faulty heater switch, heat sensor, or heater.

9. Blood roller pumpdoes not operate: Blown fuse or faulty motor control circuit.

10. Blood roller pump has incorrect speed: Speed control potentiometer is damaged or speed control circuitry is faulty.

Maintenance on hemodialysis machines includes weekly checks as follows:

1. Check all plumbing connections for leaks.

2. Clean salt residues.

3. Clean dust and solid debris from the drain, motor, and hoses.

4. Remove and clean dialysate tank screen.

5. Check for and replace any worn or kinked hoses.

6. Clean dialysate flow meter.

7. Test overtemperature shutoff and adjust if necessary.

8. Check and calibrate temperature controller.

16-22 Summary

1. *Blood* is defined as the fluid that circulates through the heart, arteries, veins, and capillaries, carrying nourishment, electrolytes, hormones, vitamins, antibodies, heat, and oxygen to body tissues and taking away waste matter and carbon dioxide.

2. *Whole blood* consists of *cells* (RBCs, WBCs, and platelets) and *plasma* (fluid with dissolved inorganic and organic substances, such as proteins, fibrinogen, glucose, fats, enzymes,

vitamins, antibodies, electrolytes, salts, and urea).

3. Toxic substances from metabolic processes are carried by the blood and excreted in the urine. These substances can be measured by clinical laboratory instrumentation.

4. *Blood cell tests* include *RBC, WBC,* and *platelet* count, *Hct, MHC, MCV, and MCHC.*

5. *Blood chemistry tests* include determination of acidity (pH), glucose (sugar), nonprotein nitrogen substances (amino acids, peptides, urea), lipids (fats), proteins (plasma, albumin, globulin, and fibrinogen), and enzymes and steroids.

6. Other blood tests include *serology* (agglutination), *bacteriology,* and *histology.*

7. The *medical laboratory department* includes special facilities, personnel, and equipment. Equipment is expensive and critical to accurate diagnosis of the patient.

8. A *colorimeter* or *filter photometer* is an optical electronic device that measures the color concentration of a substance in solution. Maintenance includes routine cleaning and calibration.

9. A *flame photometer* is an optical electronic device that measures the characteristic color intensity of substances (sodium, potassium) that have been aspirated into a flame. Maintenance is similar to the colorimeter.

10. A *spectrophotometer* is an optical electronic device that measures light absorption at various wavelengths for a given liquid sample. Maintenance is similar to the colorimeter except for mechanically moving parts (diffraction grating, rotating mirror).

11. A *blood cell analyzer* is an electromechanical device that measures the number of RBCs and WBCs per scaled volume. This is

accomplished by the electrical conductivity (Coulter counter) method. The Coulter counter output is in card form, on which is printed RBC, WBC, Hgb, Hct, MCV, MCH, and MCHC values.

12. A *pH/blood gas analyzer* is an electromechanical device that measures blood pH (acid-base balance, pH = $-\log H^+$), P_{O_2} (partial pressure of blood oxygen), and P_{CO_2} (partial pressure of blood carbon dioxide). PH glass electrodes can be modified to measure P_{CO_2} and P_{O_2} (Severinghaus and Clark electrodes).

13. A chromatograph is an electromechanical device used to separate, identify, and measure concentration of substances. Types include liquid column, paper partition, and gas chromatographs.

14. An autoanalyzer is an electromechanical-electronic device that measures and displays blood chemistry. The system consists of a sampler, proportioning pump (mixing coil), dialyzer, heating bath, colorimeter, and recorder. Examples are the Technicon SMA 12/60 and SMAC sequential multiple analyzers.

15. The *renal system* is composed of the *kidneys,* which perform functions of *waste excretion, body fluid balance, blood pH, blood pressure,* and *blood salt regulation.*

16. *Primary* (internal to kidneys) and *secondary* (external) renal disease can be detected by physical examination, X-ray exposures or scans, angiography, intravenous pyelograms, and examination of the urine.

17. Renal dialysis can be accomplished by *peritoneal dialysis* or *hemodialysis.*

18. *Hemodialysis* involves the removal of chemical substances from the blood by passing it through tubes made of *semipermeable membranes.*

19. The *hemodialysis machine* usually consists of the following systems: power, control panel light, dialysate circulatory drain, bath delivery, temperature, blood pump, and positive/negative pressure monitor.

20. *Electrical safety* is important in hemodialysis systems due to the wet areas, direct patient bloodstream connection, and the use of electrically operated devices.

21. *Typical faults* and *troubleshooting* procedures on hemodialysis machines involve burned-out lamps, blocked fluid circulation, leaking fluid, faulty pumps, heater inaccuracies, and no-heat conditions.

22. Weekly *maintenance* includes plumbing checks, cleaning, hose and clamp replacement, and temperature calibration.

23. It is important to avoid overdialyzing a patient, especially during high-flux/high-efficiency procedures.

16-23 Recapitulation

Now return to the objectives and self-evaluation questions at the beginning of the chapter and see how well you can answer them. If you cannot answer certain questions, place a check mark next to each and review appropriate parts of the text. Next try to answer the following questions using the same procedure. When you have answered all of the questions, solve the problems.

Questions

1. Blood is defined as that _____ which circulates through the _____, _____, _____, and capillaries carrying nourishment, _____, _____, _____, antibodies, heat, and _____ to the body tissues, and taking away _____ _____ and _____ _____.

2. Whole blood is composed of _____ and _____ blood cells and _____ fluid, which consists of proteins, nutrients, _____, _____, antibodies, and metabolic _____.

3. Blood spun in a centrifuge is composed of _____ percent RBCs and _____ percent plasma.

4. Blood cell tests include counts for _____ and _____, volume of _____, and color intensity of _____.

5. Blood chemistry includes _____ (acidbase balance), _____ (sugar), _____ (fats), _____ (protein), and enzymes.

6. Blood antibody agglutination evaluation is known as a _____ test and organism growths as a _____ test.

7. The importance of the medical laboratory department rests ultimately with the _____ of disease.

8. Since the medical laboratory has high volume, good record keeping helps to prevent mixup in a patient's _____.

9. State the purpose, uses, operation, calibration, and maintenance for colorimeters (include a block diagram/schematic).

10. State the purpose, uses, operation, and maintenance for a flame photometer (include a block diagram/schematic).

11. State the purpose, uses, operation, and maintenance for spectrophotometers (include block diagram/schematic).

12. State the purposes, uses, operation, and maintenance for blood cell counters (include block diagram).

13. State the purpose, uses, and maintenance for pH/blood gas analyzers (include a diagram and description of a pH glass electrode).

14. State the purpose, uses, operation, and operation for chromatographs (include the different types).

15. State the purpose, uses, and maintenance of autoanalyzers (include system block diagram).

16. The renal system is composed of the _____ and performs functions of _____ of waste products and regulation of body _____, blood _____, and blood _____.

17. Renal disease and failure can be detected by _____, _____, _____, and examination of _____.

18. Define hemodialysis, including high-flux/high-efficiency types.

19. List eight subsystems of a hemodialysis machine and draw a block diagram.

20. Why is electrical safety important in hemodialysis machines?

21. List 10 hemodialysis faults and their usual causes.

22. List eight weekly maintenance checks on hemodialysis machines.

Problems

1. Refer to Figure 16-4b. Given $V_1 = +1.5$ mV with reference cuvette and $V_1 = +35$ mV with reference and sample cuvettes, $R_2 = R_3 = 2.5$ kΩ, *calculate* the voltage read on the meter display for both conditions of V_1.

2. A nurse reports that a *colorimeter* that was previously working is now giving very low transmittance reading for all blood samples. Which portion(s) of the device would you check first?

3. A medical technologist reports that the *Coulter counter* model S in the clinical lab gives correct RBC, WBC, Hct, and Hgb readings but incorrect MCV, MCH, and MCHC readings. What checkout procedure would you use to identify the trouble source?

4. A nurse in the neonatal nursery cannot obtain accurate readings with an isolette *oxygen monitor*. Which portion(s) of the device would you check first?

5. A medical technologist reports that a *pH meter* in the clinical lab has an output that wanders about an apparently correct pH value. What part of the device should probably be replaced?

Suggested Reading

1. Crouch, James E. and Robert J. McClintic, *Human Anatomy and Physiology*, Wiley (New York, 1976).

2. Henry, R. J., D. C. Cannon, and J. W. Winkelman, *Clinical Chemistry, Principles and Techniques*, Harper & Row (Hagerstown, Md., 1974).

3. Lee, W. L., *Elementary Principles of Laboratory Instruments*, C. V. Mosby Company (St. Louis, Mo., 1970).

4. Jacobson, Bertil and John G. Webster, *Medicine and Clinical Engineering*, Prentice Hall, Inc. (Englewood Cliffs, N.J., 1977).

5. Geddes, L. A. and L. E. Baker, *Principles of Applied Biomedical Instrumentation*, Wiley (New York, 1968, 1975).

6. Laughlin, Alice, *Roe's Principles of Chemistry*, C. V. Mosby Company (St. Louis, Mo., 1976).

7. Nave, Carl R. and Brenda C. Nave, *Physics for the Health Sciences*, W. B. Saunders Co. (Philadelphia, 1976).

8. Hendrich, William L. Editor, Principles and Practice of Dialysis, 2nd Edition, Hemodialysis, Kidney Failure, Complications, Therapy, Williams & Wilkins (Baltimore, 1999).

9. McNaught, Ann B. and Robin Callander, *Illustrated Physiology*, Churchill Livingstone (New York, 1975).

10. Sullivan, Lawrence P. *Physiology of the Kidney*, Lea & Febiger (Philadelphia, 1974).

11. Geschickter, Charles F. and Tatinana T. Anlonovych, *The Kidney in Health and Disease*, Lippincott Co. (Philadelphia, 1971).

12. Kincaid, Owings W. and George D. Davis, *Renal Angiography*, Year Book Medical Publishers (Chicago, 1966).

13. Hamburger, Jean, Jean Crosnier, Jean Dormont, and Jean-Francois Bach, *Renal Transplantation—Theory and Practice*, Williams & Wilkins Co. (Baltimore, Md., 1972).

14. Boen, S. T. *Peritoneal Dialysis in Clinical Medicine*, Charles C Thomas (Springfield, Ill., 1964).

15. Hampers, L. Constantine and Eugene Schupack, *Long-Term Hemodialysis*, Grune and Stratton (New York, 1973).

CHAPTER 17
Medical Ultrasonography

17-1 Objectives

1. Be able to discuss the physics of ultrasound.
2. Be able to describe the operation of ultrasonic transducers.

3. Be able to list and describe the operation of ultrasonic instruments.
4. Be able to inspect and evaluate the performance of ultrasonic instruments.

17-2 Self-evaluation questions

These questions test your prior knowledge of the material in this chapter. Look for the answers as you read the text. After you have finished studying the chapter, try answering these questions and those at the end of the chapter.

1. What is the range of frequencies designated as *ultrasonic* in medical systems?

2. How does a 2500-kHz ultrasonic signal differ from a 2500-kHz radio signal?

3. What is the principal types of transducer used in ultrasonic systems?

4. A frequency suitable for use in Doppler flowmeters is _____ mHz.

17-3 What is ultrasound?

The term *ultrasound* refers to *acoustical waves* above the range of human hearing (frequencies higher than 20,000 Hz). Many electronics text-books arbitrarily list as ultrasound only those frequencies between 20 and 100 kHz. There is no reason, however, for placing the upper limit at 100 kHz or any other frequency. Indeed, medical ultrasound systems operate at frequencies of up to 10 MHz or more. The principal issue is not the frequency but rather the nature of the wave used. An ultrasonic wave is acoustical; i.e., it is a mechanical wave in a gaseous, liquid, or solid medium. Such mechanical waves consists of alternating areas of higher and lower pressures, called *compression* and *rarefaction* zones, respectively. Although medical applications currently are limited to about 10 MHz and below, if someone were to design a transducer for higher frequencies, then those frequencies could be used as ultrasound by anyone who had a need for them. Ultrasonic imaging is used in medicine, engineering, geology, and other scientific areas.

Most textbooks today list frequencies in the high kilohertz (kHz) and megahertz (MHz) region as *radio* waves. Although the same frequencies may be used both in medical ultrasound and in high-frequency radio systems (2 to 10 MHz), there is a distinguishing difference: Radio signals are *electromagnetic waves,* while medical ultrasound signals are *acoustical.* If an alternating current (ac) oscillation of, say, 2500 kHz, were connected to an appropriate antenna, then an electromagnetic (radio) wave would be launched. But if that same 2500 kHz ac signal were applied to an ultrasound transducer, then an acoustical signal would be launched. The acoustical signal requires a medium in which to propagate, while the electromagnetic signal can propagate in outer space, where no known medium exists.

17-4 Physics of sound and ultrasound waves

Ultrasound waves are vibrations or disturbances consisting of alternating zones of compression and rarefaction in a physical medium such as gas, liquid, or solid matter. Although some animals are able to hear frequencies above the average range of human hearing, which is about 30 Hz to 20 kHz, none are believed capable of hearing waves in the range above 500 kHz, at which medical ultrasound devices operate.

17-4-1 Wavelength, frequency, and velocity

All waves, including both acoustical and electromagnetic (or ocean waves, for that matter) possess three related attributes: *frequency* (F), *wavelength* (λ), and *velocity* (V). Other relevant properties of

ultrasound waves include *amplitude, power,* and *propagating wave type.*

Frequency is defined as the number of complete *cycles per unit of time.* Figure 17-1 shows one complete cycle. In terms of alternating current, the cycle consists of one entire positive excursion followed by one complete negative excursion of the voltage or current. In terms of sound and ultrasound waves, the cycle consists of one complete zone of compression followed by one complete zone of rarefaction. The basic unit of cycles is the *hertz* (Hz), which equals one cycle per second (1 Hz = 1 cps); the superunits are *kilohertz* (1 kHz = 1000 Hz) and *megahertz* (MHz).

Wavelength is the distance traveled by one cycle propagating away from the source and is expressed in *meters* (m), or subunits *centimeters* (cm) or *millimeters* (mm). The wavelength is also the distance between successive identical features on successive cycles. In the example shown in Figure 17-1, one wavelength is expressed as the

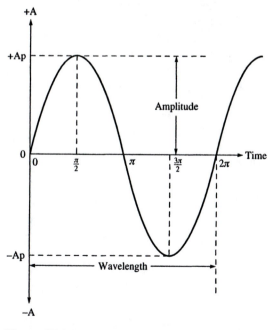

Figure 17-1
Frequency is defined as cycles per unit of time.

distance between positive-going crossings of the zero baseline. It could also be expressed in terms of the distance between two positive peaks, between two negative peaks, or between negative-going crossings of the zero baseline.

Velocity is the speed of propagation of the wave. In radio signals, the velocity is the speed of light (c), or 300,000,000 m/s. In human tissue, ultrasound propagates at a much slower rate, i.e., around 1500 m/s.

For all forms of wave, the relationship between frequency, wavelength, and velocity is:

$$V = F\lambda \qquad (17\text{-}1)$$

where

V is the velocity of the wave in meters per second (m/s)

F is the frequency in hertz (Hz)

λ is the wavelength in meters (m)

The *period* of the wave is the time required to complete one cycle and can be measured in terms of either time (T) or angle (one cycle = 2π radians). Equation 17-1 is sometimes written in the alternative form of Equation 17-2, which expresses the relationship in terms of the period of the wave rather than its frequency, where period is measured in units of time (T) and is defined as the reciprocal of frequency (T = 1/F). We may therefore write Equation 17-1 in the form:

$$V = \frac{\lambda}{T} \qquad (17\text{-}2)$$

The figure 1500 m/s as the velocity of ultrasound in human tissue is accepted as an average for devices operated in the 2- to 3-MHz range. But we also find that the actual velocity depends on other factors that are properties of the transmission media (e.g., density, stiffness), as well as frequency (Table 17-1).

The *amplitude* (A) of the wave is the difference between the zero baseline and either peak. In terms of the cycle shown in Figure 17-1, the positive amplitude is $+A_p$ and the negative amplitude is $-A_p$. In a symmetrical wave, the two peaks are the same, so $\text{ABS}(+A_p) = \text{ABS}(-A_p)$. The amplitude of the ultrasonic wave used in medical applications is usually measured in megapascals (Mpa), where 1 Mpa is a pressure of 10 atm). This definition is in terms of the compression and rarefaction pressures. Typical values for medical ultrasound devices are 4 Mpa for Doppler systems and 3 Mpa for peak positive and 2 Mpa for peak negative amplitudes.

The amplitude of the ultrasonic signal is directly related to its power, which is expressed in *watts* (W), or subunits *milliwatts* (mW) and *microwatts* (μW), and is related to the electrical signal applied to the transducer, efficiency of the transducer, and efficiency of the coupling between the transducer and the tissue. The *energy* level of the signal is measured in *joules* or *watt-seconds,* in which 1 J = 1 W-s.

The *wave type* refers to the method of propagation. The two forms are *longitudinal propagation*

Example 17-1 _____

An ultrasonic wave in human tissue has a frequency of 2,500 kHz and a wavelength of 6×10^{-4} m. Calculate its velocity of propagation.

$$V = F\lambda$$

$$V = \left(2500 \text{ kHz} \times \frac{10^3 \text{ Hz}}{\text{kHz}}\right)(6 \times 10^{-4}\, m)$$

$$V = (2.5 \times 10^6 \text{ Hz})(6 \times 10^{-4}\, m) = \mathbf{1500 \text{ m/s}}$$

TABLE 17-1   TRANSMISSION VELOCITY OF ULTRASOUND IN DIFFERENT MATERIALS

Material	Density (g/cm²) @ 25°C	Sound velocity (m/s)
Air	0.001	330
Bone	1.85	3360
Muscle	1.06	1570
Fat	0.93	1480
Blood	1.00	1560

and *transverse propagation*. In the longitudinal form, the waves propagate in the same direction as the zones of compression and rarefaction. In transverse propagation, the waves propagate in a direction orthogonal (at right angles) to the direction of the zones of compression and rarefaction. Transverse propagation occurs when the wave propagates along the surface of the medium, as on the surface of a container of water or the surface of a bone. In medical ultrasound both forms are seen. While the main mode is longitudinal propagation, a *mode conversion* to transverse propagation can occur. Mode conversion is associated with a significant loss of signal level.

17-4-2 Reflection, refraction, diffraction, and scattering phenomena

Reflections, refraction, diffraction, and scattering are phenomena affecting all waves and, in fact, define wave behavior. These phenomena occur when the waves impinge on a surface or boundary between zones of materials of different density. We are most familiar with these phenomena for light waves. For example, reflection is observed when we see ourselves in a mirror. People who fish are familiar with refraction (light rays bending at the water-air boundary) because it makes a fish *appear* to be at a location that is somewhat different from its actual location. Rarely does one phenomenon occur in isolation, i.e., without at least one of the other phenomena. Figure 17-2 illustrates the situation for reflection and refraction. At the boundary between two zones of different density, some of the wave energy is *reflected* back into the original medium, and some propagates into the second medium but is *refracted* (i.e., changes its direction of travel).

By convention, refraction and reflection angles are measured as an acute angle to a line *normal* (perpendicular) to the boundary surface at the point where the incident wave strikes the boundary.

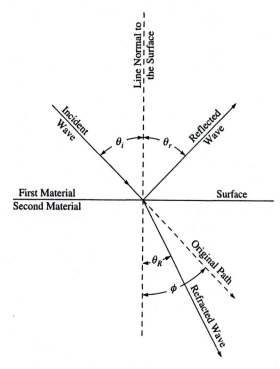

Figure 17-2
Reflection and refraction of waves.

In reflection, we know that the *angle of incidence* (θ_i) and the *angle of reflection* (θ_r) are equal to each other:

$$\theta_i = \theta_r \qquad (17\text{-}3)$$

where

θ_i is the angle of incidence

θ_r is the angle of reflection

If the incident wave impinges on the surface or boundary at an angle of 90 degrees (i.e., it is coincident with the normal line), it will be reflected back on itself. But if the angle is other than 90 degrees, then the reflected wave will travel away from the *surface at the same angle*.

Refraction phenomena affect the portion of the incident wave that enters the second medium. We may infer the behavior of ultrasound waves from the behavior of light waves in an optical medium.

The *index of refraction* (n) is defined as the ratio of the velocity of the wave in air (or in a vacuum, for electromagnetic waves) to the wave velocity in the medium, that is:

$$n = \frac{V_{AIR}}{V_{MED}} \qquad (17\text{-}4)$$

Table 17-2 shows the index of refraction for several common forms of material.

The *relative index of refraction* between two media (n_{2-1}) is found by measuring the *angle of incidence* (θ_i) and *angle of refraction* (θ_R) in the two media:

$$N_{2-1} = \frac{\sin \theta_i}{\sin \theta_R} \qquad (17\text{-}5)$$

The relative index of refraction is also equal to the ratio of the wave velocity in the two media:

$$N_{2-1} = \frac{V1}{V2} \qquad (17\text{-}6)$$

where

N_{2-1} is the relative index of refraction

θ_i is the angle of incidence

θ_R is the angle of refraction

$V1$ is the velocity of the wave in the first medium

$V2$ is the velocity of the wave in the second medium

TABLE 17-2   INDEX OF REFRACTION FOR DIFFERENT MATERIALS

Material	Value of N
Water	1.33
Ethyl alcohol	1.36
Quartz	1.46
Flint glass	1.66
Sodium chloride	1.53
Polyethylene	1.5–1.54
Air	1.00 (by definition)

Because Equations 17-5 and 17-6 both describe the relative index of refraction, we may write a new equation that relates the angles of incidence and refraction to the two velocities:

$$\frac{\sin \theta_i}{\sin \theta_R} = \frac{V1}{V2} \qquad (17\text{-}7)$$

From Equation 17-7 we may infer something about the behavior of ultrasound waves in the human body. In general, and with only a few exceptions, waves tend to have a higher velocity in denser materials than in less dense materials.* From Equation 17-7 we may conclude that:

1. θ_R is less than θ_i when incident waves cross into denser material.

2. θ_R is greater than θ_i when incident waves cross into less dense material.

Diffraction (Figure 17-3) is a bending of the direction of propagation that occurs when a wave impinges on an object of different density embedded within, and surrounded by, the incident media. Depending on the size of the object and the wavelength of the incident wave, a *shadow zone* (where little or no signal exists) may be created on the distal side of the object. Diffraction can distort the direction information of the signal.

17-4-3 Specular reflection, diffuse reflection, and scattering

The type of reflection discussed above and depicted in Figure 17-2 is somewhat idealized. A single incident ray resulting in a single reflected ray is termed *specular reflection* (Figure 17-4a). In medical ultrasound systems this rarely occurs because it requires a flat surface that is large compared with the wavelength of the signal (as when an ultrasound wave strikes a large bone, especially at a high angle). In most situations, however, the surface is rough and thus so produces *diffuse re-*

---

*An exception: The velocity of sound is slower in lead than in aluminum, even though lead is much denser than aluminum.

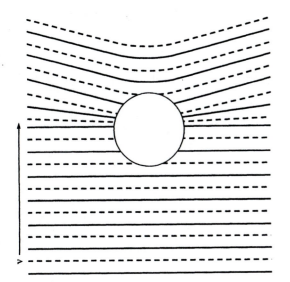

Figure 17-3
Wave diffraction.

flection (Figure 17-4b) rather than specular reflection.

Diffuse reflection gives rise to *scattering;* i.e., the light signal is sent in several directions rather than just one. Scattering also occurs when the wave impinges on small areas of greater density within tissue. Although both scattering and diffrac-

tion can occur in that situation, scattering predominates when the object is small compared with the wavelength of the signal.

Multipath phenomena (Figure 17-5) are also seen in medical ultrasound. The ultrasound transducer serves as both the receiver and the transmitter. A pulse is generated (Figure 17-6), and the system then "listens" for the echo as it reflects from underlying structures. Each pulse is one or more cycles of ultrasound energy. The time between successive pulses (T) describes the maximum distance that the system can image or, in medical ultrasound, the maximum depth in tissue. The *width* of the pulse (τ) is usually small compared to the interpulse space ($\tau < < T$), and pulse width limits the resolution available.

In Figure 17-5 we see that multipath problems can account for spurious signals reaching the transducer during receive time. The direct signal is propagated from the transducer to object A. The incident signal will be reflected back along the same path to the transducer. When this occurs, that signal is available to make the image. But note also that the signal may reflect to another object (B), especially if scattering takes place (which means that the surface of A is rough). That signal may have the correct angle under some circumstances to also be reflected into the receive

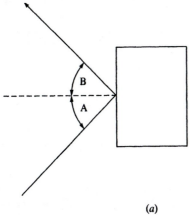

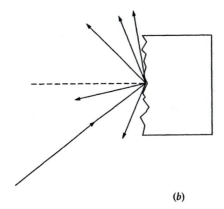

(a)

(b)

Figure 17-4
(a) Specular reflections. (b) Diffuse reflections.

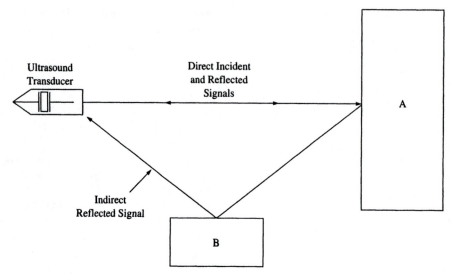

Figure 17-5
Multipath phenomenon.

transducer. When this occurs, a separate target is seen because the transducer cannot distinguish the direct and multipath reflections.

In pulse ultrasound systems, it is possible to limit the effect of multipath by using a *first-pulse*

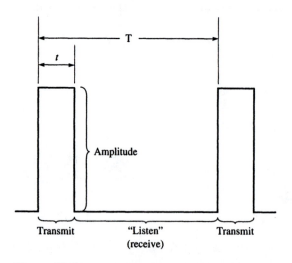

Figure 17-6
Ultrasound system transmits and then listens for pulse.

arrival circuit. The receiver will see two pulses, one from the direct reflection and one from the multipath. The direct path is shorter, however, so by accepting only the first pulse to arrive after the incident pulse is transmitted, we can eliminate most multipath. Two situations occur to mar this solution, however. The first is obvious: when the direct and multipath routes are approximately the same length. The second is rarely seen in medical ultrasound but is occasionally seen in geological ultrasound instruments, sonar, and other uses of ultrasound: when the multipath route is so much longer than the direct path that a reflected pulse arrives within the receive period of a successive transmit pulse.

17-4-4 Acoustical impedance

The *acoustical impedance* (Z_a) of a material is a measure of its opposition to the propagation of sound waves. It is sometimes characterized as a measure of the efficiency with which the signal propagates in the material. The unit of acoustical impedance is the Rayl, in which 1 Rayl = 1 kg/m^2s or 1 Rayl = 0.1 g/cm^2s.

Acoustical impedance is described by:

$$Z_a = \zeta V \qquad (17\text{-}8)$$

where

Z_a is the acoustical impedance in Rayls

ζ is the density of the medium in grams per cubic centimeter (g/cm^3)

V is the velocity of sound in the medium in centimeters per second (cm/s)

Example 17-2

Calculate the acoustical impedance of water if the velocity of sound in water is 1450 m/s and the density of water at body temperature (37°C) is 0.99 g/cm^3.

Solution

$$Z_a = \zeta V$$

$$Z_a = \left(\frac{0.99\, g}{cm^2}\right)\left(\frac{1{,}500\, m}{s} \times \frac{10^2\, cm}{m}\right)$$

$$Z_a = \left(\frac{0.99\, g}{cm^2}\right)\left(\frac{1.5 \times 10^5}{s}\right) = \frac{148{,}500\, g}{cm^2 - s}$$

Table 17-3 shows the acoustical impedance for a number of materials.

17-5 Ultrasound transducers

Recall from the earlier discussion that a transducer is a device that converts energy from one form to another for purposes of measurement or control. In ultrasound, two transducer functions are recognized: (1) conversion of ac oscillations into acoustical vibrations and (2) conversion of acoustical oscillations back into electrical oscillations. These two functions are the *transmit* and *receive* transducers, which in pulse systems can be combined into one element.

Several types of devices can be used to transduce ultrasonic energy. At lower frequencies, at which certain industrial and home ultrasound devices operate, the job can be done by dynamic microphone elements and certain capacitor assemblies. At higher frequencies, the ultrasound transducer is the *piezoelectric resonator,* sometimes called a *crystal resonator* or *crystal.*

The phenomenon of *piezoelectricity* is found in certain crystalline structures, such as natural *quartz, barium titanate, Rochelle salts,* and *lead zirconate titanate;* the latter is often used in medical ultrasound, although quartz and the other materials may also be used. Piezoelectric elements are those that *either produce a voltage across their two surfaces when deformed* or *deform if a voltage is placed across the element* from those same surfaces.

The piezoelectric element (Figure 17-7) consists of a slab of the material with electrodes connected to wires mounted on the surface of the element. In the circuits shown in Figure 17-7 the wires lead to a voltmeter, but in ultrasound devices they would lead to other forms of circuitry. When the crystal is at rest (Figure 17-7a), no voltage is produced. But if the element is deformed to the left, the voltage swings to one polarity (negative in this case), as in Figure 17-7b. Similarly, when the element is deformed to the right (Figure 17-c) the same amount, the same voltage is generated but with the opposite polarity. If a vibration of the same frequency as the resonant frequency of the crystal is used to repetitively deform the crystal, then it will oscillate back and forth, producing an alternating voltage. If, on the other hand, an alternating voltage is applied to the crystal at its resonant frequency, it will vibrate at that frequency. Because of the *resonance effect,* these operations tend to occur only at the natural resonant frequency of the crystal.

TABLE 17-3 ACOUSTICAL IMPEDANCE FOR DIFFERENT MATERIALS

Material	$Z_a(10^6$ Rayls)
Air	0.0004
Fat	1.38
Water	1.48
Muscle	1.70
Liver	1.65
Other soft tissue	1.63
Bone	7.80

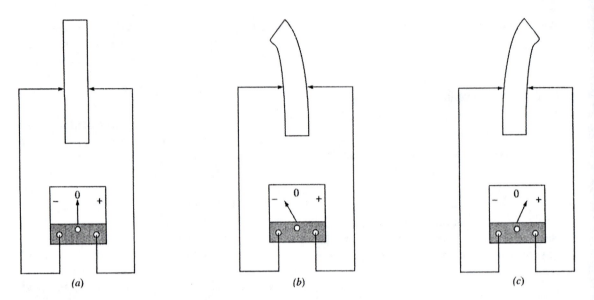

Figure 17-7
Piezoelectric element. *(a)* At rest. *(b)* Deflected left. *(c)* Deflected right.

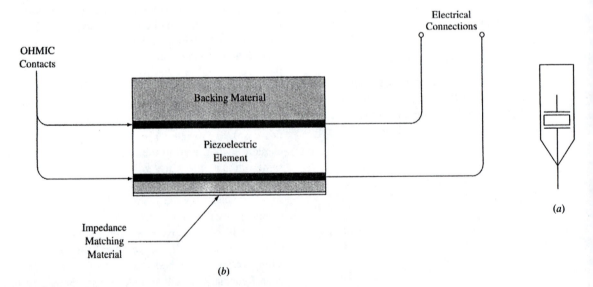

Figure 17-8
(a) Symbol for ultrasonic transducer. *(b)* Transducer structure.

Figure 17-8*a* shows a symbol for an ultrasonic transducer. Although other symbols are used in other texts, this one will be used in the rest of this chapter. The structure of the transducer is shown in Figure 17-8*b*. The piezoelectric crystal element is sandwiched between two metallic ohmic contacts, which are used for the electrical connections. Because the acoustical impedance of the crystal differs markedly from the acoustical impedance of the human body, an impedance matching layer is needed to interface with the patient. Maximum power transfer occurs only when the load impedance matches the source impedance. Also, a backing material is used to absorb energy from any direction within the assembly that is not directed toward the patient. This material prevents errors from internal transducer reflections.

If you are familiar with radio antenna theory, then much ultrasonic transducer theory will be familiar to you, even though it radiates acoustical rather than electromagnetic waves. Figure 17-9 shows a simplified unidirectional radiation pattern from an ultrasonic transducer. In close, the transducer interface surface is the *Fresnel zone,* in which the beam does not disperse very much. This region is similar to the *near field* of the radio antenna. Farther away is the *Fraunhofer zone,* in which the beam disperses proportionally to the square of the distance.

The power density of the signal at any distance is the total power divided by the area of the wavefront (disc area in Figure 17-9) and is measured in W/cm^2. As the distance increases, the area of the wavefront increases as the square of the distance, but the power remains constant. As a result, the power density drops according to the square of the distance. This is called the *inverse square law,* which states that power density, or intensity, drops off as the reciprocal of the square of the distance. In other words, attenuation $\alpha = 1/D^2$.

The *beamwidth* of the transducer (Figure 17-10) is the angle between points on the main lobe at which the power drops by half, i.e., −3 dB, relative to the maximum power point (0 dB, relative to the maximum power point (0 dB in Figure 17-10).

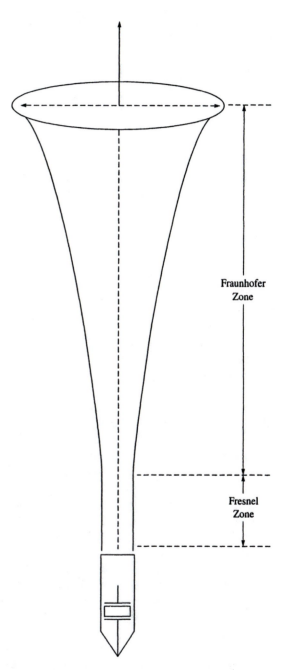

Figure 17-9
Simplified unidirectional radiation pattern.

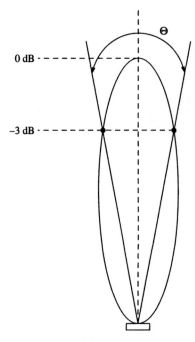

Figure 17-10
Beamwidth pattern.

The *resolution* of the ultrasonic signal is a function of two factors: the pulse width (τ) and the beamwidth. The pulse width sets the maximum *longitudinal resolution,* also called *range resolution* in radar terminology. The beamwidth sets the *azimuthal* or *angular resolution.* In some cases, you might see the *cross-range resolution* mentioned, which is the chord length between the −3 dB points on the main lobe.

The beam patterns shown thus far are somewhat idealized. In the real world things are not so clean as they are in theoretical discussions. For example, real transducers produce not only the main lobe, which does the imaging, but also spurious *sidelobes* (Figure 17-11*a*). These sidelobes sometimes send and receive pulses; thus, spurious echos can perceived as valid targets. These echos result in clutter in the image and are not valid signals. The sidelobes tend to be balanced, so they appear at angles of ±Θ from the center line of the main lobe. Figure 17-11*b* is a cartesian projection of the

transducer pattern. It shows that more than one pair of sidelobes appear with the main lobe in actual transducers.

17-6 Absorption and attenuation of ultrasound energy

A number of mechanisms cause loss of energy in the transmitted ultrasound signal. We have seen the loss due to beam spreading. Because the beam is not coherent (as in a laser), the signal level attenuates at a rate determined by the inverse square

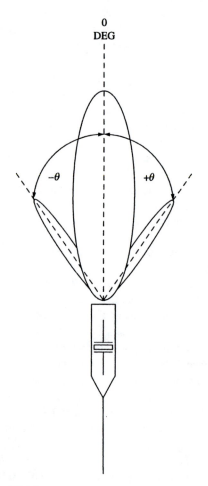

Figure 17-11
Transducer sidelobes. *(a)* Polar plot.

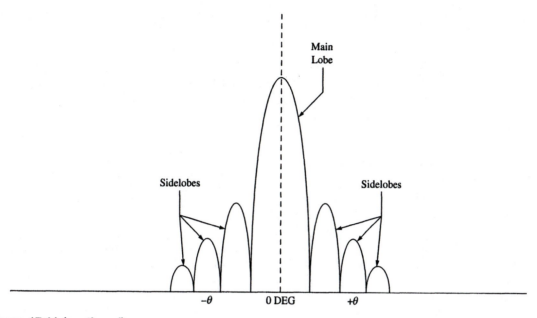

Figure 17-11 (continued)
Transducer sidelobes. *(b)* Cartesian plot.

law. There is also attenuation due to interaction with biological tissue, and it is related to the acoustical impedance of the tissue. Finally, there is also some loss due to scattering of the signal. The total attenuation is:

$$\alpha = BW + S + A \qquad (17\text{-}9)$$

where

α is the attenuation coefficient in decibels per centimeter (dB/cm)

BW is the beamwidth loss

S is the scattering loss

A is absorption loss

The value of attenuation by absorption depends on both the acoustical impedance and the frequency used. Figure 17-12 shows how soft-tissue absorption losses rise with frequency. At frequencies near 2 MHz (0.5 to 1 dB/cm), the attenuation loss is relatively small, but it climbs rapidly as frequency increases to 5 dB/cm. As a result, there is an upper limit near 10 MHz, where ultrasound can be used for medical purposes. Because the resolu-

tion of the imaging system is partially dependent on the operating frequency (the higher the frequency, the better the resolution), there is always a design trade-off between operating frequency for best resolution and minimum attenuation. Typical values for α are shown in Table 17-4. Note that

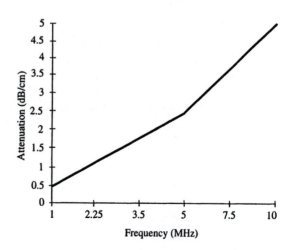

Figure 17-12
Soft-tissue absorption losses vs. frequency.

TABLE 17-4   TYPICAL VALUES FOR α

Medium	α(dB/cm)	Relationship
Air	12	F^2
Water	0.002	F^2
Bone	15	F
Kidney	1	F
Soft tissue	0.7	F
Fat	0.63	F
Blood	0.18	F

most mediums exhibit absorption that has a linear relationship with frequency ($\alpha \propto f$), but air and water exhibit absorption that has a quadratic relationship to frequency ($\alpha \propto f^2$).

Scattering losses are caused by reflected energy being sent in directions other than back to the receive transducer and include both absorption in the target (refraction loss) and reflection from the target. In any system in which both reflection and refraction take place, the energy of the incident wave is divided between the reflected and refracted products:

$$U_i = U_r + U_R \qquad (17\text{-}10)$$

where

U_i is the energy of the incident signal

U_r is the energy of the reflected signal

U_R is the energy of the refracted signal

The percentage of energy U_i that is reflected is given by the *coefficient of reflection,* also called the *intensity reflection coefficient* (some texts use Γ, others use R; we use Γ because it is more consistent with common engineering and physics practice), which is:

$$\Gamma = \left(\frac{Z1 - Z2}{Z1 + Z2}\right)^2 \qquad (17\text{-}11)$$

where

Γ is the intensity reflection coefficient

Z1   is the acoustical impedance of material 1

Z2   is the acoustical impedance of material 2

To express the reflected energy in *percentage,* multiply Equation 17-11 by 100%.

Example 17-4 _____

Calculate the intensity reflection coefficient (Γ) at the boundary between air (Z1 = 50 g/cm^2-s) and tissue (Z2 = 150,000 g/cm^2-s).

$$\Gamma = \left(\frac{Z1 - Z2}{Z1 + Z2}\right)^2 \times 100\%$$

$$\Gamma = \left(\frac{50 - 150,000}{50 + 150,000}\right)^2 \times 100\%$$

$$\Gamma = (-0.9993)^2 \times 100\% = \mathbf{99.9\%}$$

Note in Example 17-4 that almost all of the incident energy is reflected from the boundary between the two materials. This example illustrates a problem that exists in medical ultrasound: The vastly different impedance of air and tissue results in a poor transfer of power. Medical ultrasound transducers are coupled to the patient's skin through a special gel that provides an air-free path for the ultrasound waves.

Let us rework Example 17-4 using the impedance of the jelly rather than the impedance of air to see what difference the impedance-matching jelly makes to the transfer of energy. The impedance of the jelly can be taken to be approximately 1.48×10^5 g/cm-s.

$$\Gamma = \left(\frac{Z1 - Z2}{Z1 + Z2}\right)^2 \times 100\%$$

$$\Gamma = \left(\frac{148,000 - 150,000}{148,000 + 150,000}\right)^2 \times 100\%$$

$$\Gamma = (-0.0067)^2 \times 100\%$$

$$= (0.000045)(100\%) = \mathbf{0.0045\%}$$

Notice that when there is a large mismatch in the acoustical impedances, nearly all of the energy is reflected, and little is absorbed into the tissue. But when the impedances are matched, the opposite occurs, and nearly all of the energy is absorbed.

Many medical ultrasound instruments rely on pulse operation, in which the reflected wave is ex-

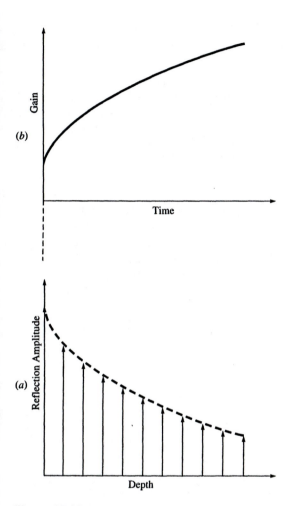

Figure 17-13
(a) Deeper targets return weaker signals. *(b)* Time-gain compensation curve.

the tissue is weaker than it would be from the same object closer to the surface. This effect is seen in Figure 17-13*a.* To overcome this problem, ultrasound machines have a receiver gain that varies with time after the pulse is fired (Figure 17-13*b*). The gain rise with time is called *time-gain compensation* (TGC), and the curve is selected to mirror the attenuation curve. This feature is also called *depth-gain compensation* (DGC) in some machines. Using TGC, the same target will produce the same amplitude response on the screen of the ultrasound monitor, regardless of its depth into the tissue.

17-7 Scan modes and scanning systems

To derive information about structures inside the body, the ultrasound device uses several different scanning modes: *A-scan, B-scan, M-mode* (once called *T-M-mode*), and *real-time mode.*

The A-scan mode (Figure 17-14) is the oldest scanning mode, dating back to the primitive radar units used in the 1930s. Whether in radar, sonar, or medical ultrasound, the A-scan mode uses a stationary transducer to fire a pulse into tissue. The oscilloscope or hard-copy readout scans time along the horizontal axis and plots the signal amplitude along the vertical axis. A large spike at the left corner (unless it is suppressed) represents the transmit spike. The tissue at the interface with the transducer will produce some near-field scatter immediately to the right of the transmit spike. Other spikes represent reflections from targets within the tissue.

The B-scan mode (Figure 17-15) may use the same time base as the A-scan but plots the strength of the returning signal as changes in brightness, i.e., a strong reflection is brighter than the weaker reflection. When the transducer is mechanically scanned back and forth, successive images are built up, allowing a two-dimensional (2-D) view of the underlying structure. Again, the strength of the reflection is graphed by the brightness of the cathode ray tube display.

amined. If the structure causing the reflection is acoustically dense compared with surrounding tissue (e.g., bone), then the reflection coefficient is large and the reflection is strong. But when the target tissue density is close to the surrounding tissue density, then only a small amount of energy is reflected and the signal is weak.

17-6-1 Time-gain compensation

The ultrasound signal attenuates as it penetrates the tissue, so reflections from an object deeper in

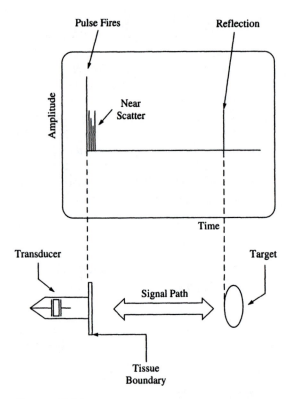

Figure 17-14
A-scan mode.

ure 17-17*b*. This particular scan is of the heart, and has the electrocardiograph waveform superimposed on the readout.

A real-time scan is provided by a B-scan system in which the scan rate of the transducer is fast enough to capture the movements of the organs being imaged. This type of system can capture the beating heart on the screen, allowing the physician to observe its motion.

An alternative 2-D B-scan system is shown in Figure 17-18. In this arrangement, an array of transducer crystals is aligned in a semicircular arc about the center line. This configuration is a crude form of electronically scanned array (ESA). An electronic switch rotates the oscillator signal from one crystal to another. This method is somewhat practical but has problems that make it not

Scanning back and forth, as shown in Figure 17-16, is not always very practical in medical ultrasound (although it is used in industrial ultrasound and was once used in medical imaging). A modified 2-D B-scan is shown in Figure 17-17*a*. In this method, the transducer is at a fixed location but mechanically scans back and forth, producing a V-shaped scanned region. This scan system is similar to the plan position indicator (PPI) display used in radar. In shipboard and land-based radar, the PPI is circular because the antenna can scan through 360°, but on airborne radar the antenna typically scans ±30° or ±60°, so it produces a scan region very similar to that in Figure 17-17*a*. An example of this form of scan is shown in Fig-

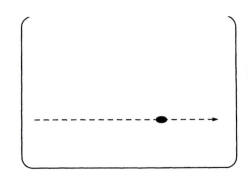

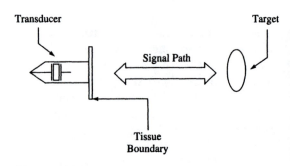

Figure 17-15
B-scan mode.

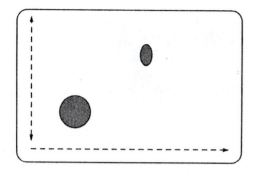

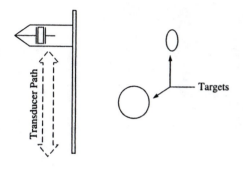

Targets

Figure 17-16
Back-and-forth scan method.

very popular. A better approach is the electronically scanned phased array transducer (discussed below).

The *time-motion* (T-M) mode is now usually called the *M-mode*. This mode is essentially an A-scan but with successive looks at the target created by scanning the time base vertically (Figure 17-19a). In machines that provide a paper readout, the vertical scanning can be produced mechanically by pulling the photosensitive paper in front of the 1-D transducer. Each instantaneous position in the scan produces depth information on one axis, time information on the other, and intensity information in the brightness of the display. Some modern color displays go one step further by color coding the flow direction. Figure 17-19b shows an example of a time-motion M-scan from an echocardiograph (heart imaging) machine. The patient's ECG signal is superimposed on the tracing.

17-7-1 Electronically scanned phased array transducers

The scanning systems discussed thus far are based on mechanical scanning, or a crude electronic scanning in which an electronic switched array is used. There is, however, a class of transducer that uses an array of transducer elements in a phased array scheme that permits passive scanning of the beam by electronic means: the *electronically scanned phased array (ESPA)* transducer.

Figure 17-20 shows a simple four-element phased array transducer. Four separate transducer elements (A1, A2, A3, and A4) are arranged in a

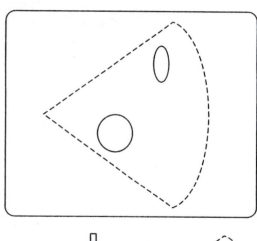

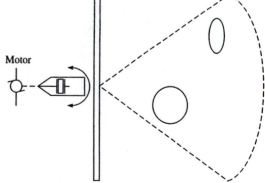

Motor

Figure 17-17
(a) 2-D B-scan.

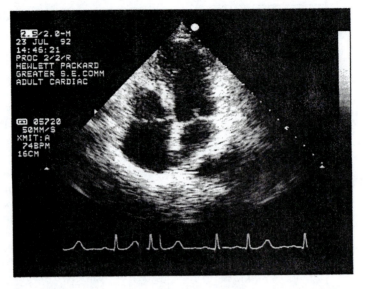

Figure 17-17 (continued)
(b) Two-dimensional B-scan of heart.

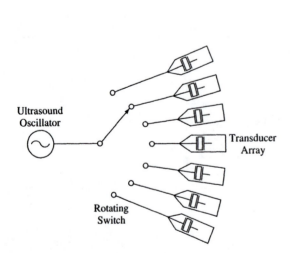

Ultrasound Oscillator

Transducer Array

Rotating Switch

Figure 17-18
Alternative two-dimensional B-scan.

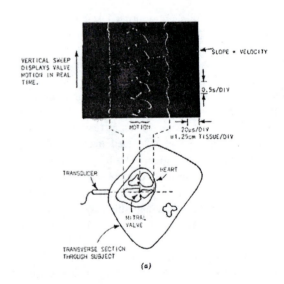

Figure 17-19
(a) Time-motion or M-mode.

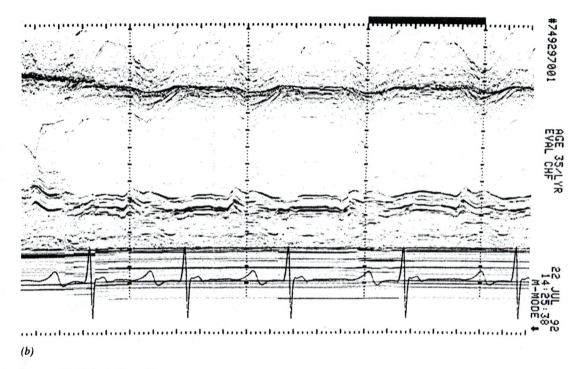

Figure 17-19 (continued)
(b) Echocardiograph plot.

linear array (curvilinear is also possible but is harder to analyze at this point in our discussion). Each transducer element is spaced a distance (*d*) apart. Although the ESPA can be used identically in both receive and transmit modes, we will begin our discussion with the receive mode. In Figure 17-20 an advancing wavefront, as from the reflection from a target, approaches the ESPA at an angle Θ_o. The phase of the signal at each element (A1 − A4) is:

$$\Psi = \frac{2\pi d}{\lambda} \qquad (17\text{-}12)$$

where

Ψ is the phase at each element

d is the interelement distance

λ is the wavelength of the impinging signal

The four individual transducers are connected such that their respective output voltages are combined into one signal, V_A. For an array of *N* transducer elements, the output voltage of the array is:

$$V_A = \sin\left(\frac{2\pi}{\lambda}t + (N-1)\frac{\Psi}{2}\right)\left(\frac{\sin(N\Psi/2)}{\sin(\Psi/2)}\right)$$

$$(17\text{-}13)$$

where

V_A is the combined output voltage

N is the number of elements in the array (e.g., 4 in Figure 17-20)

λ is the wavelength of the signal

Ψ is the phase of the signal arriving at each element at angle Θ_o

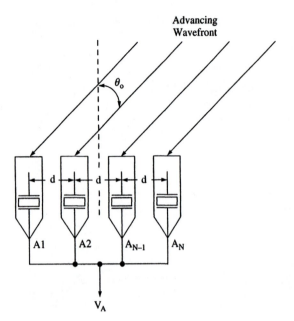

Figure 17-20
Four-element phased array transducer.

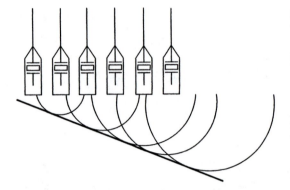

Figure 17-21
A common wavefront propagates from the array at an angle determined by element spacing.

If a signal is applied to the elements of the array in-phase (the phase of the signal is the same at all elements), then the troughs and peaks of the wavefront from each element will interfere to form a common wavefront that propagates away from the array at an angle that depends on the spacing (Figure 17-21). The advancing wavefront is created by the algebraic sum of the wavefronts of the individual elements of the array.

A steerable scanning system can be made by adding a phase shifter to each element ($\Delta\theta$ in Figure 17-22). By adjusting the phase shift at each transducer element, we can alter the direction of the combined wavefront that propagates away from the array. A *beam steering computer* sends commands (θA1 through θA4) to the transducer elements in the array. This type of system provides a sweeping 2-D B-scan without moving parts. In addition, the beamwidth of the signal is reduced because of the mutual effect of the transducer elements.

A problem with the ESPA is that the beamwidth is not constant throughout the range of scan. It is

minimum (producing better resolution) orthogonal to the array's front plane and maximum at the highest scan angle. Resolution is therefore a function of scan angle.

Another problem is *grating lobes* (Figure 17-23). Each element of the array has its own main lobes and side lobes. These combine to form the main lobe of the array, but the minor lobes do not disappear; they will appear in the final beam of the array as grating lobes.

The grating lobes appear at angles that satisfy Equation 17-14:

$$\sin\theta_g = \sin\Theta_o \pm \frac{n\lambda}{d}$$

where

θ_g is the angle at which grating lobes appear

Θ_o is the angle of the wavefront with respect to the normal line

λ is the wavelength of the signal

n is the number of elements in the array

d is the spacing of the elements within the array

When $d = \lambda/2$, the first grating lobes do not appear because $\sin\theta > 1$. The first grating lobes appear at 90° when $d/\lambda = 1$.

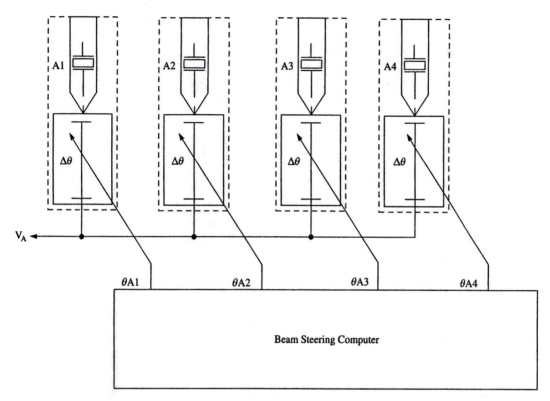

Figure 17-22
Steerable scanning system realized by adding phase shifters to each element.

Figure 17-23, only two elements are shown, for simplicity's sake. The grating lobes will cause spurious returns to be displayed. Some suppression is possible, especially based on signal strength (returns from the grating lobes tend to be weaker than returns from the main lobe).

17-8 Biological effects of ultrasound

The increased use of ultrasound monitoring, therapeutic, and diagnostic equipment has led to some concern over the possible hazard levels. Thus far, no definitive information exists concerning safe levels. Most clinical and research instruments are designed to produce power output levels between 5 and 50 mW/cm^2 at the transducer. Unfortunately, the measurement of ultrasound power levels is difficult, and there is no well-established standard accepted by all for the measurement of power levels.

Several factors are believed to have importance in the biological interaction of tissue and ultrasound waves: *frequency, irradiation time, beam intensity,* and *duty cycle.*

The principal biophysical effects of ultrasound are *thermal, cavitation, shearing action,* and *intracellular motion.*

The thermal effects are caused by sonic agitation of cells and are affected by the nature of the tissue, blood flow, and thermal conduction losses. In general, we can state that heat created is the

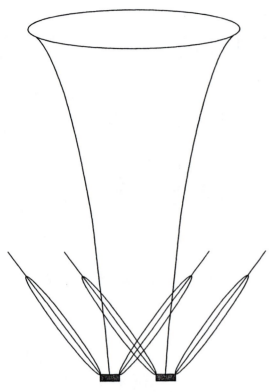

Figure 17-23
Grating lobes from phased array.

shear forces by generating eddy currents in the medium.

Intracellular movement is created when cell membrane vibrations take place under the influence of the ultrasound waves. These movements often take the form of twisting action.

17-9 Doppler effect

The Doppler effect is a change of frequency that occurs when the receiver and transmitter move relative to each other. You can observe this effect when a fire engine or police car approaches with its siren wailing. As the vehicle speeds toward you, the pitch rises an amount proportional to the relative velocity between you and that vehicle. As the vehicle with the siren passes you, the pitch abruptly shifts lower and descends as the vehicle moves away. Medical ultrasound devices can use the Doppler effect to detect motion. Figure 17-24 shows a situation in which blood or some structure in the body moves relative to the ultrasound transducer. The frequency shift is determined by:

$$f_d = 2 \, v \cos \theta \qquad (17\text{-}16)$$

product of the applied power intensity (I) in W/cm^2 and the absorption coefficient dB/cm.

$$U_h = \alpha I \qquad (17\text{-}15)$$

where

U_h is the heat energy in watts (W)

α is the absorption coefficient in cm^{-1}

I is the beam intensity in W/cm^2

The cavitation phenomenon is rather complex but can be described as the creation of gaseous bubbles in the fluid medium due to agitation by the ultrasonic waves. Cavitation is also the mechanism by which ultrasonic cleaners work.

Shear forces operate in media of low viscosity that are able to flow. The ultrasound waves create

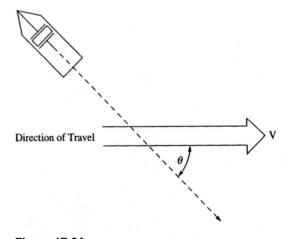

Figure 17-24
Motion of object relative to wavefront creates Doppler shift.

where

f_d is the Doppler frequency

v is the relative velocity

θ is the angle between source and receiver

Continuous wave Doppler ultrasound uses two crystal transducer elements, one each for receive and transmit. A *pulse Doppler* system uses a single crystal for both receive and transmit.

17-10 Transcutaneous Doppler flow detectors

Transcutaneous flow detectors are designed to use the Doppler effect to detect the flow of blood in arteries close to the surface of the body. An example of a commercial flow detector and several different transducers is shown in Figure 17-25.

Figure 17-26a shows the basic configuration of a Doppler flow detector. Two crystals, one each for transmit and receive functions, are placed in a plastic housing that is positioned over a peripheral artery. A frequency near 10 MHz is usually selected for these instruments to take advantage of the natural attenuation of high ultrasonic frequencies in tissue. Such frequencies also permit better focusing and a larger frequency change for any

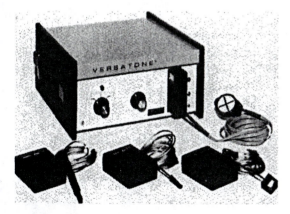

Figure 17-25
Ultrasound flowmeter. (Photo courtesy of Medsonics, Inc.)

given amount of motion. Reflections of significant amplitude from underlying tissues are therefore attenuated, while reflections from blood vessels near the surface are stronger.

The back-scatter reflections from the moving blood will have a slightly different frequency than the incident wave due to Doppler shift. If the blood were motionless, the frequency shift would be zero, so the return wave frequency will be identical to the incident wave frequency. But moving blood produces a shift that is proportional to the blood velocity. A frequency shift of approximately 200 Hz at 10 MHz corresponds to a blood velocity of approximately 6 cm/s.

The 10-MHz oscillator in Figure 17-26a excites the transmit crystal and, in some models, one port of the detector in the receiver section of the instrument. The incident wave will be shifted $\pm \Delta F$ by the flowing blood, and this frequency excites the receive crystal. The signal at the output of the receive crystal is amplified and then fed to a detector. The output of the detector is the $\pm \Delta F$ component. In most instruments the filtered output takes the form of a low-frequency hiss.

The audio output, through earphones or a loudspeaker, gives the surgeon a subjective yet accurate indication of blood flow. In a few models, an integrator circuit is used to produce a dc voltage that is proportional to the flow value. This voltage, however, is difficult to calibrate accurately but does serve as a relative flow indicator.

A probe-type flow transducer is shown in Figure 17-26b. In this assembly, two crystal elements are positioned side by side but are separated by a barrier with a high acoustical impedance.

17-11 Flowmeters

There are two general types of flowmeters. One type depends on the velocity difference between upstream and downstream sound waves. The second uses the Doppler shift of scattered waves from the moving medium (i.e., blood).

Figure 17-27a shows a transit time ultrasonic flow transducer. Two piezoelectric crystal elements

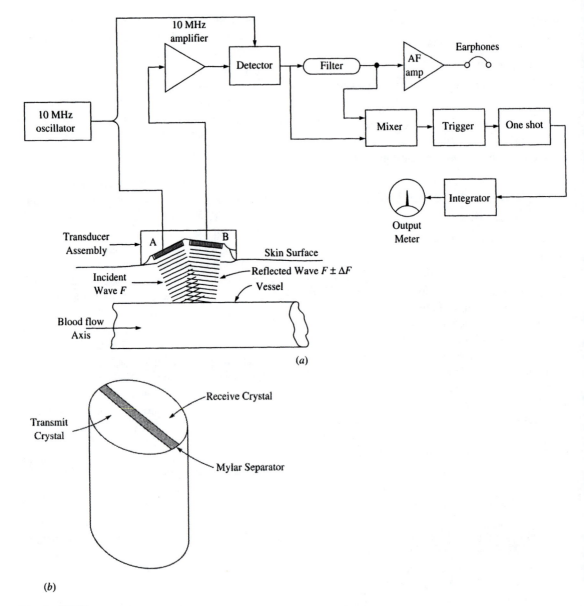

Figure 17-26
Ultrasonic flowmeter transducers. (a) Regular. (b) Pencil probe.

are aimed at each other obliquely across the flow path. The axis between these crystals has length D and forms angle θ with the flow axis.

The crystals in Figure 17-27b serve both transmit and receive functions. When measuring the downstream transit time of an ultrasonic pulse, crystal A is the transmitter, while crystal B is the receiver. When measuring the upstream time, however, the roles of the crystals are reversed; A becomes the receiver and B is the transmitter.

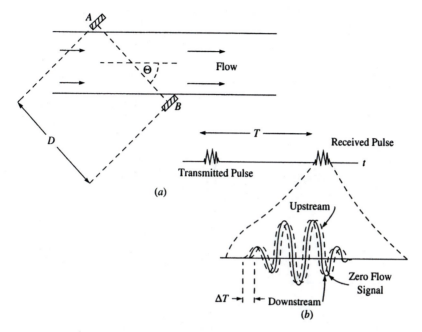

Figure 17-27
Ultrasound flowmeter capable of yielding numeric data. *(a)* Transit time ultrasonic flow transducer. *(b)* Combined waveforms. (From R. S. C. Cobbold, *Transducers for Biomedical Measurements*, John Wiley & Sons, New York, 1974.)

The difference between upstream and downstream transit times (ΔT) is measured in an electronic circuit and is then used to solve the expression

$$\overline{V} = \frac{C^2 \, \Delta T}{2 \, D \cos \theta} \qquad (17\text{-}17)$$

where

$\overline{V}$ is the average flow velocity of the medium

C is the speed of sound in the medium .

ΔT is the difference between upstream and downstream transit times

θ is the angle between the crystal axis and the flow axis.

Example 17-5

An ultrasonic flow transducer is designed to measure the mean velocity of a gaseous medium such as respiratory air. The crystal axis makes a 30° angle with the flow axis, and the crystals are spaced 1.25 cm apart. Calculate the air velocity if the transit time is 8.6×10^{-9} s. (*Hint:* The speed of sound in air is 335 m/s.)

Solution

$$V = \frac{C^2 \, \Delta T}{2D \cos \theta} \qquad (17\text{-}18)$$

$$V = \frac{[(335 \text{ m/s}) \times (100 \text{ cm/m})]^2}{(2)(1.25 \text{ cm})(\cos 30°)}$$

$$V = \frac{9.6 \text{ cm}^2/\text{s}}{2.2 \text{ cm}} = \textbf{4.4 cm/s}$$

Note in Figure 17-27*b* that the quantity ΔT tends to be very small. When analog circuits are used to measure ΔT, then matters such as noise and drift become very important. As a result, many instruments based on transit time differences use phase detection techniques rather than actual timing techniques.

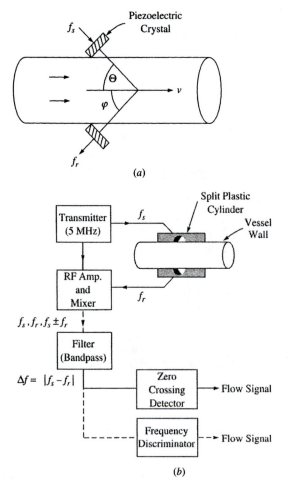

(a)

(b)

Figure 17-28
Doppler flowmeter. *(a)* Transducer. *(b)* Block diagram.
(From R. S. C. Cobbold, *Transducers for Biomedical Measurements,* John Wiley & Sons, New York, 1974.)

A Doppler flow transducer is shown in Figure 17-28*a*. This transducer uses the frequency change of a wave scattered from particulate matter flowing in the vessels. It has been shown that the change in frequency, ΔF, is given by:[†]

$$\Delta F = \pm F_s(\cos\theta + \cos\phi)\frac{v}{c} \quad (17\text{-}19)$$

where

ΔF is the frequency shift in hertz (Hz)

F_s is the transmitter frequency in hertz (Hz)

θ is the angle of the transmit crystal axis to the flow axis

ϕ is the angle of the receive crystal axis to the flow axis

A minus sign is used in Equation 17-19 when the flow is toward the crystal faces; a plus sign denotes flow away from the faces.

The block diagram for an ultrasonic flow detector based on Equation 17-19 is shown in Figure 17-28*b*. In this instrument the signal from the receive crystal F_r (i.e., $F_r = F_s \pm \Delta F$) is mixed with F_s in a radio frequency (RF) amplifier/mixer stage. A band pass filter is used to ensure that only the *difference* frequency ($F_s - F_r$) is actually used.

Two alternative output stages are shown in Figure 17-28*b*. One type uses a zero-crossing detector to produce spike pulses at each point where ΔF goes through zero. If these pulses are integrated, we obtain a dc flow signal. Alternatively, the output pulses could be processed in a digital circuit that is designed to recognize the repetition rate of the pulses.

The alternative technique is to use a frequency-sensitive discriminator to produce a flow signal.

The flow signal that is obtained from an instrument such as the one shown in Figure 17-28*b* represents the *mean flow velocity* in centimeters per second of the fluid (i.e., blood) in the tube (i.e., vessel). Both liquid and gaseous flowmeters are using this technique.

The data from the instrument does not represent volumetric flow (i.e., mL/s) rate. Only velocity data can be discerned from the output of the transducer unless the cross-sectional area of the vessel is known, in which case volumetric flow is proportional to the product of area and velocity.

[†]Richard S. C. Cobbold, *Transducer for Biomedical Measurements,* Wiley (New York, 1974), p. 280.

17-12 Ultrasonic blood pressure measurement

Ultrasonic techniques can be used to measure arterial blood pressure indirectly. Both manual and automatic (Figure 17-29) models have been manufactured.

Figure 17-30 shows how such a system operates. Piezoelectric crystals are placed between the patient's arm and a blood pressure cuff (Figure 17-30*a*). The ultrasonic circuits measure the Doppler shift caused when the incident wave reflects from a moving wall of the underlying brachial artery. The frequency of the reflected signal is proportional to the instantaneous velocity of the vessel wall. When the brachial artery is occluded, the Doppler shift is near zero. But when the arterial pressure is able to overcome the cuff pressure, the occlusion will snap open, causing a Doppler shift in the 200- to 500-Hz range.

Two Doppler events occur during each cardiac cycle (Figure 17-30*b*). When the arterial pulse pressure rises to cuff pressure, the opening event is characterized by the 200- to 500-Hz Doppler shift. But as the arterial pressure recedes back toward the diastolic, the vessel will close (i.e., reocclude) once the arterial pressure is less than the cuff pressure. This event produces a low-frequency Doppler shift in the 25- to 100-Hz range.

When blood pressure is measured, the cuff pressure is allowed to bleed down at a fixed rate. The systolic pressure is indicated by the onset of high-frequency Doppler shift sounds. At that time, the high- and low-frequency components are almost coincident (Figure 17-30*b*). But as the cuff pressure drops below systolic, the occurrence of the two events becomes further apart, until the cuff pressure drops to the diastolic pressure. At that point, the low-frequency component signifying the closing events becomes almost coincident with the high-frequency component of the *next* cardiac cycle. In a manual blood pressure instrument, these events are audible in a loudspeaker, and the operator uses them as if the instrument were a stethoscope, the ultrasonic audible events being analogous to the Korotkoff sounds in sphygmomanometry.

A simplified block diagram of an automatic ultrasonic blood pressure measurement system is shown in Figure 17-31. This instrument consists of three sections: pneumatic subsystem, control system, and ultrasonic section. The operation is as follows (the control section coordinates all events):

1. The pump turns on and inflates the cuff to the predetermined level set by the *cuff pressure* control on the front panel.

2. The bleed valve (V_1) opens to allow the cuff to *slowly* deflate, while the ultrasonic section looks for the high-frequency tones indicating systolic pressure.

3. When the cuff pressure has bled down to the systolic pressure, the electronic circuit will receive the high-frequency tones. When this occurs, the systolic hold valve (V_2) is closed, causing the systolic manometer to remain at the systolic pressure value.

4. When the cuff pressure drops to the diastolic value, the control system closes valve V_3, holding the diastolic manometer at the diastolic pressure.

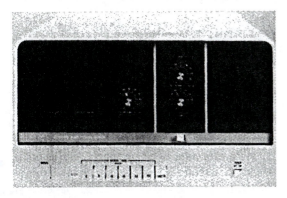

Figure 17-29
Ultrasonic blood pressure monitor. (Photo courtesy of Roche Medical Electronics, Cranbury, N.J.)

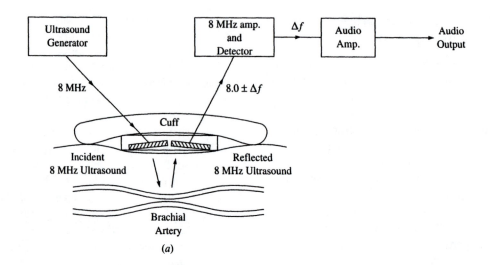

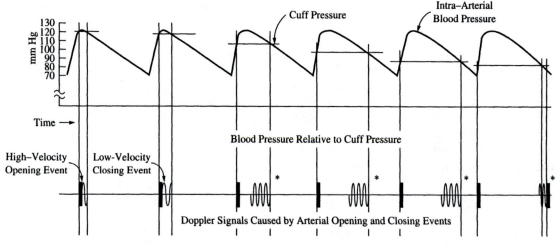

* Note approach of closing event to successive opening event as cuff pressure decreases.

(b)

Figure 17-30
Ultrasonic pressure system. (a) Transducer placement and block diagram. (b) Timing.

5. Following determination of the diastolic pressure, the control system opens valve V_4 to vent the cuff to atmosphere. The manometers, however, remain at the diastolic and systolic pressure values, respectively.

The ultrasonic blood pressure device has demonstrated an ability to measure the pressure of normal patients to within ±2.5 mm Hg, and on hypotensive patients it can obtain a valid response when auscultation is difficult or impossible. The automatic version allows continuous, noninvasive monitoring of blood pressure during surgical procedures or in the ICU/CCU.

The updated version shown in Figure 17-28 replaces the mercury manometers with electronic

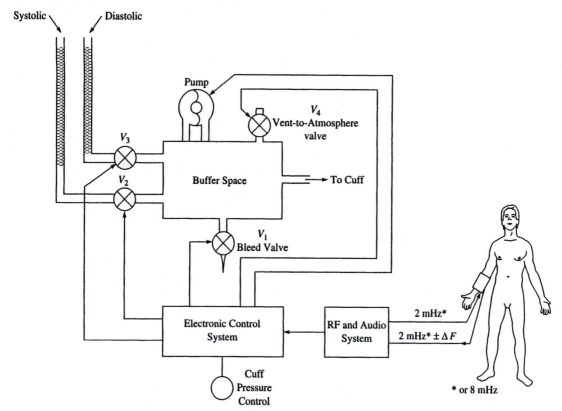

Figure 17-31
Pneumatic system for ultrasonic pressure monitor.

measurement of the chamber pressure. Such a scheme eliminates the need for valves V_2 and V_3 in Figure 17-31. If electronic pressure measurement is used, the systolic or diastolic display can be updated at the instants dictated by the control system.

17-12-1 Fetal Monitors

Fetal monitors fall into two different categories. One type is essentially an electronic stethoscope and uses ultrasonic Doppler shift to detect the fetal heart sounds. The other type is more complex and measures the fetal ECG (through scalp electrodes) and pressure of the amniotic fluid.

The simple A-scan shows time-versus-amplitude, wheras the linear B-scan is an intensity modulated display. The time-motion (T-M) plot detects motion of the heart known as echocardiography.

17-13 Echoencephalography

Echo ranging can also be used to probe the brain, and it forms the basis for an ultrasonic device called the *echoencephalograph*. Figure 17-32 illustrates the basic principle of an A-scan echoencephalograph. This diagram shows two transducer locations for the comparison of results.

The echoencephalograph will fire 1-μs bursts of 2 to 3 MHz ultrasound energy at a repetition rate of 500 bursts per second. An oscilloscope connected for A-scan will show traces such as those

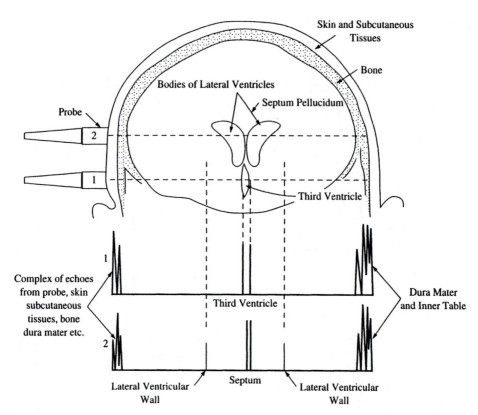

Figure 17-32
Echoencephalograph transducer placement and patterns generated. (Reprinted courtesy of
Hewlett-Packard)

shown in Figure 17-32. The left-most reflection corresponds to the skull wall nearest the transducer. The right-most feature is the reflection from the far side of the patient's skull. The features between the skull wall reflections depend upon transducer placement and certain other factors.

The midline feature is caused by reflections from the lateral ventricles, the third ventricle, and the septum pellucidum between the lateral ventricles. Ordinarily, the septum lies within ±2 mm of the center line of the skull, and its reflection on the CRO screen, will be located exactly midway between the spikes representing the third ventricle in Figure 17-32. A shift of more than ±3 mm from the correct position is often considered to be pathological and may indicate the presence of a tumor or other lesion.

One form of echoencephalogram uses two determinations of midline locations, one each for right-to-left and left-to-right paths. Figure 17-33 shows such a presentation. The procedure is as follows:

1. A good R-L path display is obtained on an oscilloscope and then photographed on an oscilloscope camera. The film is *not* advanced at this time.

2. The transducer is moved to the other side of the skull (or another transducer is used), and an L-R display is obtained.

3. The L-R display is photographed on the same photographic plate for comparison with the R-L display.

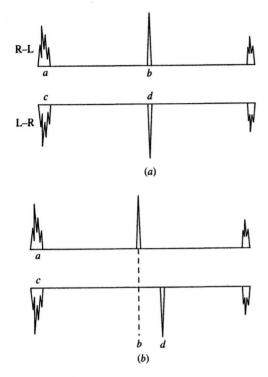

Figure 17-33
R-L and L-R patterns. *(a)* Normal. *(b)* Displacement of midline. (Reprinted courtesy of Hewlett-Packard)

Figure 17-33*a* shows a normal display, in which the R-L and L-R presentations of the midline structures coincide. But in Figure 17-33*b* the structures do not coincide because some midline shift is present.

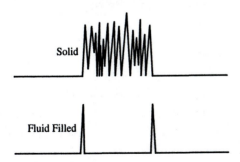

Figure 17-34
Displays of solid and fluid-filled masses. (Reprinted courtesy of Hewlett-Packard)

The locations of tumors, aneurysms, and other lesions can be determined by multiple scans to find the distance from the skull walls at different angles.

Note that solid and soft (fluid-filled) tumors produce radically different echo responses, as shown in Figure 17-34.

17-14 Summary

1. Ultrasound uses acoustical waves in the range above 20 kHz. Medical ultrasound tends to use frequencies in the 2- to 10-MHz region.

2. Ultrasound waves obey the reflection, refraction, diffraction, and scatter rules of ordinary wave behavior.

3. Several factors affect biological interaction with ultrasound: frequency, irradiation time, beam intensity, and duty cycle.

4. Most ultrasound transducers are piezoelectric crystals.

17-15 Recapitulation

Now return to the objectives and self-evaluation questions at the beginning of the chapter and see how well you can answer them. If you cannot answer certain questions, place a check mark next to each and review appropriate parts of the text. Next, try to answer the following questions using the same procedure. When you have answered all of the questions, solve the problems.

Questions

1. Define in your own words the meaning of *ultrasound.*

2. A 2-MHz signal will be a(n) _____ wave if radiated by an antenna and a(n) _____ wave if radiated by a piezoelectrical crystal.

3. Ultrasonic waves are _____ in a liquid, gas, or solid medium.

4. Ultrasound waves exhibit both _____ and _____ phenomena, characteristic of all wave behavior.

5. When waves bend around an obstruction, it is called _____.

6. Wavelength is the quotient of velocity and _____.

7. List two types of wave propagation in ultrasound systems.

8. A measure of a medium's opposition to the propagation of ultrasound waves is called _____ _____.

9. The percentage of energy reflected at any interface between media is given by the _____ of _____, also called _____ _____.

10. Impedance matching of the path between an ultrasonic transducer and the patient's skin surface requires the use of a _____.

11. Reflection in which a single incident ray produces a single reflected ray is called _____ reflection.

12. Reflection in which a single incident ray produces multiple rays is called _____ reflection.

13. List four factors affecting the interaction between ultrasound waves and biological tissue.

14. The Rayl is a unit of _____ _____.

15. The dimensions of the Rayl are such that 1 Rayl = _____/m^2-s.

16. Most diagnostic ultrasound instruments limit output at the transducer to the range _____ mW/cm^2 to _____ mW/cm^2 (true or false).

17. List four biophysical effects of ultrasound waves in tissue.

18. Most ultrasound transducers used in medical instruments are _____ crystals.

19. List two types of crystals that might be used as ultrasonic transducers.

20. The _____ of a transducer is measured between the half-power points, i.e., the points at which the power density falls off -3 dB from the maximum value.

21. The resolution of a pulse ultrasound is a function of _____ and _____.

22. The approximate ultrasound absorption of air is _____ dB/cm.

23. The approximate ultrasound absorption of soft tissue is _____ dB/cm.

24. Air and water have an F/F^2 attenuation relationship.

25. A transcutaneous blood flow detector uses the _____ effect to detect the presence of blood flowing in arteries.

26. A transcutaneous blood flow detector is a(n) noninvasive/invasive technique.

27. Most transcutaneous flow detectors use frequencies in the _____-MHz range to take advantage of the natural attenuation of tissues.

28. Draw a block diagram of a transcutaneous flow detector.

29. List two methods for making flow measurements using ultrasound.

30. Most flowmeters measure _____ flow velocity.

31. Ultrasonic blood pressure monitors use Doppler shift components to detect _____ and _____ points.

32. The systolic pressure causes Doppler shifts in the _____-Hz range.

33. Ultrasonic fetal monitors use Doppler shift to detect fetal _____ _____.

34. What is an A-scan display in ultrasonic terminology?

35. What is a linear B-scan? Compound B-scan?

36. An echocardiograph uses a(n) _____ display to detect motion of the mitral valve.

37. Depth and gain information in an echocardiograph is displayed on _____ _____ _____ curve.

38. The echoencephalograph probes the _____ using an ultrasonic A-scan.

Problems

1. Calculate the velocity of a 5-MHz ultrasound signal in water if its wavelength is 6.8×10^{-3} cm.

2. Calculate the frequency of an ultrasound signal in tissue if its velocity is 1500 m/s and the wavelength is 7.6×10^{-3} cm.

3. Calculate the wavelength of a 7-MHz (a) ultrasound wave in tissue (V = 1500 m/s), and (b) electromagnetic wave (V = 3×10^8 m/s).

4. An ultrasound wave impinges on a boundary between media at an angle of 28°. Find the angle of reflection.

5. Calculate the angle of refraction if the incident angle is $3'°$ and the relative index of refraction is 1.33.

6. Calculate the index of refraction for tissue if the ultrasound wave travels at 1500 m/s. (*Hint:* V_{air} = 335 m/s.)

7. Find the relative index of refraction at interface between two mediums if sound travels at 1500 m/s in one and 970 m/s in the other.

8. An ultrasound wave impinges on the interface in problem 17-7 at an angle of 29°. Calculate the angle of refraction.

9. Find the acoustical impedance if sound travels at 1250 m/s in a medium with density of 1.6 g/cm^3.

10. The density of material A is 1.2 g/cm^3, while the density of material B is 0.88 g/cm^3. The velocity of sound in material A is 1500 m/s and in B, 1000 m/s. Calculate the coefficient of reflection.

11. A transit time blood flowmeter uses crystal faces 1.8 cm apart, forming an angle with the flow axis of 32°. Find the mean flow velocity of the blood if the velocity of sound is 1100 m/s and the transit time is 9×10^{-9} s.

12. A Doppler flowmeter uses two crystals, one at 40° *to* the flow axis and the other at 30° *from* the flow axis. Calculate the Doppler shift in hertz of a 5-MHz signal if the flow velocity of blood is 6 cm/s and the speed of sound i 1000 m/s.

Suggested reading

1. Atles, Leslie R. and Scott Segalewitz, *Affinity: Reference Guide for Biomedical Technicians,* Kendall/Hunt Publishing Co. (Dubuque, Ia., 1995).

2. Cobbold, Richard S. C., *Transducers for Biomedical Measurements,* Wiley (New York, 1978).

3. Halliday, David and Robert Resnick, *Physics Parts I and II,* Wiley (New York, 1966).

4. *7215A Echoencephalograph Applications Notes,* Hewlett-Packard applications note AN-708 (Waltham, Mass., 1969).

5. Jacobson, Bertil and John G. Webster, *Medicine and Clinical Engineering.* Prentice-Hall (Englewood Cliffs, N.J., 1977).

6. Meire, Hylton B. and Pat Farrant, *Basic Ultrasound,* Wiley(Chichester, U.K., 1995).

7. Nave, Carl R. and Brenda C. Nave, *Physics for the Health Care Sciences,* W. B. Saunders Company (Philadelphia, 1975).

8. Schwartz, Morton D. and Dominic De Cristofaro, "Review and Evaluation of Range-Gated, Pulsed, Echo-Doppler," *Journal of Clinical Engineering* 3(2):153-161 (April-June 1978).

9. Strong, Peter. *Biophysical Measurements,* Measurement Concepts Series, Tektronix, Inc. (Beaverton, Ore., 1970).

10. Veluchamy, V., "Medical Ultrasound and Its Biological Effects," *Clinical Engineering* 3(2):162-166 (April-June 1978).

CHAPTER 18
Electrosurgery Generators

18-1 Objectives

1. Be able to describe the principles behind the electrosurgery machine.
2. Be able to draw the principal electrosurgery machine waveforms and the circuitsused to generate them.
3. Be able to describe the correct procedure for the safe handling of electrosurgery machines.
4. Be able to state how to test electrosurgery machines.

18-2 Self-evaluation questions

These questions test your prior knowledge of the material in this chapter. Look for the answers as you read the text. After you have finished studying the chapter, try answering these questions and those at the end of the chapter.

1. What is the range of frequenciesused in electrosurgery?

2. The *patient plate* is considered the _____ electrode.

3. A _____ RF ammeter can be used to make rms power measurements of electrosurgery machine output.

4. A dummy load is a resistorused to test electrosurgery machines. This resistor must be a _____ type so that the impedance is purely resistive.

18-3 Electrosurgery machines

An electrosurgery machine is an ac source that operates at a radio frequency (RF). Typical electrosurgery devices operate in the range of 300 to 3000 kHz. The surgeon uses the electrosurgery machine to cut tissue and cauterize bleeding vessels.

Figure 18-1 shows the basic principle behind the electrosurgery machine. Two electrodes are connected to the rf power generator. One electrode

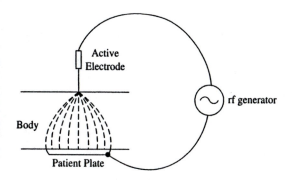

Figure 18-1
Basic principle behind the electrosurgery machine.

is said to be *active* and has a very small cross-sectional area (a few square millimeters) with respect to the other electrode. The active electrode is usually fashioned into the form of a tool or probe and is manipulated by the surgeon.

The *passive electrode* has a much larger area than the active electrode, on the order of 100 cm^2 or larger. In the past, the passive electrode was a metal surface called a *patient plate*. It was positioned beneath the buttocks or thigh. More recently, however, many hospitals have switched to a disposable electrode pad that attaches to the patient's thigh by adhesive.

Regardless of the type of passive electrode, the operating principle (Figure 18-1) remains the same. The current flowing into the patient plate is the same as the current flowing into the active electrode. But since the active electrode has a far smaller cross-sectional area than the passive electrode, the *current density* in amperes per square meter (A/m^2) is far greater. As a result of the difference in current density between the two electrodes, the tissue underneath the passive electrode heats up slightly, while the tissue underneath the active electrode is heated to destruction.

The heating of tissue is due to the power dissipated in the tissue, which is found from the expression:

$$P = \rho V I_d^2 \qquad (18\text{-}1)$$

where

P is the power in *watts (W)*

ρ is the resistivity of the tissue in *ohm-meters* (Ω-m).

V is the volume in *cubic meters* (m^3)

I_d is the *current density* in *amperes per square meter* (A/m^2)

Example 18-1

Calculate the power dissipated in 0.2 m^3 of tissue that has a resistivity of 1.6×10^3 Ω-m if the current density is 0.36 A/m^2.

Solution

$$P = \rho V I_d^2 \qquad (18\text{-}1)$$

$$P = (1.6 \times 10^3 \ \Omega\text{-m})(0.2 \ \text{m}^3)\frac{0.36 \ \text{A}^2}{\text{m}^2}$$

$$P = (1.6 \times 10^3 \ \Omega\text{-m})(0.2\text{m}^3)\,(0.13 \ \text{A}^2/\text{m}^4)$$

$$P = 41.6 \ \Omega\text{A}^2 = \textbf{41.6 W}$$

Sometimes the surgeon may elect to use a *bipolar electrode* that does not require a passive electrode. This designation is actually something of a misnomer because all RF generators, indeed all electrical current sources, require two poles. In the so-called *unipolar* systems the two electrodes are the active and passive electrodes described earlier. In the bipolar system both output terminals of the RF generator are connected to the handpiece used by the surgeon. The RF current flows between the two electrodes in the handpiece. The current density at each electrode, therefore, is quite high.

18-4 Electrosurgery circuits

The first electrosurgery machines were developed in an era when the electrical spark gap was the only means for generating significant amounts of RF power. Ships, radio-telegraph stations, and amateur radio operators used spark-gap transmitters for radio communications. The first electrosurgery machines, therefore, used spark-gap technology.

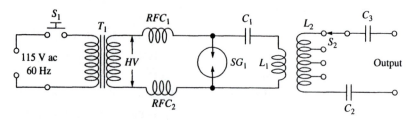

Figure 18-2
Spark-gap RF generator.

Interestingly enough, although modern solid-state machines have largely supplanted the spark-gap and vacuum tube models, it is still possible as of this writing to buy a *new* spark-gap machine. Many spark-gap machines are still in service and are likely to remain in service for several more years.

Figure 18-2 shows the circuit to a classical spark-gap machine. This circuit was common until the early 1980s but has fallen into disuse except in some physician offices and in some veterinary clinics where older human medical equipment is used. It consists of a high-voltage 60-Hz ac transformer (T_1), the spark gap (SG_1), and a series resonant tank (C_1/L_1).

Transformer T_1 increases the line voltage from approximately 115 V ac to a potential that is capable of ionizing the air in the space between the tungsten points of the spark gap (about 0.006 in. of air). Most generators use a potential of about 2000 to 3000 V ac for this job.

When the gap begins to arc, it does so in an oscillatory manner that is rich in RF components. These currents set up an oscillation in the tank circuit (C_1/L_1), which is coupled to the output circuit by induction (L_1/L_2).

The power output level applied to the patient is selected by switch S_2, which connects the active electrode to different taps on inductor L_2. Depending on design and applied voltage, spark gaps produce output power levels between 25 W and several hundred watts.

The frequency spectrum produced by the spark gap generator is centered about the resonant frequency of L_1/C_1 but contains significant compo-

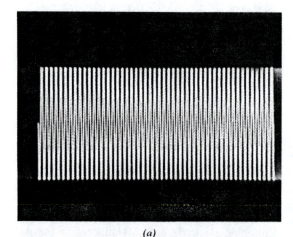

(a)

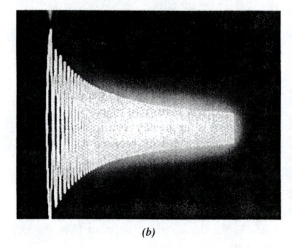

(b)

Figure 18-3
Electrosurgery waveforms. *(a)* Sine wave cut.
(b) Damped coagulation waveform.

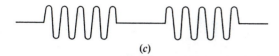

(c)

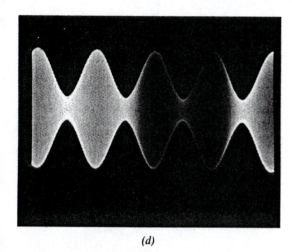

(d)

Figure 18-3 (continued)
Electrosurgery waveforms. *(c)* Chopped cut waveform. *(d)* Modulated (60-Hz) cut waveform.

nents at frequencies far removed from the center frequency. A 500-kHz spark-gap signal is audible on radio receivers tuned to frequencies well into the VHF region.

The RF chokes (RFC_1 and RFC_2) are used to prevent RF energy from getting into the power supply, thereby being radiated through the power lines. Some models delete the RF chokes but use instead a capacitor in parallel with the secondary of T_1.

The principal use of the spark gap generator is in *coagulation* or *cauterization* of bleeding vessels. Most machines offer two modes, *cut* and *coagulate,* selectable by a footswitch. The *cut* waveform is a pure, continuous sine wave (Figure 18-3*a*); the coagulation mode produces a spark-gap waveform, damped oscillation (Figure 18-3*b*), or chopped sine wave (Figure 18-3*c*), depending on which technology is used to generate the signal.

The waveform in Figure 18-3*d* is a *cut* waveform produced on a machine that does not use a smoothing filter in the high-voltage dc power supply circuit, a common practice. The use of pulsat-

ing dc produces the amplitude-modulated waveform shown in the illustration.

18-4-1 Solid-state electrosurgery generator circuits

Solid-state technology progressed to the point some years ago when transistorized electrosurgery machines could be produced at a reasonable cost (an example is shown in Figure 18-4). Today, all newly purchased instruments are solid-state models.

The circuit to a solid-state RF power amplifier is shown in Figure 18-5. This basic type of design is similar to the power amplifier stages in a number of different models. The circuit is push-pull/parallel. There are two banks of three transistors each ($Q_1 - Q_3$ and $Q_4 - Q_6$). The transistors within each bank are parallel connected, while the two banks are connected in push-pull with each other. The transformers used for input and output coupling are usually wound on a toroid-shaped ferrite core. This technique is preferred over other types of construction because the toroid shape limits the magnetic field of the coil to the immediate vicinity of the winding, thereby limiting the types of problems that are caused by mutual induction and other forms of coupling.

The RF signal is created in an oscillator circuit such as the one in Figure 18-6. When

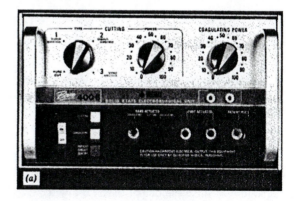

(a)

Figure 18-4
Electrosurgery machine (solid state).

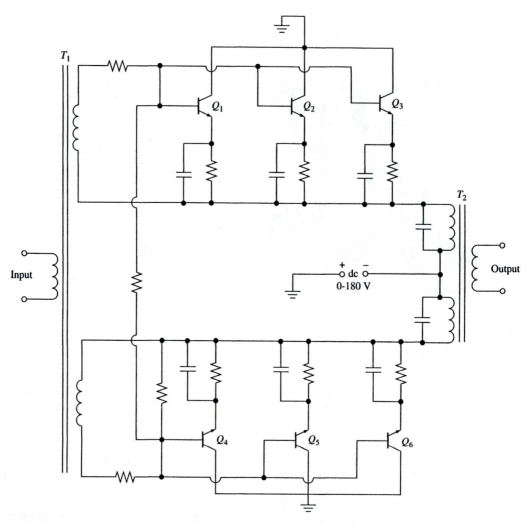

Figure 18-5
An RF power amplifier (solid state)

transistor Q_1 is forward biased, the stage will oscillate at an RF frequency determined by the circuit constants.

Transistor Q_2 operates as a switch to control
Q_1. When Q_2 is turned on, then the bias network
for Q_1 (R_3) is grounded, causing Q_1 to be forward
biased into oscillation. In the *cut* mode Q_2 remains
forward biased, so the output of the oscillator is a
sine wave. But in the *coagulation* mode, a square
wave is applied to the base of Q_2, causing it to
switch into and out of conduction. This causes a

chopped sine wave output from the oscillator (see
Figure 18-6b).

Other manufacturers use different techniques,
but most are variations on the chopped sine wave
technique shown in Figure 18-6.

18-5 Electrosurgery safety

The electrosurgery machine is a high-powered RF
generator and, as such, can pose a threat to users
and patients alike if misused or abused. When used

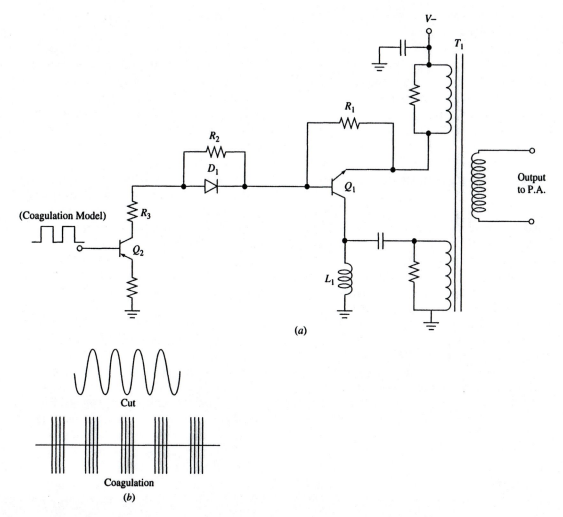

Figure 18-6
Solid-state oscillator. *(a)* Circuit. *(b)* Cut and coagulation waveforms.

in the manner intended by the manufacturer, however, the machine is considered safe, but misuse is potentially dangerous.

The most common injury to patients involves burns at inappropriate points on the body. Perhaps the most likely problem in this respect is a damaged or misapplied patient plate. Recall from Section 18-3 that burning at the patient plate site is eliminated by keeping the current density low. Local hot spots of high-current density can be accidentally formed, however, by placing the plate over a bony prominence instead of the fleshy portions of the buttocks or thigh. Hard bony regions place a more firm pressure point on the plate, thereby decreasing the contact impedance and increasing the current density.

The problem of patient burns can also be caused by dents, creases, or bends in the surface of the patient plate; the plate must be perfectly flat. Anomalies in the surface can create the local hotspots of increased current density that cause burns. In most cases, damaged patient plates should be discarded instead of repaired, so that the efficacy of the repair cannot be challenged in a malpractice suit.

An electroconductive gel or paste is used to decrease the likelihood of burns to the patient. This gel is smeared over the surface of the plate that contacts the patient's skin and is similar to the gels and pastes used in ECGand defibrillator electrodes.

A third mechanism for patient burns is the inadvertent ground path, fortunately more common on older machines than on present machines. In older designs one side of the output circuit is grounded. The patient plate on those models was usually connected to the chassis, which was in turn connected to the ac power mains ground. If a point on the patient's body became grounded with a significantly lower resistance, a major current would be diverted to the spurious ground. If the current density through the point that is grounded is high enough, burns will occur.

Danger to the surgeon using an electrosurgery machine is minimal. But if there are even microscopic holes in the surgeon's gloves, then there is a possible shock hazard. Surgeons from time to time request that a machine be inspected after they have experienced a tingling sensation.

It is possible for severe damage and electrical shock to occur if any liquids are spilled into the machine. Operating rooms are usually very crowded, so it is tempting for the staff to use the flat top of an electrosurgery machine as a table. This practice often leads to spillage of liquids into the machine, often with spectacular results, and so should be strongly discouraged. Many of the solutions used (blood, saline, Betadine) in operating rooms are quite conductive.

When testing the electrosurgery machine in the shop or lab, be sure to observe practices that prevent your injury. In section 18-6, we discuss some testing procedures and the criteria for test equipment that reduce the possibility of electrical shock or burns. In general, however, common sense will dictate the use only of secure fixtures that are well insulated and are isolated from ground.

18-6 Testing electrosurgery units

A traditional (but no longer seriously considered) method for testing electrosurgery machine output was to buy a piece of beef and then cut it with the machine. This technique is now used mostly by salespeople who wish to dramatize the effect of their product. But engineers and technicians generally prefer a more objective and quantitative testing procedure.

Almostall manufacturers of medium- to high-power electrosurgery machines recommend the test unit shown in Figure 18-7a for checking the RF output. This circuit uses a *dummy load* resistor (R_1) to simulate the patient and an RF ammeter to measure the current applied to R_1 by the machine. The resistor should have a resistance between 200 and 500 Ω, as specified by the manufacturer of the electrosurgery machine. A "universal" test box should use a 500-Ω resistor, although one will not be able to use the same output current figures as supplied by the manufacturer. In that case, establish normal values when the machine is know to be in good working condition, and then attempt to use these to test the unit in the future. The meter should have a 0- to 1.5- or 2-A full-scale range for high-power machines, and 0 to 500 mA for low power levels. In all cases, however, the meter must be a *thermocouple RF ammeter.*

When constructing the testing shown in Figure 18-7a, or any of the other circuits, care must be taken to prevent RF coupling to the metal shielded enclosure. It is the usual practice to mount the components inside a box or prefabricated enclosure. If the enclosure is metallic, then the meter should be mounted on a piece of plastic, which is in turn mounted on the front panel. Allow at least a half inch all around the meter, or isolation from the chassis will be insufficient. Similarly, corona arcing and other problems often occur if the resistor, input jacks, and wiring are not also isolated from the chassis.

The thermocouple RF ammeter is inherently a root-mean-square (rms) reading device, so it provides a true picture of the actual output level.

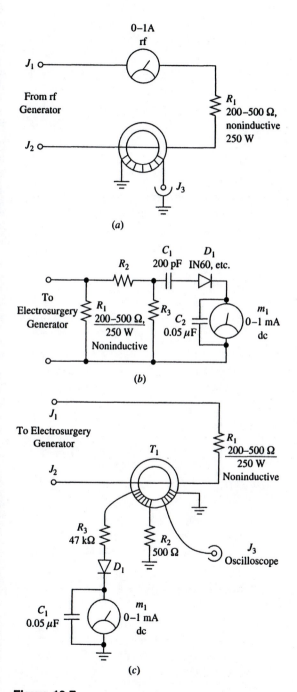

Figure 18-7
Simple electrosurgery testers. *(a)* Toroid transformer oscilloscope output. *(b)* Voltage divider. *(c)* Toroid current transformer.

Peak-reading devices are also sometimes used, but these give a true picture of output level only when sine wave cut mode is used or when the levels have been previously calibrated against an rms-reading device.

However, we find two major problems with the thermocouple RF ammeter: (1) They are more expensive than other types of meter movement and (2) the thermocouple RF ammeter does not have a linear scale; it is more crowded on the low end of the range than at the top. As a result, it is often very difficult to read low power levels on the 1.5- or 2-A movement, necessitating two meters with different ranges.

Transformer T_1 in Figure 18-7a is used to sample the RF waveform for display on an oscilloscope. It is dangerous to try connecting the oscilloscope directly to the load unless the correct probes are used, so a toroid current transformer is used. Viewing the waveform did not matter on older machines, but many of the solid-state models require adjustment of timing circuits using a cathode-ray oscilloscope display of the output waveform.

A slightly different test box is shown in Figure 18-7b. This circuit uses resistor voltage divider R_2/R_3 and a diode rectifier (D_1) to develop a dc level to drive a 0- to 1-mA dc meter movement. The circuit here is essentially a peak-reading device and so can be calibrated in watts only by comparison to an rms device such as the thermocouple RF ammeters.

Another peak-reading circuit that has found popularity is shown in Figure 18-7c. This circuit employs a toroidal current transformer, but with two windings. One winding is connected to J_3 for display of the waveform on an oscilloscope, while the other drives a dc meter movement through a rectifier diode. The circuit in Figure 18-7c is particularly useful when testing electrosurgery machines of low power rating (microcoagulators and ophthalmic and laparoscopy machines).

There are several commercial electrosurgery testers available. Specific brand names often appear as "recommended" models in the service manuals of the electrosurgery machines.

18-7 Summary

1. An electrosurgery machine is an RF power generator used to cut and cauterize tissue during surgical procedures.

2. Two output electrodes are used, a small cross-sectional area *active electrode* and a larger *passive electrode*.

3. The electrosurgery machine cuts at the active electrode, but not at the passive electrode, because of the difference in the cross-sectional areas.

4. Burns can occur to the patient if any pressure point against the passive electrode, or patient plate, has a substantially lower contact impedance than surrounding points.

18-8 Recapitulation

Now return to the objectives and self-evaluation questions at the beginning of the chapter and see how well you can answer them. If you cannot answer certain questions, place a check mark next to each and review appropriate parts of the text. Next, try to answer the following questions using the same procedure. When you have answered all of the questions, solve the problems.

Questions

1. An electrosurgery machine is an ac current source operating at RF frequencies between _____ and _____ kHz.

2. The passive electrode is also called the _____ _____ and must have an area not less than _____ cm².

3. Describe in your own words how an electrosurgery machine cuts tissue.

4. Early electrosurgery machines, some of which are still in use in veterinary clinics, used a _____ _____ to create the RF oscillations.

5. Describe the principal difference between the cut and coagulate waveforms.

6. Many solid-state electrosurgery units produce a _____ sine wave in the coagulate mode.

7. List three mechanisms by which accidental burning of a patient can occur. Also discuss the methods for preventing these burns in each case.

8. What instrument should be used to measure the rms power produced by an electrosurgery machine in the coagulate mode?

9. List a principal design feature of an electrosurgery machine tester that enhances *your* safety.

10. What range (in ammeters) is suitable to test (a) low-power, (b) high-power electrosurgery machines?

Problems

1. Find the resistivity in ohm-meters of an object whose volume is 0.6 m³ if an electrosurgery unit delivers 56 W and a line current of 600 mA.

2. Find the output power in watts of an electrosurgery machine that produces 1.2 A of RF current in a 300-Ω noninductive dummy load.

3. Find the rms power of an electrosurgery machine that delivers 500 mA into a 200-Ω load.

4. Calculate the peak RF voltage produced by the electrosurgery machine if 450 W is dissipated in a 500-Ω load while using the cut mode.

CHAPTER 19

Care and Feeding of Battery-Operated Medical Equipment

19-1 Objectives

1. Be able to describe the different kinds of batteries used in medical equipment.
2. Be able to describe the charging protocols for common batteries.

3. Be able to state the limitations of batteries.
4. Understand the maintenance of battery-operated equipment.

19-2 Self-evaluation questions

These questions test your prior knowledge of the material in this chapter. Look for the answers as you read the text. After you have finished studying the chapter, try answering these questions and those at the end of the chapter.

1. The usual protocol for charging nickel-cadmium (NiCd) batteries and cells is to charge at a rate of _____, to a level of _____% of fully charged.

2. NiCd batteries are said to possess _____ because they will adjust the fully discharged level if shallow-cycled too many times.

3. List three different forms of batteries used in medical equipment.

4. The charge available to a battery is rated in units of _____.

19-3 Introduction

Much medical equipment uses batteries of one sort or another. The "care and feeding" of batteries is a critical element in keeping the equipment ready for use and is thus especially problematic in emergency equipment. Batteries are used for many reasons. Some equipment is battery-powered for portability. A defibrillator, for example, might be needed almost anyplace; heart attacks do not always occur near an electrical outlet. Although most defibrillators are ac-powered (or dual-powered), a number are purely battery-powered models. Some patient monitors also run on batteries.

These devices are used to keep track of ECG and blood pressure as the patient is transferred between units (e.g., from the emergency room to the intensive care unit). Still other devices use batteries for patient safety. A cardiac output computer, for example, makes measurements based on a thermistor inserted into the heart. Small amounts of ac leakage current could be fatal, so batteries are used to completely isolate the instrument from the ac power line.

19-4 Cells or batteries?

The cell is the most basic element in a battery and sets the minimum voltage for that sort of device. Additional voltage is gained by connecting the cells in series, and extra current is available by connecting them in parallel. To be strict, we would refer to single entities as *cells* and multiple-cell entities as *batteries*. But in common usage, it is usually acceptable to be less than rigorous, so all cells and batteries are called batteries.

19-5 Nickel-cadmium cells and batteries

In this section we will discuss mostly the nickel-cadmium (NiCd) cells and batteries that are commonly used in portable electronics equipment. These batteries have a nominal terminal voltage at full charge of 1.2 V, except immediately prior to turn-on after a fresh charge (at which time the open-terminal voltage is 1.4 V). Shortly after turn-on, however, the open-terminal voltage drops from 1.4 V to the nominal value of 1.2 V for the duration of the operation. As the stored energy is used up, however, the terminal voltage drops lower.

NiCd batteries are rechargeable and will typically sustain a charge-discharge cycle life of 1000 times before becoming unusable. In most cases, manufacturers rate a battery as unusable when the capacity of the battery drops below 80% of its original specified value.

19-6 Battery capacity

The capacity of a battery is measured in *ampere-hours* (A-H) (i.e., the product of current load, in amperes, and the time required to reach the designated discharge state). The NiCd battery is capable of delivering tremendous currents. For example, the size D (4 A-H) and size F (7 A-H) can deliver short-duration currents of 50 A or more. That is why they are used in medical defibrillators and why certain medium-powered portable radio transmitters can use them. As a result of their ability to deliver large currents, NiCd batteries should be fused to protect printed wiring tracks, wires, and other conductors. We have seen copper foil printed wiring board tracks and an on/off switch vaporized by a shorted capacitor across the dc line.

The amount of time that a battery will last is a function of the discharge time, which in turn is determined by the amount of current drawn. Figure 19-1 shows two different discharge scenarios: one for a current of one-tenth the A-H rating and one for a current equal to the A-H rate. In Figure 19-1*a* the battery will be fully discharged in 10 hours, while in Figure 19-1*b* discharge will occur in 1 hour. This particular chart is derived from the data published for a size D NiCd cell rated at 4 A-H.

As you can see in Table 19-1, the AA cells are found in three ratings from 400 to 700 mA-H, depending upon the manufacturer and style. You will find a lot of variation from this chart, especially among consumer product NiCd batteries. Some size C cells are rated at both 1 and 1.2 A-H, and size D are rated at 2 A-H. Suspect that these are actually lesser cells dressed in size C and size D packages. One manufacturer's representative actually admitted to me that the consumer D cells were actually size C cells inside a D package.

This difference is of little practical consequence to most consumer electronics users and actually results in a lower-cost product. But if you use or service commercial, medical, or communications equipment, make sure that you get the correct ampere-hour rating. A heart patient's chance of survival can be reduced by replacing 4 A-H NiCd

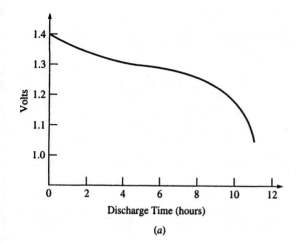

(a)

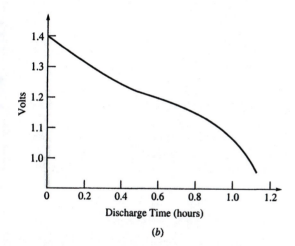

(b)

Figure 19-1
Charge/discharge curves for NiCd batteries.
(a) Charging curve. *(b)* Discharging curve.

cells in the defibrillator with a collection of 2 A-H consumer replacements intended for power toothbrushes and portable radios. *Be sure of the rating of replacement batteries and cells.*

Rating games are also played by some distributors by quoting different discharge rates. One standard method of measuring A-H capacity is the current required to discharge a cell to 1.0 V in 1 hour. Some makers, however, define it in terms of the 10-hour discharge rate normalized to ampere-

TABLE 19-1 STANDARD CELL RATINGS FOR NiCd BATTERIES

Battery size	Ampere-hour rating
AA	0.4, 0.5, 0.7
C	2
D	4
F	7

hours. From analyzing Figure 19-1*a* and 19-1*b*, you can see how this might result in a false feeling of full capacity.

19-7 Battery-charging protocols

The charging protocol for the NiCd battery depends somewhat on application and manufacturer. In general, though, the charge current must be at least A-H/20, and in many commercial consumer battery chargers it is often A-H/15. For most applications in which you can control the charge rate, it is safe to use a charge rate of A-H/10. That is, charge the battery at a current not greater than one-tenth the ampere-hour rating. In addition, the battery must be charged to 140% of capacity, so a charge time of 14 hours at A-H/10 is mandated. The general rule is: Charge at 1/10 ampere-hour rating for 14 hours.

Some chargers are designed to fast charge the battery in as little as 1 hour, with most being 3 to 4 hours. Fast charging should not be done unless the battery maker recommends it. Even then, be a little cautious about fast charging (cells can explode from charging too fast). NiCd batteries can be dangerous, so do not ad lib: Follow the manufacturer's recommendations rigorously.

NiCd batteries can also lose energy from merely sitting. Some users find that a battery charged up and then stored is unusable when it is eventually turned on. Figure 19-2 shows a storage discharge curve for a typical NiCd battery. The solution for this type of problem is a trickle charge at a rate between A-H/30 and A-H/50. Some commercial battery chargers have a switch that allows

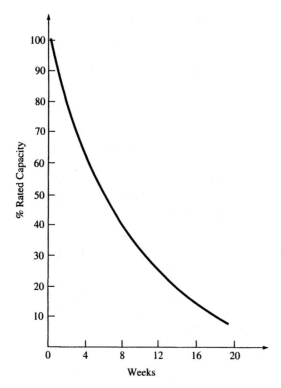

Figure 19-2
Percentageof full-rated charge versus storage time.

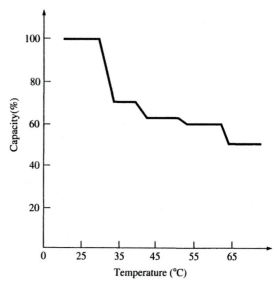

Figure 19-3
Operating capacity versus temperature curve.

either an A-H/10 regular charge rate or an A-H/30 trickle charge.

Another problem with NiCd batteries is the operating temperature and its effects on available capacity. As shown in Figure 19-3, the available current capacity is a function of temperature. As the temperature increases above room temperature (25°C), the available capacity diminishes.

19-8 NiCd battery memory

A running debate in the industry is whether NiCds do or do not have a memory problem. *Memory* means that a battery will not allow deep discharge after repeated shallow discharges. For example, if a battery is repeatedly discharged in some particular application to only 80% of full capacity, after a while it will "remember" the 80% level as the fully

discharged point. The battery will then exhibit the fully discharged potential when the charge level is only 80% of fully charged. That makes the battery look like a premature failure. A NiCd battery with memory problems can sometimes be reformed by repeatedly fully charging it and then immediately deep discharging it. After a while, the memory phenomenon may work itself out.

19-9 Battery maintenance

When equipment is subject to routine maintenance, it is possible to keep the batteries healthy by following a certain routine. For most equipment the manufacturer recommends that the batteries be periodically discharged and then recharged. The protocol for most is as follows:

1. Fully charge the battery or cell.

2. Discharge it fully with a resistor that draws a current of A-H/10 for 8 to 9 hours for multicell batteries and 10 hours for single cells.

3. Recharge the battery at the A-H/10 rate for 14 to 16 hours.

A phenomenon called *polarity reversal* might result if the battery is fully discharged. The cause of this problem is that not all cells have the same terminal voltage at any given time. It might occur that one cell will become charged backwards by the others in the series chain. For this reason, multicell batteries are only discharged to 10% to 20% of capacity.

Do not leave the battery in a discharged condition for a long period; it may develop interelement shorts. Little metallic or oxide "whiskers" called *dendrites* grow internally from plate to plate and cause a short circuit. The cell potential drops to zero or near-zero, and the cell will not accept a charge. In some cases, we would have to regard the cell as lost and replace it. Some cells, however, can be salvaged from short circuits. In medical devices, though, good engineering practice requires replacement with a new cell rather than salvaging the defective cell.

Figure 19-4 shows a revitalization circuit for shorted NiCd cells. It works by vaporizing the internal dendrites that short the plates together. A known-good cell of the same type is placed across the shorted cell through a pushbutton or spring-loaded toggle switch. It is important to use this type of switch instead of a regular switch—you do not want to keep the circuit closed for too long (battery explosion could result). Press the switch several times in succession, and then measure the terminal voltage. If the current from V_1 successfully vaporizes the dendrites inside of V_2, then the terminal voltage will rise.

A word of caution for people using this method: Be sure to wear safety goggles or glasses when performing this operation. NiCd batteries have been known to explode under high current, and explosion could happen when deshorting a cell. Most equipment maintenance technicians have never seen it happen under this circumstance, but it could.

Revitalized batteries and cells should not be regarded as reliable and should only be used for short terms, under emergency conditions, pending obtaining new batteries or cells for proper replacement.

19-10 Charging NiCd batteries

There are two basic forms of charger for NiCd batteries: *constant current* (CI) and *constant voltage* (CV). Regardless of the type, it is important not to use a charging current greater than A-H/10, unless specifically instructed to do so by the battery manufacturer (not the equipment maker, for errors are frequent). The A-H/10 rate is one-tenth of the ampere-hour rating. For a 500-mA-H AA cell, for example, a charging current of 50 mA is used. Similarly, for a 2 A-H size C cell use 200 mA, and for the 4 A-H size D cell use 400 mA. Be cautious not to overcharge batteries using other A-H ratings.

Figure 19-5 shows the basic circuit for a constant current charger of simple design. The transformer secondary voltage should be 2.5 times (or more) the cell or battery voltage. A resistor in series with the rectifier has a value that limits the output current under short-circuit conditions to the official A-H/10 charging rate. This circuit is the basic circuit for most low-cost chargers.

Figure 19-6 shows two electronic constant current chargers based on three-terminal integrated circuit (IC) voltage regulators. A variable circuit is shown in Figure 19-6a, and it is based on the LM-317 (up to 1 A) or LM-338 (up to 5 A). Both circuits require a filtered dc input voltage several volts higher than the battery or cell potential. The actual value is not critical as long as it is high enough to turn on the circuit (in general, V_{in} must

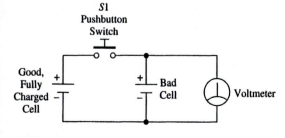

Figure 19-4
Flash revitalization circuit.

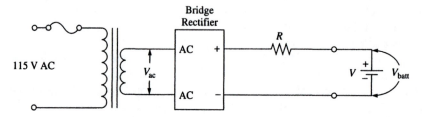

Figure 19-5
Basic circuit for a constant current charger.

be equal to or greater than V_{batt} + 3 V). We can set the charge current by setting the value of resistor R. For example, for a 400-mA charger for 4 A-H size D cells, we would use a resistor value of $1.2/I$ = $1.2/.4$ = 3 Ω. Charging currents down to 10 mA can be accommodated by the circuit in Figure 19-6a, so both regular and trickle chargers can be designed.

The circuit in Figure 19-6b will charge batteries up to 4 A-H with terminal voltages up to 12 V dc. It is similar to the circuit of Figure 19-6a but is based on the 5-V fixed regulator such as the LM-309, LM-340-05, or 7805 devices.

A constant-voltage charger is shown in Figure 19-7. The output voltage of the charger is set by

the ratio of R_1 and R_2 and is determined by the equation:

$$V_o = (1.25 \text{ V})\left(\frac{R_2}{R_1} + 1\right) \qquad (19\text{-}1)$$

A series resistor, R_3, prevents the current from exceeding the A-H/10 value and is set to allow the short-circuit current to that value. The required charger output impedance must be the resistance V_o/I_{max}, where V_o is the open-terminal battery voltage and I_{max} is the maximum permissible charging current. For a 12-V, 4 A-H battery, for example, the required impedance is 12/(4/10) = 12/0.4 = 30 Ω. We can solve the equation in the figure for R_3 and place that resistor value in series with the

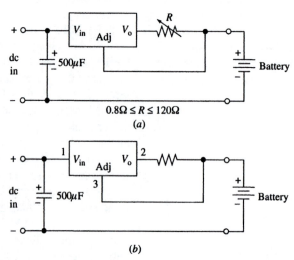

(a)

(b)

Figure 19-6
Electronic constant current chargers. (a) Variable. (b) Fixed.

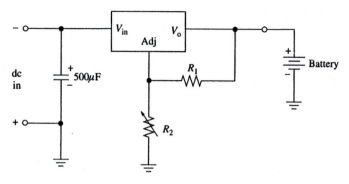

Figure 19-7
Constant voltage charger circuit.

output of the regulator. The power rating of the resistor must be $V_o I_{max}$.

19-10-1 Using bench power supplies

A bench power supply should not be used to charge NiCd batteries unless it has both a variable output voltage control and a current-limiting control. Set the output voltage precisely to the full terminal voltage of the NiCd battery, and adjust the current limiter for a short-circuit current equal to the A-H/10 value. Disconnect the output short from the power supply and connect it across the battery.

19-11 Multiple-cell batteries

A large number of multiple-cell batteries are used in electronic equipment. Most are typically 6-, 12-, or 24-V models. In most cases, these batteries are made up of individual AA, C, D, or F cells. It is possible to take apart the original battery packs and replace individual cells to restore the battery to normal operation. Some battery packs are put together with screws or snaps, while others are glued together.

When selecting cells for replacement in a multiple-cell battery, keep several factors in mind. First, of course, is the right size (AA, C, D, F) and the right A-H rating (not all C and D cells are cre-

ated equal). Also keep in mind whether regular cells or solder-tab cells are needed. Some consumer NiCd cells are in nonstandard packages. One brand of AA cells is a millimeter or so shorter than standard AA cells. As a result, intermittent operation sometimes occurs when these replacement cells are used. To avoid the necessity of shimming these cells or retensioning the contact spring, avoid buying them and use the standards instead. Medical equipment is too critical for those batteries.

19-12 Other batteries

Several other types of batteries are used in medical equipment: *lead-acid, carbon-zinc,* and *alkaline dry cells, mercury, gel cell,* and *lithium.*

19-12-1 Lead-acid batteries

For mobile (e.g., ambulance) and some high-power portable applications, the lead-acid automobile battery is often preferred. This is the familiar battery used to start automobile engines. Very heavy, and dangerous because of the wet-cell acid content, they are nonetheless popular because they are generally reliable and easily available. In addition, many radio communication sets are designed to operate from the nominal 13.6-V dc produced by the typical automobile battery.

In addition to the 13.6-V (also called 12-V) battery, 6, 24, 28, and 32 V lead-acid batteries are also available on the market. Some of these are marine (boat) batteries, others are military batteries (28 V dc), and still others are truck batteries. The terminal voltage can be increased by connecting batteries in series, while current availability is increased by connecting batteries in parallel.

Mobile operation is usually carried out with the vehicle battery. But in certain cases, it is wise to have a separate battery for the equipment in the event of main vehicle power supply failure. Some users might want to consider the type of system shown in Figure 19-8. This system is common in recreational vehicles to power the creature comforts separately from the vehicle battery. The point is to keep your capability, even if you accidentally discharge the vehicle battery by leaving the lights on or incur some other problem. The backup battery could then be used to start the vehicle or summon help (depending upon the situation).

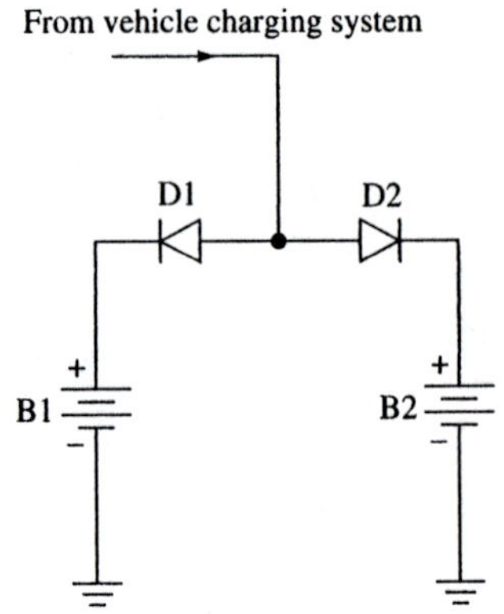

The charger will be a generator or an alternator installed on the vehicle. Although the ideal system would be to have separate charging and regulating systems, that ideal is not always achievable for certain practical reasons. Thus, we have a single charger and voltage regulator for two (or more) batteries. Isolation between the batteries is provided by a pair of large-current silicon diodes (D_1 and D_2). The rating of these diodes should be at least 1.5 times the maximum charge rate of the charger. In most cases, large stud-mounted diodes are used for D_1 and D_2, and they are mounted on a finned heat sink. Keep in mind on vehicular installations that ambient temperature is high in some locations, and that will affect diode reliability.

For portable operations, some means must be provided to charge the lead-acid battery. In most cases, a small generator powered by a gasoline or kerosene engine (called a *light-plant* in some catalogs) is used to provide battery power. In some cases, an auto-parts-store type of battery charger is

Figure 19-8
Dual battery charging system.

needed to convert the ac output from the generator to dc for the battery. It is increasingly common, however, to find small 500- to 2000-W generators that include a "12-V" output that provides from 6 to 35 A for purposes of powering radio equipment or charging batteries.

Maintenance of lead-acid batteries is relatively easy but is needed. The water level in each of the cells must be checked periodically. For people with a critical need for the battery, the level should be checked weekly. Although distilled water works best (because of the lack of additional chemicals), ordinary tap water will work in the cells. There are vents in the caps that cover the cells, and these holes must not be blocked. If dirt clogs the opening, then either replace the cap or clean it.

Warning: Lead-acid batteries produce hydrogen as a normal byproduct. If you fail to observe proper procedure, this hydrogen may blow up the battery and cause serious injury to people and damage to equipment. First, never allow the battery to become overcharged. Second, turn off all circuits connected to the battery (especially the charger) before disconnecting the wires to the battery. If current is flowing in those circuits, a spark will occur, and that spark can create an explosion. This is not a hypothetical possibility but a real danger.

19-12-2 Carbon-zinc and alkaline dry cells

These cells and batteries are the ordinary consumer types that you are familiar with in flashlights, radios, and so forth. They are not generally rechargeable and are discarded after use. They are sometimes used in medical devices but for the most part are reserved for flashlights and noncritical devices. One of the problems that limits the usefulness of these batteries and cells is that the terminal voltage drops off over the course of discharging the battery, so device performance may vary as the battery or cell ages.

19-12-3 Mercury dry cells

Mercury (Hg) cells are sometimes used in medical devices and laboratory instruments because they possess a useful attribute: The terminal voltage remains nearly constant over the life of the battery and drops suddenly at the end of the charge life. This feature means that performance remains relatively constant. The feature also allows Hg batteries (e.g., HG-1 and HG-2) to be used for instrument calibration purposes.

As with NiCd cells and batteries, carbon-zinc, alkaline, and mercury cells and batteries should be stored in cool places when not in use. It is common practice to store batteries in a refrigerator, not a freezer, to keep them cool. This practice extends the storage life of the battery.

19-12-4 Gel-cell batteries

Another form of battery that is popular in portable equipment is the gel-cell. One of the authors has seen these batteries in commercial, medical, and radio communication equipment. Several years ago I worked with a piece of medical equipment used to transport cadaver kidneys to sites where a transplant was performedon a dialysis patient. If you have ever known end-stage renal disease (dialysis) patients, then you know the tragedy of the

loss of a donor kidney. The team kept losing kidneys because of battery failure in the transport unit. The manufacturer sent a new design internal battery charger, but it too was deficient. All of the battery chargers found were high-tech models that depended upon sensing small variations in terminal voltage to determine charge or discharge state. Unfortunately, the analog-sensing circuitry drifted enough to give bad results. In desperation, the engineer in our laboratory called the battery maker, instead of the device maker, and asked him. The applications engineer asked if we had ever heard of Kirchoff's voltage law. Allowing that we had, we let the applications engineer guide us to a solution (Figure 19-9).

The circuit in Figure 19-9 will allow charging of a gel-cell (and other forms of battery) without resort to a lot of unreliable high-tech circuitry. The charger power supply must have two features: a precisely controlled output voltage and a current-limit control. With switch S_1 open, set the output voltage to exactly the value of the full-charged

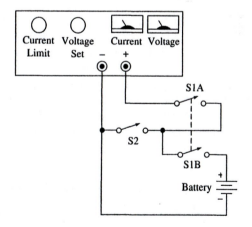

Figure 19-9
Electronic power supply for charging gel-cell batteries. S2 is used to set short-circuit output current to maximum battery charge current value when output voltage is set to minimum value. Make sure both current limit and voltage set controls are at minimum values before closing either S1 or S2.

voltage of the battery or perhaps a small amount higher (100 to 200 mV). Make sure S_2 is in the shorting position and then close S_1. Adjust the current-limit control for a short-circuit current equal to the maximum permitted charge current of the battery (A-H/10 for many batteries). After the current and voltage are set, place switch S_2 in the BATT position and charge the battery. When the battery voltage is less than the power supply output voltage, current flows into the battery. But when the battery voltage equals the power supply voltage, current flow ceases.

Batteries can provide freedom of operation for medical electronic equipment. But they can also be a nuisance if not maintained correctly. Proper maintenance of the battery will provide long and reliable life.

19-12-5 Lithium cells

These cells are typically used in computers, watches, and other digital devices as a "keep-alive" potential for CMOS memory elements. They typically last quite a long time because only leakage-level currents are drawn.

Warning: All sealed batteries and cells are potentially dangerous when overcharged, overheated, or otherwise abused. Under such conditions, the battery or cell may rupture or explode, resulting in considerable hazard. In addition, lithium batteries should not be carried aboard aircraft or otherwise subjected to reduced atmospheric pressures unless specifically designed for the purpose (consult battery manufacturer).

19-13 Summary

1. The types of cells and batteries typically used in medical equipment include nickel-cadmium, carbon-zinc dry cells, alkaline dry cells, mercury and lithium cells, and gel-cells. Lead-acid batteries are used for some mobile or high-powered portable applications.

2. The most common rechargeable battery is the nickel-cadmium (NiCd) type. They are used because they are easy to obtain yet can provide large currents.

3. NiCd batteries are typically charged at a current between A-H/20 and A-H/10 and are kept charged when not in use by a trickle charge of A-H/25 to A-H/30.

19-14 Recapitulation

Now return to the objectives and self-evaluation questions at the beginning of the chapter and see how well you can answer them. If you cannot answer certain questions, place a check mark next to each and reread appropriate parts of the text. Next, try to answer the following questions using the same procedure. When you have answered all of the questions, solve the problems.

Questions

1. Two reasons to use battery power include portability and the need to provide _____ from the patient in some instruments (e.g., cardiac output computers).

2. List four types of cells used in medical devices.

3. The _____ battery has a typical full charge terminal voltage of 1.2 V.

4. A battery is made of two or more _____.

5. An NiCd battery can typically be cycled _____ or more times when properly maintained and used.

6. A size D cell for industrial and medical use generally is rated at or near _____ ampere-hours.

7. The NiCd battery is typically charged at A-H/ _____ but can be charged at A-H/10 if properly controlled.

8. When an NiCd is trickle charged, the rate will be between A-H/ _____ and A-H/ _____.

9. Proper maintenance of _____ batteries sometimes calls for the cell to be discharged through a resistor, drawing a current of A-H/10 for 10 hours prior to fully recharging at the same rate for 14 hours.

10. Discharged NiCd cells can develop internal _____ of metal or oxide, and these can cause short circuits between plates.

11. The purpose of resistor R_3 in Figure 19-7 is _____ limiting.

12. List two features of a bench-type dc power supply that are absolutely necessary if it is to be used for charging batteries.

13. Dry cells and NiCd cells should be stored in a _____ environment to increase their storage or shelf life.

Problems

1. A constant voltage charger is made using the circuit in Figure 19-7 and requires an output voltage of 14.4 V. If $R_1 = 180 \ \Omega$, find the value of R_2.

2. If, in Figure 19-7, $R_1 = 240 \ \Omega$ and $R_2 = 2200 \ \Omega$, the output voltage, V_o, will be _____ V.

3. A 4 A-H NiCd battery is fully charged when it is connected to a load that draws 110 mA.

It has a potential life of _____ hours before becoming fully discharged.

Reference

1. Buchman, Isidor, "Meeting the Needs of the Battery" (rechargeable batteries with respect to which battery chemistry to choose, proper charging methods, and battery maintenance), *Measurement and Control Magazine,* April 1996, pp. 146-149 (Measurements and Data Corp., phone: 412-343-9666; fax: 412-343-9685; e-mail: editor@mac-med.com; mailing address: 2994 W. Liberty Ave., Pittsburgh, PA 15216).

2. Buchman, Isidor, *"Choosing a Battery that will Last,"* (Evaluation (evaluation of nickel-cadmium [NiCd], nickel-metal hydride [NiMH], and lithium ion [Li-ion] batteries as a function of life-cycling with regard to mechanical and chemical reasons for wearing down), *Medical Electronics and Equipment Manufacturing Magazine,* June, 1999 (Measurement and Data Corp., 2994 W. Liberty Ave., Pittsburg, PA 15216, phone: 412-343-9685).

CHAPTER 20
Waveform Display Devices

20-1 Objectives

1. Be able to describe the principles behind the servomechanism recorder and recording potentiometer.
2. Be able to describe the operation of the PMMC galvanometer mechanism.
3. Be able to list and describe the different types of writing system used in mechanical recorders.
4. Know how to describe the principles behind the medical CRO.
5. Be able to list the different types of CROs available.
6. Be able to describe how a *nonfade* medical CRO operates.
7. Know how to describe the principal differences between medical and engineering CROs.

20-2 Self-evaluation questions

These questions test your knowledge of the material in this chapter. Look for the answers as you read the text. After you have finished studying the chapter, try answering these questions and those at the end of the chapter.

1. Describe in your own wards a recording potentiometer.

2. Describe in your own words the operation of a PMMC galvanometer.

3. What is a *deadband*?

4. Describe in your own words the type of paper used in thermal recorders.

5. Medical CROs use _____ persistence phosphors on the viewing screen.

6. List two methods for creating two or more channels from a single CRO electron beam.

7. Typical sweep speeds for medical oscilloscopes are _____ mm/s and _____ mm/s.

8. List two different forms of sweep on a nonfade medical CRO.

20-3 Permanent magnet moving coil instruments

The chart recorder is used in medical instrumentation to make permanent recordings (hard copies) of the analog waveforms produced by the physiological measurement instruments. One of the most common types of mechanism is the *permanent magnet moving coil* (PMMC) *galvanometer.* The PMMC is very similar to the D'Arsonval meter movement. A *writing pen* replaces the meter point and is attached to the moving coil assembly that is in the field of a strong permanent magnet. Current flowing in the moving coil creates a magnetic field that interacts with the magnetic field of the permanent magnet. This will cause deflection of the pen assembly in the same manner as the meter needle will deflect in the D'Arsonval mechanism.

The tip of the pen in a PMMC assembly is positioned over a strip of chart paper that is pulled under the pen tip at a constant speed. This mechanism, therefore, will make *Y-time* recordings, in which the *Y*-axis is the deflection of the pen and the *X*-axis is the time base established by moving the chart paper at a constant speed past the pen tip. The PMMC assembly, then, will produce a chart recording of the *waveshape* of the applied waveform. These instruments are sometimes called *recording oscillographs.*

The PMMC pen assembly sweeps an arched path and so will write in a curvilinear manner, as in Figure 20-1a. The tip of the pen travels in an arc because of the rotary motion of the moving coil assembly. In some cases this may be tolerable, especially if the user will record on paper that has a special curved grid. This type of recorder is used in student instruments and when amplitude rather than waveshape is the important parameter.

The pivoted pen motor assembly of Figure 20-1*b* is a solution to the problem of curvilinear action that is used on some higher-priced ink machines. The PMMC is not connected to the pen directly, but through a mechanical link that translates the curvilinear motion of the PMMC to the *rectilinear* motion at the pen tip.

A *pseudorectilinear* writing system is shown in Figure 20-1c. In this type of recorder the pen assembly is very long compared with the width of the chart paper. The pen tip, therefore, travels in an arc, the length of which is very short compared with the radius (pen length). The trace will appear to be nearly linear in this type of recorder.

Several different writing methods are used in strip-chart recorders, but two are amenable to a special type of pseudorectilinear recording: *thermal* and *direct contact.* An example of the thermal recorder is shown in Figure 20-1d. Both of these types of recorder use a special writing stylus (rather than a pen) and a *knife edge,* also called a *writing edge.* The mark is made on the paper by the contact of the stylus on the paper along the knife edge. The stylus tip still travels in a curvilinear path, but the resulting trace is rectilinear because the knife edge is straight. This technique works because these recording methods work by contact pressure between the stylus and the knife edge. The stylus can write anywhere along its length, so by keeping the knife edge straight under the paper, we obtain the rectilinear recording that clearly shows waveshape as well as amplitude.

20-4 PMMC writing systems

Several different writing systems are commonly used on PMMC recorders: *direct contact, thermal, ink pen, ink jet,* and *optical.*

Recorders that use any type of pen (ink) or stylus (direct contact and thermal) have a relatively low-frequency response due to the inertia of the pen or stylus assembly. Most such recorders have an upper -3 dB frequency response point of 100 to 200 Hz. Ink jet and optical types, on the other hand, use lighter-weight fixtures in the writing system and so have a higher natural frequency response. An upper -3 dB point in the range of 1000 to 3000 Hz is possible in some of these instruments.

The direct contact writer uses a special type of chart paper that is chemically treated to have a carbonized back. When a pressure is applied to the

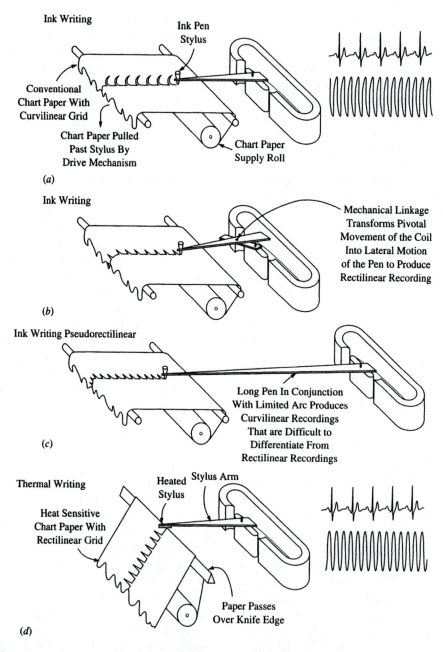

Figure 20-1
Curvilinear and rectilinear galvanometric recorder mechanisms. *(a)* Ink writing. *(b)* Ink writing.
(c) Ink writing pseudorectilinear.*(d)* Knife edge. (Courtesy of Tektronix, Inc., Beaverton, Ore.
Copyright 1970. All rights reserved.)

front of the paper, a black mark will appear through the paper. Most of these instruments have a frequency response of less than 25 Hz and so are not commonly used in medical instrumentation.

The thermal recorder also uses special paper, but in this case it is *waxed* or treated with *paraffin* so that it will turn black when heated. The thermal recorder is by far the most commonly employed in medical instrumentation, especially in cardiovascular instruments such as the ECG or pressure monitors.

The stylus in a thermal system is little more than a heated resistance wire connected to a low-voltage ac or dc power supply. Early models formed the stylus tip from a U-shaped electrical resistance element, while modern models use a resistance wire inside a cylindrical metal stylus. In both cases a low-voltage electrical power supply energizes the element, causing the tip to become heated almost to incandescence. The black mark is made at the points where the heated stylus touches the paper. Note that it takes less time to write at high temperatures than at low temperatures, so multispeed instruments typically apply a higher voltage to the heater at high speeds than at low speeds.

Ink pen writers use a hollow pen and an ink supply to write on the chart paper. In some machines the ink is pressurized by an atomizer-like (squeeze ball) hand pump. Many polygraph machines used in EEG recording use this type of writing system. Other instruments, however, are somewhat more automatic and use a thick, viscous ink in a special cartridge that is placed under pressure by a spring-driven piston. In multichannel instruments (Figure 20-2), the ink may be distributed to all pens from the same cartridge by connecting the line from the cartridge to the input side of a special *ink manifold* and the lines to the pens to the output sides of the manifold. In many multichannel machines additional pressure is applied to the ink by the solenoid-operated manifold bladder.

The high-velocity ink jet recorder is capable of higher-frequency responses than are the types

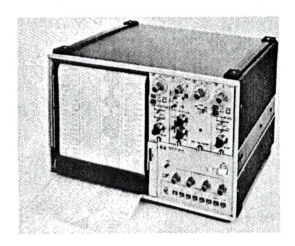

Figure 20-2
Four-channel recorder. (Photo courtesy of Hewlett-Packard)

mentioned previously. This type of recorder is popular on European instruments, of which many have found their way to the United States. In the ink jet recorder, low-viscosity ink is directed to a *nozzle* mounted on a PMMC galvanometer in place of the pen assembly. The ink jet produced by the nozzle is directed at the paper, and, when the system is properly adjusted, it will produce a recording that is very nearly rectilinear. Only a small amount of trace fuzziness due to ink splattering is apparent.

There are two types of optical recorder in common use. One is a PMMC type and uses a mirror in place of the pen or stylus. The other uses photographic paper that is pulled across a cathode ray tube (CRT) screen and is called a CRT camera recorder.

An example of the PMMC optical recorder is shown in Figure 20-3. A small, low-inertia mirror is mounted on the PMMC galvanometer in place of the pen assembly. The mirror reflects a pencil-thin beam of collimated light onto the photosensitive paper. Most of these recorders use wide paper (6 in. wide or wider) so the resolution is better than on the smaller paper widths used in pen and thermal recorders. Additionally, on a multichannel

Collimated Light Source

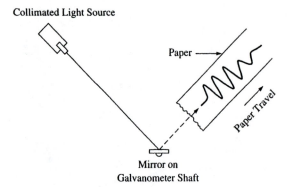

Paper

Paper Travel

Mirror on
Galvanometer Shaft

Figure 20-3
Light-beam galvanometer.

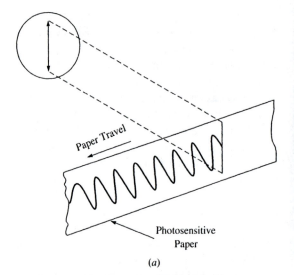

Paper Travel

Photosensitive
Paper

(a)

optical recorder, it is possible to examine the time relationships between different traces more easily because the traces can be allowed to *overlap* each other.

The paper in the optical recorder is often developed by exposure to an ultraviolet lamp as the paper comes out of the recorder, an example of *post-fogging*. The trace will fade over a long time, however, unless the paper is either wet-developed following the recording session or stored in a light-tight box.

The CRT camera recorder is shown in Figure 20-4*a;* a commercial example is shown in Figure 20-4*b*. In the CRT camera type of recorder, the CRT sweeps only the vertical axis (as many times as there are channels). The time base is provided by pulling the photosensitive paper in front of the CRT screen.

The frequency response of the CRT camera recorder is better than that ofany of the other types, being limited mostly by the writing speed of the photosensitive paper.

20-5 Servorecorders and recording potentiometers

In potentiometric measurements a three-terminal variable resistor (potentiometer) is connected to produce an output voltage that is a function of

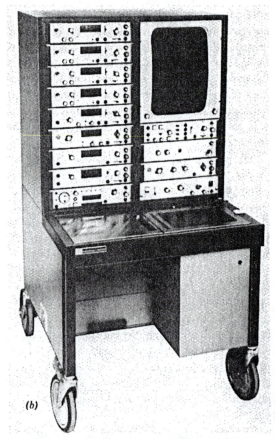

(b)

Figure 20-4
CRT camera optical recorder. *(a)* Writing system schematic. *(b)* Photograph of system.

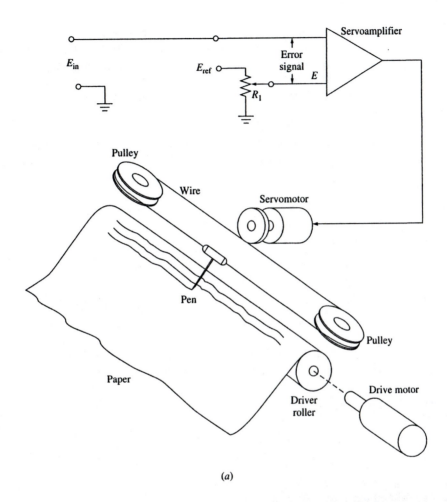

(a)

both a reference potential and the position of the variable resistor's wiper arm. A galvanometer such as a zero-center D'Arsonval or taut-band meter movement will read *zero* when the unknown voltage and the potentiometer voltage are equal. In normal operation the operator will manually null the voltage displayed on the meter and then read the value of the unknown voltage from the voltage calibration on the potentiometer dial. Figure 20-5a shows a simplified schematic for a *recording potentiometer* that is self-nulling. A *servorecorder* is a self-nulling potentiometer that records the waveshape of the applied signal on

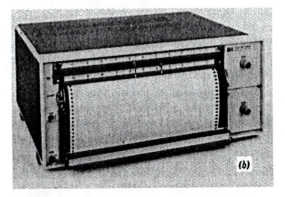

(b)

Figure 20-5
Servorecorder. (a) Simplified schematic. (b) Commercial example. (Photo courtesy of Hewlett-Packard)

graph paper. A commercial example of a servorecorder is shown in Figure 20-5b.

Figure 20-5a shows the dc potentiometer servorecorder mechanism. The pen is attached to a string that is wound around a pair of *idler pulleys* and a *driver pulley* that is on the shaft of a dc servomotor. The pen assembly is also linked to a potentiometer (R_1) in such a way that the position of the wiper arm on the resistance element is proportional to the pen position.

The potentiometer element is connected across a precision reference potential, E_{ref}, so potential E will represent the position of the pen; that is, E is the electrical analog of pen position. When the pen is at the left-hand side of the paper in Figure 20-5a, E will be zero, and when the pen is full scale at the right-hand side of the paper, E is equal to E_{ref}.

The pen position is controlled by the dc servomotor, which is in turn driven by the output of the servo amplifier. The amplifier has *differential* inputs; E_{in} (the unknown) is connected to one input, and the position signal E is connected to the other input. The difference signal ($E_{in} - E$) represents the *error* between the *actual* pen position and the position the pen *should* be in for the applied voltage. If the error signal is zero, meaning that the amplifier output is also zero and the pen is correctly positioned, then the motor remains turned off. But if $E \neq E_{in}$, then the amplifier sees a nonzero input signal and therefore creates an output signal that turns on the motor.

The motor drives the pen and potentiometer in such a direction as to *cancel* the error signal. When the input signal and position signal are equal, then the motor turns off and the pen remains at rest.

A paper drive motor forms a time base because it pulls the paper underneath the pen at a constant rate. In most servorecorders a sprocket drive is used instead of the friction rollers used in most PMMC machines. The paper used in these machines has holes along the margins to accept the sprocket teeth (Figure 20-5b).

Most high-quality servorecorders use a *stepper motor* to drive the paper supply. Such a motor will rotate only a few degrees every time a pulse is ap-

plied to its windings. A few models use a continuously running motor that drives the sprocket through a speed-reducing transmission gear box.

The stepper motor system is actually capable of very good time base accuracy because a crystal oscillator or the ac power mains (60 Hz) are used to drive the pulses used to advance the motor. Digital integrated circuit frequency dividers (countercircuits) can be used to reduce the clock frequency to the frequency required to drive the motor at the desired speed.

The reference potentiometer used to measure the position of the pen may be any of the following devices: slide-wire, rectilinear, or rotary models. The slide-wire system is often used because it can be built with less friction and no mechanical linkage. An example of a slide-wire model is shown in Figure 2-6a, while the equivalent points are shown in Figure 20-6b. A *resistance wire* and a shorting wire are stretched taut, parallel to each other and the direction of pen travel. A shorting bar on the pen assembly serves as a wiper on the

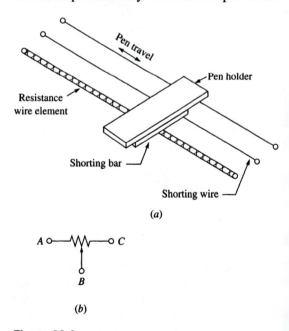

(a)

(b)

Figure 20-6
Slide-wire potentiometer. *(a)* Mechanism. *(b)* Equivalent circuit.

resistance element and also connects the shorting wire. *A, B,* and *C* in Figure 20-6*a* refer to the potentiometer terminals shown in Figure 20-6*b*. The shorting wire serves as terminal *B* of the potentiometer (the wiper).

20-6 *X-Y* recorders

The *X-Y* recorder (Figure 20-7) uses *two* servomechanisms connected to the same writing assembly, but at right angles to each other. The *X*-axis servomechanism moves the pen-bar assembly back and forth across the paper in the horizontal plane, while the *Y*-axis servomechanism moves the pen vertically up and down along the bar.

The paper itself does not move. It is held in place either by clamps or, in high-quality instruments, by a vacuum pump that is used to evacuate a hollow chamber below the paper platform. Holes in the platform create the negative pressure needed to keep the paper in place.

One advantage of the *X-Y* recorder over most other types of instruments is that almost any type

of paper may be used. One could, for example, use specially printed paper that gives units proper to, say, pulmonary function tests (see chapter 10).

The *X-Y* recorder can plot Lissajous patterns because both *X* and *Y* axes can be driven by external signals. If a *Y*-time display is required, then we can drive the *X*-axis with a linear ramp function.

20-7 Problems in recorder design

All pen assemblies will have mass, regardless of which type of drive mechanism is used. Because of the inertia produced by this mass, the pen will not begin moving from being at rest until a certain minimum signal voltage level is provided. This phenomenon, called the *deadband,* is shown in Figure 20-8. A deadband signal is the largest signal to which the recorder will *not* respond. In most recorders the deadband is approximately 0.05% to 0.1% of full scale.

The deadband can create severe distortion in low-amplitude signals (those whose amplitude approximates the deadband voltage). The solution to the deadband is to slew through it as rapidly as possible. This means that sufficient preamplification of the signal is required so that as much of the recorder's span as possible is used.

Another problem that can distort waveforms is *overshoot* and *undershoot* of the recorded trace in response to a *step-function* input signal. This problem affects all mechanical writing systems. Figure 20-9 shows the three types of responses found in recorders. In the *critically damped* case, the signal rises smoothly and quickly to the proper value with little or no curvature as it approaches the proper point.

An *undercritically damped* recorder will *overshoot* the correct point and then hunt back and forth across the correct point for a few cycles until it hones in and settles properly. If a squarewave is applied to such a recorder, the trace will show *ringing* on the waveform.

An *overcritically damped* recorder is sluggish; the pen approaches the correct position very

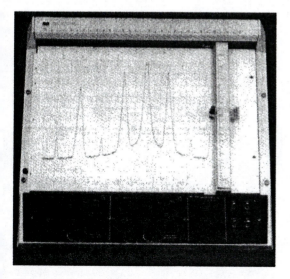

Figure 20-7
X-Y recorder. (Reprinted courtesy of Hewlett-Packard)

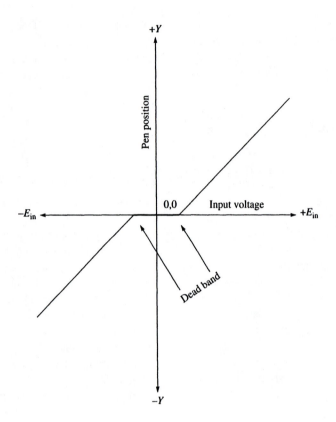

Figure 20-8
Deadband.

slowly. A square wave applied to such a system will have a rounded corner characteristic of a square wave that has been passed through a low-pass filter circuit.

The three different types of damping property are mechanical analogs of electrical frequency-selective filtering. In fact, electronic filters are often used to correct improper (overcritical or undercritical) damping. Some PMMC recorders use a *pen position transducer* inside of the galvanometer housing, and servorecorders already have a pen position signal. The *position* signal can be low-pass filtered (integrated) to vary the damping of the pen assembly.

In the PMMC recorder, the integrated position signal is fed back to the servoamplifier to be summed with the error signal.

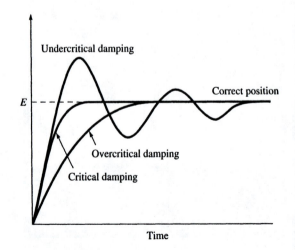

Figure 20-9
Types of responses found in recorders: critical, over-critical, and undercritical damping.

Pen assemblies are often damaged if they strike the limits-of-travel stops at a high speed. If a signal that is very large, relative to the full-scale signal, is applied to the input, then the pen may hit the mechanical stops and break.

Some PMMC recorder amplifiers use output limiting to guard against such damage. Alternatively, a pair of zener diodes connected back to back across the PMMC coil are sometimes used to accomplish the same job. The zener potential of the diodes is selected so that the diodes break over and conduct current only when a voltage greater than the normal full-scale potential is applied to the input of the amplifier.

If a PMMC *position* signal is available, then it can be *differentiated* to produce a *velocity* signal ($v = dx/dt$), and the position signal may be differentiated *twice* to form an *acceleration* signal (d^2x/dt^2). These signals can be used to apply a hard *braking* signal to the PMMC coil if either pen velocity or acceleration exceeds certain limits. The pen will still strike the stops but with considerably reduced force.

Most recorders have a *damping control* that is adjusted when a square wave (1 Hz) is applied to the amplifier input. The damping control is adjusted for best "squareness" of the tracing.

20-8 Maintenance of PMMC writing styluses and pens

There are several common faults of medical paper recorders. These are sometimes amenable to adjustment: in other cases, repair is necessary. Let's consider separately the ink pen and heated stylus types of recorder. Because they find only limited use in medical equipment, we will not consider some of the other types (even though you need to be aware of them conceptually). In this section we will discuss some common maintenance actions that do not always require trained engineering technicians.

Figure 20-10 shows how to remove an ink blockage from an ink pen recorder that has been allowed to stand too long without being used. As a

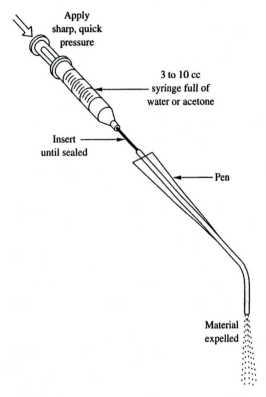

Figure 20-10
Removing ink clots from a pen recorder ink tip.

general rule, such recorders should be run for about 5 minutes or so once a week when not in regular service. Otherwise, the ink will dry up at the tip and prevent the recorder from writing. Fill a 3- to 10-cc syringe with water (or acetone, if certain types of ink are used), and insert the needle end into the ink inlet on the rear end of the pen assembly. On most recorders the pen has to be removed from the machine for this operation. The needle should be inserted up to the Luer lock hub to make a good fluid seal. Quickly, and with a single sharp motion, drive the plunger "home" so that a high-pressure jet of water or acetone is forced into the pen. The ink clot should be forced out the other end.

This procedure usually works well. Some precautions are in order, however. First, always wear protective goggles when this performing this operation. Also, wear protective clothing, as ink and water will splatter. Second, make sure that the pen tip is aimed downward into a sink. Finally, as always when dealing with needles, be careful not to stick yourself.

Keep in mind that the thick, high-viscosity ink used in these machines stains everything it touches and is nearly impossible to remove.

Ink pen tips are designed to operate parallel to the paper surface (see inset in Figure 20-11). If the pen is worn, or when a new pen is installed, it is necessary to "lap" the tip to reestablish the parallelism. The sign that lapping is needed will be either (or both) of the following: (a) a blob of ink when the machine first starts recording a waveform, or (b) a too-thick trace. In most such machines the ink should be dry before the paper leaves the paper platform at the drive roller end of the surface. If it is not dry, lapping may be needed. To lap the pen, place a piece of very fine emery cloth (a sandpaper-like material available at any hardware store) under the tip. Work the pen tip back and forth 5 to 10 times to "sand" the tip parallel to the paper.

The pressure of the stylus or pen is also important. If the pressure is not correct, then the waveform may be distorted. On medical equipment, it is possible to make a normally healthy lead-I ECG signal look as though the patient has either a heart block or a recent myocardial infarction, because of improperly adjusted stylus pressure. The manufacturer will specify a pressure in grams. The numbers vary from 1 to 10 g, depending on the machine model and year of manufacture—older models used heavier stylus pressures.

A stylus pressure gauge (Figure 20-12) is used to lift the pen or stylus from the paper, as the machine is running, until the trace just disappears. The pressure reading is then made from the barrel of the gauge. Suitable stylus pressure gauges can be purchased from ECG machine manufacturers' service or parts departments. Alternatively, the stylus pressure gauge used for phonograph tone arms is useful if the specified pressure is within their relatively limited range (usually 0 to 4 g). The stylus pressure adjustment is made using a screw that is usually located on the rear of the stylus (or pen) or the assembly that holds it in place.

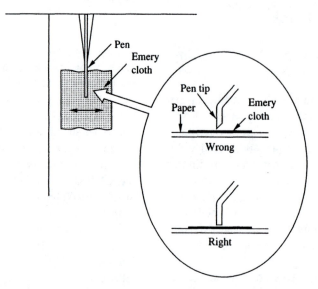

Figure 20-11
Lapping a pen tip to make it parallel to the paper.

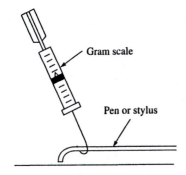

Figure 20-12
Measuring stylus or pen pressure in analog recorder.

Figure 20-13 shows several different 1-mV calibration pulses from an ECG machine. These traces can be made by pressing the "1-MV" or "CAL" button on the front panel of the machine. The ideal shape is perfectly square, as shown in Figure 20-13*a*. But this ideal is almost never achieved in practical machines because of the inertia of the pen or stylus assembly. Usually we see the slightly rounded features of the pulse shown in Figure 20-13*b*. This waveform is usually acceptable. However, the overdamped and underdamped waveforms shown in Figures 20-13*c* and 20-13*d*, respectively, are not acceptable.

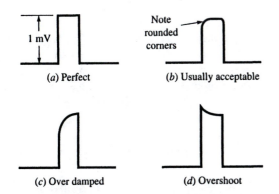

Figure 20-13
1-mV calibration pulses. *(a)* Ideal shape. *(b)* Slightly rounded figures normally seen. *(c)* Overdamped pulse. *(d)* Underdamped pulse.

On all recorders, there may be a damping control available for adjustment by a properly trained technician. This control is adjusted (usually internally to the machine) to compensate for problems. On ink pen machines, the stylus pressure can affect the wave shape, especially if it is set to too high a value (it produces the overdamped waveform). On heated stylus machines, both the stylus pressure and the heat can affect the waveform.

On some heated stylus machines, the standard procedure is to set the pressure to a specified value, set the voltage applied to the stylus heating element to a specified value (usually 5.00 or 7.00 V), and then adjust the internal damping control to produce the waveform shown in Figure 20-13*b* in response to either a square wave input or successive presses of the 1-MV or CAL button.

If the manufacturer of the machine did not provide a knob on the stylus heat control, then do not adjust it without the correct equipment (usually stylus pressure gauge and voltmeter) *and* the manufacturer's service manual.

20-9 Dot matrix analog recorders

The dot matrix printer is long familiar to users of computer equipment, even though it is now eclipsed by laser and ink jet technologies. The original dot matrix printers (mid-1970s) used a 5 × 7 matrix of dots (Figure 20-14*a*) to form alphanumeric characters.

The dot matrix machine used a print head (Figure 20-14*b*) to cause the correct dot elements to be energized to make a mark on the paper. Two different methods were once popular, although one has since faded almost to obscurity. Some of the earliest machines were thermally based. The dots were thermally connected to heating coils and could be heated when needed. Special temperature-sensitive paper was used to receive the text. This method is no longer widely used. The second method used an array of seven print hammers (actually pins). The pins would either extend or retract depending upon whether or not

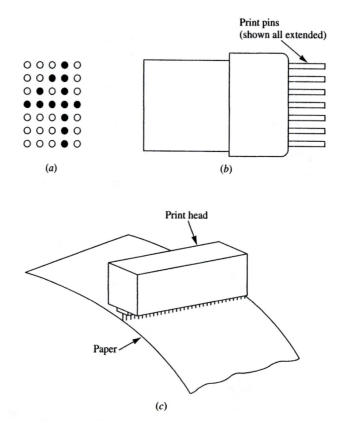

Figure 20-14
Dot matrix printer. *(a)* 5 × 7 dot matrix. *(b)* Dot matrix print head. *(c)* Dot matrix recorder system.

that particular dot was active for the character being printed. An advantage of the pin method is that ordinary paper can be used. The pins impact an inked ribbon to leave the impression. Although the original low-resolution printers were seven-pin models (Figure 20-14a and b), higher-resolution models are now available with 9-, 18-, and 24-pin print heads.

The computer world rapidly discovered that clever programmers could make a dot matrix print head do graphics as well as alphanumerics. The spate of newsletters, church and school bulletins, and other low-cost (but often creatively done) publications are a testimony to the graphics capability of modern dot matrix technology.

Dot matrix printing can be used to make analog recorders that outperform most older mechanical analog recorders. Figure 20-14c shows the concept schematically. A dot matrix print head with a large number of pins is arrayed over a platen. The action depends upon whether thermal, electro-arc, or plain strip-chart paper is used. Regardless of the particulars, however, the result is a strip-chart recording that mixes analog and digital data on the same chart.

Figure 20-15 shows dot matrix analog recordings. The digital computer backing up this system can print the appropriate grid (notice the difference between Figure 20-15a and b; these recordings were made sequentially on the same machine

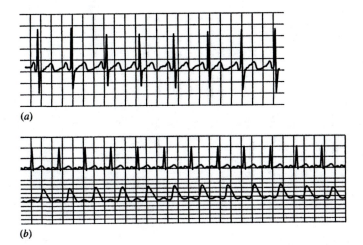

(a)

(b)

Figure 20-15
Dot matrix analog recordings. *(a)* ECG waveform. *(b)* ECG and pressure waveform.

without changing paper). Printed as alphanumeric characters along the top of the strip are data including ICU bed number, time, data. ECG lead number, heart rate, and blood pressure values.Figure 20-15*b* is similar to Figure 20-15*a* but includes an arterial blood pressure waveform along with the ECG waveform.

20-10 Oscilloscopes

The cathode ray oscilloscope (CRO) has become an elementary instrument in the sciences, engineering, medicine, and several industries. Many measurement processes can take place or are made easier by the CRO because it will display not only amplitude, but also time and wave shape relationships. Many medical instruments use the CRO to display physiological waveforms as an alternative to paper-consuming strip-chart recorders.

The heart of any oscilloscope is the CRT shown in Figure 20-16. An electron gun at the rear of the tube emits a beam of electrons that are accelerated and focused by special electrodes beyond the gun. When the accelerated electrons strike the phosphorcoated screen, they give up their kinetic energy in the form of light. With no other external influences, the beam will strike exactly the center of the screen.

Patterns can be drawn on the CRT screen by deflecting the beam up and down and left and right of its normal path. Two basic types of CRT deflection systems are in common use in medical CROs: *magnetic* and *electrostatic*. The electrostatic form is shown in Figure 20-16 and consists of two pairs of deflection plates: one each for *horizontal* and *vertical deflection*. An electrical potential applied across either set of plates creates an electrostatic field that deflects the electron beam. The *polarity* of the potential determines the *direction* of the deflection, while its *magnitude* determines the *amount* of deflection. Most laboratory and service oscilloscopes use electrostatic deflection CRTs because they can operate to very high frequencies—as high as 200 to 300 mHz in the best models.

In the magnetic deflection system, vertical and horizontal electromagnet coils are positioned around the neck of the CRT, concentric to the electron beam path. Both coils are housed in a single assembly called a *deflection yoke*. Current flowing in the deflection coils creates magnetic fields that deflect the electron beam. The inductance of the coils, plus their distributed capacitance, reduces the frequency response of the CRT system to less than 20 to 25 kHz. The frequency limitations of magnetic deflection systems prohibit their use in

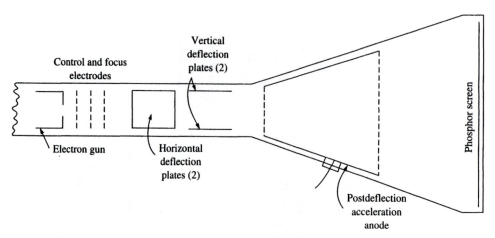

Figure 20-16
Basic CRT structures.

laboratory and service oscilloscopes. But in medical oscilloscopes, the frequency response required of the CRT is usually in the dc to 1000 Hz range or less. Magnetic deflection, therefore, is also suitable for use in medical CROs. In fact, the magnetic deflection CRT usually has a shorter neck than its electrostatic counterpart, which is an advantage in that it allows the oscilloscope to be packaged in a shorter cabinet.

Most medical oscilloscopes are of the *Y-time* type, meaning that the signal, a time-varying voltage, is applied to the *Y*-axis (vertical channel), while a sawtooth time base signal is applied to the *X*-axis (horizontal channel). This type of sweep allows us to view the waveshape of the time domain signals such as the ECG and arterial pressure waveform. The horizontal sweep speed for most medical oscilloscopes is 25 mm/s or 50 mm/s, with some with 100 mm/s as an option. On a standard 10-cm graticule, then, a 25-mm/s sweep speed requires a sweep time of

$$T = 10 \text{ cm} \times 10 \text{ mm/cm} \times 1 \text{ s}/25 \text{ mm}$$
$$T = ((10 \times 10)/25)\text{s} = 4 \text{ s}$$

which corresponds to a sweep frequency of 0.25 Hz, a distinct contrast to the megahertz sweep speeds of some laboratory oscilloscopes.

Some CRTs use only the electrodes prior to the deflection system to accelerate the electron beam to the point where it can produce light when it strikes the phosphor coating. But most medical CROs use CRTs that have a postdeflection acceleration electrode. This electrode is given a high (over 1 kV) positive potential to attract and accelerate the electron beam. The use of a post-deflection accelerator anode improves the linearity of the deflection system. Such tubes can usually be identified by the high-voltage nipple electrode on the glass bell.

20-11 Medical oscilloscopes

The medical oscilloscope differs from service and laboratory models in several principal ways: horizontal sweep speed, vertical amplifier bandwidth, and CRT phosphor persistence.

The horizontal sweep speed difference has already been mentioned. The medical CRO sweeps in the subhertz range instead of kilohertz or megahertz. This low-frequency range is consistent with the fact that physiological signals tend to have fundamental frequencies in the range of the human heart rate.

In service and laboratory oscilloscopes we look for as much vertical bandwidth as possible within the limitations of budget. We pay a heavy premium for wide vertical amplifier bandwidth. But in a medical oscilloscope, that bandwidth is totally wasted and, in fact, may be detrimental if there is a lot of high-frequency noise on the input signal. The amplifiers driving the vertical deflection system of the medical oscilloscope are purposely limited in frequency response in order to eliminate or reduce its response to artifacts. An upper -3 dB point for medical oscilloscopes is typically found in the range of 200 to 2000 Hz, depending on application.

The other principal difference is the nature of the phosphor material used to coat the viewing screen. Serviceand laboratory CROs tend to have *short persistence* CRTs, while medical CROs use *long persistence* CRTs. Persistence is the property whereby the light remains on the screen for a short time after the electron beam has swept past the point. Once generated, the light *decays* after the electron beam moves to another point; it does not turn off instantly. On the medical CRO we use long persistence CRTs because the waveforms being viewed have such low fundamental frequencies; such long sweep times are needed because if they were not used, the features of the waveform on the leading edge of the waveform would fade before the trailing edge is written onto the screen. But a long persistence CRT (P_7 phosphors) allows the entire waveform to be viewed at once.

The long persistence phosphors have an interesting light spectrum—a mixture of yellow and violet-blue. Without a filter over the viewing screen, it appears blue to violet. Yellow and green displays can be created by the use of an appropriate color filter. Both yellow and green displays, however, use the blue-violet CRT.

20-12 Multibeam oscilloscopes

There are no true multibeam CRTs, but a multitrace display can be created by certain *switching* techniques and through the use of a *gating amplifier*. Various versions of these methods are used in multichannel medical oscilloscopes.

An example of a switching system is shown in Figure 20-17. In this example, the switching function is performed by a pair of complementary metal oxide semiconductor (CMOS) analog switches such as the 4016 and 4066 devices. One side of both switches is connected to the input of the vertical amplifier. The other side of each switch is connected to the outputs of the preamplifiers, one for each input channel. The control terminals for the two switches are connected to out-of-phase square wave drive signals, so that one is turned on while the other is off. This permits only one of the two channels to be connected to the input of the vertical amplifier at one time. In most models, the switching rate is 2000 to 100,000 Hz.

Figure 20-18 shows another switching circuit, this one used by Hewlett-Packard in the model 7803C two-channel medical CRO. This circuit uses bipolar transistors Q_1 through Q_4 as an electronic switch; Q_1 and Q_2 operate channel 2, while Q_3 and Q_4 operate channel 1. Switching action is controlled by the signal from a 2-kHz multivibrator. The multivibrator is designed such that the signal applied to CR_1 is exactly 180° out of phase with the signal applied to CR_2. On one-half of the 2-kHz square wave, CR_1 will be forward biased and CR_2 will be reverse biased. Under this condition Q_3/Q_4 will be turned off, and channel 2 will be connected to the vertical amplifier through Q_1/Q_2. On the opposite half of the 2-kHz square wave, however, exactly the opposite situation occurs: Q_3/Q_4 are turned on, connecting channel 2 to the vertical amplifier, while Q_1/Q_2 are turned off. As was also true in the previous example, we alternately apply the two signal channels to the signal vertical amplifier at a 2-kHz rate.

In a gating amplifier system, the vertical axis of the CRT is scanned at a fixed rate, usually in the 15- to 25-kHz range, while the horizontal axis is swept left-to-right at a rate of 25 mm/s. This means that each successive vertical sweep will scan the CRT at a slightly different point, moving left to right with the horizontal sweep. Ordinarily, this action would produce a *raster* on the CRT screen, just as is used on the CRT

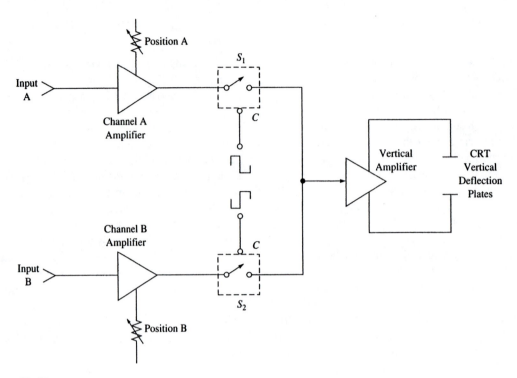

Figure 20-17
Two-channel chopper.

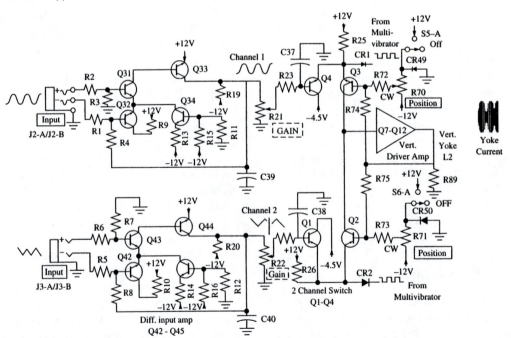

Figure 20-18
Two-channel chopper from the H-P 7803B. (Reprinted courtesy of Hewlett-Packard)

screen of television receivers. But in medical CROs, the electron beam is kept *blanked* (turned off) most of the time. The screen is unblanked at specific times by pulses from the *gating amplifier* (Figure 20-19a), which is actually a voltage-controlled pulse generator. The pulse repetition rate is controlled by the input signal voltage. An input voltage of 0 V produces a certain fixed pulse rate, while positive and negative input voltages produce lower and higher rates, respectively.

Figure 20-19b shows the operation of the gating amplifier. When the input signal is zero (upper trace), then the pulses occur at a given, fixed rate. This causes each vertical sweep to be unblanked at precisely the same point approximately in the middle of the screen. The result is a series of lighted spots that move across the CRT screen at 25 mm/s.

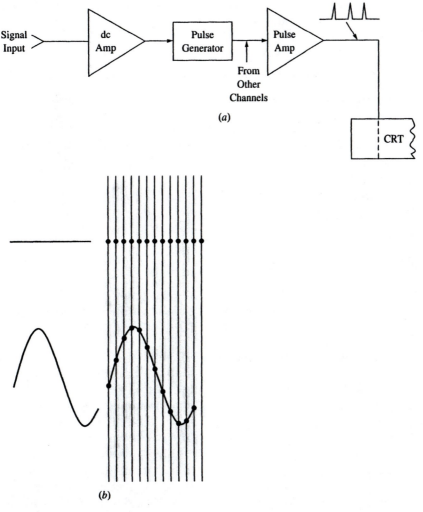

(a)

(b)

Figure 20-19
Gating amplifier system. *(a)* Block diagram. *(b)* Operation.

If a dc level is applied to the input of the gating amplifier, then the line of lighted dots will occur higher or lower on the screen, depending on the amplitude and polarity of the voltage.

Applying a voltage waveform to the gating amplifier input causes the timing of the pulses to vary according to the amplitude and polarity of the waveform. This causes the vertical sweeps to be unblanked at different times, scanning out the waveshape of the signal on the screen.

The vertical sweep frequency is on the order of 15 to 25 kHz, so the dots of Figure 20-19a actually appear to be a continuous line, an effect improved by the persistence of the phosphor and the human eye.

20-13 Nonfade oscilloscopes

The traditional oscilloscope uses a beam of electrons to sweep the screen, writing the waveform as it is deflected. Even with long persistence phosphors, however, we find that the trace vanishes shortly after it is written onto the screen. This type of CRO is sometimes calleda *bouncing-ball* display. To the medical personnel using the bouncing-ball display, it is very difficult to evaluate waveform anomalies because the trace fades too rapidly.

The solution to this problem is the *digital storage oscilloscope,* which is often called a *nonfade display.* CRT storage systems are not used in medical oscilloscopes because, at the low frequencies involved, the digital types offer a better display at competitive prices. Also, the digital type of storage oscilloscope does not "bloom" when the display is erased.

Two different nonfade formats are commonly used: *parade* and *erase bar* (Figure 20-20). The parade display is shown in Figure 20-20a. The newest data, that being written in real time, appears in the upper right-hand corner of the screen. The light beam bounces up and down at a fixed (horizontal) point in response to the vertical waveform; it does not move along the time base as in normal CROs. The old data (immediate past waveforms) moves to the left to disappear off the left-

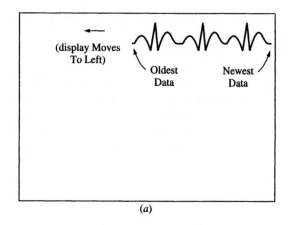

(a)

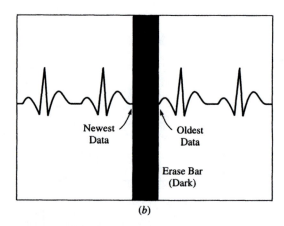

(b)

Figure 20-20
Types of nonfade display. *(a)* Waveform parade.
(b) Erase bar or cursor.

hand side of the screen. This type of display has been named the parade because the oldest waveform appears to lead the succeeding waveforms marching off the screen.

The erase bar format display is shown in Figure 20-20b. On this type of nonfade CRO, the beam of light travels left to right (it is not stationary, as on parade models). An erase bar (dark region) travels ahead of the beam, obliterating the oldest data so that new data can be written onto the CRT screen.

Figure 20-21 shows a block diagram for a nonfade oscilloscope. The principal sections are *input amplifier, analog-to-digital (A/D) converter, scratch pad memory, main memory, digital-to-analog (D/A) converter, output amplifier,* and *control logic section*. Some models also include a second D/A converter to create a horizontal time base signal that is synchronized with the memory. In many other models, however, more traditional analog methods are used to generate the horizontal sawtooth, but it is triggered by the control logic section.

The input amplifier serves both to *scale* the amplitude of the input signal to the range of the oscilloscope and to *buffer* the oscilloscope from the outside world. This stage tends to be a low-gain (A_v is usually less than 10) transistor or integrated circuit (IC) operational amplifier. The gain is usually variable so that the input signal amplitude may be scaled properly.

The A/D converter serves to create a digital binary *word* that is proportional to the applied signal amplitude. Eight- and 10-bit A/D converters are very common, although the eight-bit are probably most common. As an example, consider an eight-bit system. It might represent zero signal ampli-

tude as 00000000_2 and a full-scale signal as 11111111_2. If +2.55 V represents full scale, then each 10-mV change in the input signal will represent a one least significant bit (1 LSB) change in the digital word used to represent the voltage.

In most A/D converter designs, the operation must be synchronized with a series of pulses. The control logic section will generate a *start* pulse to initiate a conversion, and the A/D will generate an *end-of-conversion* (EOC) pulse to let the rest of the circuits know when it is finished with the conversion cycle.

The scratch pad memory is a shift register that holds one to four of the *most recent* bits of data produced by the A/D converter.

The main memory contains all of the data appearing on the CRT screen (scratch pad memory data does not appear on the CRT screen until it is transferred to the main memory). Most medical nonfade oscilloscopes use either 256, 512, or 1024 eight-bit memory locations. Each location contains a binary word proportional to some instantaneous signal amplitude. Both scratch pad and main memory are shift registers.

The D/A converter produces an analog voltage level from the binary word applied to its inputs.

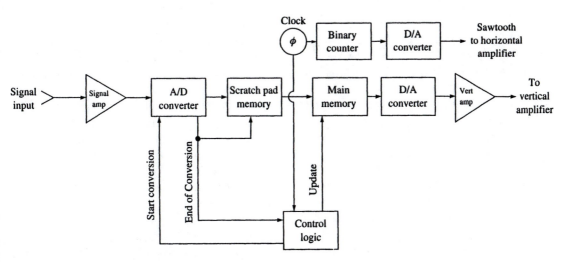

Figure 20-21
Block diagram for nonfade oscilloscope.

The output of the D/A converter is applied to the vertical channel of the oscilloscope through an output buffer amplifier.

In some models horizontal sweep is generated by a second D/A converter. A binary counter used to sequentially address memory locations also drives the horizontal D/A converter. The binary counter is driven by a clock signal, so the output lines increment by one bit for each clock pulse. The result of this action at the output of the D/A converter is that a linear ramp voltage is generated that rises a few millivolts for every clock pulse received. When the counter overflows, its output word goes from full scale (11111111_2) back to zero (00000000_2). The output of the D/A converter, then, will drop from full scale back to zero at this time, completing the sawtooth waveform needed to drive the horizontal deflection system of the oscilloscope.

In certain other nonfade models, analog circuitry is used to generate the sawtooth. Many of these models use the *Miller* integrator circuit, driven from constant reference voltage. The integrator capacitor is kept discharged by an electronic switch until a trigger pulse from the control logic section tells it to initiate a sweep. At that same instant the binary address counter is reset and then begins counting from 00000000_2.

Regardless of the sweep system used, the binary counter steps through the 1024 memory addresses as the beam is swept left to right across the CRT screen. Since this action is synchronized, each *location* in memory represents a *point* along the horizontal axis of the CRT screen. The amplitude of the reproduced signal at that point is proportional to the digital word stored in the memory location defining that point.

The waveform on the CRT screen does not fade because it is *refreshed* 64 or 128 times per second by rapidly incrementing the counter. The refresh rate is selected to allow little fading of the CRT beam between refreshes; data is constantly being rewritten onto the screen before it can be lost.

The control circuit coordinates the action of the A/D converter, scratch pad memory, main memory, and binary address counter. In most nonfade oscilloscopes the data in the scratch pad memory will replace the oldest data in memory every 4, 8 or 16 refresh cycles. In other words, the binary address counter increments through its range 4 to 16 times to refresh the CRT for every new data point entered. The sequence of events is as follows:

1. The control logic section issues a *start* pulse to the A/D converter, which then initiates a conversion cycle.

2. When the A/D converter is completed, the A/D converter issues an EOC pulse that causes the A/D data to be input to the scratch pad memory.

3. When the scratch pad memory is full (one to four words), its data is transferred to the main memory. This data replaces the four oldest pieces of data in the memory.

4. The control logicsection scans the memory to output display data 64 or 128 times per second, between those times when the scratch pad memory data is being transferred to main memory.

A large number of nonfade oscilloscopes use a simpler design, as shown in Figure 20-22. All of the other stages in this type of oscilloscope are the same as in the model shown in Figure 20-21, so only the memory is shown here. The memory is a recirculating serial shift register. Data is input on the left and will shift to the right one position (one bit at a time) each time a clock pulse is received on the shift line. As the data is output, it is also written into the input, hence the term *recirculating*. Again, data in the short-term scratch pad memory will be written into the main memory, replacing the oldest data every 4, 8, or 16 circulations.

Many nonfade models include a *freeze* capability. Such models have a front panel switch that allows the operator to transfer all of the data in the memory to an auxiliary memory of the same bit

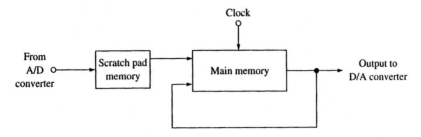

Figure 20-22
Recirculating shift register memory system.

length. The freeze memory data continues to recirculate but is never updated. As a result, the waveform on the CRT screen remains unchanged (frozen in place).

Another optional feature found on many models is the ability to *cascade* channels. A multichannel oscilloscope would require one memory chain, and possibly one A/D-D/A pair, for *each channel*. An eight-channel nonfade oscilloscope, therefore, uses eight separate memories. But when fewer than eight channels are in use, then the unused memory is wasted. If the operator selects the cascade mode, however, the output of one memory will be fed into the input of another. So when the memory for, say, channel 1 is filled, it will overflow and begin filling up channel 2.

20-14 Modern oscilloscope designs

Modern medical oscilloscopes are based on a variety of digital and analog technologies and often include a microprocessor for signals processing and control functions. Figure 20-23 shows a typical medical monitor scope used in an ICU. The pattern on the screen is physiological data. This type of monitor is used in a computer-based system that actually forms the image.

The monitor in Figure 20-23, like certain other displays, uses a *touch screen* method for the selector "switches." Figure 20-24 shows how most such scopes operate. Positioned along the edges of the display are a series of infrared (IR) sources (light-

emitting diodes [LEDs] operating in the IR region), and IR detectors. The IR light is invisible to the naked eye and so is not seen by the operator. The function labels are either painted onto the CRT by the computer (as in Figure 20-24) or affixed to the edge. When the operator touches the screen over any label, his or her finger interrupts one vertical and one horizontal beam, causing a unique pattern. For example, suppose all detector outputs are at binary low when the IR reaches the detector. The X outputs X_1-X_2 and L-L, and the Y outputs Y_1-Y_2-Y_3-Y_4-Y_5-Y_6 are L-L-L-L-L-L. And then someone touches the "self-test" label. In this case, X_1 and Y_1 are both interrupted and their respective outputs go high. Thus, the patterns become H-L and H-L-L-L-L-L. The internal

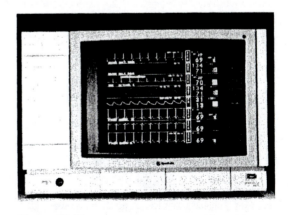

Figure 20-23
Medical monitor oscilloscope

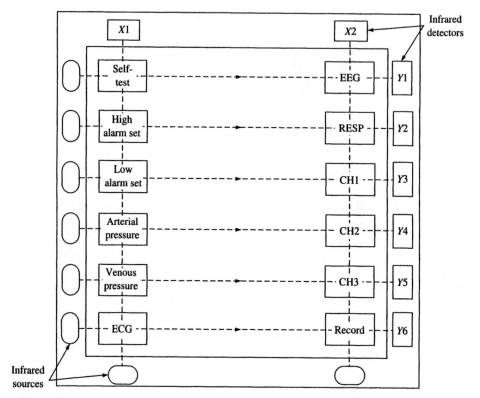

Figure 20-24
Touch screen oscilloscope

computer recognizes this as an operator command to branch to the self-test software stored in program memory.

20-15 Summary

1. Medical oscilloscopes can be classified as the *bouncing ball* design for normal *Y-T* models and *nonfade* for digital storage models.

2. Medical oscilloscopes use very low-frequency horizontal sweep (25, 50, or 100 mm/s).

3. The CRTs used in medical oscilloscopes have *long persistence* phosphors.

4. Two principal techniques are used to make multichannel oscilloscopes from single-beam CRTs: *switching* and *gating amplifier.*

20-16 Recapitulation

Now return to the objectives and self-evaluation questions at the beginning of the chapter and see how well you can answer them. If you cannot answer certain questions, place a check mark next to each and review appropriate parts of the text. Next, try to answer the following questions using the same procedure. When you have answered all of the questions, solve the problems.

Questions

1. List the principal *differences* between medical and service/laboratory oscilloscopes.

2. What property is required of the CRT in a medical oscilloscope?

3. List two general types of medical oscilloscopes, as classified by their display.

4. What is the normal sweep speed for a medical oscilloscope designed to display ECG and arterial pressure waveforms? List two other optional speeds often encountered.

5. List two different display formats found on nonfade oscilloscopes.

6. Give two different techniques for creating a two-channel oscilloscope from a single-beam CRT.

7. List two different types of CRT deflection systems used in medical oscilloscopes.

8. The use of a postaccelerator anode improves the _____ of the CRT display.

9. The upper −3 dB point in the vertical bandwidth for medical oscilloscopes is usually between _____ and _____ Hz.

10. List the principal stages found in typical nonfade oscilloscopes.

11. The output of the A/D converter represents the _____ value of the input waveform at that time.

12. The waveform on the screen of a nonfade oscilloscope does not fade because it is _____ 64 or 128 times per second.

13. Most medical ECG and arterial pressure recorders use the _____ writing system.

14. Describe in your own words the operation of a PMMC galvanometer. Draw a comparison between the PMMC and the D'Arsonval meter movement.

15. What is meant by *curvilinear recording?*

16. Describe a method by which a PMMC galvanometer can be constructed to render a *rectilinear* recording.

17. Describe in your own words, or using a picture, a pseudorectilinear PMMC writing system.

18. How does a knife edge (writing edge) render a trace rectilinear even though the stylus tip describes angular or curvilinear motion?

19. Describe a thermal writing system. Mention any special paper needed.

20. Compare the pen-and-ink and ink jet writing systems.

21. Describe the optical PMMC writing system.

22. Describe an optical CRT camera.

23. What is a *deadband?*

24. Describe *undershoot* and *overshoot.* How is it related to damping?

25. How can a position signal be used to adjust the damping of the stylus or pen in a PMMC system?

26. *X-Y* recorders use two _____ recorder mechanisms positioned at right angles to each other.

27. How can an *X-Y* recorder be made to make *Y*-time recordings?

Problems

1. Calculate the sweep frequency of a medical oscilloscope that has a 10-cm wide CRT graticule if the sweep speed is 25 mm/s.

2. An ECG oscilloscope is calibrated so that the vertical deflection factor is 1 V/cm, and an external preamplifier has a gain of X1000. How much deflection occurs if a 1- to 4-mV ECG signal is applied to the input?

3. An arterial pressure monitor is calibrated to produce an output of 10 mV/mm Hg, which is to be displayed on an oscilloscope that has a 10-cm vertical graticule. It is decided that the oscilloscope should be calibrated such that it has a scale factor of 5 mm Hg/cm. Find (a) the maximum pressure to be displayed and (b) the number of volts per division.

CHAPTER 21
Electro-Optics
(Fiber-Optics and Lasers)

21-1 Objectives

1. Be able to list the advantages of fiber-optic data/signal transmission.
2. Be able to describe the propagation modes in fiber optics.
3. Be able to describe the different types of lasers.
4. Be able to describe the physical basis for lasers.

21-2 Self-evaluation questions

These questions test your prior knowledge of the material in this chapter. Look for the answers as you read the text. After you have finished studying the chapter, try answering these questions and those at the end of the chapter.

1. List the basic advantages of fiber-optic video, data, and voice communications links.

2. Define *intermodal dispersion* as applied to fiber optics.

3. _____ is a synthetic gem material used to make red-light lasers.

4. Define an *insulating crystal laser.*

21-3 Fiber-optic technology

Fiber-optics is the technology in which light is passed through a plastic or glass fiber so that it can be directed to a specific location. If the light is encoded *(modulated)* with an information signal, then that signal is transmitted over the fiber-optic path. There are many advantages to the fiber-optic communications or data link, including:

- Very high bandwidth (accommodates video signals, many voice channels, or high data rates in computer communications).
- Very low weight and small size.
- Low loss compared with other media.
- Freedom from electromagneticinterference (EMI).

- High degree of electrical isolation.
- Explosion-proof.
- Good data security.
- Improved fail-safe capability.

The utility of the high-bandwidth capability of the fiber-optic data link is that it can handle a tremendous amount of electronically transmitted information simultaneously. For example, it can handle more than one video signal (which typically requires 500 KHz to 6 MHz of bandwidth, depending on resolution). Alternatively, it can handle a tremendous number of voice communication telephone channels. A high-speed computer data communications capability is also obtained. Either a few channels can be operated at extremely high speeds, or a larger number of low-speed parallel data channels are available. Fiberoptics are so significant that one can expect to see them proliferate in the communications industry for years to come.

The light weight and small size, coupled with relatively low loss, makes the fiber-optic communications link a very good economic advantage when large numbers of channels are contemplated. To obtain the same number of channels using coaxial cables or paired wires, the system would require a considerably larger and heavier infrastructure.

EMI has been an annoying factor in electronics since Marconi and DeForest interfered with each other in radio trials for the Newport Yacht Races prior to the turn of the twentieth century. Today, EMI can be more than merely annoying and can cause tragic accidents. For example, airliners are operated more and more from digital computers. If a radio transmitter, radar, or an electrical motor is near one of the data lines, then it is possible to either introduce false data or corrupt existing data—with potentially disastrous results. Because the EMI is caused by electrical or magnetic fields coupling between electrical cables, fiber optics (free of such fields) produce dramatic freedom from EMI (see chapter 24).

21-4 Fiber-optic isolation

Electrical isolation is required in many instrumentation systems for either the safety of the user or the health of the electronic circuits connected to the system. For example, in some industrial processes, high electrical voltages are used, but the electronic instruments used to monitor the process are both low voltage and ground referenced. As a result, the high voltage can damage the instruments. In fiberoptic systems, it is possible to use an electrically floating sensor and then transmit the data over a fiber link to an electrically grounded, low-voltage computer, instrument, or control system.

The fact that fiber optics use light beams, and these are generated in noncontacting electronic circuits, makes the fiber-optic system ideal for use around flammable gases or fumes; for example, in monitoring systems in which natural gas or medical anesthetic agents (such as ether or cyclopropane)* are used. Regular mechanical switches or relays are either on contact or when decontacting, and those sparks can create an explosion if flammable gases or fumes are present. A number of operating room explosions in hospitals occurred prior to 1980. Similarly, gasoline stations have exploded because of electrical arcs in switches.

System security is enhanced because fiberoptics are difficult to tap. An actual physical connection must be made to the system. In wire systems, capacitive or inductive pick-ups can acquire signals with less than total physical connection (i.e., no splice is needed). Similarly, a system is more secure in another sense of the word because the fiber-optic transmitters and receivers can be designed to be fail safe so that one fault does not take down the system. There was once a hospital coronary care unit data system that used parallel wire connections between the data output ports on bedside monitors and the central monitoring computer at the nurses' station. A single short circuit would

---

*These agents are only rarely used today. Since the late 1970s, when nonflammable substitutes came into widespread use, they have been considered too dangerous.

reduce the system to chaos. That is less likely to happen in a fiber-optic system.

21-5 History of fiber-optics

The basic fact of fiber-optics—that is, the propagation of light beams in a transparent glass conductor (Figure 21-1)—was noted in the early 1870s, when a man named John Tyndall introduced members of Britain's Royal Society to his experimental apparatus. An early, but not very practical, color television system patented by J. L. Baird used glass rods to carry the color information. By 1966, G. Hockham and C. Kao (Great Britain) demonstrated a system in which light beams carried data communications via glass fibers. The significant fact that made the Hockham/Kao system work was the reduction of loss in the glass dielectric material to a reasonable level. By 1970, practical fiber-optic communications were possible.

Medicine has made use of fiber-optics for more than two decades. Fiber-optic *endoscopes* can be passed into various orifices of the body, either natural or surgically made, to inspect the interior of a patient's body. Typically there are two bundles, one for viewing and one for passing a light from a (misnamed) "cold" light source into the body. For example, gynecologists can inspect and operate on certain internal organs in women using a *laparoscope* introduced through a "band-aid" incision in the abdomen. Knee surgeons can use a fiber-optic arthroscope to perform operations on the human knee with far less trauma than previous procedures. Other physicians use fiber-optic endoscopes to inspect the stomach and gastrointestinal tract. A probe is passed through the mouth or nose, down the esophagus, and into the stomach so that tumors and ulcers can be inspected without resorting to surgery. In more recent times, miniature TV cameras using charge-coupled diode (CCD) arrays have been made available, with the fiber-optics carrying the light into the stomach.

Fiber-optic inspection is used in fields other than medicine. A septic tank service company may use fiber-optics and television to inspect septic tanks; plumbers may also use fiber-optics. Other industrial and residential services also use fiber-optics to inspect areas that are either inaccessible or too dangerous for direct viewing.

Before examining fiber-optic technology, it might be useful to review some of the basics of optical systems as applied to the fiber-optic system.

21-6 Review of some basics

The *index of refraction (n)*, or *refractive index,* is the ratio of the speed of a light wave in a vacuum to the speed of a light wave in a medium (e.g., glass, plastic, water); for practical purposes, the speed of light in air is close enough to the speed in a vacuum to be considered the same. Mathematically, the index of refraction *(n)* is:

$$n = \frac{c}{v_m} \qquad (21\text{-}1)$$

where

c   is the speed of light in a vacuum ($\sim 3 \times 10^8$ m/s)

v_m is the speed of light in the medium

Refraction is the phenomenon in which a light ray changes direction as it passes across the boundary surface (or interface) between two mediums of differing indices of refraction. Consider Figure 21-2, in which two materials have indices

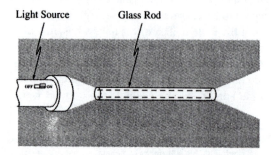

Figure 21-1
Light transmission through a glass or plastic rod.

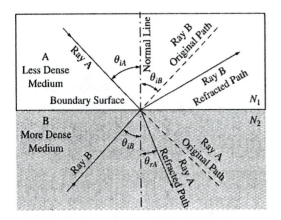

Figure 21-2
Refraction under two different circumstances.
(a) From less dense to more dense. *(b)* From more dense to less dense.

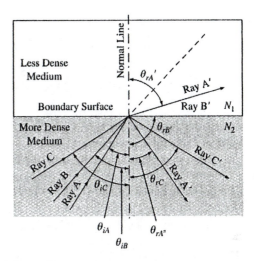

Figure 21-3
Refraction phenomenon from more dense to less dense material showing subcritical (Ray A), critical (Ray B), and supercritical (Ray C) refraction.

of refraction $n;1$ and n_2, respectively. In this illustration, n_1 is optically less dense than n_2. Consider incident light ray A, approaching the interface from the less dense side ($n_1 \rightarrow n_2$). As it crosses the interface, it changes direction toward a line normal (at right angles) to the surface. In the opposite case, ray B, the light ray approaches the interface from the more dense side ($n_2 \rightarrow n_1$). In this case, the light ray is similarly refracted from its original path, but the direction of refraction is away from the normal line.

In refractive systems the angle of refraction is a function of the ratio of the two indices of refraction (i.e., it obeys *Snell's law*):

$$n_1 \sin \theta_{ia} = n_2 \sin \theta_{ra} \qquad (21\text{-}2)$$

or

$$\frac{n_1}{n_2} = \frac{\sin \theta_{ra}}{\sin \theta_{ia}} \qquad (21\text{-}3)$$

In the particular case that concerns fiber-optics, the light ray passes from a more dense to a less dense medium. We can use either a water-to-air system or a system in which two different glasses, with different indices of refraction, are interfaced. This type of system was addressed in Figure 21-2 by ray B. Figure 21-3 shows a similar system with

three different light rays (ray A, ray B, and ray C) approaching the same point on the interface from three different angles (θ_{ia}, θ_{ib}, and θ_{ic}, respectively). Ray A approaches at a *subcritical angle,* so it will split into two portions (A′ and A″). The reflected portion contains a relatively small amount of the original light energy and may indeed be nearly indiscernible. The major portion of the light energy is transmitted across the boundary and refracts at an angle θ_{ra}, in the usual manner.

Light ray B, on the other hand, approaches the interface at a *critical angle,* $\theta_{rb'}$, and is refracted along a line that is orthogonal to the normal line (i.e., it travels along the interface boundary surface). This angle is sometimes labeled θ_c in optical textbooks.

Finally, ray C approaches the interface at an angle greater than the critical angle (i.e., a *supercritical angle*). None of this ray is transmitted, but rather it is turned back into the original media— that is, it is subject to *total internal reflection* (TIR)[†] It is the phenomenon of TIR that allows fiber optics to work.

[†]TIR is called total internal *reflection,* but it is actually a *refraction* phenomenon.

21-7 Fiber-optics

The optical fiber is essentially similar to a microwave *wave guide,* and an understanding of wave guide action is useful in understanding fiber-optics. A schematic model of fiber-optics is shown in Figure 21-4. A slab of denser material (n_1) is sandwiched between two slabs of a less dense material (n_2). Light rays that approach from a supercritical angle are totally internally reflected from the two interfaces ($n_2 \rightarrow n_1$ and $n_1 \rightarrow n_2$). Although only one bounce is shown, the ray will be subjected to successive TIR reflections as it propagates through the n_1 material. The amount of light energy that is reflected through the TIR mechanism is on the order of 99.9%, which compares quite favorably with the 85% to 96% typically found in plane mirrors.

Fiber-optic lines are not rectangular but rather are cylindrical, as shown in Figure 21-5. These components are called *clad fiber-optics* because the denser inner core is surrounded by a less dense layer called *cladding.* Figure 21-5 shows two rays, each of which is propagated into the system such that the critical angles are exceeded. These rays will propagate down the cylindrical optical fiber with very little loss of energy. There are actually two forms of propagation. The minority form (Figure 21-6a), called *meridional rays,* is easier to understand and mathematically model in textbooks because all rays lie in a plane with the optical axis. The more numerous *skew rays* (Figure 21-6b) follow a helical path and so are somewhat more difficult to discuss.

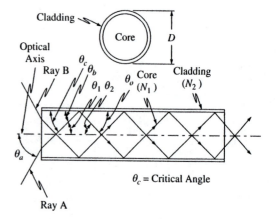

Figure 21-5
Total internal reflection forms the basis for propagation in cylindrical fiber-optics.

The light acceptance of the fiber-optic (Figure 21-7) is a cone-shaped region centered on the optical axis. The *acceptance angle* θ_a is the critical angle for the transition from air ($n = n_a$) to the core material ($n = n_a$). The ability to collect light is directly related to the size of the acceptance cone and is expressed in terms of the *numerical aperture* (NA), which is:

$$NA = \sin \theta_a \qquad (21\text{-}4)$$

The refraction angle of the rays internally, across the air-n_1 interface, is given by Snell's law:

$$\theta_{b1} = \arcsin \left(\frac{n_a \sin \theta_a}{n_1} \right) \qquad (21\text{-}5)$$

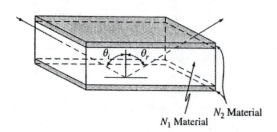

Figure 21-4
Wave guide analogy for fiber-optics.

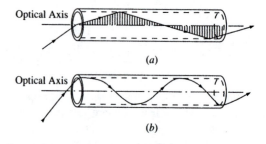

Figure 21-6
Two types of fiber-optic light propagation. *(a)* Meridional propagation. *(b)* Skew propagation.

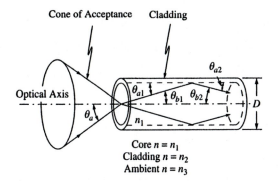

Figure 21-7
Cone of acceptance of fiber-optic.

It can be shown that:

$$\theta_{a1} = \theta_{a2} \qquad (21\text{-}6)$$

$$\theta_{b1} = \theta_{b2} \qquad (21\text{-}7)$$

$$\theta_{a1} = \frac{\theta_a}{n_1} \qquad (21\text{-}8)$$

In terms of the relative indices of refraction between the ambient environment outside the fiber, the core of the fiber, and the cladding material, the numerical aperture is given by:

$$NA = \sin\theta_a = \frac{1}{n_a} = \sqrt{(n_1)^2 - (n_2)^2} \qquad (21\text{-}9)$$

If the ambient material is air, then the numerical aperture equation reduces to:

$$NA = \sqrt{(n_1)^2 - (n_2)^2} \qquad (21\text{-}10)$$

Internally, the angles of reflection (θ_{a1} and θ_{a2}), at the critical angle, are determined by the relationship between the indices of refraction of the two materials, n_1 and n_2:

$$\theta_{a1} = \frac{\arcsin\sqrt{(n_1)^2 - (n_2)^2}}{n_1} \qquad (21\text{-}11)$$

Typical fiber-optic components have numerical apertures of 0.1 to 0.5; typical fibers have a diameter D of 25 µm to 650 µm. The ability of the de-

vice to collect light is proportional to the square of the numerical aperture:

$$\zeta \propto (NA \times D)^2 \qquad (21\text{-}12)$$

where

ζ is the relative light collection ability

NA is the numerical aperture

D is the fiber diameter

21-8 Intermodal dispersion

When a light ray is launched in a fiber-optic, it can take any of a number of different paths, depending in part on its angle of arrival (Figure 21-8). These paths are known as *transmission modes* and vary from very low-order modes parallel to the optical axis of the fiber (ray A in Figure 21-8) to the highest-order mode close to the critical angle (ray C); in addition, a very large number of rays lie between these two limits. An important feature of the different modes is that the respective path lengths vary tremendously, being shortest with the low-order modes and longest with the high-order modes. If a fiber optic has only a single core and single layer of cladding, it is called a *step index* fiber because the index of refraction changes abruptly from the core to the cladding. The number of modes *(N)* that can be supported are given by:

$$N = \frac{\left(\dfrac{\pi D\,[NA]}{\lambda}\right)^2}{2} \qquad (21\text{-}13)$$

Any fiber with a core diameter (D) greater than about 10 wavelengths (10λ) will support a very large number of modes and so is typically called a *multimode fiber.* A typical light beam launched

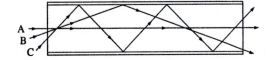

Figure 21-8
Multimode light propagation.

into such a step-index fiber-optic will simultaneously find a large number of modes available to it. This may or may not affect analog signals but has a deleterious effect on digital signals called *intermodal dispersion.*

Figure 21-9 illustrates the effect of intermodal dispersion on a digital signal. When a short-duration light pulse (Figure 21-9a) is applied to a fiber-optic that exhibits a high degree of intermodal dispersion, the received signal (Figure 21-9b) is smeared, or dispersed, over a wider area. At slow data rates this effect may prove negligible because the dispersed signal can die out before the next pulse arrives. But at high speeds, the pulses may overrun

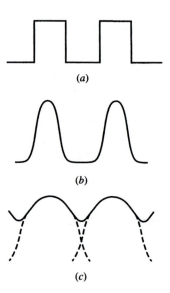

(a)

(b)

(c)

Figure 21-10
Transmodal dispersion creates problems in data fiber-optic systems. *(a)* Input data square wave. *(b)* Resultant light pulse signal. *(c)* Dispersed signal causing overriding of pulses.

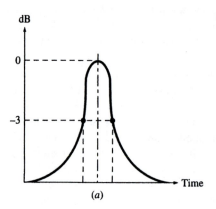

(a)

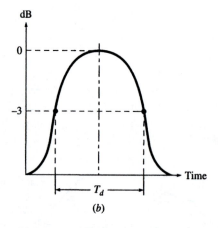

(b)

Figure 21-9
Light signal transmodal dispersion. *(a)* Input pulse. *(b)* Dispersed pulse.

each other (Figure 21-10), producing an ambiguous situation that exhibits a high data error rate.

Intermodal dispersion is usually measured relative to the widths of the pulses at the -3 dB (half-power) points. In Figure 21-9, the -3 dB point on the incident pulse transmitted into the fiber-optic is T, but in the received pulse, the time between -3 dB points is T_d. The dispersion is expressed as the difference, or:

$$\text{Dispersion} = T - T_d \qquad (21\text{-}14)$$

A means for measuring the dispersion for any given fiber-optic element is to measure the dispersion of a Gaussian (normal distribution) pulse at those -3 dB points. The cable is then rated in terms of nanoseconds dispersion per kilometer of fiber (ns/km).

The bandwidth of the fiber, in megahertz per kilometer, can be specified from knowledge of the dispersion, using the expression:

$$\text{BW (MHz/km)} = \frac{310}{\text{Disp. (ns/km)}} \qquad (21\text{-}15)$$

21-9 Graded index fibers

A solution to the dispersion problem is to build an optical fiber with a continuously varying index of refraction such that *n* decreases at distances away from the optical axis. While such smoothly varying fibers are not easy to build, it is possible to produce a fiber-optic with layers of differing index of refraction (Figure 21-11). The relationship of the respective values of *n* for each layer is:

$$n_1 > n_2 > n_3 > n_4 > n_5 > \cdots n_i \qquad (21\text{-}16)$$

The overall index of refraction determines the numerical aperture and is taken as an average of the different layers.

With graded fibers, the velocity of propagation of the light ray in the material is faster in the layers away from the optical axis than in the lower layers. As a result, a higher-order mode wave will travel faster than a wave in a lower order. The number of modes available to the graded index fiber is:

$$N = \frac{\left(\dfrac{\pi D[NA]^2}{\lambda} \right)}{4} \qquad (21\text{-}17)$$

Some cables operate in a *critical mode,* designated HE_{11} (to mimic microwave terminology), in which the cable is very thin compared with multimodal cables. As the diameter of the core decreases, so does the number of available modes, and eventually the cable becomes *monomodal;* if the core gets down to 3 to 5 μm, then only the HE_{11} mode becomes available. The critical diameter required for monomodal operation is:

$$D_{crit} = \frac{2.4\lambda}{\pi[NA]} \qquad (21\text{-}18)$$

Because the monomodal cable potentially reduces the number of available modes, it also reduces intermodal dispersion. Thus, the monomode fiber is capable of extremely high data rates or analog bandwidths.

21-10 Losses in fiber-optic systems

Understanding and controlling losses in fiber-optic systems is integral to making the system work properly. Before examining the sources of such losses, however, let's take a quick look at the notation for losses in the system, as well as the gains of the electronics systems used to process the signals applied to, or derived from, the fiber-optic system. This notation uses the *decibel* as the system of measurement.

The subject of decibels almost always confuses the newcomer to electronics, and even many an old timer seems to have occasional memory lapses regarding the subject. For the benefit of both, and because the subject is so vitally important to understanding electronics systems, we will examine the decibel.

The decibel measurement originated with the telephone industry and was named after telephone inventer Alexander Graham Bell. The original unit was the *bel.* The prefix *deci* means 1/10, so the decibel is one-tenth of a bel. The bel is too large for most common applications and so it is rarely if ever used. Thus, we will concentrate only the more familiar decibel (dB).

The decibel is nothing more than a means of expressing a *ratio* between two signal levels (e.g.,

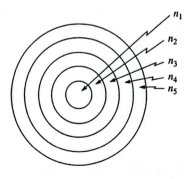

$n_1>n_2>n_3>n_4>n_5>....n_i$

Figure 21-11
Graded index fiber-optic.

the output-over-input ratio of an amplifier). Because the decibel is a ratio, it is also dimensionless, despite the fact that dB looks like a dimension. Consider the voltage amplifier as an example of dimensionless gain; its gain is expressed as the output voltage over the input voltage (V_o/V_{in}).

Example 21-1

A voltage amplifier outputs 6 V when the input signal has a potential of 0.5 V. Find the gain (A_v).

Solution

$$A_V = V_o/V_{in}$$
$$A_V = (6 \text{ V})/(0.5 \text{ V})$$
$$A_V = 12$$

Note in the preceding example that the volt units appeared in both numerator and denominator and so cancelled out, leaving only a dimensionless 12 behind.

To analyze systems using simple addition and subtraction rather than multiplication and division, a little math trick is used on the ratio. We take the base-10 logarithm of the ratio and then multiply it by a scaling factor (either 10 or 20). For voltage systems, such as our voltage amplifier, the expression becomes:

$$dB = 20 \, log \left(\frac{V_o}{V_{in}} \right) \qquad (21\text{-}19)$$

Example 21-2

In Example 21-1 we had a voltage amplifier with a gain of 12 because 0.5 V input produced a 6-volt output. How is this same gain (i.e., V_o/V_{in} ratio) expressed in decibels?

Solution

$$dB = 20 \log(V_o/V_{in})$$
$$dB = 20 \log(6 \text{ V}/0.5 \text{ V})$$
$$dB = 20 \log (12)$$
$$dB = +21.6 \text{ dB}$$

The fact that the quantity represented in Example 21-2 is a gain is indicated by the plus sign. If the quantity represented a loss (e.g., if $V_o < V_{in}$), then the sign of the result would be negative. You can see this by working the problem in Example 21-2 for the ratio 0.5/6, which results in a loss of -21.6 dB. Note that the numerical result for a loss using the same voltages is the same as for a gain, but the sign is reversed.

Despite the fact that we have massaged the ratio by converting it to a logarithm, *the decibel is nonetheless nothing more than a means for expressing a ratio.* Thus, a voltage gain of 12 can also be expressed as a gain of 21.6 dB. A similar expression can be used for current amplifiers, where the gain ratio is I_o/I_{in}:

$$dB = 20 \log \left(\frac{I_o}{I_{in}} \right) \qquad (21\text{-}20)$$

For power measurements, the important feature in light and fiber-optical systems, a modified expression is needed to account for the fact that power is proportional to the square of the voltage or current:

$$dB = 10 \log \left(\frac{P_o}{P_{in}} \right) \qquad (21\text{-}21)$$

We now have three basic equations for calculating decibels (i.e., one each for current ratios, voltage ratios, and power ratios). The usefulness of decibel notation is that it can make nonlinear power and gain equations into linear additions and subtractions. Gains (+dB) and losses (−dB) can be added to find the total gain or loss of the system.

The light power at the output end of a fiber-optic (P_o) is reduced compared with the input light power (P_{in}) because of losses in the system. As in many natural systems, light loss in the fiber material tends to be exponentially decaying (Figure 21-12a) and so obeys an equation of the form:

$$P_o = P_{in}e^{(-\Lambda/L)} \qquad (21\text{-}22)$$

where

Λ is the length of the fiber-optic being considered

L is the unit length (i.e., length for which $e^{(-\Lambda/L)} = e^{-1}$)

From Equation 21-22, and by comparing Figures 21-12*a* and 21-12*b*, you can see why decibels are used. The decibel notation eliminates the exponential notation, allowing us to add and subtract decibels in order to calculate losses in any given system.

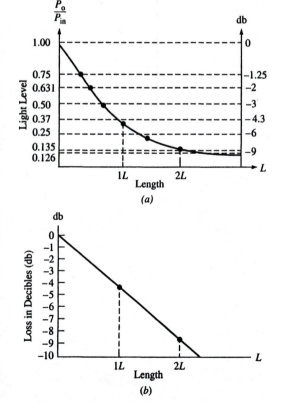

Figure 21-12
Length-dependent signal attenuation in fiber-optic. *(a)* Log-scale graph of attenuation. *(b)* Decibel scale of attenuation.

21-11 Losses in fiber-optic circuits

There are several mechanisms for loss in fiber-optic systems. Some of these are inherent in any light-based system; others are a function of the design of the specific system being considered.

21-11-1 Defect losses

Figure 21-13 shows several possible sources of loss due to defects in the fiber itself. First, in unclad fibers, *surface defects* (nicks and scratches) that breach the integrity of the surface will allow light to escape. In other words, not all of the light is propagated along the fiber. Second (also in unclad fibers), grease, oil, or other *contaminants* on the surface of the fiber may form an area with an index of refraction different from what is expected and cause the light direction to change. And if the contaminant has an index of refraction similar to glass, then it may act as if it were glass and cause loss of light to the outside world. Finally, there is always the possibility of *inclusions* (objects, specks, or voids in the material making up the fiber-optic). Inclusions can affect both clad and

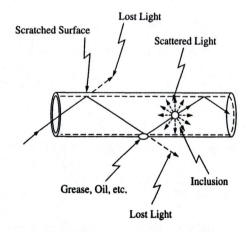

Figure 21-13
Causes of loss in fiber-optics include scratches, contaminants, and inclusions.

unclad fibers. When light hits the inclusion, it tends to scatter in all directions, causing a loss. Some of the light rays scattered from the inclusion may recombine either destructively or constructively with the main ray, but most do not.

21-11-2 Inverse square law losses

In all light systems, there is the possibility of losses due to spreading of the beam. If you take a flashlight and point it at a wall, and measure the power per unit area of the wall at a distance of, say, 1 m, and then back off to twice the distance (2 m) and then measure again, you will find that the power dropped to one-fourth. In other words, the power per unit area is inversely proportional to the square of the distance $(1/D^2)$.

21-11-3 Transmission losses

These losses are due to light that is caught in the cladding material of clad fiber-optics. This light is either lost to the outside or trapped in the cladding layer and is thus not available to be propagated in the core.

21-11-4 Absorption losses

These losses are due to the nature of the core material and are inversely proportional to the transparency of the material. In addition, in some materials, absorption losses may not be uniform across the light spectrum but may be wavelength sensitive.

21-11-5 Coupling losses

These losses are due to coupling systems. All couplings (discussed in more detail later) have loss associated with them. Several different losses of this sort are identified.

21-11-6 Mismatched fiber diameters

These losses are due to coupling a large-diameter fiber (D_L) to a small-diameter fiber (D_s); the larger-diameter fiber transmits to the lesser-

diameter fiber. In decibel form, this loss is expressed by:

$$dB = -10 \log\left(\frac{D_S}{D_L}\right) \quad (21\text{-}23)$$

21-11-7 Numerical aperture coupling losses

These losses occur when the numerical apertures of the two fibers are mismatched. If NA, is the receiving fiber, and NA, is the transmitting fiber, then the loss is expressed as:

$$dB = -10 \log\left(\frac{NA_r}{NA_t}\right) \quad (21\text{-}24)$$

21-11-8 Fresnel reflection losses

These losses occur at the fiber-optic interface with air (Figure 21-14a) and are due to the large change of index of refraction between the glass and the

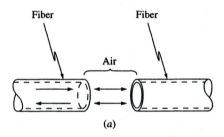

(a)

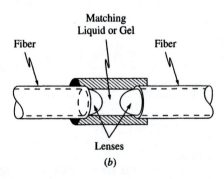

(b)

Figure 21-14
Fiber-optic coupling. (a) In air, reflections occur. (b) "Impedance-matched" coupler.

air. There are actually two losses to consider. First is the loss caused by internal reflection from the inner surface of the interface; second is the reflection from the opposite surface across the air gap in the coupling. Typically the internal reflection loss is on the order of 4%, while the external reflection is about 8%.

We may model any form of reflection in a transmission system similarly to reflections in a radio transmission line. Studying *standing waves* and related subjects in books on radio frequency systems can yield some understanding of these problems. The amount of reflection in coupled optical systems uses similar arithmetic:

$$\Gamma = \left(\frac{n_1 - n_2}{n_1 + n_2}\right)^2 \qquad (21\text{-}25)$$

where

Γ is the coefficient of reflection

n_1 is the index of reflection for the receiving material

n_2 is the index of reflection for the transmitting material

Mismatched indices of refraction are analogous to the mismatch of impedances problem seen in transmission line systems, and the cure is also analogous. Where the transmission line uses an impedance matching coupling device, the fiber-optic will use a coupler that matches the optical impedances (the indices of refraction). Figure 21-14b shows a coupling between the two ends of fibers (lenses may or may not be used depending on the system) that uses a liquid or gel material with a similar index of refraction to the fiber. The reflection losses are thereby reduced or even eliminated.

21-12 Fiber-optic communications systems

A communications system requires an information signal source (e.g., voice, music, digital data, or analog voltage representing a physical parameter),

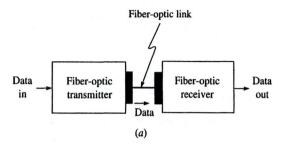

(a)

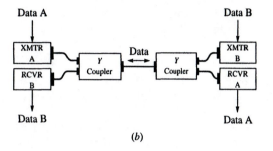

(b)

Figure 21-15
Two basic forms of communication systems.
(a) Simplex system provides one-way communication.
(b) Duplex system provides two-way communications.

a transmitter, a propagation medium (in this case fiber-optics), a receiver, and an output. In addition, the transmitter may include any of several different forms of *encoder* or *modulator,* and the receiver may contain a *decoder* or *demodulator.*

Figure 21-15 shows two main forms of communications link. In the *simplex* system (Figure 21-15a) a single transmitter sends light (information) over the path in only one direction to a receiver set at the other end. The receiver end cannot reply or otherwise send data back the other way. The simplex system requires only a single transmitter and a single receiver module per channel.

The *duplex* system (Figure 21-15b) can send data simultaneously in both directions, allowing both send and receive capability at both ends. The duplex system requires both a receiver and a transmitter module at both ends, plus two-way beam splitting *Y*-couplers at each end.

There is also a *half-duplex* system known in communications, but it is of little interest here. A half-duplex system can transmit in both directions, but not at the same time.

21-13 Receiver amplifier and transmitter driver circuits

Before the fiber-optic system is useful for communications, a means must be provided to convert electrical (analog or digital) signals into light beams. Also necessary is a means for converting the light beams from the fiber optics back into electrical signals. These jobs are performed by *driver* and *receiver preamplifier* circuits, respectively.

Figure 21-16 shows two possible driver circuits. Both circuits use light-emitting diodes (LEDs) as the light source. The circuit in Figure 21-16a is useful for digital data communications. These signals are characterized by on/off (HIGH/LOW or 1/0) states in which the LED is either ON or OFF, indicating which of the two possible binary digits is required at the moment.

The driver circuit consists of an open-collector digital inverter device in a light-tight container. These devices obey a very simple rule: If the input (A) is HIGH, then the output (B) is LOW; if the input (A) is LOW, then the output (B) is HIGH. Thus, when the input data signal is HIGH, point B is LOW, so the cathode of the LED is grounded. The LED turns on and sends a light beam down the fiber-optic line. But when the input data line is LOW, point B is HIGH, so the LED is now ungrounded (and therefore turned OFF)—no light enters the fiber. Theresistor (R_1) is used to limit the current flowing in the LED to a safe value. Its resistance is found from Ohm's law and the maximum allowable LED current:

$$R_1 = \frac{(V^+) - 0.7}{I_{max}} \qquad (21\text{-}26)$$

An analog driver circuit suitable for voice and instrumentation signals is shown in Figure 21-16b. This circuit is based on the operational amplifier (see chapter 10). There are two aspects to this circuit: the *signal path* and the *dc offset bias*. The lat-

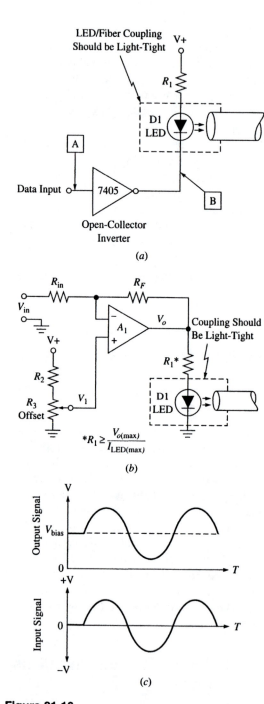

Figure 21-16
Fiber-optic communications driver circuits. (a) Digital fiber-optic driver circuit. (b) Analog fiber-optic driver circuit. (c) Effect of dc offset in preventing signal distortion due to clipping in driver circuit.

ter feature is needed in order to place the output voltage at a point where the LED is lighted at about one-half of its maximum brilliance when the input voltage V_{in} is zero. This way, negative polarity signals will reduce the LED brightness but will not turn it off (Figure 21-16c). In other words, biasing avoids clipping off the negative peaks. If the expected signals are monopolar, then set V_1 to barely turn on the LED when the input signal is zero.

The signal V_{in} sees an inverting follower with a gain of $-R_f/R_{in}$, so the total output voltage (accounting for the dc bias) is:

$$V_o = \left(\frac{-V_{in}R_f}{R_{in}}\right) + V_1\left(\frac{R_f}{R_{in}} + 1\right) \qquad (21\text{-}27)$$

Because the network R_2/R_3 is a resistor voltage divider, the value of V_1 will vary from 0 V to a maximum of:

$$V_1 = \frac{(V^+)R_3}{R_2 + R_3} \qquad (21\text{-}28)$$

Therefore, we may conclude that $V_{o(max)}$ is:

$$V_{o(max)} = \left(\frac{-V_{in}R_f}{R_{in}}\right)$$
$$+ \left(\frac{(V^+)R_3}{R_2 + R_3}\right)\left(\frac{R_f}{R_{in}} + 1\right) \qquad (21\text{-}29)$$

Three different receiver preamplifier circuits are shown in Figure 21-17; analog versions are shown in Figures 21-17a and 21-17b, while a digital version is shown in Figure 21-17c. The analog versions of the receiver preamplifiers are based on operational amplifiers (chapter 7). Both analog receiver preamplifiers use a photodiode as the sensor. These PN or PIN junction diodes produce an output current I_o that is proportional to the light shining on the diode junction.

The version shown in Figure 21-17a is based on the inverting following circuit. The diode is connected such that its noninverting input is grounded, thereby set to zero volts potential, and the diode current is applied to the inverting input. The feed-

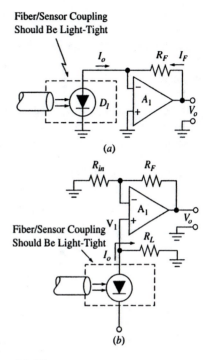

Figure 21-17
Fiber-optic receiver circuits. *(a)* Inverting. *(b)* Non inverting.

back current (I_f) exactly balances the diode current, so the output voltage will be:

$$V_o = I_oR_f \qquad (21\text{-}30)$$

The noninverting follower version shown in Figure 21-17b uses the diode current to produce a proportional voltage drop (V_1) across a load resistance, R_L. The output voltage for this circuit is:

$$V_o = I_oR_L\left(\frac{R_f}{R_{in}} + 1\right) \qquad (21\text{-}31)$$

Both analog circuits will respond to digital circuits, but they are not optimum for that type of signal. Digital signals will have to be reconstructed because of sloppiness caused by dispersion. A better circuit would be one in which the sensor is a phototransistor connected in the common emitter configuration. When light shines on the base region, the transistor conducts, causing its collector to be at a potential only a few tenths of a volt above ground potential. Conversely, when there is no light shining on the base, the collector of the transistor is at a potential close to V^+, the power supply potential.

The clean-up action occurs because the following stage is a digital Schmitt trigger. The output of such a device will snap HIGH when the input voltage exceeds a certain minimum threshold, and it remains HIGH until the input voltage drops below another threshold (snap-HIGH and snap-LOW thresholds are not equal). Thus, the output of the Schmitt trigger is a clean digital signal, while the sensed signal is much sloppier.

21-14 Lasers

Lasers can be extremely dangerous. The light produced by some lasers can cause severe, sometimes permanent, damage to eyes and skin. Even low-power lasers are dangerous and must be treated with respect. Never look directly into a laser. Even reflections can be dangerous, so be very careful when working with lasers. Become familiar with the basic safety rules provided by the manufacturers of lasers. The American National Standards Institute (ANSI), 1430 Broadway, New York, NY, 10018, publishes a laser safety standard.

Lasers are optical versions of MASERs, a concept that is used in the amplification of microwave radio signals. *MASERs (microwave amplification by stimulated emission of radiation)* were developed for amplification of very low-level signals that would normally be obscured by noise. LASERs *(light amplification by stimulated emission of radiation)*[‡] are simply optical wavelength variants on the same theme. Laser light differs from other light in several important ways. The principal characteristics of laser light are *coherency, monochromaticity,* and *low dispersion*. We will deal with these factors shortly.

[‡]Originally, *LASER* was an acronym. According to more recent dictionaries, however, by common usage *LASER* is now considered a noun and so is properly spelled *laser*.

21-15 Laser classification

Lasers can be classified according to different schemes. A common system is to use the form and material of the laser (gas, solid crystal, PN junctions, and so forth). Another method of classifying lasers is according to the safety categories published by ANSI and the Laser Institute of America (LIA), in ANSI Z136.1-1986 (consult ANSI for any current updates).

The ANSI classes are *Class I, Class II, Class III,* and *Class IV.* Class I lasers are not capable of producing biological damage to the eye or skin during intended uses by either direct or reflected exposure. These lasers may emit light in the 400- to 1400-nm region. Class II lasers emit in the visible portion of the spectrum in the 400- to 700-nm region. In Class II lasers, normal aversion responses such as blinking (~ 250 ms) are believed to be sufficient to afford protection against biological damage from direct or reflected light. For Class II continuous wave (CW) lasers, the point source power used in exposure calculations is 2.5 mW/cm^2. Class III lasers "may be hazardous under direct and specular reflection viewing conditions, but diffuse reflection is usually not a hazard." Class III lasers are typically not a fire hazard. Class IV lasers are dangerous and high-powered and may be a fire hazard and a hazard to eyes and skin from both direct and specular reflected beams, and sometimes also from a diffuse reflected beam.

Laser classes are determined by authorized laser safety officers (LSOs) according to the criteria established in the ANSI standard or its successor. Consult the latest edition of the ANSI standard (or its replacement) for current guidelines on laser safety.

21-16 Basic concepts

The concept of *coherence* is very important in understanding lasers and is responsible for much of the observed behavior of lasers. According to a dictionary, coherency infers "having a definite relationship to each other." That criterion means, in

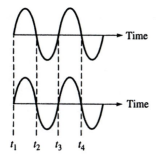

Figure 21-18
Longitudinal coherency is consistency in time phasing.

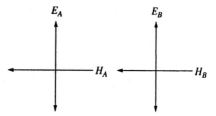

Figure 21-19
Transverse coherency is consistency across the two ways, orthogonal to the line of travel.

lasers, that points on two or more waves traveling together maintain their relationships regarding amplitude, polarity, and time phasing. In a noncoherent light source, the various emitted waves have a random relationship, so their mutual interference is also random. In lasers, there are two types of coherence: *longitudinal* and *transverse*.

Longitudinal coherence refers to a situation similar to the one shown in Figure 21-18, in which two waves of identical frequency and wavelength are propagated along parallel paths. Note that the time phasing of the two waves is the same (i.e., they both go through the zero line in the same direction and at the same time). In a laser, the phasing of such waves is so close that a laser beam split into two paths can still exhibit constructive interference when the two portions differ in overall path length by as much as 250 to 300 km. The comparable limit for noncoherent light sources is only 50 to 100 mm in path length difference.

Transverse coherency, which lasers also possess, refers to the properties of adjacent waves retaining their definite relationship when viewed orthogonal (at right angles) to the direction of travel. For an electromagnetic wave, the transverse cut would reveal similar amplitudes and alignments of the electric and magnetic fields (Figure 21-19).

The basis of laser operation is the law of conservation of energy applied to quantum systems. When an external source of energy impinges on an atom, it raises the energy level of the associated electrons, causing them to rise to a higher, but un-

stable, orbit. When the electron decays back to its ground energy state, the acquired energy is given up as light photons. The amount of change of energy state is a function of Planck's constant and the frequency of the emitted photon:

$$E = nh\nu = \frac{nhc}{\lambda} \tag{21-32}$$

where

E is the energy level

n is an integer (1, 2, 3, . . .)

c is the speed of light (3×10^8 m/s)

ν is the frequency of the emitted photon (Hz)

λ is the wavelength of the emitted photon (m)

h is Planck's constant (6.64×10^{-34} J-s)

Note in Equation 21-32 that the variables are energy level (E) and wavelength (λ). It can be inferred from this fact that laser light is monochromatic (of one color only). For any given material combination, there is only a very narrow band of possible wavelengths. For example, the common helium-neon (He-Ne) gas laser can produce a light output that is only a few kilohertz wide in the frequency domain, even though the center light frequency (analogous to the "carrier" frequency in RF systems) is 5×10^{14} Hz (or about 600 nm wavelength). Monochromaticity is one of the primary characteristics of laser light.

Stimulated emission of radiation was predicted as early as 1917 by Albert Einstein as part of his explanation of Planck's theory of energy quanta. According to Einstein's prediction, which proved out in practice, an atom can be stimulated into producing radiation when it is excited by an electromagnetic field that has the same frequency that would normally be emitted if the atom collapsed from the excited state to a lower state (usually ground state). Thus, a small excitation light source can create a larger stimulated light emission, and hence the light is amplified.

Laser action requires a process when there will be more atoms in the excited upper state than in the lower energy state, so that the probability of stimulated emission is increased. In normal situations, only a small portion of the atoms are in the excited state at any time, with the majority being in the lower or ground state. In good laser materials (or material combinations), it is possible to produce a *population inversion,* in which more atoms are excited than are not. Such materials tend to have long-lasting excited higher-energy states.

The quantum level action in typical lasers is a three- or four-stage transition, as shown in Figure 21-20. In Figure 21-20*a,* an atom at ground state (energy level U_1) is excited by an external energy source, so it raises to a pumping level state, U_3. It then undergoes fast spontaneous decay to a metastable state (U_2), and then a slower decay back to ground state (U_1). In this second decay, light photons are emitted, so this transition is sometimes termed a *stimulated emission region.* The frequency of the photons emitted is a function of the pumping energy level (Equation 21-32). In four-stage emission (Figure 21-20*b*), two spontaneous decay regions (U_{4-3} and U_{2-1}), are separated by the stimulated emission region (U_{3-2}).

21-17 Types of lasers

There are several different forms of lasers: insulating solid (e.g., ruby); insulating crystal; excimer; gas; injection (PN junction solid-state); chemical; and liquid (organic dye) lasers.

21-17-1 Insulating solid lasers

The insulating solid laser consists of a semitransparent, solid material, such as ruby, that is optically pumped into an excited state by a pulse of light from a xenon (or similar) flash tube (Figure 21-21). The ruby laser is, perhaps, the most commonly known insulating solid type of laser. Because of the xenon tube excitation system, ruby lasers are called *optically pumped, solid crystal lasers.* The ruby laser was announced by T. Maiman of Hughes Laboratories (California) in July 1960, although patent preeminence became a matter of a legal dispute. In the ruby laser, a rod of ruby material is fashioned with a fully (100%) silvered mirror at one end and a partially (a few percent) silvered mirror at the other. Surrounding the ruby rod is the xenon high-energy flash tube, which is similar to those used in photographic flash guns. Other pumping mechanisms include

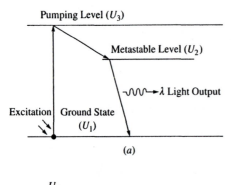

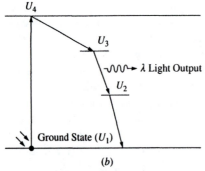

Figure 21-20
Basis for laser operation. *(a)* Three-step emission. *(b)* Four-step emission.

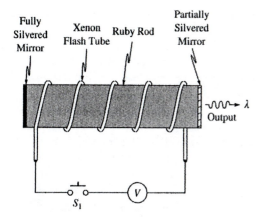

Figure 21-21
Ruby laser structure.

krypton-filled arcs and the tungsten-iodine lamps. Some lasers will lase on sunlight or room light, but this is not covered in detail here.

Rubies are a naturally occurring variety of the material *corundum* (Al_2O_3), which also includes sapphires (both of which are precious gemstones but can be produced synthetically); nongem and nonlaser uses of corundum include the grit used to form sandpaper. In rubies, the red coloring is provided by a small amount of chromium ions (Cr^{3+}) that replace some of the aluminum ions. When the xenon tube fires, it produces a short-duration, high-intensity blast of white light. The chromium ions absorb violet, blue, and green wavelengths from the white light, causing them to become pumped up to a higher energy state. The chromium ions then decay to a metastable state for a few milliseconds and then undergo the stimulated decay back to a lower energy level, emitting a photon of red wavelength (6934 Å or 693.4 nm) in the process.

The initial decay is omnidirectional, so a small fraction of the photons are directed toward the fully silvered mirror at the rear of the assembly, where they are reflected back toward the partially silvered mirror. Some photons escape from the partially silvered end, but others are reflected back toward the fully silvered end. In a short time, a number of wave fronts are reflecting back and

forth between the mirrors, building energy by mutual reinforcement; some waves escape on each reflection, forming an in-phase wave front.

Because the waves escape from the ruby rod in phase with each other, they are called *coherent,* and therein lies both the usefulness and the source of the intensity of laser light. Coherency is another of the principal characteristics of laser light. When the waves are emitted in random phase, there is a great deal of cancellation due to mutual interference, so a lot of the light energy is lost.

As a result of transverse coherence, the laser beam is very narrow and does not disperse the way random phased light does (as from a flashlight). Dispersion of less than 0.1 milliradians (mrad) is typical in lasers. The laser light beam remains very narrow over very long distances. Low dispersion is still another of the principal characteristics of laser light.

One way to designate the ruby laser is that it is an *optically pumped, crystalline solid-state laser.*

21-17-2 Insulating crystal lasers

This category of laser is very similar to the insulating solid type. Indeed, both are examples of optically pumped, crystalline solid-state lasers. Many texts place the insulating crystal lasers in the same category as ruby lasers. The insulating crystal devices differ from ruby lasers in that they use a rare earth element, such as neodymium (ND^{3+}), as a dopant to a material such as *yytrium-aluminum-garnet* (YAG), abbreviated Nd:YAG, or certain glasses, Nd:Glass.

The Nd:YAG laser typically emits a beam at infrared (1060 nm), but some are in the visible region. Energy outputs of 100 J for several milliseconds are easily obtained. Power levels on the order of 1 W CW are achieved using a krypton arc lamp for optical pumping. A multistage Nd:YAG experimental laser produced 1000 W when pumped with a tungsten-iodine lamp. In the Nd:Glass configuration, up to 10 kJ have been produced in nanosecond-length pulses. Efficiencies are typically 3%, on a 2% to 4% range.

21-17-3 Excimer lasers

An *excimer* is a molecule that does not normally exist except in the state in which the constituent atoms are excited to a higher energy state. When the extra energy of the excitation state is given up as laser output, the de-excited molecules will revert at ground state to the original constituent atoms. Typical excimer lasers mix a rare gas (e.g., argon, krypton, xenon) with active elements such as chlorine, fluorine, iodine, and bromine.

21-17-4 Gas lasers

Another common form of laser is the *gas laser;* included in this class are neutral atom lasers, ionic gas lasers, and molecular glass lasers. Gas lasers consist of a glass tube filled with a small partial pressure ($\sim$ 0.3 torr) of a gas such as He-Ne, carbon dioxide (CO_2), or argon (Figure 21-22). The end mirrors needed for oscillator behavior can be internal, but in most cases they are external, as shown in Figure 21-22, for ease of manufacture and adjustment. When external mirrors are used, the ends of the glass envelope of the tube are canted at a critical angle (α) called *Brewster's angle*. At this angle, light waves that are polarized in the correct manner will suffer no reflection losses at the two ends. Thus, reflection can take place between the two ends at a specific wavelength and phase relationship—forming the lasing action and retaining coherency and monochromaticity. In most gas lasers, the end mirrors will be spherical or parabolic, similar to the case of the crystal laser, to repeatedly reflect the light in oscillator fashion.

The gas laser works because electrons are injected into the gas chamber from a cathode electrode and are accelerated toward the positively charged anode electrode. Along the way, some of the electrons collide with gas ions (Figure 21-23), causing some of them to increase their energy state by absorbing the electron's kinetic energy. The excited state is not stable, so decay can be expected through several different mechanisms: collisions between the excited atom or molecule and another free electron, collision between excited and unexcited atoms, collision between excited atoms and the glass walls, and through the process of spontaneous emission.

He-Ne gas lasers are usually low-powered (typically 0.1 to 500 mW of output power); typically drawing $\leq$10 mA, at a potential of several kilovolts, from the dc power supply. The principal light wavelength produced by the He-Ne laser is at 632.8 nm (red region). The He-Ne laser can also produce output light lines at wavelengths of 594, 604, 612, 1150, and 3390 nm by correct design of the end mirrors. The He-Ne lasers are frequently used for classroom or hobby science demonstration projects. Some of them are in the very low

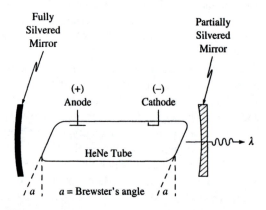

Figure 21-22
Gas laser structure.

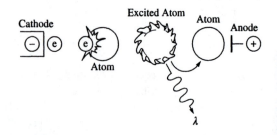

Figure 21-23
Mechanism for gas laser action: kinetic electron excites an atom. When the atom loses its excited state, it gives up a light photon.

milliwatt region, which are the types usually recommended for amateur experimental use. (*Note:* Even very low-powered lasers can be dangerous to eyesight.) Divergence of the He-Ne laser is typically ≤ 0.1 mrad. The glass tube on He-Ne lasers is typically less than 100 cm long and has a bore diameter of 1 to 2 mm. The He-Ne laser is also very low in cost compared with other lasers.

Argon gas lasers produce up to 20 W of light power at wavelengths of approximately 488 and 515 nm, in the blue and green portions of the spectrum. The typical argon laser has more gain than similar He-Ne lasers but operates at efficiencies of less than 0.1%. These lasers often require very high current densities ($\sim$100 A/cm^2) for proper operation. Special glass is needed for the outer envelope because of heating problems.

CO_2 lasers (which also contain small amounts of nitrogen and helium in addition to CO_2) are higher-powered and, indeed, can reach a very high power level (to kilowatts); CO_2 lasers can therefore be used for metal cutting and other industrial chores. The light output of the CO_2 laser has a wavelength of 10.6 μM, or about 106,000 Å, which places it in the far infrared region.

Argon and krypton gas lasers produce light in the blue and green regions and are capable of producing coherent light in two or more regions of the spectrum. These lasers find substantial application in the medical and scientific areas. Blue lasers, for example, are used for ophthalmic applications, such as "spot welding" detached retinas in the human eye.

21-17-5 Solid-state PN junction lasers

The final form of laser that we will consider is the solid-state PN junction diode laser (Figure 21-24), also called the *injection laser*. The laser diode is very similar to ordinary PN diodes and LEDs, except for the very thin PN heterojunction material (e.g., GaAs) forming the PN junction, which is sandwiched between AlGaAs sections that serve as internal resonating mirrors. Popula-

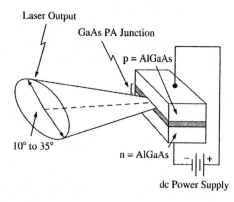

Figure 21-24
PN diode laser structure.

tion inversion, which is necessary for laser action, occurs because holes from the p-side and electrons from the n-side are forced by the applied electrical field into the junction region. The created conduction band becomes the upper laser energy level, while the valance band becomes the lower energy level.

The most common low-cost laser diodes use GaAs material sandwiched between AlGaAs and produce output lines in the 760- to 905-nm region, depending on the proportion of materials and whether a single or double heterojunction is used. In addition to GaAs, there are other material combinations. One such is iodine-gallium-arsenide-phosphorus (InGaAsP), which emits in the 1200- to 1550-nm range.

In both types of injection laser, room temperature lasing is possible, although only at low power levels and low efficiencies. For example, one AlGaAs laser diode produces 0.02 W (20 mW) CW, at 7% efficiency at room temperature. Cooling can produce a tremendous increase in both power level and efficiency. A GaAs laser diode cooled to −253°C can be as much as 50% efficient. In the pulsed mode, commonly available laser diodes can produce 3 to 10 W, drawing 10 A or so from the dc power supply. Noncooled GaAs devices produce 3 to 5 mW in some configurations and 500 mW in others.

At low current levels, the diode acts like other PN junction diodes, and at higher currents will emit a broad spectrum noncoherent light much like other LEDs. But if a certain threshold current (I_{th}) is exceeded, the laser diode will begin to lase and emit light in the direction shown. Threshold currents of 1000 A/cm^2 or more are possible, even at moderate average forward current levels, because of the very small area of the laser diode die (100 mils by 100 mils).

A stud-mounted form of laser diode package is shown in Figure 21-25a. This diode uses a threaded stud for mounting and to make the negative electrical connection. The positive electrical connection (anode) is made to an electrical terminal protruding from the rear of the mounting stud. Because laser diodes tend to be low-efficiency devices and therefore produce larger amounts of waste heat, it is often necessary to mount them on

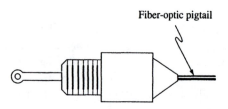

Figure 21-26
Laser diode with fiber-optic output.

a metallic heatsink (Figure 21-25b). The heatsink will carry away the excess heat that could otherwise destroy the diode. Any electrical energy that is not converted to light output goes off as heat, so the thermal condition of the diode must be a serious concern to laser diode users. A variant shown in Figure 21-26 is a stud-mounted laser diode in which the output is coupled to a fiber-optic pigtail.

21-18 Driver circuits for solid-state laser diodes

The laser diode is very much like the LED and so uses similar circuits for driving the device. Theoretically, one could use the LED-type circuit shown in Figure 21-27. In this circuit, the laser diode is connected between V$^+$ and ground, with a resistor network in series to limit current. Accord-

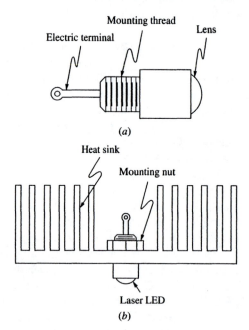

Figure 21-25
Laser diode packaging. *(a)* Typical stud-mounted laser diode. *(b)* Stud-mounted laser diode mounted on heatsink to improve heat dissipation.

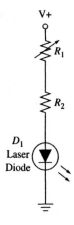

Figure 21-27
Simple laser diode driver circuit.

ing to the standard wisdom, resistor R_1 can be adjusted to vary laser diode current, and hence laser output, while R_2 is used to set the maximum current (for safety's sake) that can flow in the diode. The problem, however, is that these laser diodes tend to draw large amounts of current, so the resistors have to be 5- to 20-W types, depending on the diode (and associated voltage and current levels). As a result, it is more common on laser diodes to use a high-power transistor driver circuit to control the laser diode current.

Figure 21-28a shows a two-stage transistor direct-coupled amplifier that is used as a laser diode driver. The output transistor Q_1, is a large-power transistor such as the 2N3055. This transistor can dissipate 110-W collector power and has a collector current rating of 15 A. The beta gain of the 2N3055 is about 45. The driver transistor (Q_2) is a smaller NPN power transistor in a plastic package. It will dissipate up to +5W when heatsinked, and 1.33 W in free air, at a collector current of 1 A; the beta gain is >120.

The emitter of Q_2 is kept at a potential close to +2 V by three silicon 1-A rectifier diodes in series (although 1N4007 is shown, any of the 1N400x from 1N4001 to 1N4007 can be used). Each of these diodes has a forward voltage drop of 0.60 to 0.70 V, resulting in a total of about 2 V at the emitter of Q_2. The base voltage for Q_2 is derived from the emitter of Q_1, which is at a potential near 5 V. The voltage divider consisting of R_1, R_2, and R_3 produces a voltage near 2.6 V for the base of driver transistor Q_2, and since this voltage is partially dependent on the voltage across laser diode D_5 and series resistor R_4, it provides a bit of negative feedback.

The driver transistor excites the output transistor by varying the voltage applied to the base of Q_1. When Q_2 draws a heavy current, the base voltage of Q_1 drops, so the collector current applied to the laser diode also drops. When Q_2 draws less current, however, the collector current rises and provides more current to the laser diode.

The LED (D_4) is used as a warning indicator that power is applied to the circuit. Some laser

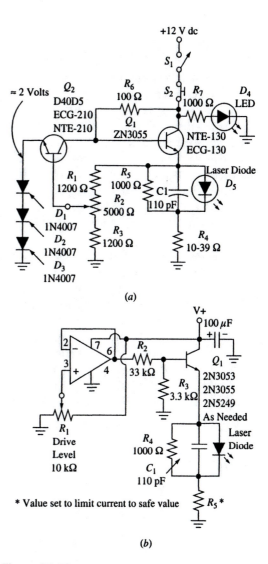

(a)

(b)

Figure 21-28
Better laser diode driver circuits. *(a)* All-transistor version. *(b)* Op-amp/transistor version.

diodes emit infrared light which cannot be seen by the human eye and are thus a danger to eyes. The LED provides a red light to warn that collector power is applied to the laser diode driver circuit.

The purpose of resistor R_4 is to limit the current available to the laser diode in the event that Q_1 shorts collector to emitter, Q_2 opens base to emitter or collector to base, or the adjustment of R_2 is too high. This resistor should have a value between 10 and 39 Ω, depending on the laser diode's maximum current, and is generally a 5- or 10-W power resistor.

Two series-connected switches are in the collector power circuit. The main power switch, S_1, is used to turn the circuit off entirely. Some users prefer to make this switch a key-operated model to limit access to the laser to those who are authorized (remember, lasers are dangerous devices). The second switch, S_2, is a pushbutton type that is used to turn on the laser when a burst of light is needed.

A variation on the circuit is shown in Figure 21-28b. This circuit uses the same type of power transistor output stage as the previous circuit, but the driver is replaced by an operational amplifier. The op-amp is connected in the unity gain noninverting follower configuration. The noninverting input (+IN) is connected to a potentiometer that sets the positive voltage applied to the +IN terminal. The op-amp output terminal is at a potential that reflects the setting of R_1, and in turn drives the

bias network for the output transistor (R_2 and R_3). Good values for R_2 and R_3 to start with in finding the correct setting are 33 kΩ for R_2 and 3.3 kΩ for R_3 (the correct values can be found empirically, or calculated if you know the beta gain of the transistor and the current range needed by the laser diode).

Another driver circuit is the *amplitude modulator* shown in Figure 21-29. In this circuit, the laser diode driver is a two-stage direct-coupled amplifier consisting of Q_1 and Q_2. The quiescent (static, no-signal) current level in the laser diode is set by adjusting potentiometer R_2. This current is modulated by applying the audio signal voltage to the base of Q_2 through dc-blocking capacitor C_4.

The audio preamplifier portion of the circuit of Figure 21-29 is an operational amplifier used as a noninverting ac-coupled amplifier. Almost any op-amp can be used for communications grade voice audio, including the 741, CA-3140, and others. To use just one dc power supply for the op-amp (instead of bipolar +V supplies), the noninverting input is biased to one-half the supply voltage by voltage divider network R_8/R_9. The audio gain of

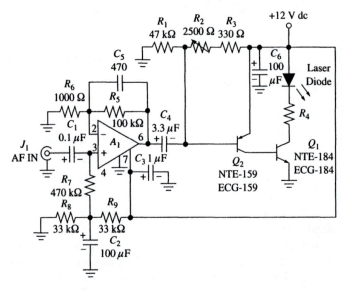

Figure 21-29
Laser diode current modulator circuit.

this circuit is set by the ratio of the two feedback resistors according to the equation:

$$A_v = \frac{R_5}{R_6} + 1 \qquad (21\text{-}33)$$

Although the gain is set to 101 in this example, it should be adjusted according to the amplitude of the audio source. The idea is to linearly modulate the current in the laser diode and so make the gain match the requirement.

The frequency response of the audio amplifier is measured between the points where the gain drops off −3 dB relative to the midband gain. The upper −3 dB point is set by capacitor C_6 shunted across R_5, while the lower-end −3 dB point is set by capacitor C_1 and resistor R_7. These points are:

$$F = \frac{1}{2\pi R_5 C_5} \qquad (21\text{-}34)$$

and

$$F = \frac{1}{2\pi R_7 C_1} \qquad (21\text{-}35)$$

where the resistances are in ohms, the capacitances are in farads, and the frequencies are in hertz.

A laser diode pulser circuit is shown in Figure 21-30. This circuit will drive only low-power laser diodes because the 555 timer (IC_1) is limited to sinking 200 mA of current. One might get away

with more because of the short duty cycle of most laser diodes, but that is not recommended practice. It would be better to use this circuit to generate a pulse that drives a circuit similar to the previous drivers shown. The pulse repetition rate (PRR) of this circuit is set by adjusting R_1, R_2, and C_1 according to the equation:

$$PRR = \frac{1.44}{(R_1 + 2R_2)C_1} \qquad (21\text{-}36)$$

The *duty cycle* is the ratio of the laser diode on-time to the off-time and can be set according to:

$$D = \frac{R_2}{R_1 + 2R_2} \qquad (21\text{-}37)$$

With the values shown, the PRR is about 270 pulses per second (PPS), while the duty factor (D) is about 19 percent. At a PRR of 270 PPS, the period of each cycle, which includes pulse on-time and pulse off-time, is 0.0037 (3.7 ms). The pulse on-time is thus 19% of 3.7 ms, or 0.7 ms (700 ns).

A *data driver* circuit is shown in Figure 21-31. This diode uses a transistor laser diode driver similar to previous circuits, but the driver is excited by a B-series CMOS digital logicIC device. In the specific example shown, the exciter is a not-and (NAND) gate, but others could be used instead.

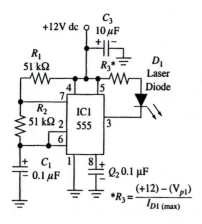

Figure 21-30
Laser diode pulse circuit.

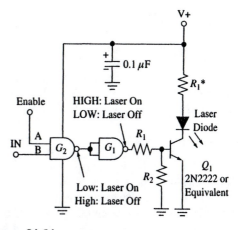

Figure 21-31
Laser diode digital driver circuit.

The B-series is preferred over the A-series CMOS because the B-series has higher drive capacity.

The terms HIGH and LOW used in Figure 21-31 are from digital electronics terminology and refer to the binary bits 1 and 0, respectively (1 = HIGH, 0 = LOW). In electronic digital circuits, it is common for LOW to be zero volts and HIGH to be a positive voltage. If the NAND gates were transistor-transistor logic (TTL) (which would require additional circuitry), then +5 V is mandatory for V+. With CMOS devices, V+ can be anything from +4.5 to +15 V. Resistors R_1 and R_2 are adjusted accordingly.

The NAND gate operates according to the following rules:

1. If both inputs are HIGH, then the output is LOW.

2. If either input is LOW, then the output is HIGH.

These rules allow us to strap both inputs together and use the NAND gate as an inverter circuit. In Figure 21-31, NAND gate G_1 is used in this manner. When the inputs of G_1 are LOW, then the output is HIGH; when the inputs of G_2 are HIGH, then the output is LOW. The laser diode is turned on when the output of G_2 is HIGH, providing a bias to Q_1 through R_1/R_2.

The data stream of HIGH/LOW bits is controlled by NAND gate G_1. Input A of G_2 is used as an active-HIGH *enable* line. In other words, when A = LOW, the output of G_2 is HIGH, disabling the laser diode output. Similarly, when A = HIGH, the output of G_2 is controlled by the other input (B). When IN = LOW, then the output of G_2 is HIGH and the laser is off; when IN = HIGH, then the output of G_2 is LOW and the laser is on.

21-19 Laser diode receiver circuits

The laser diode cannot be used in a communications circuit unless there is a receiver at the other end to recover the information transmitted. Figure 21-32 shows two laser preamplifier circuits that will pick up the varying pulse or AM-modulated

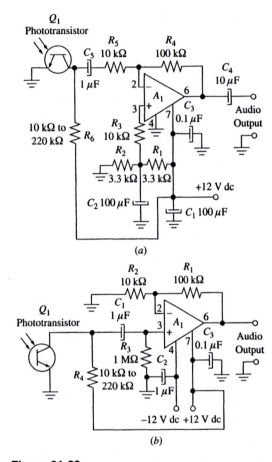

(a)

(b)

Figure 21-32
Laser diode receiver circuits. *(a)* Inverting amplifier version. *(b)* Noninverting amplifier version.

laser signal and convert it into an ac or pulse signal. In both circuits the sensor is an NPN phototransistor connected to an operational amplifier.

The circuit in Figure 21-32a uses an op-amp operated from a single dc power supply. This circuit can be used when only a single +9- to +15-V dc power supply (battery) is available. The non-inverting input is biased to one-half V+, or in this case about +6 V dc, by the action of resistor voltage divider R_1/R_2. Resistor R_3 is used to prevent charge stored in the de-coupling capacitor, C_2, from damaging the op-amp when the power is removed.

The signal gain of the op-amp is set by the ratio of R_4 and R_5. Because this circuit is essentially an inverting follower, the gain is:

$$A_v = -\frac{R_4}{R_5} \qquad (21\text{-}38)$$

The minus sign indicates that the output signal is 180° out of phase (i.e., it is inverted) with respect to the input signal.

The collector resistor supply voltage to the phototransistor can be set as low as 10 kΩ for high-frequency, high-speed operation, or as high as 220 kΩ for high-sensitivity operation. In most similar applications, the goal is sensitivity, so the resistor is set to some value between 150 and 220 kΩ.

A version of this circuit with a bipolar dc power supply is shown in Figure 21-32b. It uses V− and V+ dc power supplies rather than a single V+ dc supply (as in Figure 21-32a). The phototransistor circuit is very similar, but the output signal from the transistor is coupled through C_1 to the noninverting input of the op-amp.

A current mode receiver is shown in Figure 21-33. In this circuit, the photosensor is a photodiode that produces a current I_d, that is a function of the light level. The output voltage V_o, is found by:

$$V_o = -I_d R_1 \qquad (21\text{-}39)$$

where R_1 is in ohms and I_d is in amperes.

It is common practice to use an operational amplifier with a very high input impedance in this type of circuit to reduce the effects of input bias currents. Therefore, use a CA-3140 or its equivalent for A_1.

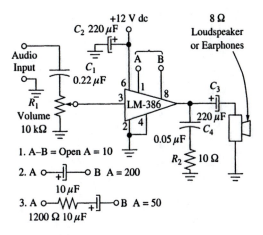

Figure 21-34
Laser diode receiver audio stage for voice communications.

For those readers interested in experimenting with laser diode communications, the circuit in Figure 21-34 provides an audio amplifier stage. It will receive the outputs from any of these receivers and amplify them to a level that will drive either a small 8-Ω loudspeaker or a pair of earphones. The basis for this circuit is the LM-386 single-chip audio amplifier. The gain of this stage can be set by the way you treat terminals A and B (which correspond to pins 1 and 8, respectively). For a gain of 10, leave A-B open (no connection or external circuitry required). For a gain of 50, however, connect a series R-C network consisting of a 1.2-Ω resistor and a 10-μF capacitor. The highest gain is 200, which is accommodated by connecting a 10-μF capacitor between A and B.

Before leaving the subject of lasers, it is prudent to reiterate the hazard warning about lasers. The coherent light from a laser, even at very low levels, is dangerous to eyes and skin. Take every step to avoid viewing laser light either directly or through specular or diffuse reflections. Read, understand, and follow all safety instructions provided by the manufacturer of any laser device that you put into operation. Before beginning to use lasers, read and understand the laser safety guidelines in the ANSI standard.

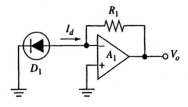

Figure 21-33
Simple laser diode receiver circuit.

21-20 Summary

1. Fiber optics is the technology in which light waves are passed through a plastic or glass fiber so they can be directed to a specific location.

2. Fiber-optics can carry light-modulated signals and are essentially free of electromagnetic radiation interference. They provide a high degree of electrical isolation and are explosion-proof.

3. Clad fiber-optics are built with a dense inner core surrounded by a less optically dense cladding layer.

4. In meridional ray propagation, all rays lie in a plane with the optical axis. In skew ray propagation, the rays follow a spiral or helical path along the fiber optic.

5. The *acceptance angle* is the critical angle for the transition from air to fiber-optic.

6. There are a number of transmission modes in a fiber-optic path. When a light beam attempts to find more than one mode, the resultant error is called *intermodal dispersion,* and it can have an adverse effect on digital signals. Dispersion problems can be overcome by using graded index fibers.

7. Loss modes in fiber-optics include surface defects (nicks, scratches), contaminants, inverse square law losses, transmission losses, absorption losses, coupling losses, mismatched fiber diameter losses, numerical aperture coupling losses, and Fresnel reflection losses.

8. Fiber-optic communications systems can be built by adding an encoder and decoder to opposite ends of the fiber.

9. Lasers produce a light beam that possesses the properties of coherency, monochromaticity, and low dispersion.

10. Lasers are classified by the ANSI and LIA standards for safety (Classes I, II, and III).

11. *Coherence* means that the light waves are in phase with each other. Lasers can offer both longitudinal and transverse coherence.

12. Types of lasers include insulating solids, insulating crystal, excimer, gas, injection, chemical, and liquid organic dye.

21-21 Recapitulation

Now return to the objectives and self-evaluation questions at the beginning of the chapter and see how well you can answer them. If you cannot answer certain questions, place a check mark next to each and review appropriate parts of the text. Next, try to answer the following questions using the same procedure. When you have answered all of the questions, solve the problems.

Questions

1. Because fiber-optic links are electrically non-conductive, they are essentially free of _____ _____ interference problems.

2. List several advantages of fiber-optics.

3. Define *optical refraction.*

4. Define the differences between *critical, subcritical,* and *supercritical* angles.

5. Express Snell's law as an equation.

6. In a _____ fiber-optic, there is an optically dense inner core overlaid with a less optically dense surface.

7. _____ rays lay in a single plane with the optical axis, while _____ rays follow a helical path.

8. Express the acceptance angle in terms of a *numerical aperture.*

9. In _____ _____, the light waves attempt to enter more than one transmission mode.

10. Any fiber with a core diameter of more than 10λ is typically called a _____ fiber.

11. A _____ index fiber consists of several layers of differing indices of refraction.

12. List several types of loss in fiber-optics systems.

13. List the elements of a fiber-optic communications system.

14. An ANSI Class _____ laser is not capable of producing biological damage to the eye or skin during intended use, by either direct or reflected exposure.

15. An ANSI Class _____ laser may be hazardous under direct or reflected situations but is not usually dangerous under diffuse reflection situations.

16. ANSI Class _____ lasers typically emit light in the 400- to 700-nm region of the spectrum.

17. Define *coherence* in your own words.

18. In _____ coherency, adjacent waves retain their definite relationship when viewed orthogonal to the direction of travel.

19. A _____ _____ is said to exist in a material when more electrons are in an excited state than are not excited.

20. List five different types of lasers.

21. Refraction occurs at a(n) _____ angle when TIR occurs.

Problems

1. Light travels in a material at 2.3×10^8 m/s. What is the index of refraction of that material?

2. A light ray in air approaches a material boundary at an angle of 18 degrees. If the index of refraction of the material is 1.75, the angle of refraction in the material is _____ degrees.

3. The acceptance angle of a fiber is 11 degrees. What is the numerical aperture?

4. What is the index of refraction of a material when the numerical aperture relative to air is 0.31?

5. A 0.51-mm fiber has a numerical aperture of 0.34. What is the relative light collection ability?

6. A 700-nm light is launched onto a 0.05-mm fiber. How many modes are possible if the numerical aperture is 0.122?

CHAPTER 22
Computers in Biomedical Equipment

22-1 Objectives

1. Be able to define basic terms (computer, input/output, data bus, hardware, software, interfacing, interrupts, ALU, CPU, controller, memory, microprocessor, microcomputer).
2. Be able to draw a simplified block diagram of a computer (organization) and describe its operation.
3. Be able to list and describe programming languages (machine, assembly, and high-level such as BASIC, FORTRAN, and COBOL, C+, PASCAL, LabVIEW).
4. Be able to draw a simplified block diagram of a microprocessor and microcomputer and describe its architecture, including word length, complexity, application, cost, memory size, program, speed constraints, and input/output.
5. Be able to describe interfacing units such as digital-to-analog and analog-to-digital converters.
6. Be able to list and describe types of large computers, microprocessors, and microcomputers in biomedical instrumentation.
7. Be able to describe a computer virus.
8. Be able to describe a neural network and how it enhances medical images.
9. Be able to describe the Internet and how it is used in health care.
10. Be able to describe the *expert system.*
11. Be able to draw a DAS in laboratory instrumentation.
12. Be able to cite some examples of computers in medical research.

22-2 Self-evaluation questions

These questions test your prior knowledge of the material in this chapter. Look for the answers as you read the text. After you have finished studying the chapter, try answering these questions and those at the end of the chapter.

1. What is the definition of a computer?

2. What is the distinction between hardware and software?

3. What are the major blocks involved in computer organization?

4. What is the difference between low-level and high-level computer languages?

5. What is the difference between a microprocessor and microcomputer?

6. How are computers interfaced to biomedical instrumentation?

7. How are computers used in biomedical instrumentation?

8. What is a computer virus?

9. What is the Internet information superhighway?

10. What is the computer expert medical system?

11. Draw a DAS laboratory block diagram.

22-3 Introduction

The following discussion is an overview of computers used in biomedical instrumentation environments. Refer to the many computer textbooks and courses that cover this subject in more detail.

In the past 50 years, the computer revolution has unfolded. The major factors contributing to this growth are curiosity, the discovery of a powerful mathematical tool, and the enormous capital invested by Western civilization. Modern times have witnessed its use in nearly every area of human life. Computers have become commonplace in transportation systems (automatic fare collection and scheduling), department stores and supermarkets (electronic computerized cash registers and inventory control), automobiles (energy control), military (peacetime and war machines), small business (record keeping devices), and medicine (diagnostic, therapeutic, and record systems). Hand-held calculators continue to permeate the public scene. The future will bring even greater uses for computers, as their diversity is expanding almost daily.

The history of computers is as interesting as it is fast and furious. Within the past 50 years, the digital computer has been structured, expanded, reduced in size, and developed for amusement, business, and scientific endeavors. Essentially, computers have transitioned from the ancient mechanical type to the gear type through the vacuum tube and transistor systems to the small-, medium-, and large-scale integration microprocessor and microcomputer. The first known computer was the *abacus,* invented between 4000 to 3000 B.C. It is a mechanical device consisting of beads that can be moved along a wire to add, subtract, multiply and divide. A skilled operator can perform calculations with amazing speed. Other mechanical machines include the rotating wheel mechanical calculator, invented in 1642 by Blaise Pascal, and a more elaborate one invented in 1671 by Baron Von Leibnitz. These gave rise to the mechanical desk calculator used by large numbers of people in the seventeenth and eighteenth centuries. Charles Babbage, a Cambridge University mathematics professor, proposed his "analytical engine" in the early nineteenth century, and this eventually led to computational machines with stored programs.

Herman Hollerith conceived the idea of the punched card in 1890 to store data, and manufacturers soon adopted this technique. While calculators were becoming motor driven in the 1930s, George Stibitz was developing the complex calculator at Bell Telephone Laboratories finalized in 1937. Howard Aiken of Harvard University generated the Mark I Automatic Sequence Controlled Calculator in 1937, and in 1944 it became operational as a general-purpose mechanical digital computer. The Bell V followed in 1946, and the Harvard Mark II and IBM 604 in 1948.

Following the age of mechanical computers, *four generations* appeared. These include *vacuum tube, transistor, integrated circuit,* and *large-scale integrated microprocessor/microcomputer.* In the 1940s, John Von Neuman proposed a general-purpose computer. UNIVAC and IBM designed and built numerous versions of vacuum tube models, but in 1958 the National Cash Register Corporation delivered the first commercial digital computer, followed by the CDC 7604 and IBM 7090 in 1960 and the CDC 6600 in 1964. In 1964, IBM announced the new 360 series, and by the mid-1970s, the advanced 370 series. Since 1977 the "computer on a chip" has been produced by such companies as Intel (8080A and Z80) and Motorola (6800).

The early computer pioneers were divided into two camps. Some of them wanted to build special-purpose computers that were optimized for a specific job (like artillery). But the other faction, in one of the greatest insights and most far-reaching visions of the twentieth century, decided to build a *programmable* digital computer. The concept is simple, but at the time it was revolutionary: a single processor that would obey instructions that were stored in a memory bank (along with data). By writing a *program* (i.e., a set of instructions that tell the computer what to do), the user could make the same machine do a lot of different chores. Thus, the same IBM-AT class machine that controls the patient monitoring system in an ICU can also be used by the administrator's secretary as a word processor, by the administrator as a management information system, by central supply staff as an inventory and processes controller, and by the biomedical engineer to keep preventive maintenance records. When the work day is over, one can run games like *Flight Simulator*® on the same machine. All of this is possible because the computing machine is now a kind of universal analytic engine. That is, it can be reprogrammed to perform a wide variety of chores.

Only four decades ago the computer was a large mainframe unit sold by industrial giants such as IBM and Honeywell. These machines took up entire rooms (sometimes more than one) and were housed in a series of large metal cabinets. They were used for large-scale data processing chores only and were not well suited for smaller tasks. In fact, at one hospital where we worked—a university medical center—the only computers used in the 1960s were the IBM-1401 and later an IBM-360 down the street at main university data processing. The same institution now uses computers of several sizes extensively and employs its own in-house programmers.

In the 1960s a new form of computer appeared on the market. The *minicomputer* was housed in a single cabinet that was 19 inches wide and about 7 feet high. The unit still required special facilities, such as a separate high-current electrical circuit and a large-capacity air conditioner to carry off the large amount of heat generated by the machine.

In 1972 a quiet revolution took place in California's now-famous Silicon Valley. The Intel Corporation was contracted to build a small digital processor integraged circuit *(chip)*. That simple unit was the start of the *microprocessor* industry. A microprocessor is a chip that contains all of the arithmetic and logic elements required for a programmable digital computer. All the designer needs to do to make a real computer is add external memory and input/output circuits. A *microcomputer* is a small desktop computer that is based on a microprocessor chip. Today, one can buy microcomputers that sit on a desktop—with plenty of room left over—and still have substantially more computing power than the roomful of equipment that we used in engineering school in 1967. In fact the abilities of the IBM-AT and Pentium that the authors used to write this chapter are considerably greater than the computers they used as engineers in past decades.

The microcomputer has literally revolutionized medical (and other) instrument and control system design. Whereas designers were once strictly analog engineers, the instrument designer today has to be a synergist who can integrate the principles of sensor selection, analog circuit design, computer hardware selection and/or design, and software. Today, even small instruments are based on microcomputer chips, and for that reason, we are going to consider these devices in some detail.

Computers in medicine began with the processing of hospital business and billing information. In the 1960s, ECG and EEG signals were analyzed. In addition, respirator function was evaluated. Computerized medical screening began during this time, and automated analysis of blood and urine was emerging. Dedicated minicomputers of modest cost allowed the generation of computerized patient monitoring, and fixed microprocessors gave rise to instantaneous analysis within the bedside unit. Currently, automation and instant analysis of medical events are requiring that computers be integrated into modern medical instrumentation.

22-4 Computer hardware and software

Computers can be classified as analog (continuous time signal) or digital (discrete step-time signal). An *analog computer* is an electronic (or mechanical) device that can perform continuous mathematical operations, such as addition, subtraction, multiplication, division, scaling, integration, and differentiation. Its accuracy is on the order of 0.01% of full scale, and while it can perform many parallel operations at high speed, it is very limited in making logical decisions. Programming is accomplished by drawing block diagrams with feedback loops and then patching the front panel with cables. However, most computers in use today, especially in biomedical instrumentation, are digital.

A *digital computer* is an electronic and electromechanical device that can perform a sequence of *arithmetic* (addition, subtraction, multiplication, division, and combinations of these) and *logical* (conditional) operations. The device can solve mathematical problems or can search, sort, and arrange information according to stored instructions. The computer program is the sequence of instructions and is known as *software*. The electronic and electromechanical portion comprises the physical part and is known as *hardware*.

The hardware is organized into various sections (Figure 22-1), including the following components:

1. *Input unit*—keyboard, network, modem, CD-ROM.

2. *Input control*—to control input data on its way to memory.

3. *Memory unit*—internal memory (composed of cells) such as random access memory (RAM), hard drive, case, floppy drive, optical drive to store data, instructions, and results of arithmetic or logic manipulation. External memory, such as magnetic tape, stores large programs and data. Magnetic tape has the longest access time but is the least expensive in terms of data quantity per size of device. Hard drive is faster but more expensive, and RAM is the fastest and the most costly. These are *nonvolatile,* or will hold information after the power has been removed.

4. *Instruction unit and controller*—to interpret or decode computer program instructions and control operations of the computer via the control signal generator.

5. *Arithmetic logic unit* (ALU)—to perform addition, subtraction, multiplication, and division and return the calculation results to the memory. An *accumulator* temporarily holds intermediate results during calculations. Essentially, all calculations are sequential in a digital computer (i.e., multiplication is repeated addition) and can require considerable time for completion. The binary (two-state) logic makes the hardware simple (and repetitive) but time-consuming for arriving at final answers. On today's market this trade-off is very successful.

6. *Output control*—to control data on its way to the output unit.

7. *Output unit*—CRT display printers, network, and modem. High-speed printers are available that can produce more than 1200 lines per minute.

The *central processing unit* (CPU), or central processor, is that part of a computer system that contains the main or internal memory, arithmetic logic unit, and special registers to provide

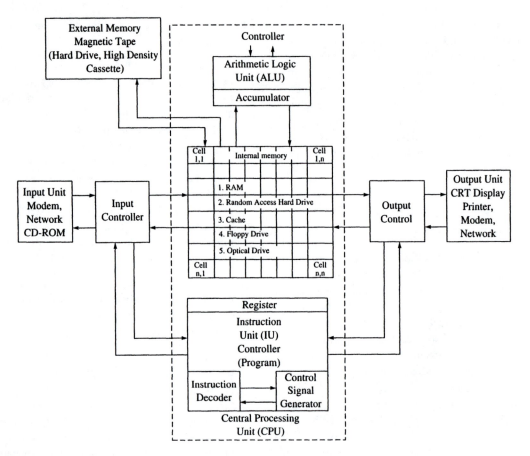

Figure 22-1
Simplified block diagram of a digital computer.

instruction processing, timing, and other house-keeping operations.

Digital computers operate in binary. Binary numbers are represented only by ones and zeros. That is, a one can be a switch that is turned on, and a zero can be a switch that is off. This allows the hardware to be simple (a two-state switch) versus a decimal number system in which a 10-position switch is required. The term *bit* is derived from *binary digit* and indicates a single character of the binary number system.

The *signal flow* through a computer (Figure 22-1) takes many paths. First, a program is written (software), and instruction and data are keyed in through the input device to be processed by the computer machine (hardware). Some keyboards contain an ASCII (American Standard Code for Information Interchange) code generator that produces a 7-bit binary number for each key pressed. Therefore, the code for the equation of a straight line could be placed into the memory via the input control, as shown at the top of the next page (the asterisk means "multiply"). Hardware accomplishes the software, and they are linked together.

The ASCII code will typically be converted into a 16- or 32-bit binary word in large computers or an 8-bit word in some microcomputers and microcontrollers. Instructions and data share the same signal path.

Character	Y	=	M	*	X	+	B
	1	2	3	4	5	6	7
ASCII Code	101 1001	011 1101	100 1101	010 1010	101 1000	010 1011	100 0010

After the linear equation is written, data can be placed in the memory as well. For example, if M is assigned as 2, X as 2, and B as 1, Y can be calculated as 5 (calculate instruction) in the arithmetic logic unit (ALU). The result, through the accumulator register, can then be stored in the memory. Later, data can be taken from memory and printed (write instruction) on the output CRT. The following shows a simple program:

Instructions

Read	Y = M * X + B	Input equation
Read	M = 2, X = 2, B = 1	Input data
Calculate	Y = M * X + B	Perform arithmetic calculation
Write	M, X, B, Y	Print or display data on CRT

The output on the CRT is as follows:

$$2 \quad 2 \quad 1 \quad 5$$

As part of the software, a flowchart (Figure 22-2) is usually generated first, and lines of code are written to accomplish the desired result. An IBM standard for flowcharts is ellipse for start/stop, parallelogram for read/write, rectangle for calculate, and diamond for decision. A flowchart for the linear equation problem is shown in Figure 22-2.

The loop is activated only if Y is not less than 4. Hence, M is assigned 1, X is 0, and B is 0, and the new Y will be 0, which is less than 4. Thus, the program stops. This simple example shows how data is manipulated inside a computer and how equations can be solved. Digital computers can do this much better. Those in biomedical instrumentation are constantly receiving updated information (data) and calculating results to be displayed for diagnostic purposes. A minicomputer and large computer system are shown in Figure 22-3.

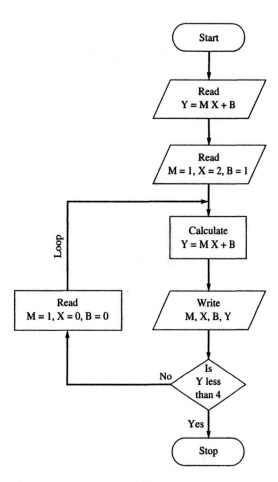

Figure 22-2
Software flowchart.

22-5 Computer programming languages

Computer programming languages represent the sequence of instructions by which the computer operates. They are classified as machine, assembly, and high level. *Machine language* is the actual binary number string that is keyed in by

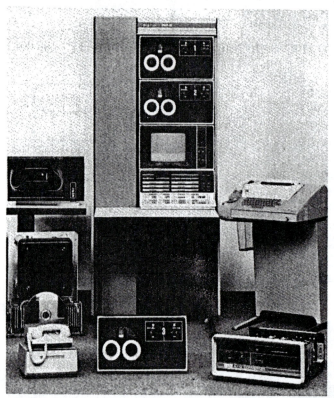

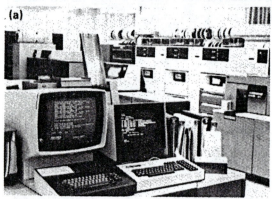

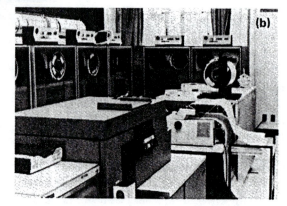

Figure 22-3
Computer systems. (a) Minicomputer. (b) Large computer.

means of switches on the computer front panel in older machines and through code translators in newer ones. In a 32-bit computer, 32 switches would have to be set for data and instruction input along with another set of address switches. Numerous instruction books that describe the instruction set of a specific computer are available (see suggested readings).

Assembly language is a symbolic code of alphabet and number characters, called *mnemonics,* that replace the numeric instructions of machine language. It has a one-to-one correspondence with an assembly program, which directs the computer to operate or perform its designated operations. Programming in this language is extensive, but knowledge of the specific instruction set of a machine is not necessary.

High-level languages are symbolic representations of alphabet, number, and special characters that are problem- or function-oriented. A single statement, close to the needs of the problems, may translate into a series of instructions or subroutines in machine language. Programming is relatively easy since a *compiler* converts symbolic instructions to machine language. Some commonly used languages are BASIC (beginners all-purpose symbolic instruction code), C-Language, PASCAL, FORTRAN (formula translation), and COBOL (common business-oriented language). Numerous texts and manuals explain these languages.

22-6 Microprocessor and microcomputer systems

A *microprocessor* is a large-scale integrated (LSI) electronic digital circuit that contains the control, pressing, and holding registers of a microcomputer (small computer system). Metal oxide semiconductor (MOS) circuits are used for lower power consumption. The microprocessor unit (MPU) handles arithmetic as well as logic data in bit-parallel fashion under control of a program.

The microprocessor is used in a system as shown in Figure 22-4a. Essentially, input signals are received (sense stage), processed (decide stage), placed in memory (store stage), and presented as output lines (act stage). The processor is surrounded by input/output (I/O) and memory. The microprocessor, as shown in Figure 22-4b, must handle address and data lines as well as clock, timing, and control lines. The entire processor is contained in a single integrated circuit package called a *chip.*

A *microcomputer* (an example is shown in Figure 22-4c) is a general-purpose computer composed of standard LSI components built around a CPU. The CPU or microprocessor is program-controlled with arithmetic and logic instructions and a common or parallel I/O bus. A microcomputer contains an MPU as well as memory circuits and interface adapters for I/O devices. The MPU has a fixed *instruction set,* which is used during programming.

Data and address enter and leave the MPU via a common bus. The lines that make up the bus are connected together through *tristate driver/receivers.* They take on three states: logic one, logic zero, and high impedance. In this way data or address can be targeted to a particular destination. For example, by disabling (high impedance) the tristate circuits in the memory and enabling those in the interface adapter, data or address can be steered to the I/O device. Although this method is slow, only one set of lines is required, thus reducing the hardware.

Storage of information is in either random access or read only memory. *Random access memory (RAM)* is a read/write memory in which data can be stored (written) at a particular address and then retrieved (read) out from the same address. This allows temporary storage of data or instructions and easy access when needed for manipulation. *Read only memory (ROM)* contains previously stored information impressed at the time of manufacture and can only be retrieved or read out. This device contains fixed program or control details for operation of the microcomputer. It can be called upon but cannot be altered. Special programmable ROMs (PROMs) are available, however, but must be erased with ultraviolet light and reprogrammed in a special device. All of these memories contain an array of flip-flops that are enabled during write and held during readout.

Newer types of memories include *magnetic bubble memory (MBM)* and *charged coupled devices (CCD),* CD-ROM (computer disc optical), and magnetic-optical tape or platter. *MBM*

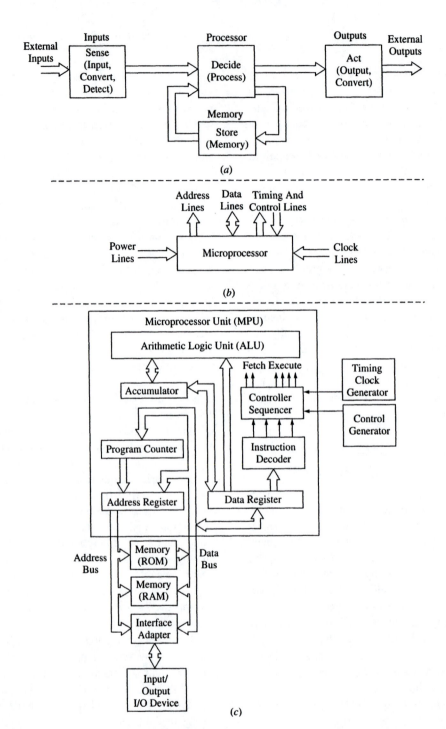

Figure 22-4
Simplified block diagram of a microprocessor/microcomputer system. (a) Basic system.
(b) Processor signals. (c) Microcomputer system block diagram.

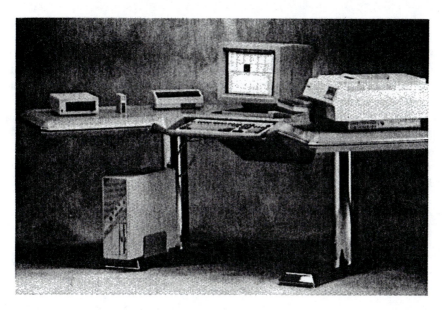

Figure 22-5
Microcomputer-based medical monitoring system.

contains microscopic magnetized areas located on a thin magnetic film. A pulsating signal current generates a moving bubble or logic one. Stored data is read out by a resistive element array that changes value when a bubble passes below a particular detector. Access time can be as long as 1 ms but is many times faster than disc and less expensive considering total storage capacity versus space. *CCD* memories are faster still but cost much more. Small capacitive charges store the bits of information and are circulated back to the input of each path. These charges change or are refreshed as they recirculate and can be read out in parallel in several microseconds. However, this memory is volatile. The CD-ROM stores information by cutting grooves in an optical platter in which a laser beam from a laser diode reflects light onto a photodiode. Magnetic-optical tape uses a laser diode and high-speed photodiode array to quickly read back data. Newer technologies bring different and unique memories. This is but one area of growth in the age of microcomputers.

An example of a biomedical instrument system that is based on a microcomputer is shown in Figure 22-5.

22-7 Interface between analog signals and digital computers

Biomedical instrumentation usually transduces, amplifies, filters, and displays *analog signals* obtained from the human body. These signals are variable amplitude and frequency waveforms continuous in time. Since digital computers require binary numbers, a converter device is required before analog signals can be accepted and processed in digital machines. Similarly, *digital signals* must be converted to analog before they can be displayed on biomedical instrumentation.

An *analog-to-digital converter (A/D)* is a device that accepts an analog signal (continuous in time) and produces a binary number (discrete in time). A 4-bit number (more commonly 8, 12, and 16 bit) can represent one of 16 possible voltage levels. In the example (Figure 22-6a), a 3-bit number represents eight levels. If the input signal were a constant +0.571 V (with a maximum of +1.000 V), the output would be 0100, which represents the fourth voltage level excluding zero. Since the output is in discrete steps, some information is lost and the resolution is 14.3% with 0.143 V per step. The resultant sequence of changing 3-bit binary numbers with time can be used as data input to a digital computer. This data can be presented in *parallel* (all 3 bits at once) or *serial* (1 bit for each computer clock time). Data can, thus, be processed and analyzed for diagnostic purposes.

A *digital-to-analog converter (D/A)*, shown in Figure 22-6b, is the reverse of the A/D converter. It accepts, in this case, a sequence of 3-bit binary numbers and produces a continuous analog waveform in time. This device must smooth out the discrete steps in the input signal, and hence some information is lost. For this D/A converter (A/D as well), the 14.3% resolution is rather coarse. An 8-bit D/A has 256 levels and approximately 0.4%

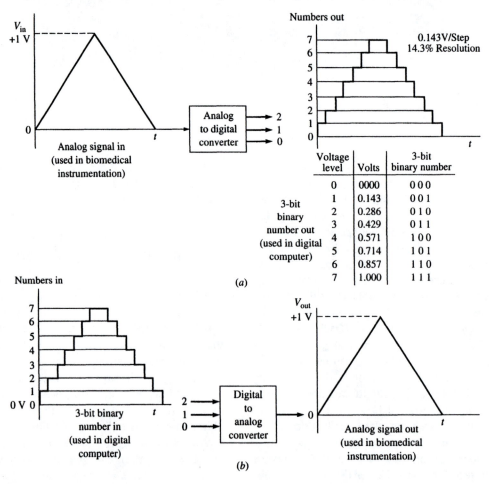

Voltage level	Volts	3-bit binary number
0	0000	0 0 0
1	0.143	0 0 1
2	0.286	0 1 0
3	0.429	0 1 1
4	0.571	1 0 0
5	0.714	1 0 1
6	0.857	1 1 0
7	1.000	1 1 1

Figure 22-6
(a) Analog-to-digital converter. (b) Digital-to-analog converter.

resolution, and a 12-bit D/A has 4096 steps and approximately 0.025% resolution. This is more acceptable for biophysical signals. For example, the accuracy of a blood transducer is 1%.

To help you more fully understand the use of computers in medicine, we will discuss the following areas in some detail: (1) hardware, (2) software, (3) firmware, (4) laboratory instrumentation, and (5) biomedical equipment. Although great advances have been made in hardware, the discerning observer knows that in most cases software makes the instrument useful.

22-8 Hardware, software, and firmware

Hardware is the physical computer with its electronics, keyboard, display, interface, and enclosure.

Software is the programs that operate a computer. It is composed of low-level and high-level types. Low-level software includes machine operating code (disc operating system, DOS, one and zero code). It can also be complex machine language (assembly language) that instructs elements of the computer system to do something, such as store data in a particular location or move data from one place to another.

However, the user typically thinks of software as: (1) fundamental programming languages (BASIC, C-Language, PASCAL, FORTRAN, COBOL), (2) high-level application programs (word processors or spreadsheets), (3) drawing programs (picture, sketch, or schematic construction), (4) graphic programming software (graphic design of a DAS with inputs, outputs, interconnections, and executable software buttons), or (5) other programs that are used to perform a specific task such as directly operate an instrument (HP-IB electronic instrument control bus).

Firmware is the combination of hardware and software that works together to make a machine operate in a specific way. They both need each other to be functional, whereas generic software will work with any computer, provided it has the right operating system.

Today, most software is easily operated by pull-down menus, which was adopted by the *Macintosh* in the 1980s. *IBM* or *DOS* machines now use *Windows* 3.0, for example, which is similar to the Macintosh approach but uses DOS to operate the computer. This uses more memory and is somewhat slower than the Macintosh. To make Windows faster with more utility and more robust against software crashes, Microsoft Corporation created Windows 95, which is now widely used. Like the Macintosh, DOS machines can now easily exchange and manipulate data and information in a more user-friendly environment.

Because choosing medical software is a great challenge; the American College of Physicians (ACP) clinical information management department provides information to guide medical professionals. The flagship document is the *Medical Software Reviews, Healthcare Computing Publications, Inc. (HCP)*. It provides state-of-the-art medical software and hardware applications in the areas of management, personal computing, continuing education, therapeutic support, portable computing devices, and the Internet (Osheroff, 1995).

22-9 Modern communications

Communications will be vastly different in the future. Combined multimedia technologies will provide voice, color fax (T-30 standard), and video-on-demand, for example. *Digital simultaneous voice and data (DSVE)* allows full duplex or simultaneous two-way communication. In the field of health care, real-time information services will alter medical education. Today basic voice mail, such as the Meridian system, has already improved productivity by permitting communication anytime, day or night. However, we have to be wary of voice mail "jail" and endless loops of nonhuman, unfriendly contacts. To make progress we must manage the problem of information overload.

Switching is the heart of telecommunication systems. The microprocessor provides management and control through a high-speed data bus (Figure 22-7). These systems use the ST-BUS,

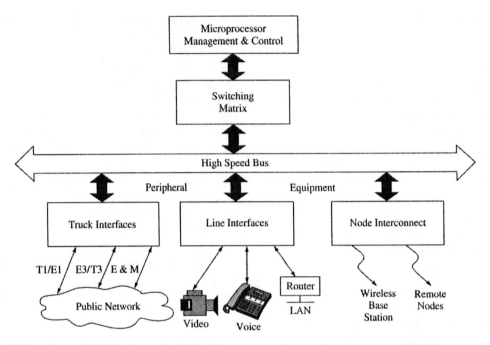

Figure 22-7
High speed synchronous serial bus telecom system. Used with permission from Mitel Corporation.

which is a high-speed, synchronous serial bus that transports voice, data, or video or a mixture of each. The T1 line shown operates at 1.544 Mbps (megabits per second) and E1 at 2.048 Mbps. Both connect central offices together, where 24 to 30 voice lines are grouped into one digital pipe. Today, higher-capacity fiber-optic cable transfers the backbone of communications with T1/E1 serving as a building block or as an attachment to the backbone.

The *distributed intelligence* revolution is now being accomplished through embedded processing. Here, dedicated processors work on specific parts of a system. You could call it information processing with on-board intelligence. Some applications include security systems for home and hospital. In particular, great advances have been made in voice and pattern recognition, permitting verbal and fingerprint identification.

Today, *wireless* or *mobile communications systems* download information through telecomputers

that do not directly use telephone wires. Some applications are video conferencing and transception of physiological data to and from ambulances. We are in the age of the mobile office and field laboratory. This is made possible by hardware (physical computer), software (programs), and firmware (combination).

Hardware telecommunications has advanced in recent years with the invention of high-bit-rate digital subscriber line (HDSL) systems. The objective is to interconnect voice and digital data users. The components of this telcom system are transmitter side and receiver side.

The transmitter includes PBX or telephone exchange, telephones, and terminals that communicate to the remote hub via the HDSL copper telephone lines, local-central office switching systems, and the toll interexchange switching systems that drive into intertoll trunks via microwave or fiber-optic transmitters.

The receiver consists of a toll interexchange that feeds a local-central office system that drives the telephone equipment of a private residence or an organization.

HDSL has the surprising advantage of being able to transmit relatively high-speed digital data over a voice-grade copper wire link. More speed also means multiple telephone lines can be put on the same wires that used to handle just one telephone. Why is this possible? The answer is *technology*. Today's electronics can restore signal integrity by compensating for distortion in copper runs. Hence repeaters, previously spaced every kilometer, can now be spaced at about 5 km. High-speed 2 Mbps carriers can be put on relatively low bandwidth copper wires. Just think about it—we can now use digital data and many voice channels without rewiring the system.

A further advance is the asymmetrical digital subscriber line (ADSL), which is capable of 6 Mbps. Using fiber-optic cable, the synchronous optical network (SONET) can achieve gigabytes of bandwidth, but new physical lines must be run at great expense. A distinct advantage of fiber is high speed and low noise. The bit error rate (BER) is as low as one error in 10,000 megabits, which is better than that attained on copper. It's a matter of performance versus cost. Also, fiber is more secure because optical systems are more difficult to break in to.

Virtual reality is also enhancing modern communications. The goal is to integrate the human with the computer. For example, great advances have been made in helping quadriplegics with physical therapy. Also, those who could not previously talk can now communicate freely.

22-10 Modern microprocessors

New microprocessor architectures have evolved rapidly in recent years. As a result of keen competition between a handful of key computer companies, only a few computer architectures have evolved. Now more than ever, hardware and software engineers work closely together on the whole

system to trade off advantages. One might ask why there are different architectures, and which computer, based on which microprocessor, would be best to use. The answers are left to the designers of biomedical equipment and are based on internal company history and policy or on availability of modern processing power. Today's predominant desktop microcomputers are either *Intel*-processor-based (IBM PC DOS/Windows) or *Motorola*-processor-based (Apple Macintosh/inherent pull down menus). Others include Compaq, Hewlett-Packard, and Sun systems.

The deficiencies of the original 8-bit data bus processors have given way to the *32-bit bus*, which can quickly address giga bytes of memory. Not everyone predicted that such powerful microcomputers would be located on the desks of average technical and nontechnical persons. This was driven by low cost through volume production. IBM, Motorola, and Apple teamed up in Austin, Texas, to invent the third generation power personal computer processor, called *MPC604*. It quadruples the number of instructions that can be executed per clock cycle. This processor is compatible with the two big computer architectures of Intel and Motorola. This allows software created in either environment to be read by the same computer. Its block diagram appears in Figure 22-8.

Meanwhile, Intel invented another powerful processor, the *Pentium*. It is similar to the 80486 in programming; however, it can execute two instructions per clock cycle because its internal architecture has two five-stage pipelines. A pipeline splits the instruction fetch, decode, and execution into independent stages to eliminate waiting. This speeds up processing dramatically, allowing clock speeds of 450 MHz and higher. It can even handle the 64-bit wide data bus. Figure 22-9 shows the Pentium. Many new IBM and similar microcomputers now use the Pentium platform. In fact, speed has become an obsession, doubling about every 2 years. The limit relates to the semiconductor process and how quickly signals travel in wires. One of the newest computers uses the POWER PC440, which has a 32-bit core processor

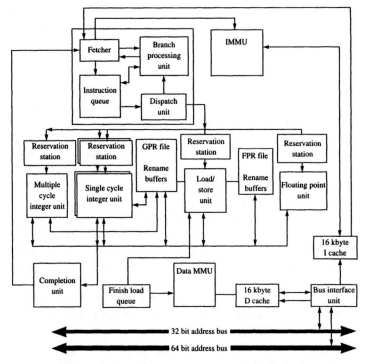

Figure 22-8
MPC604, third generation powerPC from joint IBM-Motorola-Apple design team. Used with
permission from *Microprocessor Architectures RISC, CISC, and DSP,* 2nd ed, published by
Butterworth Heinemann Newnes © 1995.

design running at a 550 MHz-clock rate. More and
more, IBM is using ASIC (application specific integrated circuits, or custom chips) to satisfy the
demands of servers, wired and wireless systems,
as well as storage and Internet installations, which
are called "pervasive computing."

In the race to produce even faster microprocessors, IBM plans to develop a 64-bit processor,
called the Power4, made with copper interconnects
and silicon-on-insulator wafers. It's an integration
of two 1-GH processors with 170 million transistors on a chip, geared toward the early decades of
the new century's computer servers, used for the
Internet and other systems. It has more than 100
gigabytes per second of bandwidth, which is
enough speed to move data between chips at
speeds greater than 500 MHz. Bandwidth between

Power4 devices is going to be greater than 35 gigabytes per second.

Also, Motorola produces a family of integrated
MC68000 processors that bridge the gap between
the 8-bit microcontroller (simpler form of a microprocessor) and the 16/32-bit M68000 families.
These are used by General Motors in automotive
applications (ignition control, fuel injection, anti-
lock braking, dash-board instrumentation). Their
advantage is clear—microprocessors allow finer
control of system parameters. They can compensate for mechanical wear, thus making a better-
performing car that is safer and lasts longer. These
microprocessors are also used in smart peripherals
that have many industrial and medical applications. Apple Macintosh microcomputers use the
68000 series platform. These are known as *embed-*

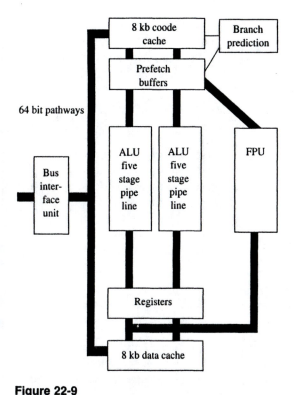

64 bit pathways

Figure 22-9
The Intel Pentium. It has additional control register
and the system management mode register that first
appeared in the 80386SL. Used with permission from
Microprocessor Architectures RISC, CISC, and DSP
2/e published by Butterworth Heinemann Newnes ©
1995.

ded computers because they perform dedicated
tasks for the environment they are connected to.

Hardware tools used to develop embedded systems have typically been in-circuit emulators (a
device that imitates another). These contain CPU-
specific debugging tools including real-time trace
code timing and performance checkers. As explained in Embedded Systems Programming Magazine (Vereen, 1998) a new approach taken by Motorola consists of adding a debug controller
directly onto the CPU chip. This allows direct access to the CPU core and uses joint test access
group (JTAG) test points for tapping into the data
path. Adding to logic analyzers, Hewlett Packard

now provides background debug mode (BDM),
where data can be traced through the embedded
system to be sure it's working properly.

Software tools for embedded systems have developed similarly to the hardware. They evolve
more slowly than that of the desktop PC tools. One
of these evolutions is special EC++ software,
similar to the C++ computer program. It has provided some relief in reducing the huge risks of un-
tried ideas on the part of design engineers. You can
imagine some medical instrument taking much
longer to bring to market if the software doesn't
work properly.

Firmware is used by the smart manager of embedded systems to produce a coding, testing, and
validation before cranking out lines of computer
code. This way the computer within the computer
works much better when it's inserted into biomedical equipment.

22-11 Microcontrollers

Microcontrollers are simpler and cost less than microprocessors. They have rudimentary functions,
such as measure, sequence, and control. Some applications are clocks, refrigerators, automobiles,
and medical incubators, where they perform basic
repetitive functions.

22-12 Digital signal processors (DSPs)

Digital signal processors (DSPs), have also advanced in the last decade. These are dedicated circuits that perform specific functions, such as mathematical operations or special data processing or
analysis. One goal of DSPs is to *off-load* the microprocessor or computer, which allows faster
through-put processing. Also, smaller computers
can sometimes be used when DSPs are present.

In *Medical Electronics Manufacturing Magazine*
(Spera, Gabriel, 1998), Spera says "the average
high-tech consumer probably touches a DSP-en-
abled product every 10 minutes." This indicates how

popular DSPs are in the modern world. They appear in wireless communications; personal electronics, such as CD players; cell phones; and digital cameras. Not surprising, modern medical instrumentation uses DSPs to perform their most common task, multiply-accumulate (MAC). Here, digital filtering is accomplished. This augments analog or hardware filtering by further limiting the bandwidth or shaping the signal of interest before it is displayed on a monitor or passed on to another computer.

DSPs often contain specialized I/O interfaces, also called on-chip peripherals, that communicate with ADCs, where conversion from analog signals to digital code occurs. They also contain one or more serial and parallel ports for inputting and outputting data from the DMA, which allows direct access to digital memory. This makes DSPs more deterministic. That means the number of computer-machine-clock-cycles for a particular operation is known exactly. General microprocessors, on the other hand, are more unpredictable in their cycling, because they permit extensive branching and out-of-order execution of commands.

DSPs are used in many medical systems. For example, MRI uses it to improve performance of the final display (Spera, Gabriel, 1998). This results in better diagnosis of a patient's condition. Even in consumer medical equipment, such as portable blood pressure devices, DSPs interpret user variations to give more accurate results. There is a bright future for these local add-ons to medical microcomputers.

22-13 Capabilities of microcomputers versus mainframes

The computer revolution transcended the mainframe computer, which was built of vacuum tubes and filled an entire room. Now transistors and solid-state electronics have shrunk powerful computers to fit on a desktop and even in the palm of your hand. This localized calculating, processing, and storage capability has changed our culture.

The benefits are lower cost and instant information. This allows more time to be creative and solve medical and equipment problems, for example. It leads to improved health care delivery.

22-14 The power of interactive data bases

In an interactive data base, data or information can be manipulated after it is stored in specific fields or memory locations. You can perform many basic and advanced operations, such as retrieve, print, sort, rearrange, and analyze. One commonly used program is Lotus Notes, which allows a group of users to independently input and share data, similar to a party line.

22-15 Impact and limitations of computers

Computers have changed the way we work. For example, one can write a paper while toting around a portable computer to the various sites where information is gathered. Our habits and attitudes have changed, too. We are more information-oriented because we have access to data on a floppy disk or a CD-ROM. Now, encyclopedias on CD-ROM offer us the ability to exercise creative search routines. We can find detailed information located in multiple places within seconds.

Computers have not only had an impact on individuals but have also changed institutions. Companies now have workers on-line, and libraries have dial-up researchers. At the end of the day, however, someone has to read or listen to the information extracted and do something with it. This is left up to us. Human factors are paramount. We should remember that "to err is human, but to create a real mess takes a computer." The computer is an unemotional, noncaring machine with no drive to do anything but what it is programmed to do.

No matter how hard we try, we cannot seem to create flawless software, just as we cannot seem to build fail-safe hardware. Computers are a product of the twentieth century, and they have limitations.

One surprising, but extremely important, limitation arises from fundamental changes in computer system architectures as they progressed from one generation to the next. The *Y2K (year2000) problem* is one of these sticky issues. Essentially, it is a "year-date" compatibility conflict between older computer systems and new ones. In the 1950s, it was decided to use two digits to specify the year. A main reason was a limitation of physical room on mechanical paper punch cards. These were utilized to write (create) and input (read) lines of code into the computer. Some computer specialists of the day knew computer technology would move very fast, and they knew the date would become a future problem. They may have conjectured computers will be so different by the year 2000 that it really didn't matter. Many people figured computer engineers would be forced to work out the date problem as a process of evolution. Maybe some just put off the decision for the next generation of technologists. Nevertheless, it certainly was easier to use just two digits for the 20th century, e.g., "99" to represent the year 1999.

The Specifics of the Y2K Date Problem After December 31, 1999, the digits 99 became 00. Unfortunately, this meant the year 1900 to some computers, and this can play havoc with some (date-based) computer programs, particularly financial accounting and recordkeeping software. The real-time clock rolled over incorrectly in older machines due to problems in their BIOS (basic input/output system). To solve the problem, a change in hardware was invented. This required the BIOS chip on the motherboard inside the computer to be changed to handle four digits. This chip allows the hardware to work with the software and run floppy disks (FDD) and hard disks (HDD). Networking PCs adds additional complications to the problem. The BIOS boots the computer through a basic set of instructions and performs all tasks at start-up time and also interfaces to underlying operating system hardware through interrupt handlers. For example, when a key is pressed, the CPU creates an interrupt to read the key. Some older PCs cannot synergistically operate with all modern hardware. To fix the problem, you replaced the BIOS or installed a device driver for the hardware.

Routinely, new computers are manufactured with this new integrated circuit, which keeps track of the date and other functions. Along with some changes to software for recognizing the new four-digit year, the problem is solved. Older hardware and software must be updated or one can fall victim to the old adage: "pay now or pay later." Also, older computers can be updated with new chips and software. In any case, the date does not matter for many computer operations, and we might be able to live with the date problem to some extent. On the other hand, embedded microcomputers that read the year 2000 incorrectly could pass on bad information and, hence, cause some systems to "crash," or create numerous errors.

The solution to achieve Y2K compliance involved diagnosing, fixing, and testing using special tools generated for this purpose. Medical and other institutions, including industry, business, education, government, and the military furiously readied themselves in the late 1990s. In a way, they were making up for not focusing on the Y2K problem earlier.

Even though computer experts do their best, unforeseen problems will undoubtedly unfold as the year 2000 progresses. Interestingly, the next date problem will be December 31 of the year 9,999 if we still use this type of calendar. Then we'll need five digits for 10,000. But, just as engineers decided to use two digits for the year in the middle of 1990s, we have decided to use four digits now. Anyway, who can predict what type of computers, if any, we will be using in the year 10,000? Maybe we will not need computers to operate biomedical instrumentation or run our health care system. Long-term predictions are uncertain.

22-16 Computers can cause health problems

While computers are part of the health problem solution, they can also cause ailments. For example, pain and numbness; carpal tunnel syndrome is becoming increasingly more common as people spend more time using the keyboard. However, the computer can also help alleviate the condition by periodically reminding us to stop and do some relief. Exercises. There are also documented cases of eye strain, headache, and general fatigue from staring at a screen for too long. The computer should be our ally, but we should be cautious not to become its slave.

22-17 Computer viruses

Similar to *human viruses* that attack living body cells, *computer viruses* attack software cells (stored in hardware memory locations) and alter their content. This disturbs or destroys the normal operation of computer programs. Unlike biological viruses, which try to perpetuate themselves in nature, computer viruses are the vehicle of malicious persons who violate our morals and laws. Examples range from mild to severe. Some just irritate you by changing information you originally entered, and some wipe you out by erasing your entire memory. With education you can see some of them about to infect you, but others are disguised as normal information. One trick is to put a so-called *program update* on the Internet to lure you into downloading it into your computer, where it promptly attempts to obliterate all information on your hard drive. *Virus checking programs* can alert you ahead of time and even correct for viruses already in your computer. Like a cat-and-mouse game, the computer criminal tries to outsmart the protection program. In military language, we invent countermeasures to avoid the virus, and the enemy invents counter-countermeasures to defeat the countermeasures. Once the game is started, it continues for a long time, until our culture changes enough to render the virus unimportant or until one group is annihilated. Immense harm can come to patients and health care professionals through the corruption of information or disruption of biomedical equipment operation.

22-18 Supercomputers

Today, supercomputers engage in high-performance computing to solve problems that we could not solve before. These computers are super fast (hundreds of megahertz) and super big (hundreds of gigabytes of memory). They are not routinely used in biomedical instrumentation but may be used in the research and design of instrumentation. One such immense computer is the Cray computer.

22-19 Neural networks and computing applications

Advances in computers have resulted in better hardware and software that achieve faster, more powerful results. But a more sophisticated advance—the *neural network*—involves a whole new way of thinking about computing.

The *neural network* is a multidisciplinary concept arising from neuroscientists, psychologists, and engineers. It has re-emerged from work done in the 1950s. A neural network is a computational system, made up of either hardware or software, and contains a large number of simple interconnected artificial neurons (nerve cells). They mimic biological systems in their computational abilities. The neural network has three characteristics: structure, dynamics, and learning. The neural network is essentially an adaptive learning system that self-organizes information. Like the human brain, it has many parallel processing paths. The biological processor in our heads creates representations (symbols) of the physical world (distinct features in the presented data). The self-organization feature allows us to generalize. Similarly, the neural network can respond appropriately even when presented with new situations. Neural networks are like learning machines that invent creative solutions to difficult problems using the human-made computer.

A closely related concept that accounts for the thinking nature of the brain (neural network) is chaos theory. Essentially, the power is in the ability to go down many dead-end paths, then back out to try another path. This intuitive searching technique leads to better solutions. It seems chaotic because the random approach appears unorganized. From the standpoint of an individual search routine, it is hit or miss. It's the inherent quality of recognizing good and bad results that provides the intelligence.

Neural networks are useful for *pattern recognition* and *adaptive control.* They have high tolerance for faults because information encoding is redundant. Their adaptive-control nature has been used by the military for recognizing targets and for robotic motion control in guiding machines around objects. Also, they can be used for texture analysis to determine the nature of an object's surface.

Neural networks have many clinical applications. For example, they are more accurate than attending physicians in diagnosing heart attacks in patients with frontal chest pain. Imaging, waveform analysis, outcome prediction, and inspecting pathological tissue specimens are other areas in which neural networks excel. ECG and EEG tracings, mammograms, and chest radiographs are read with uncanny accuracy. Soon artificial intelligence and diagnostic support systems will be embraced by medical professionals with greater vigor. Application of neural networks is described by Baxt, William G. (1995).

A specific biomedical application of neural networks is the boundary contour system (BCS), which can be used to produce an enhanced image of the human brain and hence better diagnostic quality. C/T scans can be displayed with more definition (Wasserman, 1989).

22-20 The Internet

The Internet is making a huge impact on the way people communicate and access information internationally.

The Internet is essentially a group of shared computer interconnections that allows any person to log on-line and browse through categories of information, download files, or interactively engage in discussions with other individuals who are also logged on. Individuals or groups can establish their own *Web page,* through which they display their wares by building a Web application. The *World-Wide Web,* which can be thought of as a matrix of randomly accessible data, contains information about organizations, institutions, and companies and is available anytime, day or night. It's no longer necessary to wait for traditional working hours to search for information.

In specific terms, the Internet is an *internetwork connection* of computers (or workstations or smart terminals) that allows any computer to communicate with any other computer. The so-called new *information superhighway* is the conduit through which information is transferred. Information is knowledge and wisdom arising from intelligence. It can be fact or fiction and covers all subjects, including art, religion, politics, science, and biomedical instrumentation.

Actually, the information highway is not new. In 1843 Morse code messages were communicated through electrical lines installed along the first U.S. railway system, which was built in 1830 between Washington, D.C., and Baltimore, Maryland. Information could then be transported over the same route that carried people, animals, and material.

The Internet as we know it today arises from the U.S. government and military systems established after the second World War. Its goal was to provide a shared data base of information on national security.

The modern approach for easy use of the Internet is accomplished through *browsing software.* Two dominant programs are *Navigator,* by the Netscape Company, and *Internet Explorer* by Microsoft Company. Like the Morse code, bits of information are used in the computer, but the operator manipulates a typewriter-like keyboard plus mouse, with pull-down menus instead of a click-switch. Although you don't have to learn the code, you do have to learn the software. The saving grace is that a reasonably educated person can communicate with relative simplicity in English or any other language.

In the arena of business, *ethical and legal considerations* are not always clear, and problems often arise. For example, Microsoft and Netscape companies have engaged in a legal battle for domination of the Internet. Both know that personal computing on the Internet can bring them billions of dollars in revenue. This winner-take-all approach is described by C. Ramo, (1996). Ramo asserts that these two companies "are competing not against each other so much as against their own obsolescence. The victor will not be the company with the best browser but the team that can run the longest on this insanely fast product-development treadmill."

The information highway system is composed of two parts: hardware/software and information. The *hardware* is made up of computers, servers and their interfaces, telephone copper and fiberoptic landlines, radio frequency and microwave systems, direct laser transceivers, and earth-satellite links. There are future possibilities of planetary and stellar locations. The software is composed of browsers. The real work on the Internet is performed by a device known as a *server*. Microsoft uses Windows NT Server, and Netscape uses Fast-Trak. Servers are giant computers that accept Web browser commands, such as *http://* and then route data to and from the appropriate places. But the most important part of the information highway is the *information* being communicated. This comes from humans, not computers. It arises from our imagination. Imagine doing something useful with Internet information, such as building superior biomedical instruments.

22-21 Internet and medical computer information

The Internet a very useful tool in health care and in the advancement of biomedical instrumentation. For example, *on-line searches* of books and journals from medical libraries can easily be accom-

plished through the Colorado Alliance of Research Libraries (CARL). Also, MEDLINE is used by physicians and health care workers for searching and retrieving the latest medical research and clinical techniques. Shared information through computers is creating a knowledge explosion around the world.

The *wide area network (WAN)* and *local area network (LAN)* are gaining enormous popularity in converting us to a *paperless communication society*. The difference is the geographical area covered. Some hospitals can now transfer medical records (worldwide) via the Internet. But others, for security reasons, do it via a WAN or LAN. This is confined to a limited number of users over a private link; it is not accessible from outside the users' group. This intraoffice/organization/company approach is sometimes called the *intranet*. In many cases, the only permanent storage of information is in the form of computer or digital memory. For this purpose, super *mass storage devices* have been invented to archive thousands of gigabytes of data. The storage media will probably survive in the form of optical-magnetic tape or disc. Finding someone to fix the playback equipment is another matter.

The *confidentiality problem* that threatens patients from unauthorized access to their medical records is described by Beverly Woodward (1995), who states that loss of privacy could cause people to avoid seeking care or to alter what they tell doctors. Although ethical and legal considerations are clear enough, problems with computer access are ever present.

On the other hand, the use of computers in medical care is not always so controversial. The computer can be used to prescribe drugs and make decisions with the help of CD-ROM or on-line services. Jeremy Wyatt and Robert Walton describe improvements in decision making (1995).

To extend the impact of the Internet, the *Internet telephone* might be used to conduct voice conversations through the Internet computer data link. For example, Intel is now developing a new *voice quality connection,* via special software, called

Netscape. To allow higher signal quality without broken or garbled speech, the Internet circulatory system will need more electronic bandwidth. A true multimedia environment greatly enhances biomedical communication using voice, data, and pictures. One excellent source of consumer health information can be found at the Internet address http://onhealth.com/ch1/index.asp. It provides discussions on subjects such as mind and body, nutrition, wellness, pediatrics, surgery, aging, genetics, diseases, and weight control.

22-22 PC, CD-ROM, and Interactive, Palmtop, and Laptop Computing and Health Care

The use of computers, particularly personal computers (PCs), are aiding in *home health care*. The "Computer Chronicles," a television program on the Public Broadcasting System (PBS), Newport, New Hampshire (May, 1996), aired a review of consumer medical software. Described were programs such as home diagnostic tools in which blood pressure is taken via software and hardware (blood pressure cuff and interface) that is registered by the Food and Drug Administration for accuracy. Animated graphics show step-by-step instructions. A medical fact section describes generally how to read the results. A graph routine shows long-term trends.

Another package, called *Doctor's Program of Home Remedies,* depicts the patient-doctor relationship. The patient and doctor ask questions of each other to arrive at diagnosis and treatment. The doctor, representing recognized authorities, appears in animated form with digitized voice. The patient can conduct a routine search on medical terms and subjects or ask "What can I do to treat high blood pressure?" Another group—the American Academy of Family Healthcare Physicians, describes wellness, nutrition, and disease.

Also, computer programs on exercise graphically depict body muscles. This allows one to work specific muscle groups. Action on the screen shows how to perform the exercise; results can then be reviewed.

PC-based health care programs are also used in management of pain. In a Stanford University Clinic study, 2000 patients loaded occurrences of pain through a special touch screen. This allowed medical care providers to help them manage their pain as it happened.

In addition, the Internet now offers balance and fitness for consumers. Suggestions for healthier living are covered, including cardiovascular and chiropractic help. Even the World Health Organization (WHO) provides information on the Internet.

Language is also no barrier, because a multimedia medical language translator (MLT) will translate terms and commonly asked questions in 43 languages (Gunby, 1995). This system includes a CD-ROM that operates on a laptop Windows-compatible computer and has voice-recorded messages.

Clearly, the World Wide Web is shifting from the marketplace to the marketspace, in which computer memory space is allocated on the Internet for health information and products.

The modern trend is toward more interaction between the user and the computer, where patient simulations are so good that one can communicate directly with animated images on the screen. For example, Edward Doyle (1996), in an American College of Physicians report, states that a new program extends hundreds of color images and video clips that allow physicians to interact with the computer. They can ask questions and receive instant answers for quickly assessing correctness. This is a high-end computerized continuing medical education (CME) credit system. Some say it is more powerful than conventional educational sources, such as textbooks and publications. The reason given is simple: It's easier to assimilate facts when put in context. Of course, textbooks are still essential in providing basic education to many, if not most, students. Simulations, however, allow a newcomer or working professional the opportunity to exercise and extend their mastery of the fundamental principles.

The next step beyond CD-ROM is Internet Online that is accessible from many locations with automatic updates as new material and techniques arise. One of the problems to overcome is the painfully slow information and image transfer. This can be cured, at least in part, by high-speed (wide bandwidth) fiber-optic to the house or satellite links, which use radio waves to directly connect the computer to the an overhead synchronously orbiting relay station. It is still debatable whether or not a physician or other technical professional will want to acquire all their educational credits via computer. In some areas, the touch and feel of books and live instructors provides the humanness required for superior education.

Another modern computer invention is the Palmtop, or personal digital assistant (PDA). This is a handheld device with a small screen, some pushbuttons, keyboard, and a writing pen. It offers flexibility in storing, sorting, and transferring patient information. According to Brickell Research, Inc., (1999), palmtop computing is making its way into the medical profession, and they provide software to handle these applications as described in their quarterly newsletters. PDAs, manufactured by companies such as 3-Com, continue to provide versions which are thinner, smaller, and faster. They are also easier to access and have more memory. They are protected with a flip-top cover, and hence, medical professionals find it a safe and accurate way to gather patient data right on the hospital floor. It's also easy to download appointments, notes from hospital rounds, and sketches into a larger computer. This becomes a permanent part of the patient's record. Brickell Research produces the QuickMed/PalmPilot Interface Module to accomplish this. There is one note of caution, however. Apparently people view the world through mental image pictures. Because endless computer listings are contrary to the spatial or object orientation nature of humans, many medical professionals find it challenging to find information quickly. Also, the relatively small screens permit only a small view of the big picture, similar to an ant searching the ground for food. For people,

written notes or books are sometimes more satisfying and perhaps less frustrating. Obviously, computers offer better (more accurate and permanent) memory and extensive search capability. Palmtops attempt to help this by allowing a person to write notes directly on the screen. Afterwards, it often becomes part of a big computer document, and this constitutes technological development that is here to stay.

Laptop computers are complete microcomputers that fit on a person's lap or on a small space in the corner of a desk. They often contain all the necessary programs and memory (now many gigabytes) for performing major tasks, such as word processing, spreadsheet analysis, data base search-sort, graphics, and imaging. The advantage of Palmtops over laptops is mainly size and cost. Where laptops have a distinct place in the hierarchy of computers in medicine, they are too large to carry around the hospital floor. Both palmtops and laptops can now be networked into main computers for efficient use of time and effort.

22-23 Expert system

Expert System (ES) is a computer-based program comprised of the writings of trained and experienced professionals who consult with the user through simulation. It uses a knowledge base and inference-ruled procedures that simulate the decision-making process of an expert. Figure 22-10 shows the architecture of such a system.

Computer-aided diagnosis and decision making on how best to handle a patient is now commonplace.

Telemedicine on Wheels is a method of delivering medical care to rural communities. It consists of a mobile clinic including video cameras and video-equipped medical instruments. A physician can deliver care through live, interactive telecommunication lines and satellite broadcasts. Even telesurgery is possible. Operating through *virtual reality,* computers create pictures that can guide a surgeon's robotic knife. This system at the Konawa Community Health Center in Oklahoma is described by Greg Borzo, (1996).

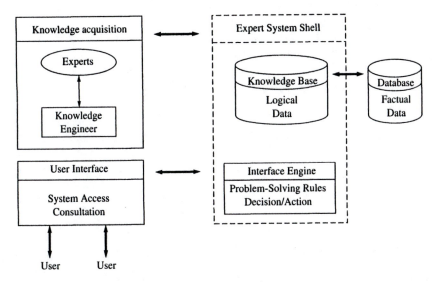

Figure 22-10
Architecture of expert systems (Permission granted from *Health Management Information Systems: Theories, Methods, and Applications,* Chapter 8, p. 249, by Joseph K. H. Tau.
© 1995 Aspen Publishers, Inc.)

22-24 Computer-based patient record

One obvious application of computers in medicine is in gathering, maintaining, and retrieving medical records. Advantages include elimination of illegible handwriting, easy tracking of a medical chart, and finding the answer to a simple question concerning a patient's condition. Computerization not only solves problems but expands use to new functions, including coordination of patient information, important clinical decision making concerning adverse drug reactions, and adherence to health policy and hospital management. Joseph Norman, (1995) details the recordkeeping system.

22-25 Computer workstations

The computer workstation has gained acceptance despite the proliferation of microcomputers on everyone's desk. For example, Groth et al. (1996), describe an instrument workstation that depicts advanced services that complement basic services

in a laboratory information system. In the modern world of *workflow management,* it is essential to carefully consider instrument and user interfacing, quality control, calibration, patient result validation, faulty diagnosis, and maintenance. Figure 22-11 shows an advanced instrument workstation diagram. In this approach, both local and decentralized instruments are accessed by the technician, engineer, nurse, and physician.

To make repair of mainframe and minicomputers more efficient, remote *instrument telemaintenance* systems over a LAN are being more widely used. Computer-aided troubleshooting is now used to reduce repair time and avoid instrument down time through predictive methods. Lower cost of computerized laboratory hardware allows quick rerouting or replacement of faulty units. Centers of repair have the advantage of more information and experience concerning failures. Artifical neural networks and knowledge-based systems diagnose problems and, if necessary, alert a human expert to intervene and fix the problem (Laugier, et al., 1996).

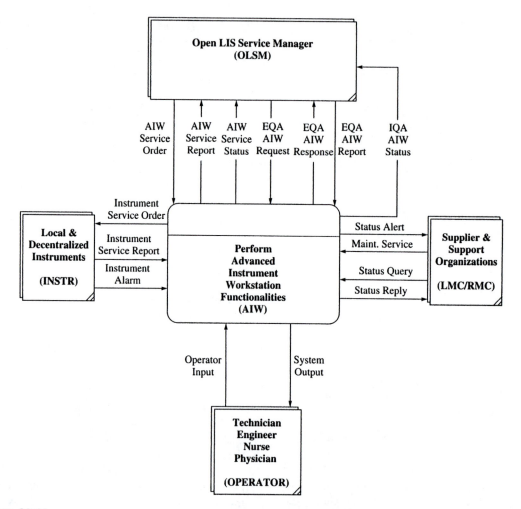

Figure 22-11
Advanced instrument workstation. (Reprinted from *Computer Methods and Programs in Bio-medicine,* Vol. 50, No. 2, July 1996, T. Groth et al. "Open Labs Advanced Instrument Worksta-tion Services," Figure 2, p. 149, © 1996 with kind permission from Elsevier Science Ireland Ltd., Bay 15K Shannon Industrial Estate, Co. Clare, Ireland.)

22-26 Computers in laboratory instrumentation

Modern laboratory instrumentation uses *standard interfaces* to exchange data with host computers. This permits interchangeability through computer buses, such as *Fieldbus* for industrial systems and *Medical Information Bus (MIB)* for medical equipment. Essentially anyone can use the pull-down menus to direct the system to perform three functions: (1) acquire sensor data, such as temper-ature, pressure, pH, humidity, fluid flow, and ECG; (2) process or analyze data; and (3) display the results. The equipment that does this is called a *data acquisition system (DAS)*. A block diagram of a commercially available multifunction board DAS is shown in Figure 22-12. It is software pro-grammable for selection of 16 single-ended or 8

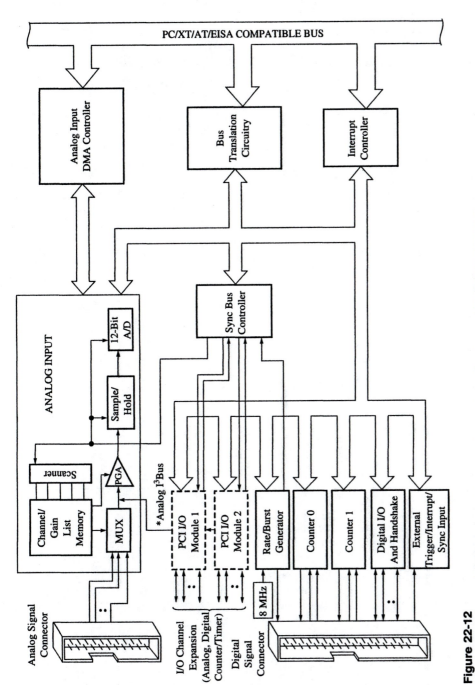

Figure 22-12
PCI-20098C Series block diagram, data acquisition system. (Courtesy of Intelligent Instrumentation, A Burr-Brown Company, 1996).

differential input channels as well as for gain through the programmable-gain amplifier (PGA). Analog inputs are digitized through the sample/hold amplifier and 12-bit A/D converter. Also, it supports direct memory access (DMA) to speed up interaction. Standard bus translators allow compatible bus connection.

Portable instrumentation used in laboratories includes hardware (computer, amplifiers, and plug-in boards), software (programs), and interface (interconnections) for hardware and software.

Accuracy in a DAS relates to the analog side of continuous signal levels and digital side of discrete steps. Notice in Figure 22-13 that there are 2^{12} or 4096 steps at the output of the 12-bit A/D converter. The smallest step, known as an LSB (least significant bit), is just 1/4096, which is equivalent to 0.024%. Therefore 1/2 LSB is 0.012 percent. Picture each step being 2.4 mV at the input to the A/D converter since the full scale is 10 V. Therefore, 1/2 LSB is 1.2 mV. This means that if the input signal steps up or down by more than 1.2 mV and as high as 2.4 mV, the converter will step up or down by one code. In conclusion, the system shown will measure an analog signal to *99.976% accuracy,* or to within 0.024% error, provided noise and nonlinearity errors are low enough. Notice that these errors are budgeted as

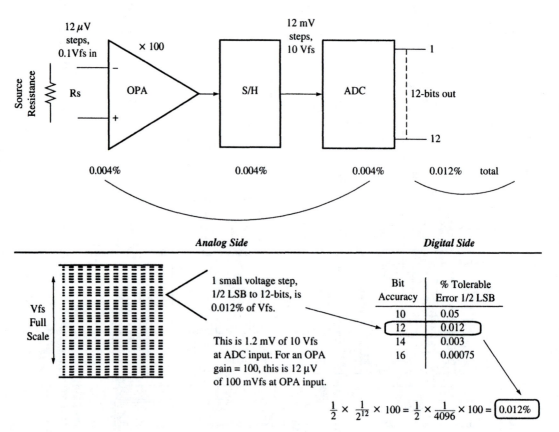

Figure 22-13
Digitization of analog signals.

the signal goes through various stages. Also, some errors, such as dc offset, add linearly. Other errors that are random, such as noise, add as the square root of the sum of the squares of each error. Since the instantaneous levels of uncorrelated noise sources are not predictable, rms or energy levels must be added to determine total noise.

Sensor electronics is changing. Most have an analog output. However, today the *digital output sensor* is becoming a reality, as shown in Figure 22-14. Here the serial output bus allows connection and communication between a number of so-called *smart sensors* and the host computer. Although the protocol is more complex, this approach allows for tremendous system flexibility and reconfigurability. Calibration can be done so that any random sensor can be connected to any electronic circuit unit. Also, the remote computer can query any sensor channel for information and tell any sensor to perform some specific task. Sensors, with their dedicated electronics, can self-

calibrate for zero, gain, and nonlinearity and check themselves for faults. Hence the term "smart." Smart sensors are used most often in industrial environments but can be used in medical equipment as well. For example, in an ECG machine, it is possible to use one A/D converter or digitizer for each electrode and then use just two wires to transmit all electrode signals to the ECG machine. Self-checking for misconnected or malperforming electrodes can be done by the dedicated electronics hooked to the ECG pad. The advantage is simple cabling that is easy to electrically isolate.

The modern phenomenon in laboratory instrumentation is called *plug and play*. This means that the hardware, software, and firmware are designed to work so closely together that anyone can use the computer without having to know anything about the computer's operating system. For example, a medical laboratory professional can use *graphical programming* software to design a DAS

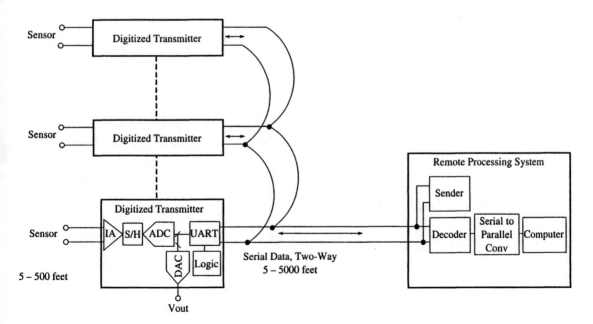

Figure 22-14
Smart digitized output transmitter with multi-drop, serial communication bus.

for monitoring physiological parameters such as body temperature, ECG, and the like. The trick is the *automatic code generator,* which creates computer codes or instructions when you type some higher-level command, such as "select channel 1." It empowers the user because it eliminates syntactical details. The most popular underlying programs are BASIC, C-Language, and PASCAL, which are time-consuming and difficult to learn. Today's laboratory instrumentation graphical software packages include Visual Designer, Signal-Analyzer, LabWindows/CVI, DISPLAY (for digital filters), ComponentWorks, VirtualBench, and LabVIEW.

Miniaturization of circuits, modules, subsystems, and entire systems has revolutionized medical laboratory instrumentation. *Plug-in printed circuit boards* have been available for some time. They insert into a microcomputer internal card slot and contain an entire DAS, including amplification, signal conditioning, digitization, filtering, timing, and interface. They are about 13 in. wide and 4.5 in. high. Another approach is the *Personal*

Computer Memory Card International Association (PCMCIA) module, which has many of the same functions in even a small space—it is about 3 inches long, 2 inches wide, and 0.5 inches high. It plugs into a connector that is external to the microcomputer. Indeed, it is the standard for the credit-card sized PC plug-in interface, which embodies optimal portability and low power consumption. This module provides a highly flexible, multichannel data acquisition addition to an already powerful computing and processing system, the laptop computer. It is universal because it has a *standard IEEE488 electrical interface* and standard mechanical connections.

Robotics and automation are also used in the laboratory. One system used robotics to measure deoxyribonucleic acid (DNA) genetic material from capillary electrophoresis in bone marrow grafts. This was from the recipient before the graft, the donor, and the recipient after the graft. This allowed quick and accurate detection of any rejection that occured (see Merel, P., et al, *Cancer Biotechnology Weekly,* August 14, 1995, p. 19).

22-27 Brief glossary of computer and laboratory instrumentation words

Computer terms will help you understand these new systems more completely (see detailed glossary at the end of this textbook).

accuracy

ADC = analog-to-digital converter

ALU = arithmetic logic unit

ANSI = American National Standards Institute

ASIC = application-specific integrated circuit

Asynchronous

ATE = automatic test equipment

bandwidth

baud rate

BIOS-Basic Input/Output System

bipolar

block-mode

bit

break-before-make

bus

byte

cache

compiler

computer

conversion time

cross talk

DAC = digital-to-analog converter

DAQ = data acquisition

DAS = data acquisition system

data flow

dB = decibel

DCS = distributed control system

DDE = dynamic data exchange

delta-sigma (sometimes called sigma-delta)

differential input

DIO = digital input/output

DLL = dynamic link library

DMA = direct memory access

DNL = differential nonlinearity

drivers

dynamic range

EEPROM = electrically erasable programmable read only memory

encoder

EPROM = erasable programmable read only memory

emulator

Fieldbus

FIFO = first-in-first-out

fixed-point

floating point

gain

GPIB = general-purpose interface bus

GUI = graphical user interface

hardware

hierarchical

IAC = interapplication communication

IMD = intermodulation distortion

INL = integral nonlinearity

Interactive = Two way interaction person and computer

interpreter

I/O = input/output

isolation voltage

linearity

listener

LSB = least significant bit

laptop

MIB = Medical Information Bus

MIPS = millions of instructions per second

MMI = man-machine interface

modulating ADC

multitasking

mux

MXIbus = Multisystem eXtension Interface bus

noise

Nyquist sampling theorem

operating system

overhead

PDA = personal digital assistant (palmtop)

parallel bus

PCI = peripheral component interconnect

PCMCIA = Personal Computer Memory Card International Association

PID control

pipeline

peripheral device

PLC = programmable logic controller

plug and play ISA

port

propagation delay

protocol

quantization error

RAM = random access memory

real time

relative accuracy

resolution

ROM = read only memory

SCADA = supervisory control and data acquisition

(continued on p. 594)

SCPI = standard commands for programmable instruments

single-ended

self-calibrating

sensor

S/H amplifier

SNR = signal-to-noise ratio

software

SPC = statistical process control

simultaneous sampling

successive-approximation ADC

synchronous

syntax

THD = total harmonic distortion

THD + N = total harmonic distortion plus noise

throughout rate

transfer rate

UART = universal asychronous receiver transmitter

unipolar

VXI open instrumentation standard

word

windows applications

Y2K = year 2000

22-28 Computers in medical research

Medical research depends heavily on computers. For example, hypoglycemia is described by Heger, et al. (1996). The researchers discuss recording EEG, heart rate, peripheral pulse, skin temperature, respiratory movements, skin impedance, arterial blood pressure, and cognitive performance during hypoglycemia. A future outcome from this research could be the indirect detection of hypoglycemia using body sensor technology. Computers were used to acquire physiological data, record streams of information, and analyze results.

Brain glucose using H NMR spectra is describe by Gruetter, et al. (1996). The authors describe the difficulty in measuring *resonances of glucose* with concentrations between 3.2 and 3.9 ppm within the human brain. The problem is the glucose signature is masked by overlapping peaks from more concentrated metabolites. A future outcome from this research could be the the noninvasive quantification of glucose in the brain. Computers played an important role in the basic operation of the nuclear magnetic resonance system, which is now called magnetic resonance imaging.

One of the most impressive uses of computers in medical research is in searching computer data bases for similar DNA sequences to understand how certain genes relate to disease. This is described by Boguski, Mark S., in an article entitled "Molecular Medicine: Hunting for Genes in Computer Data Bases" (*New England Journal of Medicine,* Vol. 333, No. 10, p. 645, Sept. 7, 1995). A future outcome could be to reveal genetic causes of diseases and, eventually, possible treatments. Special computer data bases in this application help reveal DNA disease connections that would not otherwise be discovered.

22-29 Computers in biomedical equipment

Computers are widely used in modern biomedical equipment. The following is a brief description of some of the major applications. All applications must consider techniques for *data acquisition,* ability to *store and retrieve* data, a process of *data reduction or transformation* to a usable form, *calculation* of variables, *recognition of patterns* in the endless waveforms, establishment of *boundaries or limits, statistical analysis* of variable signals, and *presentation formats* for the data.

The following is a list of large-scale and micro-computer applications.

1. *Computers in automated medical information systems* (MIS)—computers have been playing a large role in automated medical information systems. Financial recordkeeping as well as patient billing and medical history are stored in large memory banks. Pharmaceutical inventory is also computerized in large hospitals. However, computerized patient records have caused controversy involving confidentiality of medical diagnosis. Nevertheless, computers and information go hand in hand, and computer hardware is likely to evolve in health care facilities and organizations.

2. Computer analysis of the ECG—algorithms or fixed analysis sequence programs have been used in recent times to interpret ECG parameters (see chapters 2 and 3). These include detection of all peaks (*P,Q,R,S,T*), establishment of baselines, measurement of abnormalities such as PR segment depression, and determination of arrhythmias. Although sophisticated large-scale computers have been used in statistical analysis, many cardiologists seem to distrust the results. They usually read patient ECGs by eye even if a computer is used, because computer-read ECGs are questionable in about 20% of all runs.

3. *Computer analysis in patient monitoring*— most large modern hospitals use some type of computer system in ICUs and CCUs. CCU bedside monitors use microprocessor-based systems, and the central station uses a larger microcomputer to analyze and display short- and long-term trends in ECG waveforms, pressure signals, respiration rate and depth, and temperature variations. A/D and D/A converters are common. The information

derived is useful in determining response to treatment and the severity of disease. Figure 22-15 shows a computerized ECG management system.

4. *Computer analysis of cardiac catherization parameters*—cardiac catherization in the laboratory or operating room requires measurement of intracardiac blood pressures, especially across heart valves. Wedge pressures and vascular resistance are also important. Abnormalities can more easily be detected with computer programs that calculate stroke volumes and catheter effectivity and display results instantly. Catheters can then be placed more accurately.

5. *Computer averaging in electroencephalographic evoked response*— evoked responses to light flashes and tone burst show very little change in the ongoing ECG waveform. Special-purpose computers are currently being used to average evoked responses to obtain a useful display of peaks and valleys. Minicomputers and microcomputers are then used to statistically analyze time periods and relative peak amplitudes. The diagnosis of visual and hearing impairment in young children and adults has been made using such systems.

6. *Computer analysis of pulmonary function*— recently, equipment has appeared on the market that will analyze pulmonary function. Breathing rate, depth, and variations are displayed along with arterial blood gas changes. This offers a fast and accurate indication of a patient's condition. A system appears in Figure 22-16.

7. *Computer evaluation of clinical laboratory chemical tests*—computers blend naturally into the high-volume clinical laboratory tests of blood, urine, and other body fluids. Autoanalyzers and continuous analysis equipment systems use minicomputers and microcomputers to aid with data acquisition

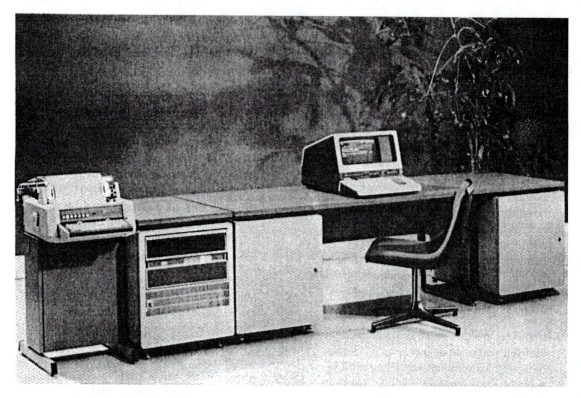

Figure 22-15
Coronary care monitoring computer system. (Photo courtesy of Hewlett-Packard)

and processing. Test results are accepted, lists are prepared, calculations are performed, and reports issued automatically. Remote terminals make the data available to the medical staff almost instantly, allowing easier and more rapid diagnosis of disease.

8. *Computed tomography (CT)*–CT scanners originated through the use of computers. X-ray images obtained from pencil beam scans at various angles are stored in and analyzed by a minicomputer. The computer then redraws the picture on a CRT. Fine differences in tissue density and tumor outlines can be readily shown (even enhanced by color). *Pattern recognition* is the key to accurate results. *Algorithms,* a problem-solving set of

rules or processes, are used to analyze and interpret data. This aids tremendously in diagnosing disease without surgery. Figure 22-17 shows such a system. Modern improvements in CT scanners arise from better analog and digital electronics. Andrew Wilson, in *Vision Systems Design Magazine* on robotics (1999) states that General Electric Corp., Milwaukee, WI, is building a new CT/i (Computer Assisted Tomography) system that produces images with 1280×1024 pixel resolution. It uses an Imagraph Corp. 9-bit accurate PC board and software, which temperature stabilizes gain, jitter, and phase in both the analog front-end and the phase-lock-loop. Usually analog integrators in the system proceed a frame-capture device, and the goal

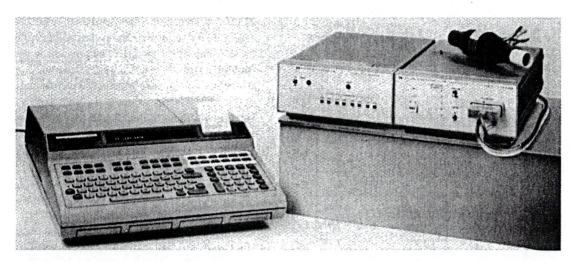

Figure 22-16
Microprocessor-based respiratory analyzer. (Photo courtesy of Hewlett-Packard)

is to add as little degradation as possible. Figure 22-18 shows a diagram of the system. Frames are grabbed by capturing the red-green-blue (RGB) and horizontal and vertical synchronization signals from the display controller output. A superior frame grabber, such as one made by Imagraph Technology, Chelmsford, MA, advances the state-of-the-art. It's a PCI-based Hi*Def Accura type, which allows CT imaging data to go to a film printer via the computer's serial or parallel ports. Another application of higher resolution frame grabbers is early diagnosis of glaucoma, or increased pressure within the eye. Physicians can treat conditions sooner and prevent vision loss and blindness.

9. *Magnetic resonance imaging (MRI)*—formally known as nuclear magnetic resonance, MRI systems operate on the principle of resonating hydrogen atom nuclei (protons) with intense radio frequency energy. The resonance concept can be understood by considering a proton as a tiny magnet that processes or moves about an axis in the same way a spinning top does as it traces a cone-shaped surface. By pushing a proton with just the

right natural radio frequency, it can be made to re-emit a radio wave of the same frequency. MRI machines utilize two types of fields. A coil generates a very strong constant or dc magnetic field at 1 tesla that lines up hydrogen atoms within the OH radical of water (H_2O or H^+OH^-). Another coil creates a weaker, changing, or ac radio frequency

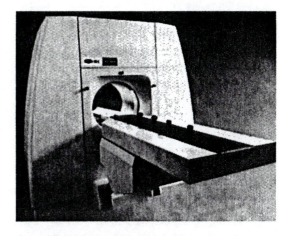

Figure 22-17
Computed tomography system. (Photo courtesy of Pfizer Medical Systems, Inc.)

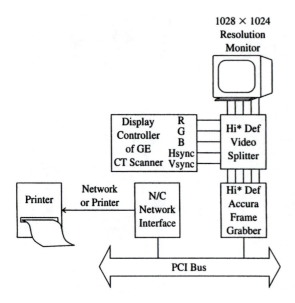

1028 × 1024
Resolution
Monitor

Display Controller of GE CT Scanner — R G B Hsync Vsync

Hi* Def Video Splitter

Printer

Network or Printer

N/C Network Interface

Hi* Def Accura Frame Grabber

PCI Bus

Figure 22-18
CT (Computed Tomographic) scanner: new fast, higher-resolution frame-grabber system by GE.

field, at about 16 kHz, which moves across the area of the body to be imaged. This resonates hydrogen nuclei to re-emit energy. This energy is picked up by a sense coil. MRI machines are very effective at imaging fine gradations in tissue density, particularly where tumors meet healthy tissue. They accomplish this by measuring how much water (hydrogen) is in the tissue. An enlarged tumor has more water, and hence shows up as an enclosed image. C/T images, on the other hand, pass X-rays through the tissues and measure how much gets through. They measure tissue density but not water density and are effective but not as good as MRI at imaging tumors that are hard to see. Both use computers to analyze and reconstruct images.

10. *Positron emission tomography (PET)*—PET systems operate by injecting a short-lived, positron-emitting radionuclide of carbon, oxygen, nitrogen, or fluorine into the body.

These substances are measured as they are taken up by target organs. As the radionuclide decays, positrons are annihilated by electrons, producing gamma rays. By simultaneously detecting and analyzing the radionuclide and gamma rays on opposite sides of the body, images of organs are produced. (A *positron* is a positive electron or any positively charged subatomic particle having the same mass and charge magnitude of an electron. It is the antiparticle of a negative electron. Radionuclides are atoms that disintegrate by emission of electromagnetic radiation.) PET imagers are useful in studying brain and heart functions, biochemical processes in these organs (such as glucose metabolism and oxygen uptake) and blood flow and volume. They use computers to analyze and reconstruct the image.

11. *Computer analysis of nuclear medicine results*—scintillation detection and gamma ray camera displays are analyzed by computer in some large hospitals. Counts are statistically analyzed, and data is presented on a CRT. Diagnosis of marginal organ function is made more reliable.

12. *Digital radiology*—a prime new application for computers. Here high-resolution digital imagery is replacing conventional X-ray films, which uses wet chemicals. John Haystead of *Vision Systems Design Magazine* (1999), states that General Electric Corp., Milwaukee, WI, is producing digital detector technology using one large integrated circuit having a 50 × 50 cm (2048 × 2048 pixels) glass substrate. The array contains 4 million high detective quantum efficiency (DQE) photodiodes, each with 10-μm diameter. This can reveal sizes of 200 μm for chest and 100 μm for breast images, and essentially rivals film pictures. Their new amorphous silicon/cesium iodide (CsI-based) sensor captures more than 80% of the original image information. This is an improvement over

charged-coupled devices (CCDs), which gather about 40%. In October, 1998, the U.S. FDA gave approval to GE to use this for chest examinations. After being digitized with a bank of high-speed 14-bit ADCs (without needing to wait for film development), the image can be analyzed more extensively and accurately than the human eye. Many visible shades of gray reveal subtle outlines of tumors. Computer-aided diagnosis is also used for full-field-mammography (FFDM) and will undoubtedly reduce deaths from breast cancer. The result is faster, lower cost screening for diseased conditions. Routine dental X-ray pictures can also be taken and evaluated quickly. This modern approach is superior to digitizing photographic X-ray films.

13. *High-resolution imaging*—this can now be done on brain tumors to pinpoint exactly where they are. Charles J. Murray, of *Design News* (1998), describes Dr. Mary Beth Dunn, a brain surgeon, who uses a special computer to precisely image a brain tumor in a 5-year-old girl, prior to cutting a 2-inch diameter hole in exactly the right place on her cranium. It is essentially a computer image-guided technique for improving surgical accuracy and enables patients to recover more quickly, because exploratory procedures are unnecessary. These clinical advances are made possible by modern, lower cost computers with more digital bits, operating at higher clock speeds. Super computers would make the cost prohibitive in "common or routine" surgeries.

14. *High-speed imaging*—now used in medical research to better understand blood flow in diseased heart vessels. According to Lawrence J. Curran, of *Vision Systems Design Magazine*, (1999), Dr. Timothy Liem of the University of Missouri School of Medicine, is using it to record images inside arteries of humans and animals that have been removed and bathed in oil of wintergreen (methyl

salicylate). A high-speed digital video system, working with a 400-MHz Dell Dimension XPS-R Pentium II PC computer, digitizes images at 500 to 1000 frames per second. Faster cameras with 8000 frames per second and shutter speeds of 10 μs will give better results, because more data will be gathered. Slow motion playback constitutes a "simulation" of what was happening to the flow in an effort to better understand abnormal conditions. This technique can be used to analyze atherosclerosis, a form arteriosclerosis (deposition of plaques, containing cholesterol and lipids on the innermost wall layer of large and medium arteries). The object is to measure impaired hemodynamics, or blood circulation, which is the major cause of heart attack. Flow-visualization systems, such as this one, measure pressure differences and shear stresses along specific portions inside blood vessels. Perhaps this information will be used to prevent or treat coronary artery disease.

15. *Biotelemetry*—another area where computers have pushed the frontier of performance and possibilities. For example, John W. Hines, et al., of Ames Research Center, California, (1999) have shown that a small transmitting unit encapsulated in a biocompatible silicone rubber housing, can be used to remotely monitor key physiological parameters of a fetus while still in the uterine environment. The object is to know when to administer proper medical treatment by detecting the onset of labor before the expected time (preterm). This system consists of an RF transmitter utilizing pulse-interval modulation (PIM) with carrier frequencies between 174 and 214 MHz. The interval between two pulses at a 1- to 2-Hz repetition rate indicates pressure. The interval between the pairs is proportional to temperature, measured with a thermistor (temperature sensor) inside the implanted housing. Intrauterine contractions

are measured at a range of 3 to 10 feet away. Two silver oxide batteries, lasting 4 to 6 months, provide power to the unit that consumes less than 40 μW. Computer processing is done by LABVIEW (registered trademark of National Instruments Corp, Austin, TX) software, where pressure and temperature are displayed as a function of time. Peaks detected assist the pediatric surgeon in an effort to deliver more healthy babies. Biotelemetry is also used to measure ECG (heart), EEG (brain), BP (blood pressure), and other bodily functions from remote locations, including one's own home via telephone connections. Allowing patients to remain ambulatory (free to move about) when possible is a big part of their diagnosis and recovery in the world of modern medicine. Because the person's whereabouts are known, quick action can be taken to deliver proper medical treatment should emergencies arise.

16. *Computers in other biomedical equipment*—a myriad of other uses for computers in biomedical equipment are becoming evident in the modern world of analysis and automation. Bedside ECG monitors as well as respiratory servoventilators have microprocessors embedded within them. Even the delivery of anesthesia is a target for a microprocessor-controlled patient-machine feedback system. Naturally, great distrust has arisen. Furthermore, microprocessor systems are being considered for ultrasonic scanning analysis. The future of computers in medicine will be considered on diagnostic merit, availability, and cost.

22-30 Summary

1. The *computer revolution* has unfolded in the past 50 years, and after four generations of computer hardware, medical systems show widespread use.

2. A *digital computer* (versus an analog device) is an electronic and electromechanical device that can perform a sequence of *arithmetic* and *logical* operations according to stored instructions. It can be used to solve mathematical problems or can search, sort, and arrange information to be displayed or printed.

3. The computer program is known as the *software* and the physical portion is the *hardware.*

4. A *computer system* consists of an input unit, input control, memory, instruction control unit (IU), arithmetic logic unit (ALU), output control, and output unit. The central processing unit (CPU) contains the main or internal memory, ALU, and IU, along with special registers, timing, and other housekeeping operations.

5. A *flowchart* is written to structure a problem, and program lines of code are written to solve the problem. The *signal path* through the computer takes many turns but always must involve the memory unit.

6. *Computer programming languages* include machine and assembly as well as high-level BASIC, C-language, PASCAL, FORTRAN, and COBOL, among others.

7. A *microcomputer* is a general-purpose computer composed of standard LSI components built around a central processing unit (CPU). The CPU or microprocessor is program controlled with arithmetic and logic instructions and a common or parallel I/O tristate bus system for data and address. Memory includes RAM, ROM, floppy drive, MBM, CCD, and CD-ROM (optical).

8. Combined multimedia technologies provide voice, fax, and video-on-demand through computer systems.

9. Wireless mobile communication systems allow transception of data in an ambulance, for example.

10. Modern microprocessors, such as the Pentium, have evolved to 32-bit buses operating at clock rates greater than 166 MHz.

11. *Microcontrollers* are simpler forms of microprocessors.

12. Interactive data bases, such as Lotus Notes, allow users to share, search, and sort information easily.

13. Computers have limitations in their hardware and software reliability and because they don't think.

14. A *computer virus* is a destructive tool used by criminals to damage or destroy computer software and possibly hardware.

15. A *neural network* is a computational system that has parallel processing paths. It can be used to enhance medical computer images or accurately recognize patterns in ECG tracings, for example.

16. The Internet is an interconnection of shared computers that allows communication via the World Wide Web. The *information superhighway* is the conduit through which individuals, organizations, and companies exchange information. The *server* or bank of giant computers accepts and routes data to and from the proper places.

17. The *wide area network (WAN)* and *local area network (LAN)* are being used to create a paperless communication society.

18. PC-based computer health care systems including CD-ROMs are enhancing health care by allowing more people access to medical information in a multimedia and interactive way.

19. *Expert System* is a computer-based program comprised of the writings of trained and experienced professionals that allows users access to their knowledge no matter where they are located.

20. To make repair of mainframe and minicomputers more efficient, remote instrument telemaintenance systems over a LAN are being used more widely.

21. Modern laboratory instrumentation uses standard interfaces to exchange data with host computers. This permits interchangeability through computer buses, such as *Fieldbus* for industrial systems and *Medical Information Bus (MIB)* for medical equipment.

22. Portable instrumentation used in laboratories includes hardware (computer, amplifiers, and plug-in boards), software (programs), and interface (interconnections) for hardware and software.

23. Accuracy in a data acquisition system (DAS) relates to the analog side of continuous signal levels and digital side of discrete steps. Percent errors in the analog signal become least significant bits (LSBs) in the digital word through the analog-to-digital (A/D) converter.

24. *Smart sensors* have dedicated electronics, can self-calibrate, and check themselves for faults.

25. Plug-in printed circuit boards and Personal Computer Memory Card International Association (PCMCIA) modules have helped to miniaturize the electronics of laboratory instrumentation. They contain an entire DAS, including amplification, signal conditioning, digitization, filtering, timing, and interface.

26. Computers are used in medical research that can someday become clinically useful.

27. *Interfacing* biomedical instrumentation to digital computers requires A/D and D/A converters.

28. *Computer applications* in biomedical equipment include automated information systems, analysis of ECG, patient monitoring, cardiac catheterization, averaging in EEG-evoked responses, pulmonary and respiratory function, clinical laboratory results, C/T scanners, MRI, PET, nuclear medicine scintillation counting, and other bedside and automated processes.

22-31 Recapitulation

Now return to the objectives and self-evaluation questions at the beginning of the chapter and see how well you can answer them. If you cannot answer the questions, place a check mark next to each and review appropriate parts of the text. Next, try to answer the following questions using the same procedure.

Questions

1. Four generations of computers are _____, _____, _____, _____, _____, and _____.

2. A digital computer is an _____ and _____ device, which can perform a sequence of _____ and _____ operations. It can solve _____ problems or can _____, _____, and arrange information according to stored _____.

3. The main sections of a computer system are the _____ unit, _____, _____ unit, _____ decoder, _____ logic unit, _____ control, and _____ unit.

4. The central processing unit (CPU) contains the _____ memory, _____ logic unit, _____, and housekeeping _____.

5. The computer programs made up the _____ and the physical portions make up the _____.

6. Write the ASCII code sequence for X = M + B.

7. What is a computer program flowchart?

8. Name two low-level and three high-level computer languages.

9. What part does the microprocessor perform in a microcomputer?

10. Why are tristate bus lines useful in a microcomputer?

11. How is a RAM different from a ROM?

12. What is the resolution of a 16-bit analog-to-digital converter?

13. What is a multimedia computer system?

14. Approximately how often do microprocessors double in speed?

15. What types of functions do microcontrollers perform?

16. A computer virus can _____ or _____ software programs.

17. A neural network can enhance a medical image but cannot recognize EEG trace patterns. (True or false)

18. For security reasons, some hospitals use a WAN or LAN instead of the _____.

19. The Expert System is repaired by an expect, such as a biomedical engineer or technician. (True or false)

20. Modern portable laboratory instrumentation incorporates (a) _____, (b) _____, and (c) interface.

21. 0.0076% accuracy in an analog circuit equals _____ LSBs in a 16-bit A/D converter.

22. Miniature PCMCIA modules contain _____ acquisition circuitry in a small space.

23. Medical researchers make use of the computer and the DAS because they can gather information and _____ results.

24. What differences exist in computer systems used for medical information and records processing compared with bedside and central station CCU monitoring?

25. Why is a computer-averaged, EEG-evoked response signal easier to analyze than a raw signal?

26. What advantage is a computer in the automated clinical laboratory?

27. Does C/T scanning produce better results than a two-dimensional chest X-ray picture, or than MRI or PET?

28. Are computer systems always applicable in biomedical equipment?

Suggested Reading

1. Acharya, Raj S. and Bmitry B. Goldgof, eds., *Biomedical Image Processing and Biomedical Visualization, IS&T, The Society for Imaging Science and Technology and SPIE,* The International Society for Optical Engineering (Washington, D.C., 1993).

2. Baxt, William G. "Application of Artificial Neural Networks to Clinical Medicine," *Lancet,* Vol. 346, No. 8983, p. 1135 Oct. 28, 1995.

3. Boguski, Mark S, "Molecular Medicine: Hunting for Genes in Computer Data Bases," *New England Journal of Medicine,* Vol. 333, No. 10, p. 645, Sept. 7, 1995.

4. Borzo, Greg, "Telemedicine on Wheels" (method of delivering medical care to rural communities, system at the Konawa Community Health Center in Oklahoma) *American Medical News,* Vol. 39, No. 5, p. 3, February, 1996.

5. Carr, Joseph J., *Microcomputer Interfacing: A Practical Guide for Technicians, Engineers and Scientists,* Prentice Hall (Englewood Cliffs, N.J., 1991).

6. *Computer Chronicles, PC Based Health Care,* broadcast May 26, 1996, on Public Broadcasting System (PBS) (computers in routine health, home diagnostics and remedies, exercise, management of pain, internet balance and fitness), Software Publishing Association (Newport, N.H., 1996).

7. "Data Book on Plug-In Computer Equipment used in the Laboratory, (1) "LabVIEW," (2) "LabWindows/CVI." (3) "ComponentWorks," and (4) "VirtualBench," National Instruments, (Austin, Tex., 1996).

8. Davis, Michael W. *Computerizing Healthcare Information* (developing electronic patient information systems), Probus Publishing Company (Chicago, 1994).

9. Dick, Richard S. and Elaine B. Steen, ed. *The Computer-Based Patient Record* (an essential technology for health care), National Academy Press (Washington, D.C., 1991).

10. Deutsch, Tibor, Ewart Carson, and Endre Ludwig, *Dealing with Medical Knowledge* (computers in clinical decision making), Plenum Press (New York, 1994).

11. Donaldson, Molla S. and Kathleen N. Lohr, *Health Data in the Information Age* (use, disclosure, and privacy), National Academy Press (Washington, D.C., 1994).

12. Doyle, John D., *Computer Programs in Clinical and Laboratory Medicine* (cardiac, pulmonary, renal, trauma/resuscitation, therapeutics, drug dosing) Springer-Verlag (New York, 1989). www.Instrument.com.

13. Freedman, Alan, *The Computer Glossary, The Complete Illustrated Desk Reference,* 5th ed., Amacom (American Management Association), (New York, 1991).

14. Frisse, Mark E. ed. *16th Symposium on Computer Applications in Medical Care* (conference of the American Medical Informatics Association; critical care computing, biomedical imaging, standards, ambulatory care, information access and retrieval, clinical data, learning process,

clinical decision support, linking databases, interfaces, patient management, laboratory research, nursing education, medline, speech recognition), McGraw-Hill, Health Professions Division (New York, 1992).

15. Gelfaud, Michael J. and Stephen R. Thomas, *User of Computers in Nuclear Medicine* (acquisition, computer processing, and reading images), McGraw-Hill (New York, 1988).

16. Groth, T., et al. "OpenLabs Advanced Instrument Workstation Services," and Laugier, A., et al, Article "Remote Instrument Telemaintenance," *Computer Methods and Programs in Biomedicine,* Vol. 50, No. 2 p. 148 July, 1996.

17. Gruetter, Rolf, et al, "Observation of Resolved Glucose Signals in H NMR Spectra of the Human Brain at 4 Telsa," *Magnetic Resonance in Medicine,* Vol. 36, No. 1, July, 1996.

18. Gunby, Phil, "Computer-Based Medical Translator System helps Bridge Language Gap Between Physician, Patient," *Journal of the American Medical Association,* Vol. 274, No. 13, p. 1002, Oct. 4, 1995.

19. Heath, Steve, *Microprocessor Architectures.* (RISC [reduced instruction set computer], CISC [complex instruction set computer], DSP [digital signal processor], Motorola MC68060, 68300 and Intel 80486, Pentium microprocessors) (Clays Ltd. St. Ives Place, 1995).

20. Heger, G., et al, "Physiological Measurement" (monitoring set-up for selection of parameters for detection of hypoglycemia in diabetic patients), *Medical and Biological Engineering and Computing,* Vol. 34, No. 1, January, 1996.

21. Hwang, Kai, *Advanced Computer Architecture* (parallelism, scalability, programmability, computer science series-electrical and computer engineering, computer organization and architecture), McGraw-Hill (New York, 1993).

22. *Informationweek* Weekly Magazine, Evans, Bob, Editor-In-Chief, Internet Address: bevans@cmp.com, Letters to Editor Address: iweekletters@cmp.com, May 20, 1996, Informationweek (600 Community Drive, Manhasset, NY 11030, 1996)

23. *Intel 6-/32-Bit Embedded Processor Handbook,* Intel Corporation, Microcomputer Company (Mt. Prospect, Ill., 1990).

24. *Internet World* Monthly Magazine (ISSN 1064-3923), Neubarrh, Michael, Editor-In-Chief, Internet Address: neubarrh@iw.com, June, 1996, Mecklermedia Corp (20 Ketchum St. Westport, CT 06880, 1996).

25. Kain, Richard Y., *Advanced Computer Architecture: A System Design Approach,* Prentice Hall (N.J., 1996).

26. Katzir, Abraham ed., *Proceedings of Biomedical Fiber Optic Instrumentation,* Society of Photo-optical Instrumentation Engineers (Washington, D.C., 1994).

27. "Laboratory Instrumentation Data Book on Plug-In Computer Equipment used in the Laboratory, (1) "Visual Designer," (2) "Signal Analyzer," (3) "DSPLAY" for digital filters," Intelligent Instrumentation Inc., Burr-Brown Corporation, (Tucson, Ariz., 1996). www.Instrument.com.

28. Lacanette, Keery, "Silicon Temperature Sensors: Theory and Applications" (including digital output sensors used in computer environments), *Measurements and Control Magazine,* Vol. 30, No. 2, 176, April, 1996.

29. Laugier, A., et al. "Remote Instrument Telemaintenance," *Computer Methods and Programs in Biomedicine,* Vol. 50, No. 2, p. 158 July, 1996.

30. Ledley, Robert S., *Computers in Biology and Medicine,* Pergamon Press (New York, 1993).

31. Lorenzi, Nancy M. and Robert T. Riley, *Organizational Aspects of Health Informatics* (computers in health care, managing technology change), Springer-Verlag (New York, 1995).

32. Maj, S. P., *The Use of Computers For Laboratory Automation,* Royal Society of Chemistry (Cambridge, England, 1993).

33. Maren, Alianna J., Craig T. Harston, and Robert M. Pap, *Handbook of Neural Computing Applications* (history, structures, hardware implementation, optical, pattern recognition, fault diagnosis, business, data communications, sonar, medical diagnosis, neural networks for man/machine systems, predictions beyond the year 2000), Academic Press, (New York, 1990).

34. *Medical and Healthcare Marketplace Guide,* Book and Computer CD-ROM, 12th ed. (in-depth information and marketplace guide on more than 5500 manufacturers in the health care industry; includes trends, future outlook and financial data by company, geography, products, and services; can be used to determine job opportunities), IDD Publication (Circulation Department, 18th Floor, 2 World Trade Center, NY, NY 10277-0516, Phone: 212-432-0045, Fax: 212-321-2336, 1996).

35. Merel, P., et al, "Robotics and Automation in the Laboratory" (system measures D NA genetic material from capillary electrophoresis in bone marrow graphs from the recipient before the graft, the donor, and the recipient after the graft), *Cancer Biotechnology,* p. 19, August 14, 1995.

36. Mitchell, H. J., *32-bit Microprocessors,* 2nd ed., (AT&T, Inmos, Intel 80346, Motorola MC69030, National Semiconductor Series 32000 Microprocessors, Oxford Blackwell Scientific Publications (London and Boston, 1991).

37. *Mitel Analog/Digital Telecom Components* (analog switches, signalling, CODECs, digital phone, voice compression, echo cancellation, interfaces, timing, control) Mitel Corporation, (Kanata, Ontario, Canada, 1995).

38. Morell, Jonathan A. and Mitchell Fleischer, *Advances in the Implementation and Impact of Computer Systems,* JAI Press, Inc. (Greenwich, Conn. And London, 1991).

39. *Motorola Microprocessor Data,* Vols. 1 and 2, Motorola Processor Products Group, Microcontroller Division (Austin, Tex., 1988).

40. Murray, Katherine, *Introduction to Personal Computers* (How-to manual for computer novices, computer basics for IBM and Mac [speed, memory, display microprocessor, memory, expansion, floppy/hard drives, keyboard, mouse, printer, modem], software review [spreadsheets, word processing, data management, integrated programs, desktop publishing, graphics, communications, educational, recreational], Que Corporation (Carmet, Ind., 1990).

41. Norman, Joseph, "Building the Computer-Based Patient Record," *Journal of the American Medical Association,* Vol. 273, No. 13, p. 1063, April 5, 1995.

42. "Operator Interfaces and Workstations," Measurements & Data Corporation (2994 W. Liberty Ave, Pittsburgh, Pa. 15216, 1996)

43. Osheroff, Jerome A., *Computers in Clinical Practice* (managing patients, information, and communication), American College of Physicians (Philadelphia, Pa. 1995).

44. Palmer, Philip E. S. and Thure Holm, "The Basics of Diagnostic Imaging," *World Health,* Vol. 48, No. 3, p. 12, May-June, 1995.

45. Ramo, Joshua C., "Winner Take All" (epic battle between Microsoft (Internet Explorer) and Netscape (Navigator) companies on Internet Browser software), *Time Magazine,* p. 56, September 16, 1996.

46. Ruffin, Marshall, "The Wonderful Evolution of Personal Computers," *Physician Executive,* Vol. 22, No. 5, p. 41, May, 1996.

47. Sabot, Gary W., *High Performance Computing* (problem solving with parallel and vector architectures), Addison-Wesley Publishing Company (New York, 1995).

48. *Seventh Symposium on Computer-Based Medical Systems,* IEEE Computer Society Press (Washington, D.C., 1994).

49. Shabot, Michael M. and Reed M. Gardner, *Decision Support Systems in Critical Care* (computers in medicine, data links, clinical alerting tools), Springer-Verlag (New York, 1994).

50. Sobel, David S. and Tom Ferguson, "Magnetic Resonance Imaging," *The People's Book of Medical Tests,* 1st ed. p. 385, Summib Books, New York, 1985.

51. Tau, Joseph K. H., *Health Management Information Systems* (theories, methods, and applications, state-of-the-art technologies, artificial intelligence, the new paradigm of total quality management (TQM), road map to the 21st century), Aspen Publishers, Inc. (Gaithersburg, Md. 1995).

52. Tan, Lenny, K.A., "Medical Imaging in Modern Medicine," *World Health,* Vol. 48, No. 3, p. 8, May-June, 1995.

53. Walker, Henry M., *The Limits of Computing* (problem solving, hardware reliability, software correctness, human factors, security issues), Jones and Bartlett Publishers (Boston and London, 1994).

54. Wasserman, Philip D., *Neural Computing* (theory and practice, fundamentals of artificial neural networks, backpropagation, statistical methods, bidirectional associative memories, optical neural networks, recognition, biological neural network), Van Nostrand Reinhold, New York, 1989.

55. Williamson, Michael R., *Essentials of Ultrasound* (physics of ultrasound and reading images), W. B. Saunders Company (Philadelphia, 1996).

56. Woodward, Beverly, "The Computer-Based Patient Record and Confidentiality," *New England Journal of Medicine,* Vol. 333, No. 21, p. 1419, Nov. 23, 1995.

57. Wyatt, Jeremy and Robert Walton, "Computer Based Prescribing: Improves Decision Making and Reduces Costs." *British Journal,* Vol. 311, No. 7014, Nov. 4, 1995.

Further Readings

1. Doyle, Edward, *"Computerized CME (Continuing Medical Education) Makes Strides with new Features-Patient Simulations and Instant Feedback,"* CD-ROM version of previous MKSAAP extends hundreds of color images and video clips that allow physicians to interact with the computer to ask questions and receive instant answers for quickly assessing correctness, (American College of Physicians Magazine-American Society of Internal Medicine, ACP-ASIM, Observer, 1996).

2. Brickell Research, Inc., *"Palmtop Computing,"* (Computers in Medicine (sm) Online Quarterly Newsletter on computer applications for the medical profession, 2nd Quarter Edition, 1999, cmeditor@brickellreserach.com).

3. Clifford Pickover, Ed., "Future Health: Computers in Medicine in the 21st Century", (St Martin's Press, NY, November 1997).

4. Morse, Gary and McCormick, Kathleen A., The Consumer Search of Health Information on the Internet (computer assisted instruction video recording), advantages and disadvantages of the existence of consumer information on the Internet, Health & Sciences Network, division of PRIMEDIA Healthcare (1998).

5. Slack, Warner V., Forward by Ralph Nader, Cybermedicine: how computing empowers doctors and patients for better health care, Jossey-Bass Publishers (San Francisco, 1997).

6. *Embedded Systems Programming Magazine,* Lindsey Vereen, Editor-In-Chief, Ivereen@mfi.com, November, 1998, Vol. 11, No. 10, Buyers Guide Issue, software and hardware, and firmware tools for embedded systems development, integrated circuits, and plug-in boards, (reprints 415-905-2591, subscribe 847-647-8602, Chicago, IL, www.embedded.com 1998).

7. *Embedded Systems Development Magazine,* Halligan, Editorial Director, thalligan@penton.com, November 1998, Embedding the Internet, hardware and software fault tolerance, (Penton Media, Inc., 611 Route #46 West Hasbrouck Heights, NJ 07604, 201-393-6060, 1998).

8. Spera, Gabriel, "DSPs: A Growing Option for Medical Applications," discusses improving digital signal processor (DSP) architectures, which handle more instructions at higher speeds, minimizing board space, development time, and overall project cost, *Medical Electronics Manufacturing Magazine,* Buyers Guide Issue, Spring, 1998, (Canon Communications LLC Publisher, 3340 Ocean Park Blvd, Suite 1000, Santa Monica CA 90405, 1998).

9. Curran, Lawrence J., Contributing Editor, "Medical Researchers Apply High-Speed Imaging To Simulate Blood Flow," Dr. Timothy Liem, vascular surgeon at University of Missouri School of Medicine, Columbia, MO, uses high speed imaging to look at blood flow in diseased arteries with atherosclerosis (a form of arteriosclerosis), *Vision Systems Design Magazine,* PenWell Publishing Co., 1421 S. Sheridan, Tulsa, OK 74112, 918-832-9257, www.vision-systems-design.com, April, 1999).

10. Haystead, John., Contributing Editor, "Medical X-rays and Digital Radiology Advance Image Diagnostics", General Electric Medical Systems (GE), Milwaukee, WI, use of new amorphous silicon/cesium iodide bank of photodiodes to produce digital X-ray images, *Vision Systems Design Magazine,* PenWell Publishing Co., 1421 S. Sheridan, Tulsa, OK 74112, 918-832-9257, www.vision-systems-design.com, April, 1999).

11. Wilson, Andrew., Contributing Editor, "Technology Trends: Dual-PCI-bus Computer Increases I/O Bandwidth," Microdisc Corp., Yardley, PA has produced a high speed computer chip set using a 400-MHz Pentium Xeon processor that allows faster scan rates using the peripheral component interconnect (PCI) in camera and other systems, *Vision Systems Design Magazine,* PenWell Publishing Co., 1421 S. Sheridan, Tulsa, OK 74112, 918-832-9257, www.vision-systems-design.com, April, 1999).

12. Wilson, Andrew, Contributing Editor, "Technology Trends: Robots and Vision Systems Handle Packaged Seeds," General Electric Medical Systems (GE), Milwaukee, WI builds a new CT/i (computed tomography)

system that produces images with 1280 ×
1024 pixel resolution using an Imagraph
Corp. a 9-bit accurate PC board and software
which stabilizes gain, jitter, and phase in both
the analog front-end and the phase-lock-loop,
Vision Systems Design Magazine, PenWell
Publishing Co., 1421 S. Sheridan, Tulsa, OK
74112, 918-832-9257, www.vision-systems-
design.com, November, 1998).

13. Murray, Charles J., Senior Regional Technical
    Editor, "Computers Pinpoint Brain Tumors-
    image-guided techniques improve surgical
    accuracy and enable patients to recover more
    quickly," describes Dr. Mary Beth Dunn, brain
    surgeon, who uses a special computer to
    precisely image a brain tumor in a five-year
    old girl, prior to cutting a 2-inch diameter hole
    in exactly the right place on her cranium,
    Design News magazine, Vol. 53, No. 11, June
    8, 1998 (Cahners Business Information
    dn@cahners.com, 275 Washington Street,
    Newton, MA 02158, 617-964-3030,
    www.designnews.com, 1998).

14. Hines, John W. Ames Research Center and
    Somps, Christopher J., Ricks, Robert D., and
    Mundt, Carsten W. of Sverdrup Technology,
    Inc., "Biotelemetry Using Implanted Unit to
    Monitor Preterm Labor-pressure changes are
    telemetered to the outside and analyzed to
    detect intrauterine contractions," Refer to
    ARC-14280, *NASA Tech Briefs Magazine,*
    May, 1999, (Ames Research Center, Moffett
    Field, CA, 650-604-5104, www.nasatech.com,
    1999).

CHAPTER 23

Radiology and Nuclear Medicine Equipment

23-1 Objectives

1. Be able to list uses of diagnostic and therapeutic X-ray and nuclear medicine equipment.
2. Be able to describe the origin and list the properties and measurements of X-rays (atomic and nuclear physics).
3. Be able to describe the nature of radioactivity, including types of nuclear radiation.
4. Be able to list the dangerous effects to health from X-ray and nuclear radiation exposure.
5. Know how to draw a diagram of an X-ray tube and describe the production of X-rays.
6. Know how to draw a simplified block diagram of an X-ray machine and describe its operation, including generation, detection, and display on a photographic plate.

7. Be able to list the external controls and their use in X-ray machines (MA, kV, and exposure time settings).
8. Know how to draw a simplified block diagram of a fluoroscopic machine and describe its operation, including detection by fluorescence and display on a CRT.
9. Know how to draw a simplified block diagram of a nuclear medicine system and describe its operation, including detection by scintillation crystals, amplification by photomultiplier tubes, and display on a CRT.
10. Be able to describe computer systems used in X-ray and nuclear medicine equipment.
11. Be able to list calibration, typical faults, troubleshooting, and maintenance procedures on X-ray and nuclear medicine equipment.

23-2 Self-evaluation questions

These questions test your prior knowledge of the material in this chapter. Look for the answers as you read the text. After you have finished studying the chapter, try answering these questions and those at the end of the chapter.

1. What equipment is used to diagnose bone fractures, view functioning organs, and measure organ activity?

2. What type of equipment is used to treat (therapeutic function) cancer by irradiation of tumors?

3. Describe the nature of X-rays and nuclear radiation.

4. List the dangers to health from X-rays and nuclear radiation exposure.

5. How does an X-ray tube produce X-rays?

6. From a simple block diagram, describe the operation of an X-ray machine, including external controls (generation, detection, display).

7. From a simplified block diagram, describe the operation of a fluoroscopic machine (generation, detection, and display).

8. From a simplified block diagram, describe the operation of a nuclear medicine system (injected substances, detection, amplification, display).

9. What purpose do computers serve in X-ray and nuclear medicine equipment?

10. Describe general troubleshooting and maintenance procedures for X-ray and nuclear medicine equipment.

23-3 Types and uses of X-ray and nuclear medicine equipment

X-ray machines are devices that generate exceedingly *high-frequency* (short wave-length), high-energy *electromagnetic waves* that penetrate the body during medical procedures. They are used in the radiology department. These machines serve diagnostic (measurement) and therapeutic (treatment) purposes. X-ray equipment has been used for many years to produce pictures of bodily tumors and skeletal fractures or deformations. While they are part of quality medicine in the modern world, they can be extremely *dangerous* (over the short and long term) causing nausea, vomiting, dizziness, sterility, burns, genetic mutations, cancer, and death if used incorrectly or in excess. All personnel operating the equipment should stand behind a lead wall or wear a protective powdered iron apron.

X-rays are high-energy waves (0.01 to 100 Å) that pass through the body and indicate relative tissue density on a photosensitive plate. Essentially, bones are dense and pass less X-ray than soft tissues, such as blood vessels, organs, and muscle. The X-ray that does not pass through (transmitted) is absorbed and stored within the body in accumulating doses. High accumulated doses over the long term represent a health hazard.

X-ray machines generally fall into the following *categories:*

1. *Diagnostic still picture* X-ray is used to examine bones and internal organ and tissue structures. The wavelengths are usually 0.01 to 1 Å, and energy levels vary with tissues to be observed. Broken bones and tumors can be detected.

2. *Diagnostic continuous picture* X-ray *(fluoroscopy)* is used to examine organ systems as they are functioning. Contrast substances (opaque to X-rays) fill bodily cavities and show anatomical shapes. The wavelengths are usually similar to still picture exposures, but the energy levels are considerably less due to the long exposure times. Tumors and blockages can be observed.

3. *Diagnostic motion picture* X-ray *(angiography)* is used to examine circulatory systems as they are functioning. Contrast fluids (opaque to X-rays) are introduced, for example, into the blood circulation of the heart (cardioangiography), kidney (renal angiography), or brain (cerebroangiography, chapter 13). X-ray still picture exposures are then taken, one every five seconds or faster, and played back on a motion picture machine. This gives the effect of dynamic circulatory action through the blood vessels. Blockages can be visualized.

4. *Diagnostic still picture* X-ray scans *(tomograms)* are used to examine bones, organs, and tissues from many different angles. As in brain scans (chapter 13),

whole body scans are radiographs taken through successive scanning by highly collimated X-ray beams. Small contrast differences in selected planes can be seen and *provide considerably more information* than simple two-dimensional one plane or two-dimensional two plane (stereoscopy) X-ray exposures. Ultrasonic scanning is another technique using high-frequency sound waves instead of X-rays. X-ray *computed tomography* (CT) is a technique of recording and processing a set of image projections that represent a reconstruction of the object scanned. Essentially, a *thin layer* of the structure is *tomographically* (in sections) scanned with a pencil beam. The X-ray attenuation is then recorded with a *scintillation counter* in groups of parallel scans. Many-angle X-ray exposures are obtained every degree for 180°, and the projected scans (three-dimensional information) are stored in a computer. Through a complex program or algorithm, the original object is redrawn by the computer and displayed on a two-dimensional (CRT). Colors have been used to indicate various tissue densities. A scanning layout can be seen in Figure 13-2 and a tomograph of the skull (brain scan) appears in Figure 13-3.

5. *Therapeutic* X-ray is, essentially, the same as diagnostic X-ray except that the aim of therapy is to eradicate and destroy cancerous tissues and tumors. Whereas some healthy tissue is also exposed, it is hoped that it will regenerate while abnormal tissue will not. X-ray energy penetration, location, and dosage must be carefully chosen, and this can be done by using a scanning device first to pinpoint the boundaries of the tumor. Special lead forms are also used to protect surrounding healthy tissues. The wavelengths are usually long, ranging up to 100 Å, and energy levels vary according to tissue radiosensitivity.

Nuclear medicine equipment is similar to X-ray scanning machines from the standpoint of radiation detection (scintillation counters). It is somewhat different from angiography and considerably safer. Small amounts of short-lived radioactive isotopes (i.e., iodine 131 taken up by the thyroid gland) are introduced into the cardiovascular system. They accumulate in various target organs throughout the body. The concentrated radioactivity is measured with a *scintillation counter,* which responds to impinging alpha, beta, or gamma rays given off by the particular radioactive material used. The amount of substance taken up by a specific gland indicates (for diagnosis) the physiological function of the gland. Since very little radioactive substance is required and its emission life is very short, the danger to the patient is minimal. Special nuclear materials can also be used for therapy to treat tumors.

Nuclear medicine machines generally fall into the following categories:

1. *Diagnostic* low-level radiation (isotope) tracer detection devices used to measure target organ function. Radiopharmaceuticals injected and taken up by an organ are measured for concentration by gamma-ray cameras, rectilinear scanners, fixed detectors or scintillation counters, and survey instrumentation.

2. *Therapeutic* low-level localized radiation isotope source used to treat tumorous growths.

The radiology and nuclear medicine departments house the most costly equipment in the hospital or clinic. X-ray equipment gets high usage from almost every area of medical specialty because X-ray techniques allow visualization of internal body structures without surgery. X-ray is a noninvasive procedure compared with other techniques, although radiation does pass through the body. Nuclear medicine equipment is being used more frequently today and represents a minor invasive process. Since equipment demand is high and total money received from services to patients is enormous, biomedical electronic servicing specialists are called frequently to repair these machines.

23-4 Origin and nature of X-rays

The modern era of atomic and nuclear physics (twentieth century) has paved the way for understanding the origin and nature of X-ray radiation.

X-rays are actually electromagnetic waves, as are light and radio waves. The principal difference is a matter of *frequency* or *wavelength*. Figure 23-1 shows a spectrum chart giving the relationship between radio waves, light, and X-rays. Electromagnetic waves are different from other types of waves, such as sound or water. Electromagnetic waves can travel in a vacuum or in outer space. Some of the basic properties of electromagnetic waves are as follows:

1. They obey the relationship $V = F\lambda$; where V is the velocity, F is the frequency, and λ is the wavelength.

2. They propagate in a straight line.

3. They obey the *inverse square law* ($1/d^2$); their intensity falls off inversely proportionally to the square of the distance as they propagate away from the source.

4. They produce interference and diffraction patterns.

5. They are not deflected by magnetic fields.

The inverse square law can be demonstrated with the use of an ordinary flashlight. Turn on the switch and point it at a blank wall. Measure the distance between the light and the wall, and note the wall intensity with a light meter. Now move to a point exactly twice as far away and note the rapidly reducing level of illumination. Two observations are predominant. First, the intensity at any one spot has decreased to one-fourth of the previous intensity. Second, the overall area that is illuminated has increased. In fact, one will find that the increase in the illuminated area has the same factor as the decrease in spot intensity. This is because the light energy from the flashlight remained constant, while the area of illumination increased. This same phenomenon is critical in medical X-ray systems.

Essentially, three types of radiation exist:

1. *Alpha rays*—positively charged (ionized) particles of helium nuclei whose velocity is moderate (approximately 5% of the speed of light) and whose penetration depth is small (approximately 5 cm).

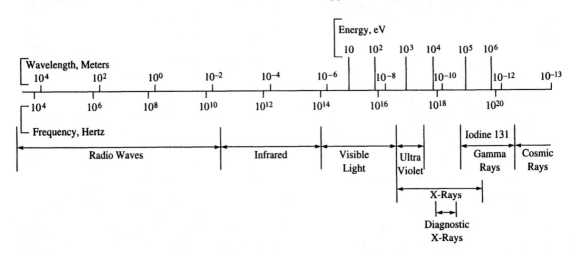

Figure 23-1
Electromagnetic spectrum chart (relative wavelengths of radio and lightwaves and X-rays).

2. *Beta rays*—negatively charged electrons of widely varying velocity (may be up to the speed of light) and whose penetration depth is small.

3. *Gamma rays* (10^{14} MHz) and *X-rays* (10^{10} MHz)—electromagnetic waves that travel at the speed of light and have high penetration depending upon wavelength (energy). The energy is expressed as:

$$E = hf \qquad (23-1)$$

where

   E is energy in joules (J)

   h is Planck's constant (6.624×10^{-34} J-s)

   f is the frequency (Hz)

The electron volt (1 eV = 1.602×10^{-19} J) is the usual expression for gamma ray radiation energy. Furthermore, the radiated wavelength (distance the wave travels in one cycle) can be calculated from the following expression:

$$\lambda = \frac{c}{f} \qquad (23-2)$$

where

   λ is the wavelength in meters, centimeters, or angstrom units

   f is the X-ray frequency in Hz

   c is the speed of light (3×10^8 m/s)

The angstrom unit (Å) is commonly used to measure wavelength.

$$1 \text{ Å} = 10^{-8} \text{ cm} = 10^{-10} \text{ m}$$

Higher frequencies (shorter wavelengths) *possess greater energy* than lower frequencies but require higher voltages to produce.

Example 23-1

Given the energy level of 6.624×10^{-18} J imparted to an electron stream by an X-ray device, calculate the frequency in MHz and wavelength in m, cm, and Å of the X-ray beam.

Solution

$$f = \frac{E}{h} = \frac{6.624 \times 10^{-18} \text{ J}}{6.624 \times 10^{-34} \text{ J-s}} = 10^{10} \times 10^6 \text{ Hz}$$

$$f = \mathbf{10^{10} \text{ MHz}}$$

$$\lambda = \frac{c}{f} = \frac{3 \times 10^8 \text{ m/s}}{10^{10} \text{ MHz}}$$

$$\lambda = \mathbf{3 \times 10^{-8} \text{ m}} \text{ (low-frequency or soft X-ray)}$$

$$\lambda = 3 \times 10^{-8} \text{ m} \times \frac{10^2 \text{ cm}}{\text{m}} = \mathbf{3 \times 10^{-6} \text{ cm}}$$

$$\lambda = 3 \times 10^{-6} \text{ cm} \times \frac{\text{Å}}{10^{-8} \text{ cm}} = \mathbf{3 \times 10^2 \text{ Å}}$$

Basically, the following quantum effects exist for electromagnetic waves (X-rays included):

1. *Photoelectric effect.* The photoelectric effect was first noted by Heinrich Hertz in 1887 and won Albert Einstein the Nobel Prize in 1905. The photoelectric effect is the emission of electrons from a clean metallic surface (phototube) when electromagnetic radiation (light waves or X-rays) falls onto that surface. Three other effects are thermionic, field, and secondary emission. Two facts have been noted about the photoelectric effect. First is that the phototube potential is totally *independent of light intensity.* Thus, the energy of the emitted electrons is not a function of light intensity. The light intensity affects only the number of electrons emitted, not their relative energy level. Second, phototube potential is *dependent on the light color.*

2. *Compton effect.* The Compton effect is a phenomenon that relates to a photon's (packet of energy) ability to transfer only a part of its energy to a charged electrical particle such as an electron in a collision. The photon still exists after the collision because only part of its energy is transferred to the electron. It does, however, exhibit a lower frequency than it had prior to the collision. This lower frequency or longer wavelength (color change) is caused by lost energy.

3. *Bremsstrahlung.* This phenomenon is especially important to the study of medical X-ray apparatus because it is primarily responsible for the generation of the radiation in the X-ray machine. The word *Bremsstrahlung* in German means *breaking radiation.* As shown in Figure 23-2, an electron with an initial kinetic energy E_i approaches and is deflected by the heavy nucleus of a nearby atom. After the deflection, the electron has taken a new (lower) energy level E_d. The law of conservation of energy in this case reveals that the energy of the deflected electron and photon equals that of the incident electron. The energy level of the incident electron minus that of the deflected electron becomes a photon, and if the loss of energy is sufficient, the wavelength of the photon will be in the X-ray region of the electromagnetic spectrum. More energy lost means higher X-ray frequency (hard X-rays).

$$E \text{ (incident electron)} - E \text{ (deflected electron)}$$
$$= E \text{ (photon)} \qquad (23\text{-}3)$$

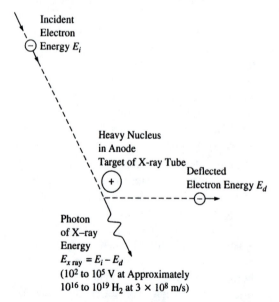

Incident
Electron
Energy E_i

Heavy Nucleus
in Anode
Target of X-ray Tube
Deflected
Electron Energy E_d

Photon
of X–ray
Energy
$E_{x\,ray} = E_i - E_d$
(10^2 to 10^5 V at Approximately
10^{16} to 10^{19} H$_2$ at 3×10^8 m/s)

Figure 23-2
Bremsstrahlung collision resulting in X-ray production.

Ionizing radiation is biologically harmful and is caused by high-energy atomic collision that produces alpha particles (helium nuclei), beta particles (electrons), and gamma rays (photons).

23-5 Nature and types of nuclear radiation

Atomic structure is extensively considered in the field of atomic and nuclear physics. Medical radiation and nuclear physics is a specialty within this field, and many texts contain detailed explanations of the theory. This discussion is directed at equipment technology, and only a brief description of nuclear medicine radioisotopes follows.

In general, radioactivity is grouped into two classes:

1. *Natural radioactivity* results from the natural atomic flux (constant motion). Some collisions within an atomic nucleus produce an impact energy that exceeds the nucleus binding energy. Subnuclear particles then escape through *disintegration.* The nuclear *decay process* produces nuclear radiation of particles (alpha and beta) and rays (gamma). Natural radiation occurs in materials involving a sequence of steps called a radioactive series. Four series currently exist: thorium (decay to stable lead 208), actinium (decay to stable lead 207), uranium (decay to lead 206), and neptunium (decay to bismuth 209).

2. *Artificial radioactivity* is the same as the natural type, except the radionuclides (radioactive nuclei) are synthetic. These artificial substances (not naturally occurring) are produced by bombarding stable nuclides with neutrons, protons, deutrons, or alpha particles in a linear accelerator or cyclotron. *Ions* (atoms with a net positive or negative charge) and *isotopes* (atoms with more neutrons than protons) are produced. Frequently used medical isotopes (radiopharmaceuticals) are shown in Table 23-1.

TABLE 23-1 SOME MEDICAL RADIOISOTOPES

Isotope	Radiological half-life	Predominant radiation half-life	Some target organs
^{2}H (hydrogen)	Stable	—	—
^{2}H (hydrogen)	12.3 years	Beta	—
^{14}C (carbon)	5770 years	Beta	Pancreas
^{24}Na (sodium)	15 hours	Beta	Blood
^{32}P (phosphorus)	14.3 days	Beta	Liver
^{42}K (potassium)	12.4 hours	Beta	Cardiovascular system
^{45}Ca (calcium)	165 days	Beta	Bones
^{85}Sr (strontium)	10.26 years	Gamma	Bones
^{51}Cr (chromium)	27.8 days	Gamma	Urinary tract
^{58}Co (cobalt)	71 days	Gamma	Urinary tract
^{82}Br (barium)	36 hours	Gamma	Intestinal tract
^{131}I (iodine)	8.07 days	Gamma	Thyroid, urinary tract, and gastrointestinal system
^{198}Au (gold)	64.8 hours	Gamma	Liver
^{197}Hg (mercury)	65 hours	Beta	Kidney
^{99m}Tc (technetium)	6 hours	Gamma	Spleen, brain, lung, and cardiovascular system

23-6 Units for measuring radioactivity

The following units are used to indicate the intensity of radioactivity. Essentially, they all indicate how many nuclear disintegrations occur in a given time.

1. *Curie (Ci)*—amount of radioactivity in one gram of radium (3.7×10^{10} disintegrations per second).

2. *Roentgen (R)*—unit of radiation exposure or amount of X-radiation that will produce 2.08×10^9 ion pairs per cubic centimeter of air at standard temperature and pressure (STP). Usable units are the milliroentgen (mR) and microroentgen (μR).

3. *Radiation absorbed dose (rad)*—One rad is the radiation dose that will result in an energy absorption of 1.0×10^{-2} J per kilogram of irradiated material. For practical purposes:

$$1 \text{ R} = 1 \text{ rad}$$

Absorbed dose in rads = exposure in roentgens $\times$ 0.834 $\times$ factor of absorbing material.

4. *Dose rate*—amount of radiation expressed in roentgens administered or produced per unit time.

5. *X-ray intensity*—dose rate per unit area irradiated.

23-7 Health dangers from X-ray and nuclear radiation

Radiological safety cannot be overemphasized. The effects of cumulative X-ray dosage of ionizing radiation may result in *mutations*—genetic changes resulting from damage to chromosomes; *physical illness*—vomiting, headache, dizziness, loss of hair, and burns; and *death*—destruction of vital physiological systems such as nervous, cardiovascular, respiratory, renal, and digestive systems and tissues.

23-8 Generation of X-rays in an X-ray tube

X-rays are generated by a high-vacuum X-ray diode tube in which electrons are accelerated to high velocities (using a high-voltage power supply up to 100 kV). Radiation intensity is obtained by varying the *high voltage, current,* and *time of exposure.* The radiation is filtered and formed (collimated) to produce optimal contrast relative to the patient dose. The *X-ray tube* (high-vacuum diode) shown in Figure 23-3 operates by emitting electrons from a heated cathode tungsten filament toward a rotating high-voltage anode disc. X-rays arise from the target disc at right angles and are focused by the collimator. Most of the energy is heat. Image *intensifier* or *photomultiplier tubes* allow greater viewing contrast and hence less required patient radiation dose. *Images* are received and viewed on an imaging device (photographic film plate or *fluoroscopic screen*). Light and dark areas on the film represent high and low tissue penetration, respectively. Dynamic (ongoing) radiographic images, when viewed on a fluoroscopic screen, are termed fluoroscopy.

Two methods are used to overcome the heat problem in X-ray tubes (the target anode must be able to withstand tremendous heat). One is to construct the target anode of tungsten alloy, which is embedded in a *large mass of copper.* A design trade-off is necessary. Maximum heat capacity results from a large target area, but the best X-ray photographic resolution results from a small target area. Forming a *bevel* on the anode contributes greatly to good heat dissipation and high resolution.

The other solution is to use the *rotating anode* shown in Figure 23-3. The spot target of the previous design is now replaced with a moving (i.e., rotating) target on the rim of a disc. The electron source (cathode) is placed so that it will impinge on only a small spot on the rim of the disc. This keeps the focal area down to a few square millimeters, yet the structure is large enough to permit the dissipation of a large amount of heat. Anodes of this type might rotate at 10,000 rpm, and the ro-

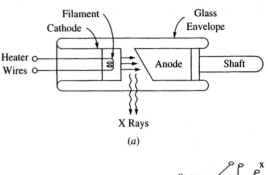

(a)

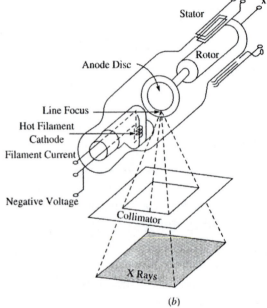

(b)

Figure 23-3
X-ray tube with rotating anode. *(a)* Basic tube. *(b)* Basic tube with X-ray output. (From *Medicine and Clinical Engineering,* by Bertil Jacobson and John Webster. Prentice Hall. Used by permission.)

tating disc shaft spins as a result of magnetic coupling through the sealed glass envelope.

The inside of the X-ray tube consists of a *vacuum* to ensure an undisturbed path for electrons and long anode life. Coefficients of thermal expansion of the glass case become important as the tube heats up. Too much heat on these tubes will burn them out quickly. Special microcomputers have been used to warn the operator of excessive anode heat.

Stationary anodes are used mostly in low-energy-level X-ray machines, while the more common rotating anodes are used in higher-energy machines.

The housing used for the X-ray tube must provide three types of protection in addition to the physical or mechanical protection:

1. High voltage—grounded metal housing with high-quality electrical insulation and oil-filled housing to withstand 10 to 150 kV.

2. Heat dissipation—properly constructed anode and oil-filled housing. If excessive heat expands oil too far, a microswitch activates a control circuit to turn high-voltage power off.

3. Radiation shielding—properly constructed metal casing.

23-9 Block diagram and operation of an X-ray machine

X-ray machines generate high-energy, high-frequency electromagnetic waves (X-rays) for use in diagnosing and treating disease and physical malfunctions. To accomplish this, X-ray machines have the following major sections, as shown in Figure 23-4:

1. *Multitap ac line autotransformer,* which allows selection of taps to compensate for incoming line variations. These also permit the operator to choose voltages for specific applications.

2. *X-ray tube filament circuit and transformer,* which transforms the ac line to supply power for heating the cathode filament. This power can be selected by taps to change filament heat (filament mA), which changes X-ray tube current (tube mA) and, hence, total X-ray energy delivered to the patient.

3. *X-ray tube high-voltage circuit, transformer, and bridge rectifier,* which transforms the ac line to supply the high dc voltage for accelerating electrons from cathode to anode. The high voltage can be selected by taps to change the kV_p (kilovolt peak) and, hence, total X-ray energy delivered to the patient.

4. *Timing circuit,* which controls turn-on, turn-off, and length of X-ray exposure delivered to the patient.

Essentially, *three basic controls* exist on X-ray machines to control patient X-ray dose (penetrating quality, quantity, and timing). These are interrelated and must be properly chosen to suit the slim or obese patient. Good photographic results are sometimes difficult to obtain. These controls are *filament heat* control (mA) for exposure strength, not depth; *kilovolt* control (kV) for penetration depth and contrast; and *timing* devices for time exposure length.

It is extremely important to observe *X-ray tube heat ratings.* Excessive heat will damage a very expensive tube, and the cost and inconvenience of replacement are equally high.

X-ray emission from the tube can be improved by using filters, stationary grids, moving grids (Potter-Buckey diaphragm), cones, cylinders, diaphragms, collimators, and intensifiers (image intensifier tube to increase brightness of the photographic image).

The *multitap ac line autotransformer,* T_1 (shown in Figure 23-4*b*), has several purposes. One is to compensate for normal input line variations by adjusting S_1. When the line is low, S_1 is set near the top until the line-voltage meter indicates normal. The line strap setting, S_2, is set by the installation engineer or technician initially (110 to 450 V ac). The autotransformer also contains switch settings for coarse (S_3, 10 kV) and fine S_4, 1 kV) high-voltage selection.

The *X-ray tube filament circuit* consists of selector switch S_5, filament transformer, T_2, and the filament of the X-ray tube T_2 provides isolation from the high-voltage transformer and an added measure of safety. *Electrocution* (see chapter 19) from as much as 150 kV is a potential danger on X-ray machines. Switch S_5 selects 25, 50, or 100 mA for filament current as adjusted by filament resistors during calibration. As X-ray tubes age, more filament current is required to achieve constant X-ray intensity. A filament current meter, M_1, shows the milliamperes in the X-ray cathode.

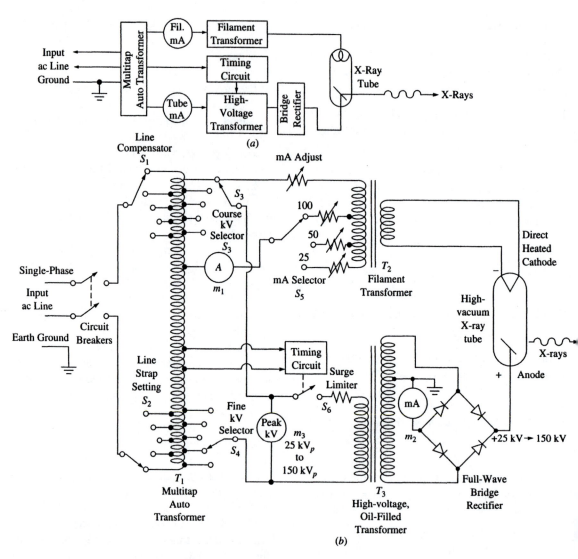

Figure 23-4
Sections of an X-ray machine. *(a)* Simplified block diagram. *(b)* Circuit diagram.

The *high-voltage circuit* is, essentially, the power supply for the X-ray machine. A separate oil-filled, high-voltage transformer, T_3, receives selectable voltages from coarse and fine kV selector switches (S_3 and S_4) and provides high voltage to the high-voltage diodes. The diode bridge provides full-wave rectified unfiltered dc voltage to the X-ray tube anode. An X-ray tube current meter, M_2, shows the milliamperes passing through the tube,

and meter, M_3, indicates the peak kilovoltage applied to the anode. Higher peak voltages (energy) produce higher-frequency X-rays and greater patient penetration capability (see Example 23-1).

Many larger X-ray machines have *three-phase power* applied. Instead of 120 peaks per second in single phase, 360 peaks per second occur from three-phase. The ripple frequency is higher and, hence, the effective high voltage is greater. Usually the primary windings are connected in the *delta* and the secondary in the *wye* configuration. This gives a more efficient system, and greater sustained energy levels can be obtained. This scheme is, however, more expensive since transformers with three windings and 12 diodes are required.

The *timing circuit* consists of a mechanical motor-driven or electronic counter that closes switch S_6 and applies high voltage to the X-ray tube anode for short periods of time (1/120 s to several seconds). A *mechanical timer* is a handwound spring of a clock. A *synchronous timer* is also *mechanical* and consists of a synchronous motor driven from the 60-Hz ac line that closes switch contacts. These contacts are protected by a surge-limiting resistor. An *electronic timer* uses an *electronic switch,* such as a transistor timed by a digital circuit.

Figure 23-5 shows a fixed X-ray machine, and Figure 23-6 shows a portable one.

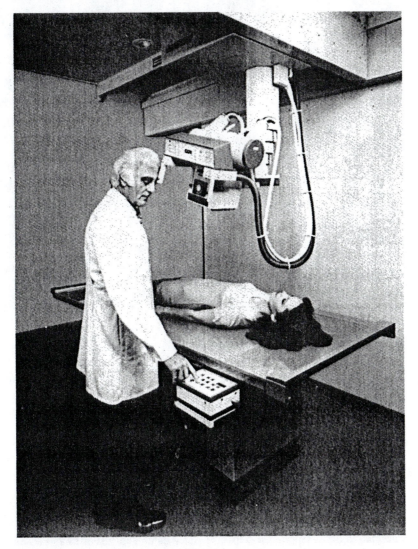

Figure 23-5
Fixed X-ray machine. (Photo courtesy of CGR Medical Corporation)

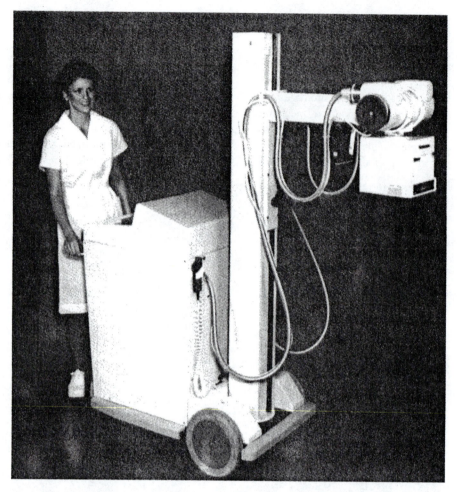

Figure 23-6
Portable X-ray machine. (Photo courtesy of CGR Corporation)

23-10 Block diagram and operation of a fluoroscopic machine

Fluoroscopic machines are X-ray machines that generate soft X-rays (reduced frequency and intensity) to produce dynamic visualizations on a fluoroscope. Internal body organs are viewed through the use of a contrast medium that is opaque to X-rays. Patient dosage should not exceed 10 R per minute. Transmitted X-rays fall upon a fluorescent plate or screen as a function of varying tissue density. Fluorescence is the emission of visible light produced when X-rays fall upon crystals in the coating of the screen.

As shown in Figure 23-7, the major sections are the X-ray machine (subsections previously discussed), fluoroscope image pickup, and CRT or closed-circuit video system. The X-ray image falling on a fluorescent grid causes a visible "light" picture to appear. This is optically focused by a lens on the film of a motion picture (automatic) camera. The film can be played back at a later date. The visual image is also focused on a phototube lens and made brighter by an image en-

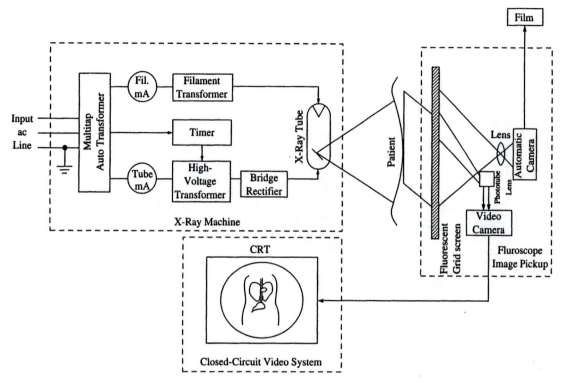

Figure 23-7
Simplified block diagram of a fluoroscope machine.

hancer. A video camera converts the light image into an electrical video signal, which is delivered to a CRT and displayed through a closed-circuit video system. This gives a real-time or instantaneous visualization. A fluoroscope machine is shown in Figure 23-8.

23-11 Block diagram and |operation of a nuclear medicine system

Nuclear medicine systems are used to count radioactive decay from isotopes that have been injected into the body in small amounts and taken up by a target organ to measure its activity. The basic components are a gamma ray camera, rectilinear scanner, fixed detector for in vitro samples, scintillation counter, and survey instrument.

As shown in Figure 23-9a, a *Geiger-Mueller tube* radiation detector counts beta particles. Beta particles passing through the gas mixture in the tube cause ionization, and the electrons are collected by the anode and the positive ions by the cathode via a high potential of approximately 1 kV. Therefore, each beta particle causes a brief pulse of current. The total number of current pulses, electronically counted over a given period of time, indicates the radiation intensity falling on the mica window.

As shown in Figure 23-9b, a scintillation crystal detector with photomultiplier tube measures gamma radiation intensity. The incident gamma rays are detected by the crystal, and flashes of light are produced and reflected onto the cathode of the photoamplifier tube. The dynodes multiply the electrical signal in a secondary emission process

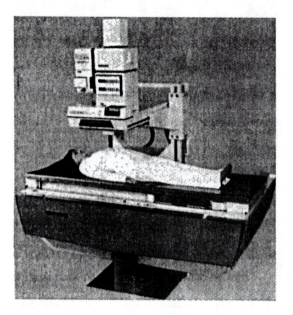

Figure 23-8
Fluoroscope machine. (Photo courtesy of CGR Medical Corporation)

by as much as 10 million to produce an appreciable current pulse. Current pulses are produced for rays striking the fixed surface area of the scintillation detector and are then counted to indicate radiation intensity (rays per second).

A *nuclear medicine system* (rectilinear scanner), as shown in Figure 23-10, consists of a detector-collimator, amplifier, analyzer, and recorder. The detector-collimator, driven by the scanner motor assembly, scans back and forth in a linear fashion. A graph or contour map of radioactivity can then be drawn indicating the amount of radioactive isotope taken up by the target organ. Improper amounts indicate organ malfunction.

The *detector-collimator* typically uses an Na-I crystal to detect the radiation collimated toward its surface. The photomultiplier tube intensifies the signal, after which it is linearly amplified. Its pulse is analyzed for comparisons between successive events. Numbers of pulses per unit of time are important. The dot scan recorder produces a map of

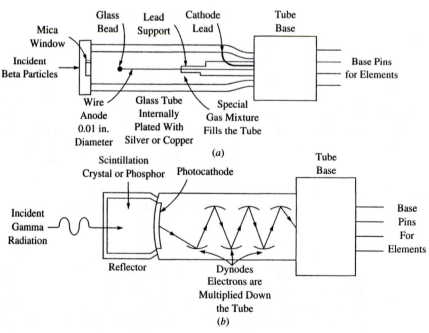

Figure 23-9
Nuclear medicine system. *(a)* Geiger-Mueller tube. *(b)* Scintillation crystal detector with photo multiplier tube.

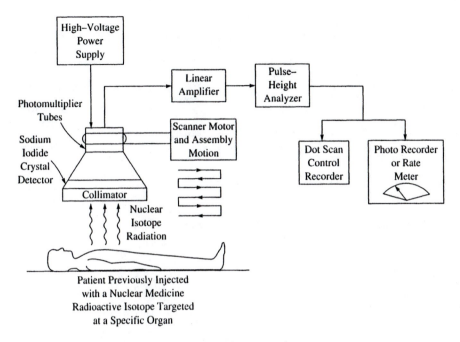

Figure 23-10
Simplified block diagram of a nuclear medicine system (rectilinear scanner).

dots or dash marks on paper representing the distribution of radioactivity. The photographic recorder produces a photograph of light flashes. Recordings move simultaneously with the scanning device to produce one line scan in unison. Figure 23-11 illustrates a nuclear medicine system.

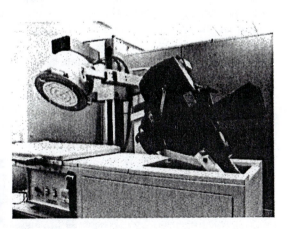

Figure 23-11
Nuclear medicine system.

The *gamma ray camera,* shown in Figure 23-12, produces an image in a different manner than that of a scanner. Gamma rays interact with a large sodium iodide scintillation crystal in the camera, and the scintillations (flashes) are observed by an array of photomultiplier tubes. Typically, 19 tubes are used, and a position analyzer evaluates the flashes from four crystal quadrants. Flashes are produced on an oscilloscope display when the gamma ray meets the pulse-height analyzer requirements. A Polaroid or 35 mm camera photographs the flashes on the oscilloscope to produce a scintiphoto. Up to 500,000 counts, for example, may accumulate for brain scans on the CRT screen.

23-12 Computer systems used in X-ray and nuclear medicine equipment

Computers serve two basic purposes in X-ray and nuclear medicine equipment: *image enhancement recording and analysis* of dynamic data. Computer

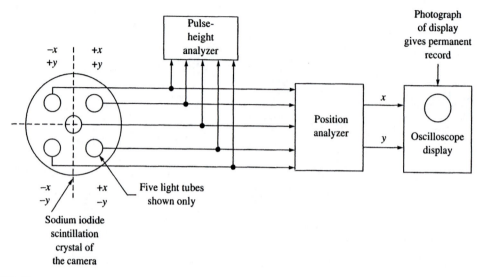

Figure 23-12
Simplified block diagram of a gamma-ray camera.

enhancement of X-ray images can be accomplished by measuring fine graduations of exposure intensity on a film or plate. However, the human eye can detect a remarkably small difference in shades of gray, and many physicians prefer to read the X-ray negative directly. Computer techniques are also useful to enhance the response of a gamma-ray camera to correct for the nonuniformity of the crystal face.

CT scanners use computer algorithms for pattern recognition. Each scan must be stored and relative intensities analyzed. For 180° scans, the computer must redraw the three-dimensional X-ray information into one two-dimensional picture. The result gives more information than could be obtained from one two-dimensional X-ray picture.

Dynamic imaging systems used to analyze results from gamma cameras involve digitally storing the information and successively analyzing the results. However, the analog analysis involved in viewing the original display may yield a diagnosis as accurate if not more so than by computer. Clearly, the computer is of tremendous value, but in the final analysis humans will evaluate results,

diagnose, and embark on a treatment procedure. In short, computers analyze, humans think.

23-13 Calibration, typical faults, troubleshooting, and maintenance procedures

Calibration of *X-ray machines* involves checking timing against known standards and verifying kilovoltage and milliampere settings on the operating panel. To verify mechanical timing for 1/120 s, observe one pulse on an oscilloscope while synchronizing to the 60-Hz ac power line. Spinning tops are used for longer durations. Special digital devices can also be used. A digital timer is triggered when the X-ray strikes a transducer. When the X-ray pulse has passed, the digital timer is placed on hold. The readout indicates elapsed time or X-ray pulse duration. A *penetrometer* (stack of different lengths of aluminum bars) is used to calibrate the kV and mA. If successive film depths produce proper shaded exposures for changes in the autotransformer taps, the machine is working properly.

Prepared plates at fixed distances should receive proper shading for proper calibration.

Calibration of nuclear medicine equipment involves verification of proper operation of the lower-level discriminator or pulse height analyzer, proper amplification, and display results. A standard nuclear radiation module can be placed under the scanning mechanism and scanned as usual. Observation on the display of a proper map is testimony of proper calibration. Adjustments in the collimator, pulse height analyzer, and synchronous scanning display unit can be made.

Typical faults in X-ray machines occur mostly in the mechanical device servo-mechanisms for positioning the patient tables. Wires break, cables snap, and jams occur. Relays become intermittent and stick open or closed. Most problems, therefore, are electromechanical, not electronic. Occasionally, high-voltage rectifiers open, X-ray tube filaments open, or rotating anodes become pitted. Replacement of the X-ray tube with oil circulation is done by factory-trained personnel. Elimination of radiation leakage paths with special instrumentation and electrical safety are of paramount significance. The electronics in modern machines are highly reliable. Finally, operator error occurs on occasion and can result in injury or death to the patient and operator. Radiation exposure is checked and minimized by periodically measuring exposure tags worn by employees.

Typical faults in nuclear medicine machines are also mostly electromechanical. The scanning mechanisms malfunction, and recorders occasionally fail. The electronics are reliable, and computers are serviced by manufacturer personnel.

23-14 Summary

1. *X-ray machines* are devices that generate high-frequency, high-energy electromagnetic waves (X-rays). These rays penetrate the body and are detected on a photographic plate. The result on the negative is an exposure or picture shown as shades of gray. Dark areas represent high exposure to X-rays (soft structures within the body). Light areas represent bones and dense structures. Internal body parts can then be observed.

2. *Types of X-ray machines* include still picture or chest type, fluoroscope, angiography, CAT scanner, and radiation therapy units.

3. *Nuclear medicine machines* are devices used to detect radiation from isotopes injected into the bloodstream that accumulate in target organs. Scintillation crystals detect the radiation, and counters measure the amount of disintegration per time. Organ activity can then be measured.

4. *Types of nuclear medicine equipment* include rectilinear scintillation scanner and isotope therapy sources.

5. Nuclear radiation involves *alpha rays* (positive helium nuclei), *beta rays* (negative electrons), *gamma rays* (electromagnetic waves), and *X-rays* (exceedingly high-frequency waves).

6. The frequency of X-rays is proportional to their energy.

7. Three quantum effects are the photoelectric effect, Compton effect, and *Bremsstrahlung*.

8. Units for measuring radioactivity include the curie (Ci), roentgen (R), rad, dose rate, and X-ray intensity.

9. Excessive short-term or long-term (accumulated) X-ray or nuclear radiation dosage may cause mutation, physical illness, or death.

10. X-rays are generated in a high-vacuum diode in which electrons are accelerated to high velocity by a high-voltage power supply.

11. The *major sections of an X-ray machine* are the multitap autotransformer, filament circuit and transformer, high-voltage circuit and transformer, and timer.

12. The *major sections of a fluoroscopic machine* are the X-ray machine, fluoroscopic image pickup, camera, and closed-circuit video system.

13. The *major sections of a nuclear medicine system* are the detector-collimator, scanner motor assembly, linear amplifier, pulse height analyzer, and recorder.

14. *Computer systems* in radiology include *image enhancement* and *recording and analysis* of dynamic data.

15. Calibration on X-ray and nuclear medicine equipment should follow manufacturers' recommendations—typical faults most often include electromechanical failures.

23-15 Recapitulation

Now return to the objectives and self-evaluation questions at the beginning of the chapter and see how well you can answer them. If you cannot answer certain questions, place a check mark next to each and review appropriate parts of the text. Next, try to answer the following questions using the same procedure. When you have answered all of the questions, solve the problems.

Questions

1. Four classes of X-ray equipment used to measure anatomical features are the _____-_____ machine, _____ continuous display, _____ or motion picture, and _____ or tomographic systems.

2. CAT scanner refers to _____ _____ _____.

3. X-rays are high-frequency _____ waves.

4. Alpha rays are positive _____ nuclei; beta rays are negatively charged _____; and gamma rays are _____ waves.

5. Higher energy levels imparted to electrons produce *harder/softer* X-rays on the X-ray tube.

6. *Bremsstrahlung* refers to _____ radiation.

7. The roentgen unit refers to the amount of radiation energy dose per _____, the dose-rate to exposure per _____, and the X-ray intensity to dose-rate per _____.

8. List the major hazards from radiation exposure including accumulated doses.

9. X-ray tubes use rotating anodes to avoid _____ and prolong tube _____.

10. Name and describe the operation of the major sections of an X-ray machine.

11. Name and describe the operation of the major sections of a fluoroscopic machine.

12. Name and describe the operation of the major sections of a nuclear medicine system.

13. In X-ray machines and nuclear medicine systems, why is calibration important? Where do most of the malfunctions occur?

Problems

1. Given an X-ray machine set to 125 kV (on the X-ray tube), which produces X-rays of wavelength 0.01 Å? Calculate the wavelength in meters and energy in joules. Are these hard (diagnostic) or soft (therapeutic) X-rays?

2. Given a 136-lb person who receives 0.3 J of radiation energy over his or her entire body, calculate the kilograms of the person and the dose of radiation (rad) absorbed.

3. Given a 136-lb person who accidentally receives a whole-body exposure of 200 mR/min dose rate for 30 min, in general, should this person avoid a chest X-ray of 0.2 rad within one year if the physician does not consider it mandatory? *Hint:* for practical purposes 1 R = 1 rad and a maximum of 5 rads per year should be observed (recommended exposure limit by the International Committee on Radiation Protection).

4. Refer to Figure 23-4, simplified block and circuit diagram of an X-ray machine. Given a short in the primary of the filament transformer, T_2, discuss the system fault symptoms from the operator's standpoint. Include meter readings, activation of X-ray machine, circuit breakers, and X-ray tube operation.

5. Refer to Figure 23-4, simplified circuit diagram of an X-ray machine. Given system fault symptoms of loud cracking sounds, discuss possible faulty components. Include all transformers, rectifier bridges, and wiring.

Suggested Reading

1. Hill, D. R. et al., *Principles of Diagnostic X-ray Apparatus,* Phillips Medical Systems (London, 1973).

2. Nave, Carl R. and Brenda C. Nave, *Physics for the Health Sciences,* W. B. Saunders Company (Philadelphia, 1975).

3. Fernando, Antonio, Conclaves Rocha, and John C. Harbet, *Textbook of Nuclear Medicine,* Lea & Febiger (Philadelphia, 1978).

4. Lange, Robert C., *Nuclear Medicine for Technicians,* Year Book Medical Publishers (Chicago, 1973).

5. Early, Paul J., M. A. Razzak, and Bruce D. Sodee, *Textbook of Nuclear Medicine Technology,* C. V. Mosby Company (St. Louis, 1975).

6. Sodee, Bruce D. and Paul J. Early, *Technology and Interpretation of Nuclear Medicine Procedures,* C. V. Mosby Company (St. Louis, 1975).

CHAPTER 24
Electromagnetic Interference to Medical Electronic Equipment

24-1 Objectives

1. Be able to define *electromagnetic interference* (EMI).
2. Be able to describe the mechanisms of EMI.
3. Be able to describe the effects of EMI on sensors and medical circuits.
4. Be able to describe the basic methods for suppressing EMI.

24-2 Self-evaluation questions

These questions test your prior knowledge of the material in this chapter. Look for the answers as you read the text. After you have finished studying the chapter, try answering these questions and those at the end of the chapter.

1. Define *intermodulation interference*. Use an equation, if needed.

2. Two transmitters operate close to the hospital. One produces a signal on 188.2 MHz, while the other operates on 146.94 MHz. Is there any danger that either the fundamental frequencies or their first two harmonics can combine to produce intermodulation interference?

3. What measures can be taken to prevent radio frequency interference from entering the equipment cabinet via the power lines?

4. What kind of filter can be used to remove a 98.7-MHz FM broadcast signal that is interfering with the operation of an ECG radio telemetry system?

24-3 Introduction

Electromagnetic interference (EMI) is a major problem in all areas of society today. Put quite simply, EMI is interference to an electronic device by electrical energy generated elsewhere. Some EMI is natural (e.g., lightning), but most of the problems discussed in this chapter are of manmade origin.

At one time, most EMI problems were military and were created by the large number of electronic devices used in that environment. The aircraft carrier *U.S.S. Forestall* had an accidental release of a rocket because of EMI, resulting in the loss of 134 sailors and 27 aircraft. Now that automobiles have a large number of electronic devices on board, EMI is a major problem. More than two decades ago the first automobile computer was used on German and Swedish automobiles. Amateur radio operators found they could not do mobile operations in those cars because EMI to the computer caused the car to stop. Anti-skid brakes have also be affected by EMI.

Similarly, problems were noted when passing a broadcast station. Airline trade organizations report more than 20 incidents a year in which electronic devices used by passengers interfere with navigation equipment. If you fly today, the cabin attendants will make an announcement on which devices can be used and under what circumstances.

Medical devices also experience EMI problems. An electric wheelchair with electronic controls, for example, may veer out of control. In tests done by the FDA, wheelchair wheels rotated at speeds up to 30 RPM with fields of only 20 V/m. Pacemakers were subject to interference by leaky microwave ovens, although that problem seems to have abated because of design changes in both pacemakers and microwave ovens. Respirators have also been affected by EMI problems ranging from extra breaths to cessation of operation, depending on design and the strength of the local interference source.

Many hospitals ban cellular telephones, and require them to be turned off altogether. Generally, studies have shown that medical devices malfunctioned when nearby cellular telephones were operated. A more refined test, using a method for measuring field strengths, found that seven of eight medical devices failed with a field of only 10 V/m (which is regarded as "normal" in an urban environment). Further, six of eight devices failed with a 3 V/m field, which is about that expected from a cellular telephone at a distance of about 2 meters. It

is common to require people to turn off their cellular telephones entirely while in the hospital. It is not sufficient to refrain from using the device because of the "polling" feature of cellular telephones. Base stations periodically poll their area to see who is present, so the system knows which phones are in its area. As a result, cellular telephones will transmit from time to time even when not in use.

Hospitals are not the only medical venue where EMI problems occur. A defibrillator manufacturer found fields of 60 V/m present in ambulances. These fields could emanate from on-board electrical equipment or from the radio communications equipment used in ambulances.

24-4 Types and Sources of EMI

Three general classes of EMI problem are: *radiated, conducted,* and *electrostatic discharge* (ESD). Radiated EMI consists of electrical fields, magnetic fields and electromagnetic fields. It is characterized by the fact that it is transmitted through space, and does not need wires to carry it. When a radio transmitter interferes with a patient monitor, that is an example of radiated EMI. Similarly, a computer printer cable radiating signal during a print operation is also radiated EMI.

Conducted EMI requires a wire or other conductor to transfer it from one place to another. When a hair dryer causes snow on the television screen it is conducted EMI. Similarly, when an electrosurgery machine transfers radio frequency energy through a patient's body (a conductor) to the ECG machine, it is conducted EMI. Another form of conducted EMI is the high-voltage lightning, capacitance charge, and switching transients arriving on the AC power lines. Some of those transients are quite long and have a high amplitude.

An "ANSI standard pulse" for the power line has a 2,000 V peak amplitude, lasts for 20 μs and has a 5% negative polarity undershoot. Electronic equipment must be able to operate through such a pulse. The "surge protector" used with desktop computers is not really for "surges" (which are relatively slow increases of voltage over several seconds) but rather for high-voltage transients. Older analog electronic equipment absorbed transient voltage spikes without any noticeable problem, but digital circuits (including computers) are sensitive to them.

Electrostatic discharge (ESD) refers to the build up of electrostatic potentials on tools, objects, and the human body caused by mechanical action, such as rubbing. The problem with many electronic circuits is that they have low dielectric strength, so potentials as low as about 80 V will cause damage. With potentials on the human body normally running to several kilovolts, damage is inevitable if precautions are not taken.

At one time it was common to use explosive anesthesia agents in operating rooms of hospitals. Ether and cyclopropane are examples. If such agents are used, it is possible for ESD to cause an explosion. The rooms where such anesthesia agents are used are kept equipotential by using conductive flooring; conductive casters on rolling stock, such as back tables; and conductive shoes or shoe covers on personnel. It was also common to see a requirement for cotton or paper garments on personnel, even down to their underwear.

24-5 Fields

Any electrical circuit can, under the right circumstances, either produce EMI or suffer from the EMI of others. The main issue seems to be the strength of the signal in the vicinity of the affected equipment. Outside of a controlled test environment it is difficult to predict field strengths. The rule-of-thumb advice is that the electric field (E) is found from the standard *dipole equation:*

$$E = \frac{K \sqrt{P}}{D} \qquad (24\text{-}1)$$

Where:

E is the electrical field in volts per meter (V/m)

P is the radiated power in watts (W)

D is the distance in meters (m)

K is the antenna factor (0.2 to 8)

Equation 24-1 is not a very good predictor because the local situation creates a variation as much as 10 to 100 times from the predicted value. For example, a large amount of material that will absorb radio or electrical energy (e.g., foliage, carbon-impregnated operating room floors) reduces the signal strength. Reflective surfaces, such as metallic objects, may increase or decrease the signal level at any given point depending on whether or not the interference of the reflected and direct signals is constructive or destructive.

The magnetic field (H) will vary with the electric field (E) such that

$$H = \frac{E}{377 \ \Omega} \qquad (24\text{-}2)$$

Where:

H is the magnetic field in amperes per meter (A/m)

E is the electric field in volts per meter (V/m)

377 ohms is the impedance of free space

The electric field falls off inversely proportional to the distance, where the power level (which is proportional to the square of the voltage) falls off according to the inverse square law ($1/D^2$). At distances of more than about one-third to one-half wavelength the *E* and *H* fields fall off about the same, so one usually uses the *E* field as the indicator of signal strength. Closer than one-third to one-half wavelength other effects are noted. The magnetic field, for example, falls off at a rate proportional to $1/D^3$ and the power at $1/D^4$. This area is known as the *near-field* of a radio antenna or other radiator. Figure 24-1 shows the distance required to maintain a 3 V/m electric field strength for power levels from 0.01 W (e.g., PCS telephones) to 1,000 W (e.g., ham radio or small AM transmitter).

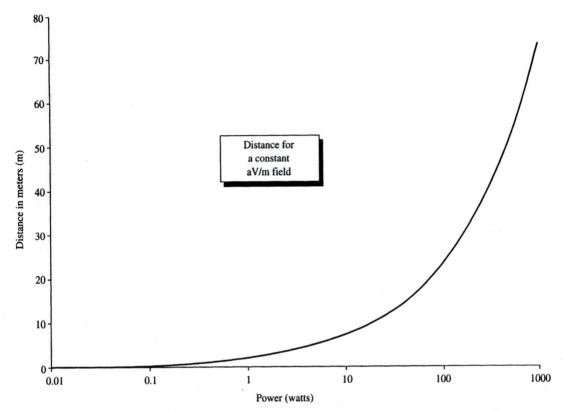

Figure 24-1
Left space for a one line caption to be supplied.

24-6 EMI Effects

The degree to which EMI affects a given piece of equipment depends on certain design factors. For example, because an ECG or EEG monitor has long, often unshielded, patient electrode wires, the pick-up of external energy is significant. The wires act as an antenna. If the wires happen to be an integer multiple of quarter wavelength (1λ, $1\lambda/2$ or $3\lambda/4$) then the effect is multiplied because the wires act like a resonant antenna (the odd multiples are usually worse than the even multiples).

The methods used for grounding the internal circuits, and the layout, affects the internal EMI of electronic equipment. It is common practice to separate audio, video, digital, small signal instrumentation, radio frequency, and large signal areas so they are not intermingled. If possible, different printed circuit boards are used, but at the very least some spatial separation is provided on the same board.

Another method is to make sure the amplifiers (including integrated circuits) used have symmetrical slew rates (i.e., the rise time and fall time of the amplifier are the same), and that the transistors are biased in the middle of their operating range. Proper use of filtering and shielding will also help immunize the circuits against EMI.

The term *electromagnetic compatibility* refers to the attributes of a piece of equipment to: 1) not cause interference with other devices and 2) not be susceptible to outside interference.

24-7 Standards, Regulations, and Laws

There are a number of regulatory issues dealing with EMI. In the United States, the FCC regulates radio and telecommunications, as well as devices that interfere with these services. The FDA Center for Devices and Radiological Health regulates medical devices, including their EMI/EMC attributes. The American National Standards Institute (ANSI), the Institute for Electrical and Electronic Engineers (IEEE), and the National Institutes of Standards and Technology (NIST) are also involved. For medical equipment, the FDA and the Association for the Advancement of Medical Instrumentation (AAMI) can advise on current standards and regulations.

The EMI situation in Europe is at least as bad as the US situation, and possibly worse because of population densities. In 1989, the European Community (EC) issued Directive 89/336/EEC to regulate EMI/EMC in most products sold in Europe (or at least that part that is in the EC). The directive gave several years grace period for compliance, but is now fully in force.

The EC recognizes the International Electrotechnical Commission as a technical standards organization. The International Special Committee on Radio Interference (called CISPR after the French version of its name) is the IEC faction that deals with EMI/EMC problems. There are also two other European organizations dealing with these problems: European Telecommunications Standards Institute (ETSI) and the European Organization for Electrotechnical Standardization (CENELEC).

The primary standards are IEC-801, which deals with compliance to the EC EMC directive. Standards IEC-801-2 deals with ESD and IEC-801-3 describes the susceptibility to radiated EMI

for industrial process control instruments. Another standard is the multi-part IEC-1000. The EC standards are called "European Standards" and are designated with an "EN" prefix, after the French for "European standard." EN-55022 came from CISPR 22 and deals with the signals emitted by digital devices between 30 and 230 MHz (30 μV/m at 10-m distances). In the United Kingdom, this standard is also known as British Standard BS-6527. Two generic standards are also used: EN-50081 for emissions of electromagnetic energy and EN-50082 for immunity to electromagnetic energy.

European manufacturers and importers of electrical equipment must ensure that the equipment neither causes EMI nor is susceptible to EMI from other devices. The "EC" mark is the manufacturers certification that testing has been done and the equipment that is marked EC is compliant with the EC regulations. This mark is normally a good mark to look for when purchasing medical equipment.

24-8 EMI Mitigation

The job of the clinical engineer (CE) and biomedical equipment technician (BMET) with respect to EMI/EMC is to: 1) ensure that equipment purchased adheres to applicable standards and regulations and 2) mitigate the effects of EMI problems in the health care facility.

Separation is one of the best methods for mitigating the effects of radiated EMI. If the goal is to maintain a field of 3 V/m or less, the following "rules of thumb" are useful (see also Fig. 24-1):

5-W walkie-talkie	6 m
600-mW cellular telephone	2 m
10-mW PCS digital telephone	0.3 m

Where separation is not possible, other means are needed to mitigate the effects of EMI. In the sections that follow, techniques are presented that have been found to work. Correct application depends on correctly diagnosing the cause of the EMI.

24-9 Intermodulation problems

There are two interrelated problems that often deteriorate radio reception in communications systems: *intermodulation* and *cross-modulation*. Although there are fine technical differences between these two problems, their solutions are about the same, so we will take the liberty of calling them all *intermod problems*. These problems result in *interference on a given frequency due to heterodyning (mixing) between two other unrelated signals.*

Heterodyning is a term that refers to the nonlinear mixing of two radio frequency signals. Consider the guitar analogy. Pick one string and make it vibrate to produce a tone. That tone has a frequency of F_1. After that tone dies out, pluck another string and cause a new tone (F_2). Now pluck both strings simultaneously. What happens? How many tones are present? The initial answer might be F_1 and F_2, but that is wrong. In an nonlinear system (such as hearing), additional frequencies are created. In addition to F_1 and F_2, there will be the sum frequency ($F_1 + F_2$) and the difference frequency ($F_1 - F_2$). It is the difference frequency, $F_1 - F_2$, by the way, that some guitar players use to tune the instrument. When two frequencies are close, but not exact, the difference frequency is very low, almost subaudible. It is this low frequency that accounts for the slow, wavering tone that one hears as the strings are tuned closer to the same pitch. Exact tune is indicated by the wavering disappearing. This is *heterodyning.*

Other combination frequencies are also produced, and these are determined according to the expression $mF_1 + nF_2$, where m and n are integers. For most purposes, however, these additional frequencies are unimportant (a distinctly important problem with these additional frequencies is discussed here; intermod problems need not work on only F_1 and F_2).

There is a hill close to where one author lives that radio technicians and engineers call Intermod Hill. It happens to be one of the higher locations in the county, so several broadcasters and AT&T have seen fit to build radio towers there. In addition, both of the two main radio towers bristle with landmobile antennas, whose owners rent space on the tower in order to get better coverage. In total, there are two 50,000-W FM broadcast stations, a 2000-W AM broadcast station, a many-frequency microwave relay station, and several dozen 30- to 950-mHz VHF/UHF landmobile stations and radio paging stations. Nearby is a major community hospital that operates its own security system radio station and a hospital radio pager system. The hospital also has a coronary care unit that uses UHF radio telemetry to keep track of ambulatory heart patients. All of those signals can heterodyne together to produce apparently valid signals on other channels.

When two or more signals (F1 and F2) are present at the input of the receiver or amplifier there is a possibility of generating additional frequencies (especially if at least one of them is a strong signal). The additional frequencies generated are:

$$F_{NEW} = m\,F1 \pm n\,F2 \qquad (24\text{-}3)$$

Where:

F_{NEW} is a new frequency generated by nonlinear combination of F1 and F2

F1 and *F2* are the two frequencies

m and n are either integers or zero (0, 1, 2, 3....n)

The *order* of the intermodulation product is given by the sum of the integer coefficients to F1 and F2 (i.e., m plus n). Given input signal frequencies of F1 and F2, the main IPs are:

Second-order:	F1 $\pm$ F2
	2F1
	2F2
Third-order:	2F1 $\pm$ F2
	2F2 $\pm$ F1
	3F1
	3F2
Fifth-order:	3F1 $\pm$ 2F2
	3F2 $\pm$ 2F1
	5F1
	5F2

Whenever an amplifier or receiver is over-driven, the second-order content of the output signal increases as the square of the input signal level, while the third order responses increase as the cube of the input signal level, which can cause serious problems. As a result, when troubleshooting a problem with interference, you must sometimes look for completely unrelated frequencies that will satisfy Equation 24-3 and thereby land on your frequency. When troubleshooting this type of problem it is necessary to eliminate or at least reduce the frequency of one of the two offenders, preferably the strongest, rather than the receive frequency. Later in this chapter an actual case of IMD problems is discussed.

The IMD problem occurs because the combined strength of the two signals drives the receiver RF amplifier or first mixer of the receiver into a deeper region of nonlinear operation. If the applied RF signal levels are low enough, no problems occur. All mixers operate nonlinearly, so we usually look to the *third-order intercept point* (called either TOIP or IP3) to determine susceptibility to IMD problems. The TOIP is usually specified in terms of dBm (decibels above one milliwatt). The higher the TOIP the better the receiver or amplifier. In general, look for numbers higher than −10 dBm, with a strong preference shown for amplifiers with at least +15 dBm when available.

If the receiver system is linear, then there is little chance for a problem. But nonlinearities do creep in, and when the receiver is nonlinear and extraneous signals are present, then intermods show up. Being in the fields of so many radio transmitter signals almost ensures nonlinearity, due to simple overload; hence intermod problems abound on and around Intermod Hill. Imagine the number of possible combinations when there are literally dozens of frequencies floating around the neighborhood!

The ability (or lack of same) to reject these unwanted signals is a good measure of a receiver's performance. A high-quality, well-designed radio receiver does not respond to either out-of-band or within-band off-channel signals, except in the most extreme cases of overload. The ability to discriminate against these spurious signals is a necessary requirement to specify when requesting quotations and estimates from industry for a new radio communications or telemetry installation.

The linearity of dynamic range of the input RF amplifier of the receiver is the cause of most cases of intermodulation interference. There are other causes, however, and one must consider anything that can cause nonlinearity. For example, a certain type of radio had problems with the automatic gain control (AGC) rectifier diode. It was leaky and would produce a situation in which the radio was easily overdriven by external signals. In some sets, the manufacturer used a pair of back-to-back silicon small signal diodes across the antenna terminals in order to shunt possible high-voltage potentials to ground. This method was especially popular a few years ago. A large signal could drive these diodes into conduction and produce severe nonlinearity.

Consider an odd intermod problem that occurred in a hospital that used a VHF radio telemetry unit to monitor patient ECGs in the PCCU, where CCU patients go to when their condition is no longer acute but they still bear watching. The portable ECG transmitters generate 1 to 4 mW of VHF RF energy that is frequency modulated with the patient's ECG signal. The signal level is so low that five or more 17-inch whip antennas, sticking down from the false hanging ceiling, are needed to cover an area that consists of two corridors approximately 150 feet in length. Each antenna is connected directly to a 60-dB master TV antenna amplifier (the VHF ECG radio transmitter channels are located in the guard bands between TV video and audio carriers of commercial VHF TV channels); one of the whip/amplifier assemblies is right over the receiver console.

One morning, about 2 A.M., a nurse called the biomedical equipment technician at home complaining that Mr. Jones's ECG was riding in on Mr. Smith's channel. Not quite believing her, the technician nonetheless went to the hospital and checked out the situation. Swapping receivers,

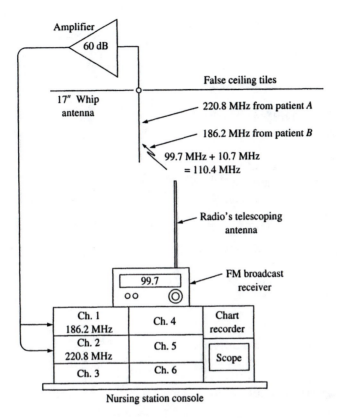

Figure 24-2
Configuration that led to an unusual intermodulation problem.

telemetry transmitters, and amplifiers did no good. Finally, after two hours of trying, he noticed the FM broadcast receiver sitting on top of the telemetry receiver cabinet less than 18 inches from the antenna/amplifier (Figure 24-2), and it was playing. On a sheer hunch, he turned off the receiver and Jones went back to his own channel. Previously, Jones's signal was showing up on both his own channel and Smith's channel, but was now only where it belonged. Turning the FM receiver back on caused the situation to return. Also, tuning the radio to another channel made the problem go away.

What happened in that situation? The FM radio is a superheterodyne model (they all are), and its internal local oscillator signal radiated and was heterodyning with Jones's signal to produce an intermod signal on Smith's channel. The situation is shown graphically in Figure 24-2. The six VHF receivers used in the system are installed in a mainframe rack that forms the nurses' station console (along with an oscilloscope and strip-chart recorder). The FM receiver was placed on top of the receiver rack such that its telescoping whip antenna was only a short distance from the telemetry receiver antenna.

Because the FM receiver is a superheterodyne, it produces a signal from the internal local oscillator that is 10.7 MHz higher than the received frequency. If the radio is tuned to the station at 99.7 MHz on the FM dial, then the local oscillator operates at 99.7 MHz + 10.7 MHz, or 110.4 MHz.

This signal is radiated and picked up by the telemetry antenna. Because of its close proximity, it is the strongest signal seen by the input of the 60-dB amplifier. The other signals impinging on the antenna are weak signals at 220.8 MHz from patient A and 186.2 MHz from patient B. The mixing action at the input of the 60-dB amplifier, then, consists of 110.4, 186.2, and 220.8 MHz.

In the case cited, it was apparently the second harmonic of the FM radio local oscillator signal (110.4 MHz × 2, or 220.8 MHz) that caused the problem. Consider the mathematics: 186.2 MHz + 220.8 MHz = 407 MHz. And, also, 407 MHz − 186.2 = 220.8 MHz. In this scenario, the 186.2-MHz transmitter signal will appear on the 220.8-MHz channel.

The general rule of thumb for which signal will appear is based on the *capture effect.* Telemetry transmitters and receivers are frequency modulated (FM). An FM receiver will generally capture the strongest of two competing co-channel signals and exclude the other. As a result, the strongest of the two signals (in this example, 186.2 MHz translated to 220.8 MHz by mixing in the 60-dB amplifier) predominates.

After that night, the hospital banned FM radio receivers, patient-owned TV receivers, and citizen's band and ham radio sets in the CCU/PCCU area for exactly the same reason they are banned on commercial airliners: interference with critical electronic equipment.

24-9-1 Some solutions

There are a number of ways to overcome most intermod problems. Modification of the receiver is possible, especially since poor design is a basic cause of intermods. But that approach is rarely feasible except for the most technically intrepid. There are, however, a few pointers for the rest of us.

First, make sure that the receiver is well shielded. This problem rarely occurs in costly modern equipment but is a strong possibility on lower-cost receivers. Most radio transceivers have adequate shielding because of the requirements of

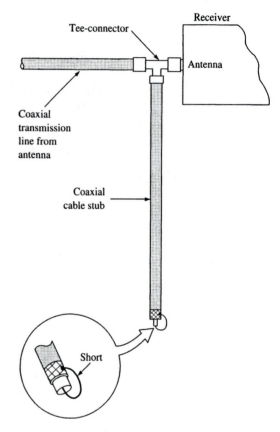

Figure 24-3
Use of coaxial half-wavelength shorted stub for EMI suppression.

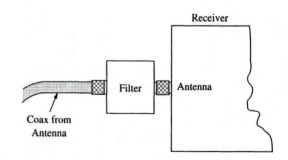

Figure 24-4
Use of a frequency selective filter to block EMI signals.

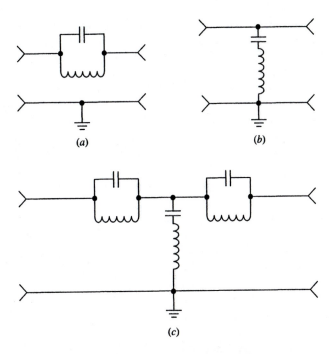

Figure 24-5
Several different wave traps. *(a)* Parallel. *(b)* Series. *(c)* Combination series and parallel.

the transmitter in the same cabinet with the receiver and FCC requirements. But if there are any holes in the shielding, then cover them up with sheet metal or copper foil. For others, the best approach is to use one of the methods shown in Figures 24-3 through 24-5. In all cases, you must identify one of the interfering frequencies or (in some cases) at least the band.

24-9-2 Halfwave shorting stub

A nonmatching load impedance attached to the load end of a transmission line repeats itself every half wavelength back down the line toward the input end. For example, if a 250-Ω antenna is attached to the load end of a half-wavelength piece of 50-Ω coaxial cable, an impedance meter at the input end will measure 250 Ω. Lengths other than integer multiples of half wavelength will see different impedances at the input end. This phenome-

non is the basis for transmission line transformers used in antenna matching. Therefore, if the end of a piece of coaxial cable is shorted (Figure 24-3), then the input end will see a short circuit at the frequency for which the coaxial cable is a half wavelength. The interfering frequency will be shorted to ground, while the desired frequency sees a high impedance, provided that the two are widely separated. The length L is found from $L_{ft} = 492V/F_{MHz}$; where L is in feet, F is in MHz, and V is the velocity factor of the coaxial cable (usually 0.66 for regular coaxial cable and 0.80 for polyfoam coaxial cable).

The method of Figure 24-3 is best suited to cases where the interfering signal is in the VHF region or lower. Because the length of the coax stub is very short relative to the HF wavelength of the desired band, some very untransmission-line-like behavior might take place when transmitting. Therefore, for transceivers, some engineers recommend adding a second antenna jack, especially for the stub, but connected to the receiver circuitry (RX CKT).

Another method (Figure 24-4) is to use a frequency selective filter. The selection of type of filter, and the cutoff frequency, is determined by the case. In a maze of frequencies like those on Intermod Hill, it might be wise to use a bandpass filter on the band of choice. Otherwise, use a low-pass filter if the interfering signal (at least one of them) is higher than the desired band, and a high-pass filter if the interfering signal is lower. For most cases, a low-pass television interference (TVI) filter is desirable on high frequency (HF), so this solution is automatically taken care of; the 35- to 45-MHz cutoff point of most such filters will attenuate most VHF signals trying to get back in.

Figure 24-5 shows some of the different types of filter configurations that might be used. The first wavetrap is a parallel resonant circuit (Figure 24-5a) in series with the signal line. A parallel resonant trap has a high impedance at the resonant frequency but a low impedance on other frequencies, so it blocks the undesired frequency. Figure 24-5b shows a series resonant trap across the signal line. The series resonant circuit is just the opposite of the parallel case: It offers a low impedance at its resonant frequency and a high impedance elsewhere. Thus, it serves much like the coaxial cable stub in Figure 24-3. Figure 24-5c shows a combination wavetrap that uses both series and parallel resonant elements.

If the interfering station is an FM broadcaster, then most video shops and electronic parts stores will carry FM wavetraps for 75-Ω antenna systems. These traps cost only a few dollars but provide a tremendous amount of relief from the interference produced by FM broadcast stations.

It might be that the interfering signal is entering the equipment on the ac power line. This situation is especially likely if you live very close to a high-power broadcasting station. If there is space inside the receiver, then it might pay to install an ac line filter. Electronic parts distributors sell EMI ac line filters suitable for equipment up to 2000 W (V-A) or so (look at the ampere rating of the filter). Also, it is possible to install ferrite blocks around the line cord to serve as RF chokes. Some computer stores sell these blocks to reduce EMI from long runs of multiconductor ribbon cable. It is sometimes possible to reduce the EMI pickup by either reducing the cord length or rolling it up into a tight coil. This solution works well when the cord is of a length nearly resonant (quarter wavelength) on the interfering signal's frequency.

24-10 Dealing with TVI

Television interference, TVI, is the bane of the radio communications and broadcasting communities. True TVI occurs when emissions from a transmitter interfere with the normal operation of a television receiver. Except for solo explorers on the North Slope of Alaska and missionaries among the Indians of the Amazon basin, all radio operators have a potential TVI problem as close as their own TV set or their neighbors' sets.

One way to classify TVI is according to the cause. All electronic devices must perform two functions:

1. Respond to desired signals.

2. Reject undesired signals.

All electronic devices perform more or less in accordance with the first requirement, but many fail with respect to the second. Often, a legally transmitted signal will be received on a neighbor's TV or hi-fi set even though the transmitter operation is perfectly normal. On some TV sets, the high-intensity signal from a nearby transmitter drives the RF amplifier into nonlinearity, and that creates harmonics where none existed before. In other cases, audio from the transmission is heard on the audio output of the set, or seen in the video, as a result of signal pickup and rectification inside the set. Improper shielding can cause signals to be picked up on internal leads and fed to the circuits involved.

Remember two rules of thumb: (1) If transmitter emissions are not clean, then getting rid of the Television Interference/Broadcast Interference (TVI/BCI) is the radio operator's responsibility; and (2) if the transmitter emissions are clean, and the TVI/BCI is caused by poor equipment design, then it is the equipment owner's responsibility to fix the problem—not the radio operator's. Unfortunately, in a society that depends too much on lawyers, the solution opted for by some ill-advised administrators is to hire lawyers to intimidate the radio owner into silent submission. Wise managers will shun the lawyers and hire an engineer to solve the problem in a manner that will allow both parties to operate compatibly.

On the other hand, radio transmitter owners must respond responsibly to EMI complaints for several reasons. First, they have a legally imposed responsibility to keep transmitter emissions clean and free of spurious or unnecessary components. They must operate the transmitter legally. Second, it makes for good neighborhood relations if they attempt to help solve the problem. After all, we live in a society in which more people seem willing to go to lawyers than to engineers to solve technical problems. The following steps should be taken:

Step 1. Make sure that the transmitter emissions are clean. Although it requires a spectrum analyzer to be sure that the harmonics are down 40 dB or more below the carrier, a few simple checks will tell the tale in many cases. An absorption wavemeter is an old-fashioned device that can spot harmonics that are way too high. Also, listening on another receiver from a long distance (1 mile or more) will give some indication of problems: At that distance, if you can hear the second or third harmonic, then it is probably real. Finally, if you own an RF wattmeter or a forward-reading VSWR meter, and a dummy load, then you can make a quick check of the transmitter by measuring the output power with and without a low-pass filter (Figure 24-6) installed in the line. If the power varies between the two readings by appreciably

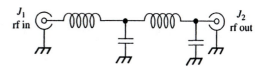

Note: Component values are a function of frequency.

Figure 24-6
Use of a low-pass filter such as this circuit and an RF power meter allows us to check for harmonics.

more than the insertion loss of the low-pass filter, then suspect that harmonics are present.

The techniques for making the transmitter clean are simple: a low-resistance earth ground and adequate filtering. In the station shown in Figure 24-7, there are three frequency selective elements after the transmitter: *low-pass filter, antenna tuning unit* (in lower-frequency stations), and a *resonant antenna*. All of these will help in reducing whatever harmonics the transmitter puts out.

Step 2. Determine whether you really have a TVI problem. Check for TVI with the transmitter turned on and turned off. Also, make sure the TV is properly adjusted.

Step 3. Try adding a high-pass filter to the TV set. These filters will only pass signals with a frequency greater than about 50 MHz and severely attenuate HF amateur or CB signals. As shown in Figure 24-8, the high-pass filter must be installed as close as possible to the antenna terminals of the TV set. Make the connection wire as short as possible to prevent it from acting as an antenna in its own right.

Advise the affected TV set owner to install an antenna that uses a coaxial cable transmission line rather than 300-Ω twin-lead. Although theory tells us that there should be no difference, it is nonetheless true that 75-Ω coaxial cable systems are less susceptible to all forms of noise, including TVI. Install a high-pass filter and a 75- to 300-Ω TV-type Balanced/Unbalanced (BALUN) impedance transformer at the TV's antenna terminals.

Many, perhaps most, TV receivers have very poor internal shielding, so signals can bypass the

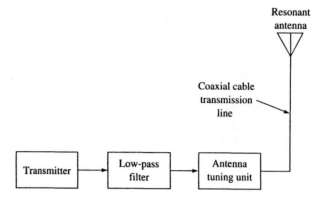

Figure 24-7
Typical transmitter installation with low-pass filter and antenna tuning unit.

high-pass filter and get picked up on the leads between the TV tuner (inside the set) and the antenna terminals on the rear of the set. This situation makes the high-pass filter almost useless. A solution for this dilemma is to mount the filter directly on the tuner, inside the set, making the lead length essentially zero.

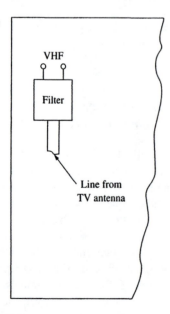

Figure 24-8
TVI filter for interference suppression.

24-11 Dealing with signal overload problems

Radio receivers are often subject to overload interference. While high-priced, high-quality telemetry receivers will handle overload conditions better than the cheaper models, the only real issue is what signal, at what strength, will cause overload problems. In this section we will explore some of the methods that might be used to overcome these problems on shortwave and scanner receivers.

Four basic types of overload problems are seen on radio receivers: *desensitization, generation of unwanted harmonics, distortion of the desired signal,* and *intermodulation frequencies.* These can also be broken into those that involve *co-channel interference, adjacent channel interference,* and *off-channel interference.* Let's take a look at each of these in turn, keeping in mind that actual situations may involve two or more combinations of both groups—and in fact probably will.

Co-channel interference involves signals on the same channel as the desired signal. Unfortunately, next to nothing can be done for these problems at the receiver. The best solution is to use a directional antenna that favors the desired station and rejects the unfavored signal. Every directional antenna has a direction of least pickup; that is, a null direction. For example, a half wavelength dipole

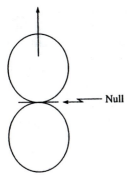

Figure 24-9
Yagi or quad antenna. Beam antenna radiation pattern.

has two nulls off the ends of the radiator element (Figure 24-9), perpendicular to the directions of maximum pickup. A Yagi or quad antenna (Figure 24-10) has the null in the direction opposite the direction of maximum pickup (or "off the back"). To overcome co-channel interference, place the null of the antenna in the direction of the interfering signal.

The null directions on beams and dipoles are relatively easy to locate. Unfortunately, many of the antennas used by shortwave listeners are either random length or long-wire types, and the nulls on

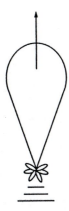

Figure 24-10
Yagi or quad intenna. Beam antenna radiation pattern.

those antennas are multiple and functions of both frequency and physical length. For those antennas, the prediction of null directions is difficult.

VHF/UHF receivers often use omnidirectional, or at least multidirectional, antennas, so the co-channel problem is particularly difficult. For those cases, a change of antenna type might be in order if receiving a particular station is important.

Adjacent channel interference is caused by stations that are on channels close to the frequency being received. In some cases, wavetraps will suffice, but for others the only solution is to have a receiver with excellent dynamic range and selectivity characteristics. We will take a look at wavetraps shortly.

Off-channel or *out-of-band* interference is caused when a strong local signal on a frequency that is unrelated, and not very near the desired frequency, causes interference. These signals are dealt with by using wavetraps, passband filters, or bandstop filters. A wavetrap will attenuate a signal frequency; a passband filter will pass the desired frequency band and attenuate other frequencies; a bandstop filter will attenuate the frequencies in the band of the offending signal, but not other frequencies.

Desensitization occurs when a strong local signal drives the RF amplifier or other front-end components very heavily, leaving little dynamic range for desired signals. The effect on the receiver is almost as if someone turned down the RF gain control. If the problem comes and goes, it might mean that the local interfering transmitter is being turned on and off. A common cause of desensitization is when the offending RF signal autorectifies in the input RF amplifier device and causes a dc bias that reduces the receiver front-end gain much like automatic gain control.

Generation of unwanted harmonics comes about because a nonlinear electronic circuit will cause even a pure, harmonic free sinewave RF signal to become rich in harmonics. This problem is found mostly when an AM broadcast station nearby overloads the RF amplifier of the receiver and drives it into a nonlinear region of operation.

Harmonics are integer multiples of the fundamental frequency (2f, 3f, 4f, 5f . . .), so one will find the AM-band station at successively higher frequencies. For example, a station at 1500 KHz AM will be found at 3000 KHz, 4500 KHz, 6000 KHz, and so forth.

Do not call the FCC or the station's chief engineer until you check out the receiver. The problem is not bad tuning or malfunctions at the radio station, but rather a normal (if undesired) response to nonlinear conditions in *your* receiver.

Rarely are more than the first three or four harmonics generated, but it is possible to find cases in which the spurious harmonics are generated well into the low-VHF band. In one case, interference existed in the 35-MHz region, but the scanner owner lived close enough to the AM station's tower to worry during hurricane season.

Distortion of desired signals occurs when a receiver lacks the dynamic range to handle a strong local signal. Not only might the audio recovered from the signal be distorted, but there might be some distortion of the RF signal that causes spurious signals to the generated. I have seen a strong FM band signal re-create itself up and down the FM band at frequency spacings that are probably explained by modulation theory. The solution is simple: Attenuate the unwanted signal.

24-11-1 Attenuators

An attenuator is a resistor circuit that will provide a loss between input and output. The ratio of the loss is usually expressed in terms of decibels from the following expressions:

$$dB = 20 \log_{10} \left(\frac{V_o}{V_{in}} \right) \qquad (24\text{-}4)$$

and

$$dB = 10 \log_{10} \left(\frac{P_o}{P_{in}} \right) \qquad (24\text{-}5)$$

for the sake of reference, a 2:1 ratio of voltage represents −6 dB loss, and a 2:1 ratio of power is a −3 dB loss.

When designing attenuators it is important to make sure that the devices are truly resistive and contain no reactive components such as inductors and capacitors. Reactive attenuators are sometimes seen but are difficult to make successfully. Second, the attenuator should input and output impedances that are the same as the antenna input impedances of the receiver system; that impedance is usually 50 Ω but in some cases is 75 and 300 Ω (the latter are used in TV systems).

Figure 24-11 shows an attenuator that is used in receiver circuits. It is designed for 50-Ω antenna systems and can be used from very low frequency (VLF) up to the mid-VHF region (≈ 200

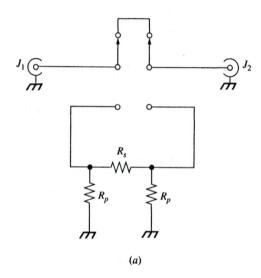

(a)

Attenuation (dB)	$R_s(\Omega)$	$R_p(\Omega)$
1	6.2	910
2	12	470
3	18	300
5	33	200
10	75	100
20	270	68

(b)

Figure 24-11
Attenuator used in receiver circuits. *(a)* Pi-network attenuator. *(b)* Resistor values.

MHz). The resistors are 1/4-W carbon composition or metal film types; it is important *not* to use wirewound resistors because of their excessive inductance.

The resistor network in Figure 24-11(a) is a pinetwork attenuator in which a single series resistance (R_s) is used with two shunt or parallel resistances (R_p). When a receiver has a single-stage attenuator with IN and OUT being the only selections, it is likely that this is the type of circuit used.

The values for the attenuator pad resistors are shown in the table in Figure 24-11b. These values cause a slight impedance mismatch, or possibly a slightly different attenuation ratio. Because this attenuator is used to reduce overload rather than to make precision signal strength measurements, we can live with this slight error in order to use commonly available resistance values.

A *double-pole double-throw* (DPDT) switch is used to connect or disconnect the attenuator from the circuit. When the switch is in the up position, the attenuator is disconnected from the circuit. Alternatively, when the switch is in the down position, the attenuator is placed in series with the signal path between jacks J_1 and J_2. The circuit is bilateral, so it does not matter which jack is connected to the antenna and which is connected to the receiver.

More than one attenuator can be connected in series to form greater attenuation ratios. Each section should be provided with its own shielded enclosure, or at least shielded section of the main enclosure, in order to prevent RF leakage or coupling from providing a ratio other than the design value.

24-11-2 Wavetraps

A *wavetrap* is a circuit that will attenuate either a single frequency or a very narrow band of frequencies. These circuits can be used to attenuate the signal from a single offending station. For example, if you have interference from an AM radio station, then it might be prudent to wipe out that

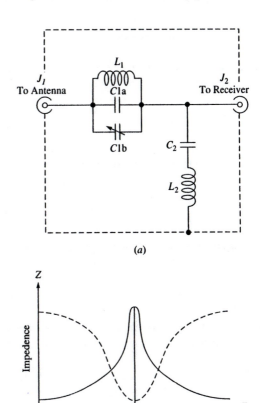

(a)

(b)

Figure 24-12
Pair of wave traps in a single shielded enclosure.
(a) Parallel and series wave traps. *(b)* Frequency response curves.

frequency in the antenna input circuitry. Figure 24-12 shows a pair of wavetraps in a single shielded enclosure. Either the parallel version (C_{1a}, C_{1b}, L_1) or series (C_2, L_2) can be used alone, or both can be used together as shown.

The wavetrap works because of the respective properties of series and parallel resonant inductor-capacitor *(LC)* tank circuits. A parallel resonant tank circuit, such as $C_{1a}/C_{1b}/L_1$, offers a very high impedance to the resonant frequency, but a low impedance to frequencies removed from resonance. Thus, when a parallel resonant tank circuit is placed in series with the signal path, as it is in

Figure 24-12*a*, then it provides maximum attenuation at the resonant frequency (solid curve in Figure 24-12*b*), A series resonant circuit, on the other hand, provides a very low impedance to its resonant frequency but not the others (dotted-line curve in Figure 24-12*b*).

In practical circuits, using both series and parallel resonant wavetraps will maximize the attenuation of a single frequency if both tank circuits are tuned to the same frequency. In some cases, however, there are two interfering stations, and it might prove necessary to make one tank circuit resonate on one frequency and the other wavetrap resonate on the other frequency. For example, suppose there are two strong AM stations: a 2000-W daytime-only station on 780 KHz, and a 24-hour 5000-W station on 1390 KHz. Both of these stations are capable of ruining the reception in the low end of the medium-wave and HF shortwave bands. A dual-frequency wavetrap is the solution to this problem.

The values of the components used in the wavetrap depend on the frequency and are found from:

$$F = \frac{1}{2 \pi \sqrt{LC}} \qquad (24\text{-}6)$$

or, because we are more likely to know the frequency to be attenuated, and we want to know the inductance or capacitance:

$$L = \frac{1}{39.5 \, F^2 L} \qquad (24\text{-}7)$$

or

$$C = \frac{1}{39.5 \, F^2 L} \qquad (24\text{-}8)$$

where F is in hertz, L is in henrys, and C is in farads. The actual values will vary from the equation values because of stray capacitances and component tolerances; at low frequencies stray inductances are not usually a factor. Examples of values from Equation 24-8 are provided for the preceding 1390-KHz example:

$L*$(henries)	C (farads)
100 μH	131 pF
220 μH	60 pF

*Selected value from catalog

The actual value of the capacitor will be somewhat less than this because of strays, so make either the capacitor or the inductor (or both) adjustable to compensate for the error.

24-11-3 Bandstop wavetrap

A bandstop wavetrap will attenuate the frequencies within an entire band. These traps are used especially when there are multiple stations in the band that overload the short-wave or scanner receiver. The AM broadcast band is a prime candidate for this treatment because of the large number of high-power signals found on the band in some metropolitan areas. Figure 24-13 shows a bandstop filter designed for the AM broadcast band. It uses components that are relatively easy to obtain and is easy to build. One rule, however: Separate the coils a couple of centimeters and place L_3, L_4, and L_5 at right angles to L_1/L_2.

24-11-4 High-pass filters

In the cases that we have been dealing with, the offending signals are usually below the desired frequency. Thus, we can use a *high-pass filter* to pass those frequencies that we want and attenuate those that we do not want.

Scanner receiver operators who worry about AM stations, HF ham stations, and CB stations (not all of which operate at 5-W legal power) might want to use a low-VHF high-pass filter such as those shown in Figure 24-14. The version shown in Figure 24-14*a* is for coaxial input receivers that require a 75-Ω impedance in the antenna circuit, while Figure 24-14*b* shows one that is for balanced 300-Ω twin-lead systems. In the

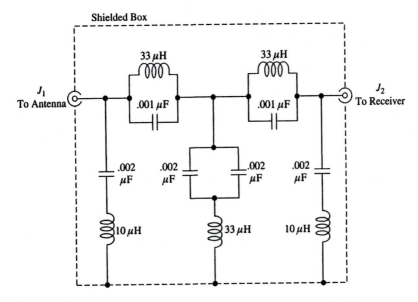

Figure 24-13
Bandstop filter for suppression of the AM BCB.

latter case, sometimes 0.001-μF, 1000-V disc ceramic capacitors are used at the points marked *X*.
These capacitors are used for receivers that do not
use a power transformer (ac/dc). Such receivers

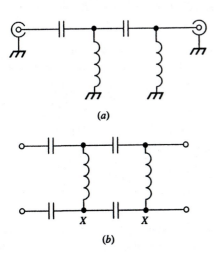

(a)

(b)

Figure 24-14
High-pass filter circuits. (a) Unbalanced.
(b) Balanced.

are too dangerous to use in a hospital environment
(electrical shock hazard is substantial).

These filters are very similar to the TV high-
pass filters used to prevent amateur radio and CB
interference. You can buy such filters for frequencies higher than 54 MHz in TV and video stores.

A universal high-pass filter is shown in Figure
24-15a. The capacitors were 0.001 μF, and the inductor was a 2.7-μH coil. The coil was actually a
10.7-MHz FM intermediate frequency (IF) coil
with the capacitor disconnected. Figure 24-15b
shows the frequency response curve for the filter.
The filter was designed to pass frequencies above
3000 KHz and attenuate those frequencies (such as
the AM band) below 3000 KHz.

The capacitors and inductors for other frequencies are found from:

$$L = \frac{R}{4 \pi F_c} \qquad (24\text{-}9)$$

where *L* is in henrys, *C* is in farads, F_c is the cutoff frequency in hertz, and *R* is the system impedance, either 50 or 75 Ω.

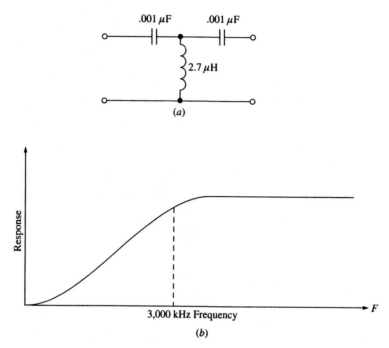

Figure 24-15
High-pass filter. *(a)* Universal high-pass filter. *(b)* Frequency response curve.

24-12 ECG equipment and EMI

Medical equipment seems especially sensitive to picking up interfering signals. The ECG electrode wires are exposed at the ends. In addition, the patient's body is basically an electrical conductor, so it makes a relatively good antenna to pick up signals that exist in the air. The solution to that problem is a low-pass filter (Figure, 24-16) that blocks radio signals but not the ECG. These filters are not like the 60-Hz filter that is used in the ECG machine to eliminate power-line artifact. That filter takes out a segment of the 0.05- to 100-Hz spectrum that is normally part of the ECG waveform and so will always affect the shape of the waveform presented to the medical person using the machine. The RF low-pass filter has such a high cutoff frequency that the ECG waveform is not affected.

24-13 EMI to biomedical sensors

Most biomedical sensors are susceptible to EMI because of the typically very low signal levels produced by those sensors. One authority points to an especially severe EMI problem with Wheatstone bridge strain gauges that typically have very low gauge factors. It is worthwhile, therefore, to review the causes of, and possible solutions for, these types of EMI problems.

Sources of EMI are the same sort of RF generators that also afflict radio receivers (discussed earlier). One cannot connect a half wavelength shorted stub across a sensor output line, however. At the low (non-RF) frequencies used by sensor signals, all shorted RF stubs are short circuits to all relevant signal frequencies—so the sensor output will be shorted into the stub along with resonant RF frequencies. To identify solutions to problems for this

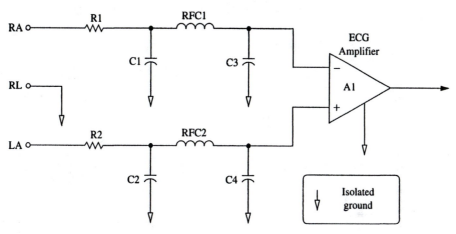

Figure 24-16
Space allowed for a one line caption to come.

type of EMI, it is helpful to know the typical routes that EMI signals follow to enter a sensor system.

There are three principal transmission paths for EMI into a sensor system: *penetration, leakage,* and *conduction.* Figure 24-17*a* illustrates penetration. In this case, the impinging electromagnetic (EM) wave cuts across the sensor and its circuit, setting up RF currents in the sensor circuitry. These RF currents become valid signals in the system. The argument is sometimes made that sensor circuits typically have such low frequency response that RF signals will not affect them. This argument is, unfortunately, largely specious because of phenomena such as *autorectification.* When this problem occurs, the RF signals rectify (detect) in the PN junctions of the semiconductor components used in the sensor electronics. This action either produces a dc bias that distorts the operation of the circuit or extracts modulation components that are within the frequency response passband of the circuit.

The solution for eliminating penetration EMI is to shield the circuit entirely in a shielded environment. A proper shield is metallic, or another conductive material, and is well sealed. Often, especially when very high frequencies or microwaves

are causing the interference, the shielded box holding the electronics must have additional shielding. In many cases, extra fasteners or screws are needed to seal the lips or edges of the shielded cabinet. The rule of thumb is that the screws should be spaced less than one-half wavelength at the highest frequency expected (or specified for that particular product).

Leakage occurs when the EM wave enters the shielded cabinet through small cracks or spaces in the shielding (Figure 24-17*b*). The standard wisdom is that a half-wavelength slot will admit RF to a shielded compartment, unfortunately, that is not always true, especially when nonsinusoidal RF waveforms are present. The wavelength of the signal fundamental frequency is:

$$\lambda_{meters} = \frac{300}{F_{MHz}} \qquad (24\text{-}10)$$

Thus, a 150-MHz taxicab transmitter creates a 2-m wavelength signal and so is not a problem in most cases because the necessary gap (1 m) is wide compared with the size of the instrument cabinet. In the microwave region, however, wavelengths drop to the centimeter and millimeter region, so these become a large problem.

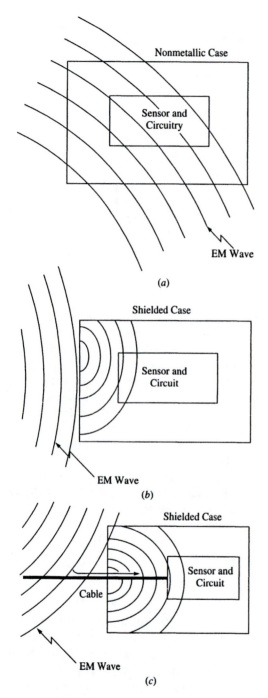

Figure 24-17
Routes for EMI interference to equipment.
(a) Penetration. *(b)* Leakage. *(c)* Conduction.

Even at lower frequencies, however, modulation or other situations can raise the number and strength of the harmonics of the fundamental, and these can cause severe interference under the right circumstances. Pulsed signals, for example, can have significant harmonics of 100 times the fundamental frequency. A 400-MHz signal has a wavelength of 0.75 m. If it is a sine wave signal, or contains linear voice modulation (or certain other forms), then there will be few harmonics. But if the 400-MHz signal is pulsed, then it might easily have harmonics to 4 or even 40 GHz. At these frequencies, the shielding must be tight.

There are two modes of leakage. The resonant mode occurs when the gap in the sensor shielding is resonant at the interfering frequency. If the gap is a half wavelength, then it will act as a slot antenna and efficiently reradiate the offending signal inside the shielded enclosure.

Conduction EMI (Figure 24-17c) occurs when a signal induces current into an exposed power, ground, control, or signal cable entering or leaving the shielded compartment. In this type of interference, the EMI signal reradiates inside the housing and is picked up by the sensor or its electronics. Surprisingly short lengths of wire will act as relatively efficient antennas in the UHF region and above.

24-13-1 Some solutions

Figure 24-18 shows two common solutions for EMI in sensor systems: *filtering* (Figure 24-18a) and *shielding* (Figure 24-18b). It is likely that both will have to be used in any given system.

The use of filtering to attenuate RF signals before they get to the sensor or electronics circuits is shown in Figure 24-18a. Each line in the system (whether power or signal) has a π-section filter consisting of an inductor element called an *rf choke* (RFC) and two capacitors. An example in Figure 24-18a is $RFC_1/C_1/C_4$ in the +Power line. The π-section filter is basically a low-pass RF filter that has a -3 dB cutoff frequency that is well below the offending signal's frequency but well above the highest frequency in the Fourier

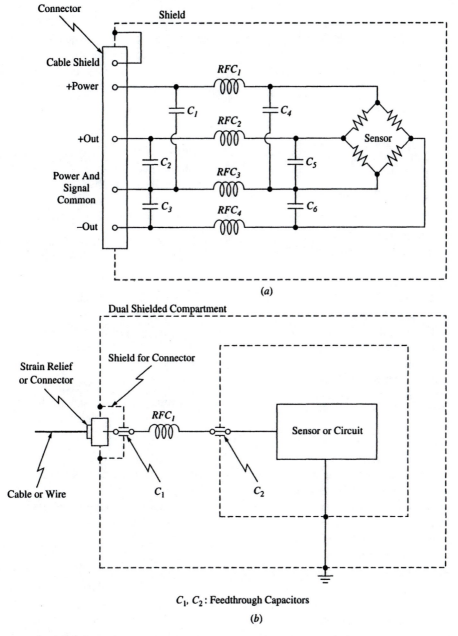

Connector

Shield

Cable Shield

+Power

RFC_1

C_1

C_4

+Out

RFC_2

Sensor

C_2

C_5

Power And
Signal
Common

RFC_3

C_3

C_6

–Out

RFC_4

(a)

Dual Shielded Compartment

Strain Relief
or Connector

Shield for Connector

RFC_1

Sensor or Circuit

Cable or Wire

C_1

C_2

C_1, C_2 : Feedthrough Capacitors

(b)

Figure 24-18
Solutions for EMI. *(a)* Filtering. *(b)* Shielding.

spectrum of the sensor output signal. A rule of thumb for the filter cutoff frequency is to calculate it from the length of exposed cable in the sensor system:

$$F_c << \frac{300}{2L} \qquad (24\text{-}11)$$

where

F_c is the -3 dB cutoff frequency of the low-pass filter

L is the length of cable in meters

For example, a 1-foot (0.295 m) cable is half-wavelength resonant at a frequency of 509 MHz. Signal interference is maximum at that frequency but is still significant at frequencies removed from F_c, especially those that are higher. The "much less than" symbol ($<<$) in Equation 24-11 can be taken to mean 1/10, so the cutoff frequency, F_c, of the low-pass filter should be F_c/10, or, in the preceding case, 509 MHz/10 = 50.9 MHz.

The filter should be installed as closed to the connector in the shielded bulkhead as possible. Otherwise, reradiation can occur from the wiring between the connector and the filter. Commercially available EMI filters usually are chassis or bulkhead mounted, so this requirement is easily met most of the time in actual practice.

If the EMI filter is installed in an ac power line, then make absolutely certain that it is of a type that is specifically designed for such service (the voltage rating is not always a sufficient indicator—look for the words *ac line* in the specification). If a filter is not specifically designed for service in 110-V ac or 220-V ac lines, then using them in that service can be dangerous.

Double shielding combined with filtering is shown in Figure 24-18*b*. The sensor is located inside an inner shielded compartment that is itself enclosed within the outer shielded compartment. An EMI filter (*RFC/C$_1$/C$_2$*) is placed between the cable strain relief and the inner shield compartment.

Artifacts in sensor data can be largely eliminated by the proper use of the techniques discussed in this chapter. While the topic is worthy of a book in its own right (and indeed, several have been written), these techniques are suitable for many—perhaps most—practical applications.

24-14 Summary

1. Telemetry systems are subject to a number of interference situations, including overload and intermodulation. There are also situations in which stations on adjacent channels and the same channel cause interference.

2. The solution for intermodulation problems is usually filtering to remove one or more offending signals.

3. Medical equipment, such as ECG units, that use exposed leads can suffer interference from electrosurgery and other RF generators. The usual solution is to remove the RF signal by filtering.

4. Filters useful for removing EMI include low-pass, high-pass, and bandpass filters. Sometimes half-wavelength shorted stubs are used.

5. EMI from a variety of sources can enter medical equipment either by direct pickup, by pickup in breaks on the shielding, and via conduction through power lines and signal lines going into the cabinet.

24-15 Recapitulation

Now return to the objectives and self-evaluation questions at the beginning of the chapter and see how well you can answer them. If you cannot answer the questions, place a check mark next to each and reread appropriate parts of the text. Next, try to answer the following questions using the same procedure. When you have answered all of the questions, solve the problems.

Questions

1. Define *electromagnetic interference* in your own words.

2. _____ interference is caused by two frequencies, F_1 and F_2, or their harmonics, mixing together in a nonlinear circuit to produce a third frequency.

3. The process of mixing together two frequencies (F_1 and F_2) to produce either the sum ($F_1 + F_2$) or difference ($F_1 - F_2$) frequencies is called _____ing.

4. Poor _____ or _____ range in the receiver is the cause of most intermodulation interference.

5. What circuit inside an FM broadcast receiver has the potential to interfere with radio telemetry units operating in the VHF region?

6. The _____ effect occurs in FM receivers and is characterized by the strongest of two co-channel signals locking the receiver to the exclusion of the weaker signal.

7. A _____ resonant wavetrap in series with the signal line will reject a signal on the trap's resonant frequency.

8. Two functions required of all electronic equipment are _____ and _____.

9. Operators of a transmitter are responsible for ensuring that the output signal is free of _____ that might interfere with other services.

10. A _____ _____ filter can be used in series with the leads of an ECG machine to reduce radio frequency EMI.

11. List four classes of overload problem seen on radio receivers.

12. _____ occurs when a strong local signal drives the RF amplifier of a receiver very heavily.

13. A receiver can generate harmonics of received signals, even when none exist in the actual signal. True or false?

14. An RF attenuator produces an output voltage of 50 μV when the input signal level is 750 μV. What is the loss in decibels?

15. A _____ _____ is a circuit that will attenuate a single frequency.

Problems

1. Calculate the intermodulation products for two signals: 432.33 MHz and 220.22 MHz.

2. A VHF telemetry transmitter operates on 174.15 MHz. In the same vicinity an FM broadcast station is operating at 88.5 MHz, and a landmobile station is operating at 478.33 MHz. Is there any likelihood of intermodulation interference to the telemetry receiver up to the third-order product?

3. It is necessary to remove a 1390-KHz AM broadcast band signal from a VHF telemetry system. Calculate the capacitance needed to resonate with a 220 μH inductor to form a parallel resonant wavetrap.

4. Calculate the electric field at a distance of 3 meters from a 2-W transmitter in which the antenna factor is 0.45.

5. Calculate the distance that a 5-W transmitter must be kept from a sensitive medical device in order to ensure that the E-field is less than 3 V/m when the antenna factor is 7.

Suggested Reading

1. AAMI. Technical Information Report. *Guidance on Electromagnetic Compatibility of Medical Devices for Clinical/Biomedical Engineers—Part 1: Radiated Radio-Frequency Electromagnetic Energy.* TIR-18-1997 Arlington, Virginia 1997. Carr, Joseph J.

Practical Antenna Handbook 3rd Edition. McGraw-Hill. New York 1996.

2. AAMI *Electromagnetic Compatibility of Medical Devices: Issues and Solutions.* FDA/AAMI Conference Report. Arlington, Virginia 1995.

3. Carr, Joseph J. *Receiver Antenna Handbook 2nd Edition.* Universal Radio Research. Reynoldsburg, OH, 2000.

4. Gerke, Daryl and Kimmel, William, *"EMI in Medical Devices,"* (Description of Five common EMI problems of ESD, RFI, power disturbances, emissions, self-compatibility, and four special medical EMI concerns of patient isolation, mixed technologies, multiple environments, cost of failure, (Medical Device Manufacturing and Technology Business Briefing Report and CD-ROM, Aspen Market Services, World Markets Research Center, Academic House, 24-28 Oval Road, London, WWI 7 DP, June, 1999, phone: +44-171-526-2400, Internet: www.wmrc.com)

5. Hare, Edward (ed.). *The ARRL RFI Book: Practical Cures for Radio-Frequency Interference.* ARRL, Newington, CT 1998.

6. Lohbeck, David. *CE Marking Handbook: A Practical Approach to Global Safety Certification.* Butterworth-Heinemann Newnes. Oxford (UK), 1998.

7. Scott, John and van Zyl Clincton. *Introduction to EMC.* Butterworth-Heinemann Newnes. Oxford (UK), 1997.

8. Watkins, Brad H. "Electromagnetic Compatibility of Strain Gage Transducers", *Sensors,* November 1989, pp. 35ff.

CHAPTER 25

Quality Assurance and Continuous Quality Improvement

25-1 Objectives

1. Understand the nature of variation.
2. Learn how to make a histogram.

3. Learn the data charting methods.
4. Understand the causes of variation.

25-2 Self-evaluation question

These questions test your prior knowledge of the material in this chapter. Look for the answers as you read the text. After you have finished studying the chapter, try answering these questions and those at the end of the chapter.

1. The _____ of variation recognizes that there is _____ in all things.

2. List two types of variation in a system.

3. The LSL and USL are related to the 3σ points. *True* or *false*.

4. Control chart is based on _____ chart concept.

25-3 Introduction

If there is any constant in life it is *variation*. Doctor W. Edwards Deming (1900–1993) spent a lifetime studying variation. His lessons were learned by Japanese industry in 1950, and formed the basis for their economic growth. But it wasn't until 1980 that they became well-known in the United States. It has been said that "failure to understand variation is the central problem of management" (Joiner, 1994). In one of Deming's teaching videos, he stated that we should export everything to foreign nations except American management style, which would be, he averred, ". . . Equivalent to an act of war." In the context of the video, Deming was referring to the profound lack of appreciation by managers for the role of variation in work systems, and how to deal with it. We are going to take a look at variation, what it means, how it is measured and how to treat it.

Variation is found in all things. Even where it looks like there is no variation in a group of like things, it is usually the case that our measurement lacks sufficient resolution to see it. With adequate measuring tools, however, we will see it. We now know two things about variation:

• It is in all things.

• It can be measured, given adequate tools.

Variation has long been understood in the scientific, medical research, and engineering fields, but (until recently) only poorly in American management circles. In other countries, notably Japan, variation in work processes is well recognized, and mechanisms are in place to overcome the problems of variation. Oddly, it was an American, W. Edwards Deming who taught the theory of variation to the Japanese. He is credited by Japanese industrial leaders as being largely responsible (in 1950) for setting the Japanese economic miracle on the path to success.

Deming is so highly regarded in Japan that the major competitive industrial prize in that country is called the Deming Prize. But, even though his theories were developed in the United States, notably at firms such as Western Electric and were the basis for the spectacular production in the USA during World War II, Deming was largely a prophet without honor in his own country until 1980. At that time, Deming's theories were the subject of an NBC television white paper titled *If Japan Can, Why Can't We?* Since 1980, Deming's theories gained popularity under the names "total quality management" (TQM), "continuous quality improvement" (CQI), performance improvement (PI) and similar titles. The acronyms "CQI" and "PI" are used most commonly in medicine but refer to the same thing as "TQM."

25-4 The theory of variation

The theory of variation recognizes that there is variation in all things: the temperature in your

work space; the throughput of the clinical laboratory; the attributes of supplies purchased; the effectiveness of drugs; the work product of individuals. Most people intuitively recognize that variation is a part of life and demonstrate it by placing a high amount of confidence in the bell-shaped normal distribution curve. Unfortunately, a little knowledge can be a dangerous thing: it is often the case that the causes of variation are misinterpreted, and incorrect (often harmful) action is taken in response to variation.

It is extremely important to understand how variation works, how it pertains to a system, and what can or cannot be done to correct it in any given situation. Lacking such insight, any management action whatsoever is likely to be incorrect and will probably exacerbate rather than alleviate the problem.

25-5 Variation in a system

A system typically has one or more inputs. It's function is to process inputs and then deliver some output product, i.e. that which is of importance to its customer. For example, a biomedical engineering department receives inputs in the form of malfunctioning equipment, executes a repair process, and then outputs repaired equipment. All systems produce variation in the results. Examples include the length of time needed to discharge the patient; the state or condition of the patient on discharge; the turn-around time for a biomedical shop, the time to response to trouble calls; and the percentage of calls completed on the first attempt.

25-6 Variation throughout history

The importance of and response to variation has differed throughout the ages. Although the Egyptians around 3,000 B.C. dabbled with the concept of making identical, interchangeable bows and arrows for their troops (Provost 1990), the principal response to variation in the ancient world was simple fitness for use. If the customer could use the product, regardless of how it was made (and how well), then it was "quality" (by definition). Pretty much the same system is found until about 1800. Throughout the Middle Ages and beyond, trained guild craftsmen turned out products. The guild controlled the training of the artisans (through apprenticeship arrangements) and the quality of their output.

But something happened at the turn of the nineteenth century that changed things forever. In the mid–1700s, a French gunsmith named Honoré Le Blanc invented the idea of making muskets according to a standard pattern that all workers copied. An American, Eli Whitney, won a government contract to make 10,000 muskets in 2 years. The two government arsenals together produced only 1,000 firearms in 3 years. Although Whitney took nearly 10 years to fulfill his first contract, in 1801 he invented an improvement on the standard pattern idea in which interchangeable parts were used to assemble the muskets. In a demonstration, President Thomas Jefferson selected a set of parts from piles of identical parts, and Whitney assembled a working gun from the selected parts.

Interchangeable parts assembly requires some means for ensuring that all parts of the same type are very nearly identical to each other: i.e., variation among the parts must be reduced. By 1823, manufacturers following Whitney's idea used "go/no-go" gauges and templates to accept or reject parts. As mechanical products became more sophisticated, the methods of quality control had to improve. In the 1890s, the "go/no-go" concept was extended to include *specification limits and tolerances.* Measurements could be made and parts accepted that fell between a *lower specification limit* (LSL) and an *upper specification limit* (USL). Inspectors were used from the mid-19th century and still are. In the 1920s, Walter Shewhart of Western Electric developed the idea of *statistical process control* (SPC), and by 1931, had published his idea of using a *control chart* to keep tabs on work processes.

25-7 Variation

There is no known situation where real things or processes do not exhibit variation. When someone claims that measurements made on a specific group of things showed no variation, it is inevitably the case that the measurement device lacked the resolution to detect the differences. Those differences were present, but the "ruler" was not up to the task of discerning it.

An example of hidden variation was seen when Ford Motor Company compared transmissions made by one of their U.S. plants with supposedly identical transmissions made for them in Japan from the same engineering drawings. When certain critical internal dimensions were measured, the Ford-made parts were all within the specification limits set by the engineers, but varied normally between the limits. The Mazda-made parts, on the other hand, showed no variation. Believing the gauge to be broken, the test engineer summoned a repair technician, who found the gauge in good working order. The normal variation expected by the engineer was, indeed, present in the Mazda-made transmissions, but it was too small to be detected by the instrument.

25-8 Types of variation

There are two basic types of variation, and they are called by different names in different situations. One type of variation is the *normal variation* that is inherent to the thing that is varying. It is the natural variation that is built into the system. Normal variation is *random* in nature, i.e., it is not possible to accurately predict one value from prior knowledge of any other value.

The other basic type of variation is *abnormal variation,* i.e., variation that is due to other than natural causes. Abnormal variation does not usually appear random, although apparent randomness is sometimes seen because of either insufficient or incorrect data.

In evaluating variation in work processes or products, the knowledge that randomness is exhibited by normal variation, but not by abnormal variation, provides us with very valuable clues as to the source of the variation.

Another way that normal and abnormal variation is expressed uses the terms *unassignable variation* for the normal case, and *assignable variation* for the abnormal case. The reason for these terms is that natural variation, being inherent in the process and random in nature, cannot be attributed to any specific cause. Abnormal variation, however, has an assignable cause—e.g., a machine tool is worn, an accounting clerk is not properly trained, or incoming material or supplies are not what was ordered—that can be sought out and corrected.

In modern quality management theory, such as that taught by W. Edwards Deming, normal (unassignable) variation is referred to as *common cause* variation, while abnormal (assignable) variation is referred to as *special cause* variation.

It is the role of both workers and managers alike to understand the differences between the two broad categories of variation so that proper action can be taken when it is found. In the past, when variation produced unacceptable results in a work process or product, managers sometimes blamed workers for not trying hard enough. This approach was characterized by the attitude ". . . if we whip the cat hard enough, it'll pull the piano up the stairs." Today, it is well recognized that workers cannot be held responsible for random variation, regardless of the outcome with respect to results, because they have no control over random processes. Deming and his disciples state that only 4% (or less) of the problems caused by variation are assignable to the worker, and fully 96% are assignable to either management or to the processes themselves; only management has the authority and resources to deal with defective processes.

25-9 Charting variation

There are several tools that can be used for charting variation in your work processes. These include: *histograms, run charts,* and *control charts.* Let's look at a practical example for handling data using these tools. Our scenario is a measurement of service quality: the length of time required to

TABLE 25-1   SERVICE RESPONSE TIME (MINUTES)*

55	56	52	54	52
49	53	54	51	53
53	50	56	51	57
52	52	55	50	52
54	53	51	55	52

*Read left-to-right, top-to-bottom.

TABLE 25-2   SORTED LOW-TO-HIGH

49	50	50	51	51
51	52	52	52	52
52	52	53	53	53
53	54	54	54	55
55	55	56	56	57

respond to an emergency service call. The data for 25 consecutive calls is shown in Table 25-1 below.

These data reflect the length of time from receiving a service request and the technician arriving on site. First, let's make a histogram. A histogram is a type of bar graph that shows the variation of the value of a single variable. (Bar graphs, on the other hand, compare different variables.) The first step is to order the data low-to-high, as shown in Table 25-2.

These data show variation from a low of 49 minutes to a high of 57 minutes. Normally, we would group these data into adjacent categories. But because these data are integers, and the range is not too large (49 to 57), we can use the values themselves to create groups of one value each. When we tally these data into the histogram, we get a pattern as shown in Figure 25-1.

Notice that these data tend to cluster around some central value (as indicated by the largest bar at 52 minutes).

25-10 Creating a histogram

The histogram is used to show the distribution of values of a single measurement. For example, if a machine cuts 250-mm steel bars from longer stock, vibration and other processes will make

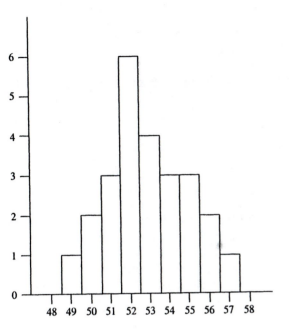

Figure 25-1

the actual lengths slightly different. For example, actual measurements on 110 rods might show lengths from 248.10 mm to 252.43 mm. A histogram can be used to see the dispersion of the actual measurements, as well as the shape of the distribution of values. To get a good snapshot of the process, one would need to take at least 30 data points. The actual number depends somewhat on the dispersion found; a wide dispersion suggests that more data points be collected. Up to a point, where the sample becomes too cumbersome and a rule of "diminishing returns" takes effect, the general rule is the more data points the better the information provided by the histogram.

The first task is to decide what to measure and how to measure it. The second task is to collect enough data to make a decent histogram. The data could be tabulated on a sheet of paper, or entered into a computer, but the job is to collect the values. Once the data are tabulated, the following steps are followed.

Step 1: Determine the range of the data. This is done by examining the tabulated data and picking out the lowest and highest values. The range (R) is maximum minus minimum. In the case of the steel bars above, the values were found to run from 248.10 mm to 252.43 mm, so R = (252.43 − 248.10) = 4.33 mm. The general rule is to make the range of the histogram slightly wider than the range of the data so that all of the data can be accommodated without ambiguity.

Step 2: Determine the number of intervals (K). To be meaningful, the data must be divided into a convenient number of intervals. There is no fixed rule as to the number of intervals, except that one must keep focused on the goal: communication of some aspect of the data. Too few intervals tends to blend things together and destroy the patterns and exceptions that the user needs to see. A grove of three trees does not make a forest. Too many, on the other hand, gets too "busy," and the forest becomes obscured by all the trees. A "reasonable number" seems to be on the order of 5 to 20 intervals, depending on the number of data points and what is being depicted. One useful guideline based on the number of data points is:

Data Points	Intervals (K)
< 50	5 to 7
50–100	6 to 10
100–200	7 to 12
200–250	13 to 16
> 250	17 to 20

Step 3: Determine the width of each interval (H). Divide the range (R) by the number of intervals (K) to find a trial interval width (H):

$$H = \frac{R}{K} \qquad (25\text{-}1)$$

In the case of our 110 steel rods from above, the table tells us to select 7 to 12 intervals to cover the range. Because we want to make the histogram range larger than the data range, we might want to use 248 mm for the lower limit and 253 mm for the upper limit, for a histogram range of 5 mm. Trying Equation 25-1 for various values of K from 7 to 12 yields:

K	H
7	0.714
8	0.625
9	0.556
10	0.500
11	0.455
12	0.417

The case for K = 10 looks good, and may well be our choice. A reason to not use it, however, is that many people find that an odd number of classes is more appealing, especially when the distribution is symmetrical. Let's use K = 9, for H = 0.556.

Step 4: Specify the boundaries for each interval. The actual interval boundaries are specified to one more decimal place than is used in the measurement to construct mutually exclusive classes.

Step 5: Make a frequency of occurrence tally sheet.

Step 6: Transfer the frequencies of occurrence from the tally sheet to a histogram.

Example 25-1 _____

An adhesives curing oven is suspected of being out of control because of the irregularity of results being obtained. A very accurate thermometer

is mounted in the oven so that the actual temperature can be compared with the set temperature of 750°F. The sorted data obtained over 15 trials are shown in Table 25-3. It is found that the actual temperatures ranged from 506°F to 989°F, with a mean of 784°F and a standard deviation of 157.

To construct our chart, we need to find the range ΔR:

$$\Delta R = T_{max} - T_{min} = 989 - 506 = 483 \qquad (25\text{-}2)$$

We next need to select the number of intervals (K) of temperatures for our chart. It is rarely useful to select as few a three intervals, or more than about twenty (which becomes too busy). For our case, let's use K = 7. The selection is sometimes almost arbitrary, but in this contrived case 483 is divisible by 7. The width of each interval is:

$$H = \frac{R}{K} = \frac{483}{7} = 69 \qquad (25\text{-}3)$$

A good general rule is to use one more decimal place for setting the intervals than are present in the data. In this case, our thermostat displays temperatures to the nearest degree, so we should use a thermometer that is accurate to tenths of a degree to set the end points. This procedure keeps us from seeing data points on the boundary between two intervals, which would make a counting error.

The lower bound of the graph is either the lowest value in the data set, or the next lowest rounded value below it. In our case, we can use 506°F as the lower bound. We then add the interval width to find the next boundary: 506 + 69 = 575. The next interval starts at 575.1, and so on. These values are shown in Table 25-4.

TABLE 25-3   TEMPERATURE DATA FROM CURING OVEN

506	517	522	538	541	550	551	583	586	599
626	635	640	664	673	680	697	699	706	728
749	782	785	791	805	835	838	851	851	858
863	875	891	895	899	906	907	938	954	955
956	963	964	965	971	972	973	981	987	989

TABLE 25-4

Interval No.	Range
1	506–575
2	575.1–644.1
3	644.2–713.2
4	713.3–782.3
5	782.4–851.4
6	851.5–920.5
7	920.6–989.6

We can then go to Table 25-5 to count the number of data points in each interval, which are:

TABLE 25-5

Interval No.	Number In Interval	Proportion
1	7	0.14
2	6	0.12
3	6	0.12
4	3	0.06
5	7	0.14
6	8	0.16
7	13	0.26
	50	1.00

The resultant histogram is shown in Fig. 25-2.

The range of temperatures along the horizontal axis is very nearly the same as before because the range of the data did not change. A convenient length of graph paper was laid out (in this case, it was chosen to be approximately equal to the horizontal axis of the previous graph). On the graph paper that I used, the length turned out to be 115 small lines, which was then divided by the 484-degree range of data, yielding a step of about 0.24 lines per degree. This factor was then multiplied by the width of each interval to find the number of lines that are required to represent the interval on the graph paper. When that was done, it became possible to lay out the scale on the horizontal axis.

The vertical axis height (H) is a measure of the relative frequency (i.e., P is the number of measurements in the interval divided by total number

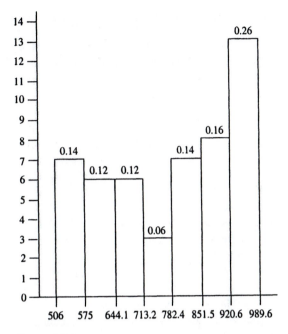

Figure 25-2

of measurements) divided by the width (W) of the interval:

$$H = \frac{P}{W} \qquad (25\text{-}4)$$

In the histogram of Figure 25-2 the value of H is placed over the bar for that interval, while the number of measurements that are within the interval are shown inside the bar.

25-11 Using histograms in quality control

Quality control specialists use histograms and other devices to monitor the "voice of the process" for producing a product or service. The shape, range, and any peaks or valleys in the data become clues to whether the process is working as it should, whether it is not performing adequately, and where it can be improved.

A key concept in quality control is that of *specification limits*. An engineer might specify that a lid for a can of soup have a 6.3-cm diameter. In an ideal world, the lid-cutting machine would produce tens of thousands of lids all with a diameter of 6.30000 cm, but in the real world the values will vary over a range. To use as many of the produced lids as possible, the engineer will specify a minimum and maximum actual diameter. Lids with less than the minimum diameter will leak and the soup will either spoil or be lost. If the lids are too large, then they will not fit onto the can. Damage to the entire can may occur (increasing loss), or the can will leak because the lid deformed when it was force-fitted onto the can.

Figure 25-3a shows the situation. The *target value* is 6.3-cm diameter that the engineer specified, while the *lower specification limit* (LSL) is the minimum acceptable diameter and the *upper specification limit* (USL) is the maximum acceptable diameter. When the data are plotted (Fig. 25-3b) it is easy to see whether the dispersion falls within the LSL to USL range.

If all of the values are within the range, then all of the product can be usable. If some product falls outside the LSL to USL range (Fig. 25-3c), that product is scrap and must be rejected.

In most cases, the target value will be midway between the LSL and USL, but that is not always true. There may be an engineering reason for keeping the tolerance tighter on one side of the target or the other.

There may also be a management reason for such an offset; for example, when the dispersion of actual value is such that the offset produces more reworkable product than scrap product (therefore less loss), then it might be prudent to shift the target towards the most economical end (assuming that no improvement is possible). For example, suppose we are cutting the 250-mm steel rods mentioned earlier. Any product above the USL can be machined to a shorter length and recovered; that material is *rework,* and although it is a loss, it may be less of a loss than the *scrap* produced below the LSL.

25-12 Interpreting QC histograms

The histogram tells us much about the process being measured. The shape and dispersion of the data are evident from the histogram. We can also

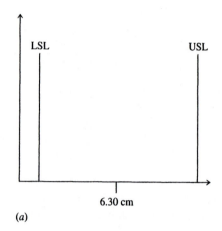

(a)

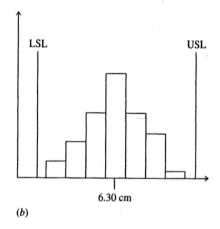

(b)

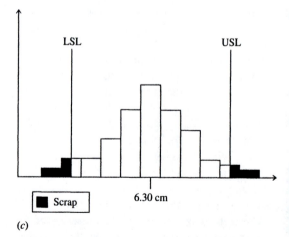

(c)

Figure 25-3

tell the location of the central peak, and how both the peak and the dispersion relate to the USL and LSL limits. If the dispersion is narrow compared with the USL and LSL, then we know that the process will tolerate a small amount of drift before either scrap or rework is produced. In this section we will take a look at some of the special cases that might arise.

Figure 25-4a shows an outlier in the data. Because the different values can occur randomly, this outlier may be completely natural, and if kept to a small frequency of occurrence, it could be ignorable. The outlier could also indicate that a measurement error occurred or that a measurement instrument needs repair or calibration. It could also indicate a disturbance to the process, in which case the person responsible for the process must determine whether it was a one-time event or part of a continuing pattern.

Another possible explanation for an outlier is that the process is trying to whisper something in your ear. The outlier could indicate the first few data points in a new cohort of data that will eventually tell you that the central peak or the dispersion has shifted above the USL.

The dispersion in Fig. 25-4b could indicate that some natural limit was reached and that no further data to the right of the peak can be obtained. It could also indicate that product above the cut-off point was culled out for some reason. The culling might be due to an inspection process, or it might be due to product being removed from the population to specify the requirements of some particular customer.

Another example of culling is seen in Fig. 25-4c. In this case, the culling was due to an inspector rejecting product that fell below the LSL. In the example of Fig. 25-4d culling is seen at both LSL and USL. This approach is "quality by inspection" and is regarded as a less satisfactory approach than designing the process to operate in the center of the range with a small dispersion. The

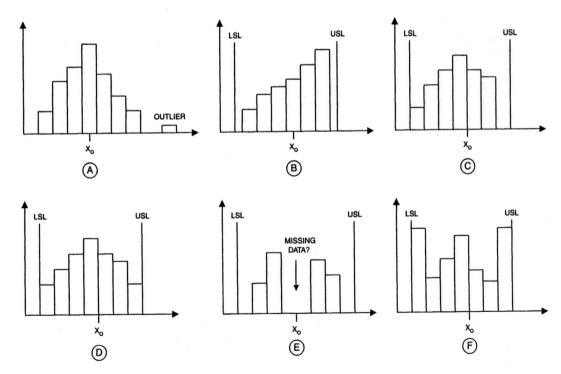

Figure 25-4

reason is that no inspection process is 100% reliable, and this situation almost surely results in some bad product reaching the customers.

The example of Figure 25-4e is a "heart cut." If too few data points are taken, then this distribution could conceivably be due to a bimodal distribution that hasn't completely filled out yet. However, a better explanation is that it is due to culling for a special customer or special project. An example was seen in the U.S. Army's Springfield Arsenal. Parts for ordinary infantry rifles were subject to the LSL/USL limits. Special, highly accurate rifles were needed by the rifle team and by snipers. These were manufactured with parts that fell very close to the target values. To have sufficient parts to make these "Five Star Springfields," all parts that fell close to the target value were culled out and set aside. When the remaining parts are measured and tallied, a "heart cut" histogram results.

The distribution in Figure 25-4f has the classes at either end of the LSL/USL range with seemingly too many occurrences. If the process was working correctly, then it is more likely that those bars would be shorter than the adjacent bars. A probable reason for this situation is flinching on the part of the inspector. For some reason, the inspector is accepting product outside of the LSL/USL limits. In the case of flinching, the outsize bars might be against either LSL, USL, or both limits (as shown).

When the situation of Figure 25-4f is found, it is necessary to figure out what is causing the problem, because customers are almost surely getting bad product. One possible cause is that the inspector has been "reprogrammed" by supervisors who question rejection decisions in an effort to get the daily production numbers up and rejection rate down. It might be a simple case of the foreman snidely asking, "You don't *really* [tone of voice change for emphasis] think this is a reject, do you?" Or it might be more overt pressure to get product out the door and let the devil take the hindmost. It doesn't take the inspector long to figure out that life will be nicer if they make close judgment calls on the side of acceptance rather than rejection . . . But the customer still gets bad product.

25-13 Control charts

Histograms are very useful, but are not the only method for graphing quality data. The control charts are based on the *run chart* concept. A run chart plots data as a function of time, or otherwise in a sequence. Figure 25-5 shows a typical run chart. This chart sometimes gives a false view regarding trends up and down. This type of error is especially likely if only over a short period of time. For example, the first four data points in Figure 25-5 show a downward trend. The question is whether or not these data show a genuine trend.

A *control chart* takes the run chart and adds three lines to it: *mean, lower control limit* (LCL), and *upper control limit* (USL). The mean is the

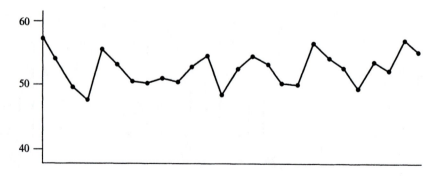

Figure 25-5

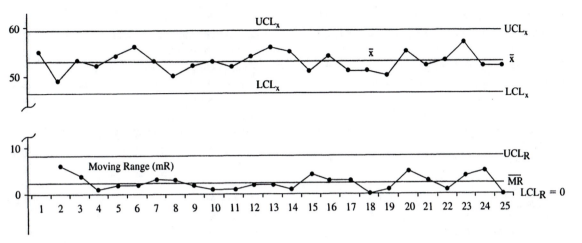

Figure 25-6

arithmetic average; the LCL and UCL are calculated from the data (and are approximations of the 3σ points on the normal distribution curve). An example of an X-mR "moving range" control chart is shown in Figure 25-6. This type of control chart plots individual measurements. Other examples of chart plot averages of samples greater than one, number defective, and percent defective. For our present purposes we will consider only the X-mR type of control chart. This particular chart was made using the data for the service response time study given in Table 25-1 at the beginning of this chapter.

Two different plots are shown in Figure 25-6. The X-plot shows the data from Table 25-1, with lines connecting the data points. This is essentially the same as in a run chart. Also added, however, are the mean ("X-bar"), UCL, and LCL lines. The

other plot is the moving range (MR) plot shown below and aligned to the X-plot. The "moving range" is the absolute value of the difference between adjacent data points, or R = ABS($X_i + 1 - X_i$). For example, let's take a look at the first six data points from Table 25-1, here in Table 25-6.

For the data in Table 25-1 we can calculate X-bar (mean average) as 52.9, and the mean for the MR as 2.46. The upper and lower control limits for the two sets of data are calculated from the equations below.

25-13-1 Moving Range

$$UCL_R = 3.2267 \times \overline{MR} \qquad (25\text{-}5)$$

$$LCL_R = 0 \qquad (25\text{-}6)$$

25-13-2 X-data

$$LCL_X = \overline{X} + (2.66 \times \overline{MR}) \qquad (25\text{-}7)$$

$$UCLX = \overline{X} - (2.66 \times MR) \qquad (25\text{-}8)$$

25-14 Analyzing control charts

If a work process results in only random variation, which indicates that the variation is inherent in the system, then all of the X and R data points will fall between the LCL and UCL for their respective

TABLE 25-6

X	mR
55	(not defined)
49	6
53	4
52	1
54	2
56	2

plots. If a data point is outside the LCL to UCL limits, then there might be a problem (which will be discussed later). Also indicating a potential problem is any pattern in the data, even though all points are inside the LCL/UCL limits. Normally, the data in a random system will more or less flip to either side of the mean value. Potential problems are indicated by:

- Six or more data points in a row on one side of mean
- Six or more consecutive data points in either a rising or falling line

What to do about these indications are discussed below.

25-15 Causes of variation

All variation is caused. There are four basic classes of variation in systems (Joiner and Gaudard, 1990): *common causes, special causes, structural causes,* and *tampering causes.* Understanding these causes, and how they operate, enables managers to correctly ". . . recognize, interpret, and react appropriately to variation. . . . (Joiner 1990)."

Common causes are the random variations in inputs, processes, and other factors that combine to produce a variation in the system output; it is the collective effect of all natural variation inherent within the system. When measurements are made of the process output, the data for common causes tends to be randomly distributed.

Special causes are those causes of variation that are *assignable,* i.e., those that can therefore be tracked down to some specific source: bad supplies, inappropriate procedures, improperly trained personnel, and so forth. Special causes tend to be nonrandom, and can be detected by patterns or extreme points in the data used to track the system.

Structural causes tend to be either periodic or due to some long-term trend. Examples of the periodic events that may affect system results might include the annual vacation periods popular with patients or surgeons, annual holidays when few surgeries are scheduled (or where there is a rush to be done before the holiday), or summertime, when

regular staff are on vacation and temps or RNs (who may be unfamiliar with operations in that unit) are used extensively.

Tampering causes are induced variation that is produced largely by management decisions or staff actions to solve the problems of the other three forms of cause, without understanding the nature of such causes. Typical of "tampering" are situations where a new rule or procedure addresses a symptom of a root cause, but does not address the root cause at all. A medical analogy might be relieving a fever with aspirin, but not treating the underlying bacterial infection with antibiotics.

Typical of tampering situations is the scenario where a tampering causes things to get better temporarily, allowing the manager to take credit for it, but then they worsen again, often to a worse state than previously, causing the manager to seek someone to blame for the recurring failure.

Tampering usually results from confusing special causes and common causes. The appropriate reactions to common and special causes are different, and confusing them results in inappropriate action and, often, a worsening of the situation rather than improvement. No amount of rebuke of staff, no amount of supervisor ranting, will ever fix a common cause problem.

25-16 Discriminating between special and common causes

The means for determining any particular form of variation is to collect data on some meaningful parameter that properly reflects what one wishes to control and then properly analyze and interpret that data. For example, one might wish to track the length of time required to return a defective instrument to service.

Once a metric on the parameter of interest is determined, e.g., time-to-repair, then the data are collected and charted. An old-fashioned and often ill-used charting method is the ordinary run chart. The metric value is plotted along the vertical axis, while the events, or time, are along the horizontal axis.

A pernicious problem with the run chart approach is the fact that it does not allow one to discern common and special causes. Managers tend to misinterpret run charts. When the average discharge time is low, then the manager will praise the staff, and when it is high they rebuke or discipline the same staff. This dizzying approach leads to serious morale problems in the worst cases because the staff is alternately praised or rebuked for things they either don't know how to change or know are beyond their control.

25-17 Common causes and special causes: detection

When a system is *stable* and in *statistical control,* all of the data points on a control chart will be: (a) within the UCL/LCL limits and (b) randomly distributed about the midline. All causes of variation in such a system are common causes.

When data points fall outside of the control limits, or when certain nonrandom patterns appear within the limits, then variation, or at least some portion of it, is due to special causes. Patterns within the limits that indicate a problem include: seven points in a row on one side of the mean, a run of seven points in a row in either ascending or descending direction, and points falling outside the control limits.

The terms "stable" and "in control" do not indicate a necessarily desirable situation. They merely indicate that all causes of variation capable of affecting the average performance are common causes, as indicated by the randomness. A system that consistently produces bad results may well be stable and in control, but is also in a state that is not acceptable. In those cases, rebuking workers will not solve the problem and may indeed make it worse. In those cases, the system solutions may be subtle and are those that either tend to move the average in a desirable direction, narrow the distance between UCL and LCL, or both.

The UCL and LCL are not "specification limits," but rather derive from calculations made on the actual data. Specification limits can be set by management or the customer, and are what are sometimes called "tolerances" in the mechanical world. That is, limits to variation between which

the product is still useful. For example, a design engineer might tell production that the dimension of a certain mechanical part must be 6.5 ± 0.010 inches. This means that the part can be used if its actual length is between 6.49 in. and 6.51 in. Another example is a specification may be set for the length of time required for a stat lab to get a blood test result back to the floor. Such a specification limit might be stated as "2 hours," meaning any time from zero to 120 minutes. In that case, the lower specification limit (LSL) is zero, and the upper specification limit (USL) is 120 minutes.

An error often made by managers who are not familiar with statistical thinking is to assume that they can order the LCL and UCL changed to get better performance. The LCL/UCL data are solely a function of the actual data (they are what they are); it's the specification limits (LSL/USL) that are open to management change (they are what the customer needs).

25-18 Responses to common and special causes

The correct management responses to common and special causes are different. A common cause can only be improved by working on the system to eliminate the root source of the problem. A special cause can be investigated, using scientific research methods where necessary, and dealt with accordingly (and "do nothing" may be an appropriate response in some cases). An example of a special cause in the "time to repair" example may be reduced staff due to the flu being prevalent in the community. Such a special cause will be transient and may need no response other than noting it. Common causes may be poor parts ordering, insufficient staff, or lack of technical manuals. Those problems can be identified and rectified.

25-19 TQM, ISO-9000, and Six-Sigma

Even a casual observer of the business scene knows that a worldwide quality movement is in progress. Billed by some as a response to the

Japanese, which is partly true, the quality movement has gathered momentum since the early 1980s when the teachings of quality gurus such as W. Edwards Deming and Joseph Juran began to receive as much attention in the West as they did in Japan.

There are two main thrusts to the global quality movement: "Total Quality Management" (TQM) and ISO-9000. While some people see these two thrusts as being at odds with each other—TQM is seen as trying to replace what ISO-9000 represents—they are actually complementary and not antagonistic at all.

25-19-1 The ISO-9000 series

The ISO-9000 series of quality standards are touted to be a "European standard," which is absolutely required to sell products in Europe these days. Neither part of this statement is totally true.

The perceived "Europeaness" of the ISO-9000 series standards is due in part to the fact that it is sponsored by the International Organization for Standards based in Geneva, Switzerland. Another element in the perceived Europeaness of ISO-9000 is the fact that it is officially adopted by the European Community (EC). The perception lends ISO-9000 a somehow foreign and inscrutable aspect that is false for at least two good reasons.

First, the ISO-9000 standard was not evolved solely by Europeans. The United States representative to the ISO is the American National Standards Institute (ANSI), who participated in the formulation of the ISO-9000 series of standards from the beginning.

Second, the ISO-9000 series has an American heritage. It embodies principles that are long familiar to American quality assurance professionals, and are deeply ingrained in much of American industry. The direct parentage of the ISO-9000 includes the British Standard BS 5750 (1979), which is in turn based, at least in part on British military standard DEF/STAN 05-8 and NATO standard AQAP-1. The NATO AQAP-1 standard was adapted from the United States Department of Defense standard MIL-Q-9858A (1959, 1963). While ISO-9000 was

promulgated by an international organization based in Europe, it is still an *international* standard in which Americans participated heavily.

The notion that ISO-9000 is absolutely essential to anyone wishing to sell products in Europe is also not totally true. The European Community Council of Ministers mandated ISO-9000 certification for *certain regulated products* sold in Europe after January 1, 1993. Such products include medical devices, communications terminal equipment, commercial scales, construction products, gas appliances, and industrial safety equipment. Other products can be legally sold with or without ISO-9000 certification.

There may also be a practical difference between what the EC laws allow and common industrial practice. Customers see ISO-9000 as a credibility factor and may tend to prefer ISO-9000 suppliers. Indeed, some customers are already putting ISO-9000 registration as a requirement on their own suppliers. You may, therefore, see a solicitation for bids or price quotes carry a requirement of ISO-9000 registration even though the product can be legally sold without it. Many American companies are requiring ISO-9000 of their suppliers, even though the ISO-9000 consciousness is only beginning here.

Some people have complained that ISO-9000 results in a heavy flow of useless paperwork. That complaint comes from people unused to documenting what they do. The truth is that ISO-9000 paperwork requirements are not nearly as onerous as some have made them out to be. In fact, ISO 9004 specifically instructs companies to not create more paper work than is necessary to control the product's quality. A typical ISO-9000 top-level quality manual is about 50 to 65 pages long. Because many companies include procedures in their quality manual, some existing manuals run hundreds of pages. Much of the paperwork is what people ought to be doing anyway in their own best interests.

Another frequent complaint is that a company can be ISO-9000 compliant and still not put quality products out the door. That is true, but it is also irrelevant, because any standard is only as good as its enforcement. If your customers, who are the chief enforcers of their own quality requirements, will accept shabby products and sloppy service, then ISO-9000 doesn't prevent them from letting you slide, although your ISO-9000 re-registration will be a problem in the future if you slough off in the present. Re-registration audits are required every 3 years, and surveillance audits are performed twice a year.

What does ISO-9000 mean to you? It is rapidly becoming the ticket to success because customers are demanding it. Besides, there may be good, sound business reasons for adopting ISO-9000, becoming registered and then "walking the walk as well as talking the talk:" ISO-9000 companies are successful. In Britain, the bankruptcy rate for non-registered companies is 7.14% and, for registered companies, only 0.2% (Johnson, 1993). Some people claim that this means that ISO-9000 gives companies a competitive edge (which it does), but a better interpretation is that well-managed firms take quality seriously, and they are: a) less likely to go bankrupt because of their good management and b) more likely to succeed at earning ISO-9000 registration.

25-19-2 Total quality management

The total quality management (TQM) movement is based largely on the works of W. Edwards Deming. A quick overview of the principals of TQM can be found in Walton (1986) and Gabor (1990). The focus of TQM is seemingly opposite that of the traditional quality effort represented by ISO-9000. While it is true that traditional quality methods rely heavily on inspection after manufacture (or following major subassemblies) by trained quality specialists, the TQM focus is on continuous inspection in process by the workers doing the work. TQM is about worker empowerment, which means tapping the knowledge, skills, and abilities of workers to the fullest. In a TQM plant, a machinist will continuously plot her results on a control chart and is empowered to shut down the machine for repairs or adjustments when the data shows that the quality is drifting off.

There has been much in the press these days about whether TQM is just another business fad that is passing from the scene, despite more than a decade of success here and several decades of success in Japan. A recent survey, "TQM: Forging Ahead or Falling Behind," shows the opposite (Crawford 1993). The survey covered 536 organizations and more than 7,000 people at all organizational levels. There is a distinct correlation between high marks for TQM and the length of time the philosophy has been in place. Those working in a TQM environment for more than 2 years reported considerably greater gains than those working at it for less than 2 years. TQM is not a bandaid or "quick fix" palliative for problems. "There is no instant pudding," intones Dr. Deming. Companies where TQM appears to have failed are most often those with a severe short-term focus (e.g., the next quarterly profit), and no 5- to 20-year strategic plan.

Other studies have shown similar results. In one study, about one-third of the companies reported outstanding success, one-third were indifferent, and one-third reported failure of TQM. A common trait was that the successful companies had the total support (not just an order to "go do it" or a memo to the troops) and personal involvement of the most senior management, while those that were indifferent or failures tended to have either no support or the kind of insipid support that issues a memo and expects miracles by next Monday. In the Department of Defense, where TQM is called total quality leadership (TQL), such lack of top management involvement is sometimes called "total quality lip service" (TQLS). Where management is committed and willing to persist for the long-term, TQM works wonders.

Here is a test for those proposing TQM for their company: If the top executive can't see fit to clear his or her plate enough to devote 15% to 20% of his or her time to quality matters, then the probability of success is low. If you are in charge of your own department or plant, then do the same: clean your plate enough to work quality. And if people above you are not inclined towards TQM, then do what you can, where you can, and wait for the dinosaur to die, move on or evolve into an eagle: one of those will surely occur.

The TQM and ISO-9000 style of quality management systems are related. The ISO-9000 provides the documentation, the standardization, the discipline, and a common language that lets everyone know what quality means in the context of your company. The TQM side provides an ethic and method of continuous quality improvement, a formalized customer focus, the use of constant measurement, statistics and long-range strategic planning. The intersection of ISO-9000 and TQM is found in the realm of customer satisfaction and the formal quality assurance system in place in the plant.

As to the charge that TQM seeks to replace the old-style quality operation, we can say a couple of things. First, the old-style quality department, with its emphasis on the police functions of inspection and sorting, simply cannot hack it today. But those people in QA/QC also possess the skills and knowledge needed to make TQM work. Under TQM their role changes from policeman to coach, teacher, mentor, and managers of a total quality system. Their role changes, expands and their prestige goes up . . . unless they fail to shift from the cop paradigm to the new paradigm.

25-19-3 Six-Sigma quality

The Six-Sigma (6σ) manufacturing concept is a lofty quality goal that only the best can achieve. The name "Six-Sigma" refers to the $\pm6\sigma$ regions of the normal distribution curve. In manufacturing terms, this means not more than 3.4 defects per million products. Ordinary quality control is often considered 3σ (2,700 defects per million) or 4σ (63 defects per million).

A number of Japanese companies are committed to Six-Sigma. In this country, one of the leading practitioners of Six-Sigma is *Motorola*. The normal kind of quality control activity represented by ISO-9000 is probably good enough to get a firm to three-sigma, and possibly somewhat beyond. But reaching Six-Sigma status is

very difficult, and requires a well-planned, long-term effort involving everyone. It is a hard job, and companies that reach it are to be commended . . . And the marketplace knows how to commend winners.

The Six-Sigma regime seems to be an area where the ISO-9000 type of quality effort and TQM become fused. According to one consultant, it is difficult and may be impossible to reach Six-Sigma without doing both expertly.

Trade press discussions indicate ISO-9000 will be amended to incorporate more of the concepts of TQM.

Firms that have reached, or are about to reach, Six-Sigma have extremely well-developed quality programs, yet are not very enthusiastic about being held to ISO-9000. Japan is reportedly negotiating with the EC to permit their own quality standards, which they claim are higher than ISO-9000, to be used in lieu of ISO-9000. Similarly, some American Six-Sigma companies are searching for ways to get the benefits of ISO-9000 registration without losing ground in their own quest for the highest standards of quality.

25-20 And the benefits . . . ?

So what does the quality movement mean to you? Several things, actually. First, it means that you must pay close attention to quality efforts to remain competitive both in the United States and abroad. If your customers demand ISO-9000 registration, then you will have to become registered to keep the customer. If your nearest competitor is registered, then you will be at a serious disadvantage when customers value that status in their suppliers.

Second, it means that many firms will have to become ISO-9000 registered to just stay in place. For some, this task will be a relatively easy drill (one company reportedly did it in 4 months), but for others it may well prove to be the first time in many years that they have taken a serious look at how they "do quality." Sources claim that 12 to 18 months is the usual time required to achieve registration.

Finally, the quality movement represents a positive business opportunity for sensors manufacturers. Much of the thrust of TQM efforts is in understanding and controlling processes to minimize variation in the product. Even the more traditional quality approaches lean heavily on understanding and controlling processes.

25-21 Summary

1. Variation occurs in all things.

2. Normal variation is random in nature, abnormal variation has a cause. This is called *unassignable* and *assignable* variation, or *common cause* and *special cause* variation.

3. Three types of charts are useful: *histograms, run charts,* and *control charts.*

4. The *upper specification limit* (USL) and *lower specification limit* (LSL) around the *target value* are the values that are acceptable.

25-22 Recapitulation

Now return to the objectives and self-evaluation questions at the beginning of the chapter and see how well you can answer them. If you cannot answer certain questions, place a check mark next to each and review appropriate parts of the text. Next, try to answer the following questions using the same procedure.

Questions

1. Variation is in all things, and it can be _____ given adequate tools.

2. Two forms of variation are _____ and _____.

3. Histograms can be used in quality control. True or false?

4. A key concept in quality control is _____.

5. The _____ specification limit and _____ specification limit bracket the _____ value and are the tolerances that the engineer is willing to accept.

6. A control chart is a _____ chart to which mean, lower control limit, and upper control limit lines have been added.

7. A variation is caused. There are four basic causes: _____, _____, _____ and _____.

8. A process can be _____ and in _____ control and not be within LCL and UCL.

Suggested Reading

1. Bureau of Business Practice (1992). *ISO-9000 Handbook of Quality Standards and Compliance.* Waterford, CT: Prentice-Hall.

2. Crawford, Kathleen (1993). "Survey Confirms TQM is a Successful Business Strategy," *The Quality Observer,* November 1993.

3. Deming, W. Edwards, *Out of the Crisis.* Massachusetts Institute of Technology, Center for Advanced Engineering Study (Cambridge, MA 1982, 1986).

4. Dobyns, Lloyd and Clare Crawford-Mason, *Quality or Else: The Revolution in World Business.* Companion to an IBM-funded Public Broadcasting System three-part series of the same name. Houghton Mifflin Co. (Boston, 1991).

5. Gabor, Andrea, *The Man Who Discovered Quality,* Random House/Times (New York, 1990).

6. Johnson, Perry (1993). *ISO-9000: Meeting the New International Standards.* New York: McGraw-Hill.

7. McKean, Kevin (1985). "Decisions, Decisions," *Discover,* June 1985, pp. 22-31.

8. Provost, Lloyd P. and Clifford L. Norman (1990). "Variation Through the Ages," *Quality Progress,* December 1990, pp. 39-44.

CHAPTER 26

Medical Equipment Maintenance: Management, Facilities, and Equipment

26-1 Objectives

1. Be able to define the different types of maintenance repair organizations.
2. Be able to define the different skill levels of medical equipment technical personnel.
3. Be able to understand the levels of capability of repair organizations.
4. Be able to describe the management approaches that are appropriate to medical equipment maintenance.

26-2 Self-evaluation questions

These questions test your prior knowledge of the material in this chapter. Look for the answers as you read the text. After you have finished studying the chapter, try answering these questions and those at the end of the chapter.

1. What are the three levels of maintenance organization capability?

2. What is the difference between a biomedical equipment technician and a registered professional engineer?

3. What is the difference between a registered professional engineer and a licensed first-class engineer?

4. What is the difference between O-level and D-level tasks?

26-3 Introduction

Several management options exist for maintaining medical equipment. An organization such as a hospital, local government emergency medical service (EMS), or medical practice can look to several forms of maintenance repair organizations (MROs) to take care of its equipment service problems. The general ground rules in this chapter assume a commercial MRO, an in-house hospital-based MRO, or a shared service MRO. Each of these organizations has several clients (or departments served, in the case of an in-house shop) served by more than two technicians. With either too few clients or such a light work load that only one or two technicians are needed, a somewhat more ad hoc work plan is needed.

Similarly, with regard to city EMS and medical practices, options are somewhat more limited because the total work load is relatively light. For them, service *à la carte*, or a service contract with each manufacturer, may prove both sufficient and cost-effective. Alternatively, a local commercial MRO may well serve your needs. While an argument can be made that hospital in-house service can be cheaper, it is rare that a small medical organization needs such staff. However, it is not unprecedented for medical practices to use either the same outside shared services MRO as the local hospital where they have staff privileges or the hospital's own in-house department.

26-4 Types of MROs

Although the makeup of MROs varies considerably, there are several important categories: manufacturers' service shops, commercial MROs, in-house hospital-based MROs, shared services MROs, in-house contractors, part-time shops, and single-employee shops. In addition, there are various levels of capability. Borrowing shamelessly from the military logistics world, we will call these levels *organizational* (O level), *intermediate* (I level), and *depot* (D level). The type of service program employed by any given organization should be tailored from these alternatives and may be a blend of several. It is important for managers and administrators to understand these distinctions in order to make solid decisions on the types of organizations employed.

26-5 Levels of capability

The concept of levels of capability is not intended to reflect on either the competence or the integrity of the people involved, but rather on the design and mission of the repair organization. For example, an organization may find it worthwhile to employ a single highly skilled electronics technician in a partially management and partially technical role. Although the technician could easily perform higher-level tasks (and indeed does on some. systems), logistics considerations (e.g., test equipment, spare parts) may preclude higher than O-level repairs despite the ability of the technician(s). The main tasks of that person would be to manage service contracts and be the decision point regarding what is either beyond capability of maintenance or beyond economic in-house repair. The person selected for this type of billet must be capable of making such decisions unemotionally. Many highly competent technical people are self-confident (and properly so), capable, and action oriented. If the logistic infrastructure is not in place, however, then such enthusiasm quickly results in an overextended employee.

26-5-1 O level

This level of capability is the most local, is least expensive, requires the smallest amount of training and support, but is also the least capable. The O-level shop, however, is not to be disdained, for it offers a first line of defense that can:

1. Determine whether a fault actually exists, or whether an operator error was the cause of an anomaly. One of the most common findings in medical equipment shops is *no fault found*. An O-level worker can reduce the incidence of this finding and therefore the lost time incurred when equipment is sent for repair when none is needed.

2. Perform module or equipment substitution to bring the medical capability back on line rapidly while the defective equipment is taken back to the shop for repair. The result is rapid return to service of the medical function involved.

3. Perform such minor technical tasks as can be trusted to on-the-job trained non-technical personnel. For example, on a lot of equipment,

nurses and paraprofessionals can perform many repair tasks such as stylus battery replacement.

4. Serve as an inventory control point for management to monitor equipment that was referred to higher-level maintenance groups.

5. Keep records pertaining to equipment maintenance histories. Such records are useful in analyzing future procurement options and for defending malpractice actions based on supposedly improperly maintained equipment. In addition, the organization may find the records useful for prosecuting product liability lawsuits or regulatory actions against the manufacture of defective equipment.

The O-level maintenance activity is almost always in-house. Higher capability levels, however, may be either in-house or out-of-house.

26-5-2 I level

This level of MRO is more highly skilled than the O-level MRO. Electronics and mechanical technicians, biomedical equipment technicians (BMETs), or even graduate professional engineers may be employed, depending upon the scope of the MRO's mission. The I-level MRO can handle any task that can be done at O level, and more. An I-level shop is one that can:

1. Test medical equipment to verify performance and adherence to specifications and safety standards.

2. Diagnose and troubleshoot equipment at least to the subassembly level. These subassemblies are sometimes called *shop replaceable assemblies* and are those that can be stocked as spare parts. For example, an I-level shop should be competent (and equipped) to replace printed circuit boards, front or rear panel components or controls, dc power supplies, and bolt-on mechanical parts (e.g., motors, pump).

3. Adjust, align, or harmonize internal controls that are not normally available to the operator.

This type of operation assumes that the I-level shop has the test equipment required to verify performance and the validity of those settings.

The I-level shop requires sufficient spare parts inventory or a blanket purchase authority with the vendor to ensure relatively quick repair action turnaround time. Often, the hospital cannot afford to have the technician go through the purchasing department to obtain parts. At least some limited trust must be placed in the person outside the system, or the hospital must be willing to accept less than rapid repairs. A competent I-level technician who lacks a replacement internal assembly is not able to perform up to the level of expected capabilities. Most locally situated MROs are basically I-level shops (although a few are depot capable).

25-6-3 D level

The depot is the highest level of repair activity. For many systems, only a major local or regional MRO will qualify. In these cases, the manufacturer's plant may be the only available depot. The D-level shop is capable of troubleshooting to the piece-part level. While the I-level shop works to a subassembly level (e.g., printed circuit boards), the D-level shop can find and replace the faulty component on the subassembly (e.g., the blown transistor of "microchip" that caused the problem).

It is frequently the case that D-level shops work not on equipment as a whole, but rather on the subassemblies that are sent in from I-level shops. In a typical scenario, an I-level technician will replace a printed circuit board to bring a piece of equipment back in service. The faulty circuit board is then sent to a D-level shop for detailed troubleshooting to the piece-part level.

26-5-4 Which level to employ

A large organization that must grapple with managing a large medical technology base faces the decision regarding level of shop capability required. Although there is a strong temptation to seek easy solutions, that approach is not always the best for any given organization. For example, a commercial MRO may propose taking over all equipment maintenance within the hospital. The facts rarely support such claims.

Similarly, in-house staff, perhaps feeling threatened by the prospect of being replaced by a contractor, may also claim capability that is not supportable by facts. The technical abilities of the employee are rarely an issue, but rather the issue is whether it is economically feasible to support such a facility.

A proper management approach is to inventory the equipment that requires support and then study the staffing and support requirements for each level of support. The decision of whether in-house support is D level, I level, O level, or none at all rests on cost versus the speed with which repairs must be performed.

26-6 Types of organization

Several broad categories of MROs have been identified. Although that list was not intended to be exhaustive, it does serve as a guide to generic types of MROs. Let's discuss each class in turn.

26-6-1 Manufacturer's service department

This class of MRO includes those owned and operated by the manufacturer of the equipment. It may be located at the factory (usually D level) or locally (usually I level). As a general rule, the manufacturer can provide among the best and most competent service on its particular equipment. They have better information, deeper experience, and more rapid access to spare parts. However, because of certain problems, the manufacturer MRO may not be the best suited to your situation.

First, there is a potential *better is the enemy of good enough* situation. The question is whether the *better* (if it truly exists) is worth the higher cost. Manufacturer's service is usually more expensive

than either in-house or commercial MRO service because the manufacturer's overhead burden is typically higher.

Second, the actual proximity of *local* service may make a sham out of any claims of rapid service. If the shop serves a region rather than a small locale, then response time may suffer.

Third, the promise of *local service* is sometimes met by placing a single technician in either a *desk space only* office or the basement of his or her own home. Whether this arrangement works out depends on the size of the service area covered and the number of clients served. One company that used this form of service also used the same people to install equipment when new installations were done. As a result, the single technician in the area was sometimes tied up on an installation and therefore unavailable for several days.

Finally, the manufacturer may not have a total commitment to service. To most manufacturers, the money is in sales of new systems and support products (electrodes, gel, supplies); service is a loss center that is viewed as a necessary evil by the company management. In those cases, the service department receives little support or resources in an effort to minimize losses. Make sure the manufacturer views service in a kindly light before committing to its service department. An indicator of the future is your experience during the warranty period, when you have no choice. If the manufacturer seems unwilling to meet warranty obligations, then do not expect it to make a sudden recovery postwarranty.

26-6-2 Commercial MROs

These shops are commercial firms that provide service on medical equipment. Some commercial MROs provide the best solution for cost-effective management of the maintenance problem. As with any type of contractor, the desirability of entrusting work to commercial MROs depends on their integrity, reputation, technical abilities, depth of their spares inventory, and ability to respond to customer demands. Each MRO must be evaluated on its own merits. There are, however, a few pitfalls to look out for.

First, the marketing claims often belie the actual capability of the company. Contract performance is at risk when the technical staff is not actually in place at the time of proposal. Too often, commercial managers shrug off their lack of staff with the promise that staff will be hired as needed. While that flexibility may exist for low-skill-level billets, it is often a pipe dream at the higher-level billets needed for many types of medical equipment service.

Second, the financial condition of the company may not be adequate to support the level of service expected. Even world-class technical staff is unable to perform well if adequate space parts, service literature, and test equipment are not available. Both the level of technology and the prospect of product liability tend to drive up the cost of medical equipment and the supporting spares. Some electronics components companies are so fearful of product liability suits that they publish a disclaimer against use of their products in medical equipment. In most cases, the price of simple components destined for medical equipment, even at the original equipment manufacturer level, is huge compared with the price of the same component for general industrial products. The same problem afflicts the local service company and increases both its own liability and the costs of the spares it sells.

Third, there is frequently an imprudent *can-do* attitude on the part of commercial MROS. Although action-oriented managers often admire such an attitude, it often conceals a lack of real ability to perform. The can-do attitude that is not backed up with real or potential capability is a dangerous illusion.

Fourth, the smaller MRO may be insufficiently covered by liability insurance. The author has seen repairs done by inexperienced commercial MRO personnel that could have been called malpractice. In one case, a defibrillator failed during a routine test. The fault was traced to inexcusably poor work practices by the commercial MRO and may have resulted in a patient death if the hospital inspector had not found it in time. If that MRO lacked coverage or the resources to self-insure, then the hospital might have had a severe liability problem.

Hospital and EMS managers are rarely equipped to evaluate the technical capability or the depth of spares inventory of any commercial MRO. However, their armamentarium is not empty if the company has a track record. Demand a list of present and past customers who can be contacted for references. A manager should be able to elicit good information about the company's past service record from his or her peers. A string of lost customers, service contract nonrenewals, or dissatisfied clients is not a good indication that the company can do a good job.

26-6-3 In-house MROs

This category of MRO is owned and operated by the organization or hospital that it serves. A properly staffed and equipped department can provide competent service in a very short response time. Experience has shown that equipment emergencies that would otherwise affect patient care can be dealt with promptly by an in-house MRO. One of the authors has repaired equipment in an operating room during open-heart surgery procedures. Although repair during a procedure is bad practice in most situations, there were several cases when the surgeon ordered it done because he believed it critical to have the instruments to bring the patient back off the heart-lung pump, and because the hospital lacked the spare equipment to back up the main system. Neither commercial MROs nor manufacturer service departments can provide that level service.

The in-house shop can also supply around-the-clock service through the simple expedient of issuing a beeper to the on-call technician. Although other types of MROs can also offer that service, the reality is often a bit different from the salesperson's claims. For one thing, odd-hours service may cost more than normal-hours service. Also, the definition of *24-hour service* may be disputed. In one contract, we understood 24-hour service to mean *around the clock at any hour of the day or night*. However, the company responded to our complaints of noncompliance with the suggestion that 24-hour service meant that they had to provide the service sometime within the next 24 hours after logging in the call from the customer. Ambiguity in a contract can be devastating.

Although cost and convenience advantages are considerable, there are also some disadvantages to in-house service. A big one is the availability of properly trained I-level and D-level technical staff. It is difficult to balance the salaries and benefits required to attract and hold good people, considering the needs to contain costs. In addition, in-house shops often lack the room for career growth for the technician. As a result, the better person leaves within a short time, often disgruntled. Alternatively, the person settles down into a long term of gray mediocrity that leads to a rut, requiring occasional management *attitude adjustment* actions.

26-6-4 Shared service MROs

Equipment maintenance is an expensive proposition, especially if full I level is required on all systems (plus D level on selected systems). Many institutions simply cannot afford their own repair facility beyond the most basic. Even large institutions with adequate resources may find it economically desirable to share the cost of such facilities with other institutions.

A shared service is an MRO that is owned and operated by two or more cooperating institutions that are also the users of the service. In some cases, the shared service is owned by one of the institutions but serves the others on contract. In other cases, the shared service is a separate entity but is owned and managed by the member institutions. The shared service is sometimes a separate corporation in which the chief officers and/or directors are also officers or directors of the member institutions.

Some shared service MROs are actually more like consortiums. Each institution has its own service facility, but each group is highly specialized in the type of work it handles. For example, one group might specialize in electronic patient monitoring equipment, another in anesthesia machines and respirators, and still another in dialysis machines. The overall capability of the consortium is greater because of nonduplicated efforts.

Shared services can be an effective and low-cost solution to the overall maintenance problem of several institutions. However, as with the other options, there are some problems to solve. Perhaps one of the most difficult problems is the tendency of one institution to dominate the resources of the shared service. Usually, the majority (or most senior) member siphons service capability that is rightfully due other members.

Another problem with shared services is the tendency to build empires. This problem especially afflicts consortiums because each hospital may want to develop local capability that would ordinarily be allocated to another shop. Service shop managers who see their career potential enhanced by accretion of duties, capability, and power may be most guilty of this practice.

If the problems can be solved and peace maintained, then shared service MROs can be a well-managed, low-cost solution to the equipment maintenance problem. However, the track record of shared services is spotty in this regard because of the aforementioned problems.

26-6-5 In-house contractor MRO

This category represents a cross between the in-house concept and the commercial MRO concept. In this arrangement, a contractor places either an entire technical and management team or a manager who oversees hospital personnel in the hospital to manage the in-house repair facility. Only a few groups of this type exist, so little can be said about them. However, the concept has worked with housekeeping management and so should work well with medical equipment maintenance.

26-6-6 Part-time shop

In this case, a small repair organization provides medical equipment maintenance for the local hospital on a part-time or ad-hoc basis. In general, it is a bad idea unless the owner of the shop (or key personnel) is familiar with the repair of biomedical equipment. In that case, it might be a good first line of defense for a rural or remote hospital. We recall one shop that normally repaired commercial video equipment and two-way radios and also repaired the equipment in the coronary and intensive care units of the local hospital. The nearest commercial MRO or manufacturer service shop was a 6-hour drive through the Nevada desert. The manufacturer of the patient monitoring system sold the hospital a stock of spare printed wiring boards and mechanical parts and trained the local shop owner to provide a minimal I-level capability. It worked in that case, but this approach is otherwise fraught with difficulty.

26-6-7 Single-technician department

In some smaller hospitals, a single repair technician is employed in plant operations (erroneously called *engineering* in most hospitals, even when no college-graduate engineers are employed there). If adequately supported with test equipment and spares, the properly trained technician can provide O-level, or even I-level, service for a limited number of in-house client departments. However, be careful to ensure the employment of an adequate technician. Many hospitals have been known to employ an electrician who thinks he or she knows something about electronics, or someone with an amateur radio license, as the electronics technician. Insist on credentials for such an employee.

26-7 Technical personnel

One of the mysteries of medical equipment maintenance for managers and administrators is the types of technical personnel involved and their level of training. Unfortunately, too many titles are less than descriptive to the uninitiated. In addition, there are titles that are shared by different people. For example, consider the title *engineer*. If you asked most medical people to define engineer, you would elicit images of a person with little education, a blue-collar plant operations uniform, and a leather tool pouch on his or her belt; the use of the term engineer by those people is illegal in some states and only tolerated by the law in others because of a long history. The title derives from the use of the word engineer to describe highly skilled steam and boiler technicians, whose city licenses often refer to them as first-class, second-class, or third-class *steam engineers*. We will discuss true engineers in this section. Various levels and categories of technicians are found in medical equipment maintenance. Some of them are highly specialized, while others are generalists. Several levels of education are common.

1. *On-the-job or self-trained.* This type of person is trained as an apprentice to others and is generally capable of limited tasking. Although there are exceptions, these workers are not generally capable of more than the simplest tasks. However, certain factors are indicators of higher than elementary achievement: status as a certified electronic technician (CET), certification as BMET, certain other industrywide certifications, and a diploma from a recognized home-study school. Although often the butt of jokes, the home-study route is an established tradition in electronics. A number of programs are well regarded in the electronics industry because they turn out knowledgeable graduates.

2. *Vocational technical school graduate.* The vo-tech school is one in which subcollege, post-high-school training is offered. Some vo-tech schools offer the last year or two of high school plus additional work that is normally beyond the high school level. These schools may be local or state government operated, or commercial. Unfortunately, a few commercial

schools are little more than diploma mills that rip off guaranteed loan payments offered to immigrants or disadvantaged people to upgrade their economic prospects (check the reputation and accreditation of the school).

Vo-tech training emphasizes the practical aspects of electronics theory and differs from the higher levels in the amount and type of mathematics employed in the curriculum. Graduates can perform O-level maintenance and many I-level tasks depending upon the quality of the school.

3. *Associate degree technicians.* The A.Sc. degree requires two years of academic training in a community college or technical institute. The level of training is more theoretical and mathematically oriented than that of the vo-tech. These graduates can handle O-level, I-level, and most D-level tasks. It is common to find bright, highly talented people in this category who prefer the technical hands-on work that requires an A.Sc. degree but who disdain the more paper-oriented tasks of the engineer.

4. *Bachelor's degree technicians.* At one time the B.Sc. degree differentiated the technician from the engineer. Today, however, there are many four-year, accredited degree programs that offer a Bachelor of Science in Electronics Technology (BSET) degree. It is perhaps fitting to refer to these people as *technologists* or something similar rather than *technicians.* They can handle all tasks and, indeed, can often manage the shop on a professional level.

5. *Biomedical equipment technicians.* The title BMET is an indicator of certification in medical equipment maintenance. Some applicants may have earned a degree or diploma in medical equipment technology and thereon base a claim to the title. However, to avoid confusion, it is perhaps best to reserve the title BMET to those who have passed the appropriate certification examinations.

6. *Engineers.* The true engineer is a graduate of a college or university engineering program or a program in a related science that leads one to the same body of knowledge that engineers require. The general rule is simple: no Bachelor of Science degree, no title of engineer, unless the state government has seen fit to issue the person a professional engineer (PE) certificate. (*Note:* Very few nondegree PE certificates still exist, although a few states still allow the old method of qualification.)

It annoys engineers to be compared with, or thought of in terms of, the plant operations engineers, because the true engineer holds a degree that is one of the hardest to earn. Indeed, a physician told the author that he switched from engineering to pre-med because he was not smart enough to survive the freshman year in engineering school. Engineers working in hospitals are often looked down on or disdained by nurses with B.S.N. degrees (or even other nurses) as somehow intellectually inferior. There is no nursing degree, even at the graduate school level, that compares in difficulty or intellectual level to even the B.Sc. level in engineering. Anyone who doubts that claim would do well to enroll in the first semester of engineering school to find out the truth. (A typical engineering school has a 45% to 55% flunk-out or quit rate at the end of the freshman year; it is not uncommon for deans of engineering schools to address incoming freshman. "Look at the person next to you . . . In June one of you will not be here—half flunk out or wisely change their major by the end of the first year.")

The Bachelor of Science in Engineering (B.S.E.) degree is the usual qualification for an engineer. Some applicants enumerate their degrees as B.S.E.E. (electrical engineering), B.S.M.E. (mechanical engineering), B.S.C.E. (civil engineering), and B.S.Ch.E (chemical engineering). In addition to these categories, there are also materials engineers, engineering mechanics degrees (a cross-disciplinary degree), and biomedical engineering degrees. In the latter case there is some doubt regarding what curriculum was followed. It is not unusual to find that these graduates are really traditional engineers with a little biology and a few medical instrumentation courses. For example, one friend of mine has a B.Sc. in biomedical engineering but took only six credit hours' fewer chemical engineering courses than a B.S.Ch.E. graduate. There are other examples of specialty engineering B.Sc. degrees, but in the main specialization beyond the basic traditional engineering disciplines is done in graduate school.

In some cases, graduates with degrees in science (particularly physics) or mathematics are accepted as engineers after a certain amount of relevant training and professional experience:

1. *Certified clinical engineer (CCE).* The CCE is a professional board engineering certification. It requires a level of education (B.Sc.) plus four years of relevant experience in a hospital or similar facility. Some older clinical engineers were "grandfathered" into the program on the basis of experience, but newer certificates require full compliance with the educational requirements.

2. *Registered professional engineer (PE or RPE).* This title indicates that the applicant possesses a state license to practice engineering. It is unfortunate that not all engineers are required to have a state license. In general, only those who are in private practice, who work on public projects, or who must routinely appear as an expert witness in court are required to possess an engineering license. Although some states legally limit those who may use the title engineer to describe themselves, there are exceptions. For example, some states exempt engineers employed in manufacturing, as junior engineers to a PE, or (in some cases) those who are employed in institutions such as schools or hospitals. There are also occupational exemptions under which railroad train drivers, crane and heavy equipment operators, and steam mechanics can call themselves engineers. A *sanitary engineer,* by the way, is not a garbage collector with a sense of humor but rather is a speciality subset of civil engineering that designs sewage systems and water treatment plants.

The PE license is based on education, two levels of examination, and four years of experience. The first level of examination, called the Engineer in Training (EIT) exam, is opened to seniors in engineering programs with 90 hours of acceptable course work completed and to all graduates of engineering programs. After four years of progressively more responsible professional experience, the engineer may take the specialty examination for the type of engineering he or she is qualified to practice. While all EITs take the same exam, the PE exam is tailored to civil, electrical, mechanical, or chemical disciplines. Although not strictly required, some people feel that major hospitals ought to employ a PE who also holds the CCE certificate as the administrator over both biomedical engineering and plant operations.

A few states allow licensing of professional engineers without a degree, or with degrees other than engineering. These states call such qualification *eminence.* If a person demonstrates the body of knowledge required, plus a 12-year record of "progressively more responsible professional experience," then the board may vote to issue the license despite the lack of an engineering school degree. This method of qualification especially benefits foreign graduates whose schools are based on the European model, wherein one "reads engineering" rather than takes specific courses.

Small departments, or the departments in smaller hospitals, can be managed by a technician with a BSET or related degree. Alternatively, with adequate training and experience, less educated people also work out well. Larger hospitals, however, should insist on filling the job of Director of Biomedical Engineering Department with a graduate engineer with a certain minimum (two years) relevant experience level. While these people are hard to find, they are also professional people who are able to relate to the medical professionals they serve.

26-8 Management approaches

Over the years, one of the authors was associated with many maintenance or repair organizations in both technician- and engineer-level positions. In addition to practical experience in the workplace, the author's insights were organized by exposure to certain modern management theories that proved themselves in a wide variety of environments.

Hospitals, and often the associated commercial vendors supplying services, are among the least-well-managed enterprises in the country. Indeed, one of the many reasons for the runaway cost of health care is that medical enterprises often have defective management. It is the responsibility of management to find and correct causes of extra or hidden costs in order to make their enterprise more economically viable.

It is not intended here to cover all of the problems in health care management, for indeed the author is not qualified to do so; rather, the problems and issues related to small unit management are discussed. Both biomedical engineering and nursing personnel would be wise to consider some of the issues raised herein.

While one is quick to recognize the inefficiencies of medical enterprise management, one must be just as quick to point out that such inefficiencies are not necessarily the fault of present managers and supervisors. Rather, they are the fault of the system that these people inherited and learned under. Part of the problem these people face is that they are professionals in fields other than management. For example, head nurses and directors of nursing are drawn from the ranks of the registered nurses, just as directors or biomedical engineering are drawn from the ranks of the engineering profession. Their training, the poorly thought-out claims of the proponents of the B.S.N. degree notwithstanding, lacks relevance to management. Yet there is hope, for those people tend to be high-quality individuals who care about the health of the organization—and the skills situation is easily correctible with training.

The principal technique of small-unit management in most industries, including health care, is also the most inadequate and least effective. In fact, it is counterproductive and often leads to exactly the opposite effect than intended. Sometimes called *theory X* management, one might be tempted to call this method the *drill sergeant* approach because coercion and intimidation rule the unit. Wherever this method is employed, the supervisor (and usually his or her superiors) operate from a set of basic premises that require elements of the following worldview:

1. People are inherently no good; they are lazy and want a free ride. Any quality resulting from their efforts is merely incidental or the result of supervisory browbeatings. This view is exemplified by a cartoon of a tabby cat pulling a piano upstairs under a whip lash: "If you whip the cat hard enough, it will pull a piano upstairs."

2. There is no pride of workmanship. That is, the lazy or incompetent worker (which includes all workers) does not want to do a good job, cannot be convinced to do a good job, and will not do a good job unless coerced.

3. A proper employee is one who keeps quiet, stays in his or her place, never makes waves or rocks the boat, and never offers any opinion or suggestion. "Just do the job, don't comment on it" exemplifies this view.

4. All—or at least the overwhelming majority—of problems in the unit, especially production-related issues, are the fault of workers who will not do their best.

These views are fundamentally flawed. The concept that all employees are lazy is often implicitly accepted by supervisors and managers, even though considerable evidence to the contrary exists. If a set of employees seems to fit the foregoing description, then it is a sure bet that some problem in management is responsible for that morale problem. Perhaps the apparent laziness or incompetence is actually due to severe demoralization brought on by irrational, inconsistent, or insensitive management.

Regarding the belief that the cat will pull the piano upstairs if whipped hard enough, experience suggests exactly the opposite—the cat will walk out. This problem is often obscured in the medical, nursing, and medical equipment industries because, in any one locality, it is often the case that other employment opportunities in the field are lacking. Perhaps that is why so many nurses claim to *burn out* so young—they are totally demoralized by the ineffective management of their supervisors.

A key factor to research when a unit has a high turnover rate is the kinds of jobs taken by those who leave. If their new jobs are predominantly career advances, then the problem is mere attrition and no action need be taken. But if the jobs tend to be lateral or dead-end positions, or otherwise not career enhancing, this is evidence that the employees are leaving because of poor management.

The only way that any organization can remain economically viable over the long haul is to be in a state of constant improvement. Management must stimulate this process, but it requires the efforts of all employees. Unfortunately, there is a tendency in management (not just in health care) to assume that employees cannot make improvements. In fact, managers often believe that employee suggestions are boat-rocking. There is even record of a head nurse who demanded that the personnel department select interviewees for a position who are "introverted and not the least bit innovative." That prescription is a blueprint for disaster. It is a simple fact that the person who does the job is the one who knows the most about it and is therefore one of the principal people who should be in on solving problems.

If an organization is in such serious trouble that innovative employees are shunned or beaten into demoralization, then theirs is a boat that does not need freedom from boat rockers, but rather needs very much to be rocked—and hard.

One of the most destructive attitudes among managers is the mistaken belief that problems in a unit are due to employees not pulling hard enough. Often accompanied by exhortative slogans, this attitude demonstrates that management does not know its business or is unwilling to think hard about the problem. According to W. Edwards Deming, in *Out of the Crisis,* the truth is exactly the opposite. In Deming's view, the overwhelming majority of problems are due to the system— which is management's responsibility—not the employee.

Problems should be solved with a view toward making the system better. One of the principal errors involves setting work standards or objectives. When you set standards, you often get exactly what you measure—and no more. Often, what you measure was selected because it is easy, not because it is relevant. Let's consider some examples.

1. In maintenance shops it is common to rate employees on the number of repair jobs completed per week, or the average amount of time spent to repair each unit. The measured parameter that affects the technician's pay next year (and self-esteem this year) is quantity, not quality. Thus, the technician is naturally directed to turning in completed *tickets* rather than ensuring that the hospital's equipment does what it is supposed to do.

2. In many hospitals, nurses are treated severely for medication errors (there is no doubt that medication errors are a serious issue). One hospital fires nurses who make three medication errors in 12 months. As a result, in response to a new nurse who wanted to formally report her medication error, a supervisor said, "On this unit, we don't have medication errors!" Which is more dangerous to patients—a system in which medication errors can be freely admitted, or one in which it is in the nurses' best interest to hide the truth and hope that no harm comes to the patient?

In both of the preceding examples, it is the superior management technique to statistically evaluate the work performance and determine if the system is stable. If the technician does not produce enough repair jobs, then perhaps training, equipment, or spare parts supplies are at fault. Similarly, if there are a lot of errors in medication, the perhaps there must be an evaluation of the system to determine how it can overcome the potential for error.

Overcontrol is the last problem we will address here. It is the habit of many supervisors to closely monitor, and frequently tweak, employee performance. An example of this occurs in word processing or data entry departments, where computers automatically record the number of keystrokes made per minute. Rather than having the desired effect (i.e., improvement of employee performance), these data actually breed resentment and poorer performance: Keystrokes up, errors up, too.

Another insidious form of overcontrol is the habit of some supervisors to make rules or take general disciplinary action on the entire unit for the sins and problems of a few—or even one. Poor managers think that every special problem that arises needs a new regulation. Of course, the new regulation will seem to work for a while, but it is soon ignored. When confronted with special problems, the supervisor needs to evaluate the situation in order to discern whether the problem is systematic or is singular. It never seems to occur to some people that events often are not systematic (the only kind that succumb to general rules) but rather are either random happenings or single-point failures that may never happen again. In the absence of evidence of a wider cause, any generalized action taken will probably be counterproductive and is definitely little more than wheel spinning.

26-9 Summary

1. There are three levels of maintenance repair organizations (MROs): organizational (O), intermediate (I), and depot (D). Each of these levels represents an increasing capability.

2. There are several different types of organizations within the three levels: manufacturer's service department, commercial MRO, in-house MRO, shared service MRO, in-house contractor operated MRO, part-time shop, and single-technician department.

3. Several levels and categories of technical personnel are used in medical equipment maintenance: those trained on the job, vocational-technical school graduates, associate degree technicians, bachelor's degree technicians, biomedical equipment technicians, graduate engineers, certified clinical engineers, and registered professional engineers. The BMET and CCE are certifications, and the RPE is a state license.

4. One of the natural roles of the clinical engineering staff in a hospital is participation in the selection and acquisition of high technology systems. In some cases, the role even includes information systems technology, although there remains some tension between the two technologies. The problem is that it is no longer clear where computerized biomedical equipment technology leaves off and the business-oriented computer systems take up. In either case, however, the management of the technology and its acquisition is critical. In Chapter 27, you will learn the most important—and most often overlooked or poorly done—part of the technology acquisition process.

26-10 Recapitulation

Now return to the objectives and self-test questions at the beginning of the chapter and see how well you can answer them. If you cannot answer certain questions, place a checkmark next to each and review appropriate parts of the text. Next, try to answer the following questions using the same procedure.

Questions

1. A(n) _____-level maintenance organization troubleshoots to the component level.

2. A(n) _____-level maintenance organization generally replaces subassemblies such as printed wiring boards and pumps.

3. The most common finding in O-level shops is _____ _____.

4. A(n) _____ _____ maintenance repair organization is owned jointly by several users (e.g., hospitals, medical practices)

5. Three technical training levels include: _____, _____ degree, and _____ degree.

6. A graduate engineer is a person who possesses at least a _____ degree or its equivalent.

7. A _____ _____ technician is a certified technical worker with experience and training in the repair and maintenance of medical equipment.

8. A _____ _____ engineer is a professional person who is especially trained, educated, and experienced in managing medical equipment maintenance activities.

9. Overcontrol is a symptom of theory _____ management style.

Suggested Reading

1. Aguayo, Rafael, *Dr. Deming: The American Who Taught the Japanese About Quality.* Simon & Schuster/Fireside (New York, 1990).

2. Amsden, Robert T., Howard E. Butler, and Davida M. Amsden, *SPC Simplified: Practical Steps to Quality,* Quality Resources (White Plains, N.Y., 1986, 1989).

3. Deming, W. Edwards, *Out of the Crisis,* Massachusetts Institute of Technology, Center for Advanced Engineering Study (Cambridge, Mass., 1982, 1986).

4. Dobyns, Lloyd and Clare Crawford-Mason, *Quality or Else: The Revolution in World Business.* Companion to an IBM-funded Public Broadcasting System three-part series of the same name. Houghton Mifflin Co. (Boston, 1991).

5. Gabor, Andrea, *The Man Who Discovered Quality,* Random House/Times (New York, 1990).

6. Noeth, Carrie A., Quality Assurance Microbiologist, Sulzer Carbomedics, *"Routine Use and Troubleshooting for the Validated Isolator,"* (setting up a preventive maintenance schedule and procedures for standard operation and environmental monitoring of biologically hazardous substances as trapped and isolated by high-efficiency particle arresting (HEPA) filters, (Medical Device Manufacturing and Technology Business Briefing Report and CD-ROM, Aspen Market Services, World Markets Research Center, Academic House, 24-28 Oval Road, London, NWI 7DP, June, 1999, phone: +44-171-526-2400, Internet: www.wmrc.com)

7. Walton, Mary, *The Deming Management Method,* Putnam Publishing Company/Perigree (New York, 1986). Paperback edition.

8. Walton, Mary, *Deming Management At Work* (six case studies), Putnam Publishing Company/Perigree (New York, 1990, 1991). Paperback edition.

CHAPTER 27
Requirements Management

27-1 Objectives

1. Be able to describe the different types of requirements

2. Understand the importance of requirements.
3. Be able to write high-quality requirements.

27-2 Self-evaluation questions

These questions test your prior knowledge of the material in this chapter. Look for the answers as you read the text. After you have finished studying the chapter, try answering these questions and those at the end of the chapter.

1. Three class of requirements are _____, _____ and _____.

2. List three symptoms of poor requirements.

3. List several functional requirements for a bedside monitor.

4. Define "requirements" in your own words.

27-3 Introduction

Managing the acquisition of the high technology systems used in modern health care institutions is

a major problem. Technology is difficult to manage, and neither nurses, administrators, or clinical engineers are particularly well-equipped to do so by either training or experience. The technology management role falls naturally to the engineer. Technology acquisition projects are often over-budget, fail to meet schedule, do not perform as expected, or worst of all, sustain all of these problems. The proportion of high technology projects that fail along one or more of these lines is high. In one study of 8,380 information system development projects, the cost overruns averaged 189%. More than 31% of the projects were cancelled before completion, and only 16.2% of the completed projects met the specifications of the purchaser. On average, of those projects that were completed but did not fully meet all of the customer's specifications, only an average of 61% of the required functionality was provided. A dismal 9% of the

8,380 projects were completed on schedule and on budget.

That health care institutions frequently fail in technology acquisition is not surprising for one reason: very few organizations, health care or otherwise, manage their technology acquisition programs very well. It is a hard job that is little understood by managers, executives and engineers. The root cause of most failures is, however, well-known. Repeated research, and the professional experiences of systems engineers over the past 30 years, has consistently yielded the same results: *the major cause of technology acquisition failures is poor requirements engineering and management* (REAM). It has been shown that the root errors leading to such failures break out as follows:

Requirements: 56%

Design: 27%

Coding: (computer programming) 7%

All other causes: 10%

Although REAM is a systems engineering discipline, it involves skills that can be learned and put into practice by other professionals.

27-4 Some definitions

The word *requirement* as used by professional systems engineers refers to a formal written statement of the needs and expectations of the customer (i.e., the health care facility buying the system). "Requirements" is the generic term that includes the entire set of capabilities, functions, behaviors, characteristics, and attributes of or constraints on a proposed system. The requirements document is your principal means of communication with the system developers (e.g., engineers or computer programmers) regardless of whether those developers are in-house employees or external contractors.

REAM is the application of a disciplined, scientific approach to eliciting, validating, specifying, and verifying requirements. Although REAM is a function of the systems engineering profession, the basic approach can easily be adopted by anyone who is responsible for acquiring technology.

Requirements documents are typically incorporated into requests for proposals, bid requests, statements of work, purchase orders, contracts, and other documents pertaining to the technology acquisition project. When made part of the contract, those documents become legally binding on both parties.

The REAM approach can be applied broadly to purchases and materials management activities, but its primary benefit is found in acquiring complex high technology systems. It is applicable to large capital investment items such as magnetic resonance imaging systems, the bedside monitoring suite for a coronary care unit, a large management information computer system, or the building to house them.

27-5 Why are requirements important?

Requirements documents are vital because they formally describe what is needed or desired in the system design and are the contractually binding guidance for the developer or vendor. Although the REAM process continues through the entire life-cycle of the system, the majority of the most important activity occurs very early. The earlier an error occurs in the development process and the later it is discovered and corrected, the more expensive it will be to correct. Requirements errors tend to occur early and be discovered late, so are typically much more expensive to fix than other problems. In terms of the level of effort required to fix problems, 82% of effort is expended in fixing requirements errors, 13% to fix design errors, 1% to fix coding errors, and all others efforts are at 4%.

Because requirements are the responsibility of the acquiring organization, the cost of correcting the problem caused by bad requirements will usually fall on them. Studies performed at various times since the 1970s have yielded similar results (Figure 27-1). If an error costs $1 to fix in the re-

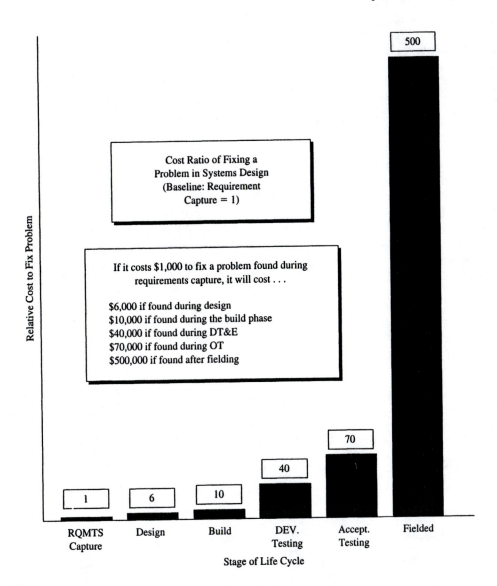

Cost Ratio of Fixing a
Problem in Systems Design
(Baseline: Requirement
Capture = 1)

If it costs $1,000 to fix a problem found during
requirements capture, it will cost . . .

$6,000 if found during design
$10,000 if found during the build phase
$40,000 if found during DT&E
$70,000 if found during OT
$500,000 if found after fielding

Relative Cost to Fix Problem

| RQMTS Capture | Design | Build | DEV. Testing | Accept. Testing | Fielded |

1   6   10   40   70   500

Stage of Life Cycle

Figure 27-1

quirements document, it will cost up to $70 to cor-
rect if discovered in the vendor's systems testing
phase and up to $500, if discovered after installa-
tion. Clearly, the greatest leverage of REAM occurs early in the process.

Another reason for the importance of requirements is that they can profoundly affect operational costs long after the system is installed. If

REAM is done poorly, then there may be excessive maintenance costs, excessive use of consumables, frequent (and very costly) upgrading or
change, and rapid obsolescence. Systems engineers recognize that the up-front acquisition
costs may loom large when capital investments
are being considered, but are only a small part of
the overall life-cycle cost of acquiring, installing,

operating, maintaining, and finally disposing of a system. REAM affects both the up-front and continuing operational costs.

27-6 What types of requirements are there?

Requirements can be classified as *functional, nonfunctional,* and *constraints* (Figure 27-2). Functional requirements are those things that the system must do. For example, a medical imaging system must be able to detect certain structures within the human body. A system designed to image kidneys, for example, fails if it cannot see kidney-sized soft tissue objects. Similarly, an in-

formation technology system that tracks material usage must be able to access a database of supplies and their prices, as well as the software that computes the patient's bill.

Nonfunctional requirements include operator or maintainer training, an availability specification (e.g., the number of hours per week the system must be available for use), or a reliability figure (e.g., mean time between failures).

Constraints may be management considerations or other limitations on the final system design. Examples of the former might include a budget ceiling or a date by which the system must be installed. A system design constraint might be a requirement that the hardware fit within a certain size of room or vehicle or be operable on certain

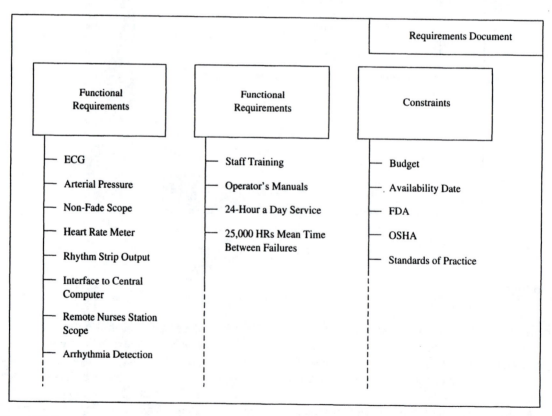

Figure 27-2

types of electrical power. Constraints may also arise from the demands of government regulatory agencies, accreditation bodies, insurance companies, or other external sources.

27-7 Scope of requirements

The particular set of requirements applicable to any given project depends on the type of project and the overall individual situation. If you are purchasing an off-the-shelf system with few possible options, then it is relatively simple to select a vendor. Indeed, in that case, selection by brand name, price, or availability may make more sense than clinical or technical matters. In other cases, however, the task is considerably more complex. If the system is entirely custom-produced (e.g., some types of management information systems) or is highly configurable from a list of available options (some of which may be standard catalog items, but others are custom-built for your project), the REAM process is more demanding.

The specific requirements for any given system in your institution may resemble those of similar organizations, but must be customized to your situation and elicited from your staff. It is usually a very serious mistake to simply copy a successful specification from another institution or department.

27-8 Symptoms of bad requirements

There are a number of symptoms of bad requirements. If project deadlines are missed or costs rise considerably over predictions, suspect poor requirements. Another symptom is that the performance of the installed system is less than or different from what was expected by the end users. End users may fail to use many of the system's capabilities, use the system in an unintended or unauthorized manner, or reject it altogether. Observe whether or not there are widespread or frequent attempts to either circumvent the system or to perform the tasks of the system with some man-

ual "work-around" method (e.g., keeping paper copies of records that should have been entered electronically).

Another symptom is that users make a large number of requests for engineering changes, issue a large number of trouble or failure reports, or demand new or different features shortly after the new system is installed. Some such dissatisfaction may be caused by legitimate changes in the actual requirements that occurred after the REAM process ended. Some dissatisfaction may also be the result of unfamiliarity with the new system or normal resistance to change. But widespread or persistent dissatisfaction deserves investigation by management.

An early symptom of an emerging bad requirements situation is that the requirements change as various vendors present their proposals to the selection committee. If there is resistance to writing and holding to a formal requirements document and you permit the resistance to prevail, you can almost guarantee that unnecessary problems will emerge.

27-9 Primary and derived requirements

Primary requirements are those that are levied on the contractor or vendor by force of contract. They represent the needs of the end customer for the system. In contractual language, these requirements are generally phrased in terms of "shall," implying a mandatory situation. For example, ". . . the system shall be transportable on a standard intravenous bag pole attached to a gurney." Derived requirements flow down from the primary requirements and reflect some attribute of the system that must be present to meet the primary requirements. Because transportability on a gurney is a primary requirement, there will be derived requirements concerning the maximum weight, length, width, and height of the system (without which it would not meet the "transportability" primary requirement).

27-10 Functional and nonfunctional requirements

Requirements may be functional or nonfunctional and may take different forms. Functional requirements are those things that the system must do. For example, a medical imaging system must be able to detect certain structures within the human body. Nonfunctional requirements are mostly constraints on the system design. For example, the medical imaging system must fit within a certain size room or be operable on certain types of electrical power. A constraint might also refer to an attribute such as reliability. For example, the medical imaging system must have a reliability of not less than 25,000 operating hours mean time between failures (MTBF).

27-11 Stakeholder and system requirements

We can also divide requirements into *stakeholder requirements* and *system requirements*. The former are the requirements of the end users of the system. System requirements are more detailed and may involve interfaces to existing environments and other factors. Both stakeholder and system requirements may have functional and nonfunctional elements.

27-12 Requirements application

The application of a requirement identifies the object of the requirement. There are two aspects: *product parameters* and *program parameters.* The former refer to things specific to the product or service being supplied and may be either qualitative (e.g., paint color) or quantitative (e.g., weight). A program parameter refers to the *activities* required to produce the product or service. These may relate to tasks, evaluation of compliance to user requirements, external regulatory requirements, or program and design reviews.

27-13 Compliance level

The compliance level specifies whether the requirement is *mandatory* (e.g., system will not be accepted without it), for *guidance* (highly desirable to implement), or *informational* (some external factor that greatly affects the design solution).

27-14 Priority

It is rare that all requirements on a system are equally important. The priority of a requirement refers to its relative importance in the overall scheme of things. The priority is highly affected by perspective, so what may not be high priority at the overall systems level may be viewed as critical at a lower tier. Priority assignment is needed because complex systems often must be designed using compromises, called "trade-offs" in engineering jargon. Without priority assignment, making trade-offs becomes much more difficult.

27-15 Requirements documents

Any document that describes properties, attributes, services, functions, or behaviors needed to accomplish the goals and purposes of the system is a requirements document. This means that the performance specification written for the request for proposal (RFP) is also a requirements document. Once the contract is awarded and system design commences, the contractor will create a number of other requirements documents for themselves, the customer, subcontractors, and vendors. The level and the usage is the difference between these documents, but all are species of requirements documents.

If all goes well, one should be able to trace the lowest level requirements to higher level requirements. Ultimately, even the most detailed low-level requirement should be a reflection of (and traceable to) some item in the highest level document.

It is unfortunate that many highly complex systems have been acquired by medical institutions with little effort expended in developing the requirements. Although the better-qualified systems developers will perform that task, it is also necessary for the customer to do some ground work and develop their own idea of what is to be acquired before soliciting solutions from providers.

27-16 What are the characteristics of good requirements?

Good requirements have the following attributes:

Necessary. Only those things that are essential to the mission and function of the proposed system should be included. "Nice to have" things may be stated as goals or objectives, but as such, carry much less weight than requirements. The "necessary" criterion *excludes* to both specification of a particular design without good reason to do so and to specification of redundant requirements. The latter are requirements that are either covered more than once or are aggregated within a set of individual requirements.

Verifiable. A requirement that cannot be verified by some objective means is not really a requirement. Verification can be performed either by *inspection, analysis, demonstration,* or some sort of *formal test.* If a draft requirement cannot be thus verified, it cannot be contractually binding. Each requirement should be verifiable by a single test. If multiple tests are needed for verification of a particular requirement, then it may be true that the requirement is actually several requirements rolled into one statement. In that case, it should be broken into the constituent subrequirements.

Attainable. A requirement that is unattainable is also not a real requirement. Unattainability may be because of some limitation of engineering technology or science, or it may be that the system cannot be provided at an affordable cost. If the return on investment is unfavorable, or if the physics are impossible, then the requirement is unattainable.

Complete. A good requirements document contains all of the information needed by the developer or provider to furnish what is needed by the customer. Incomplete requirements often result

from the fact that the developer (e.g., an engineer) is not a domain expert (e.g., a nurse) and vice versa. When a nurse, physician, administrator, or accountant specifies some requirement, they may fail to realize that the developer might not understand what they mean or may have different assumptions of what is included. Similarly, when the engineers use their technical jargon, the domain expert may not understand it.

Consistent. Requirements are usually supplied by different source groups (e.g., nurses, maintainers, physicians) and therefore may be contradictory, because of the different, sometimes opposing, interests of the source groups. These inconsistencies must be negotiated out of the document before it is submitted to the developer. Otherwise, the developer may be confused or may make implicit assumptions that are not in the best interests of the firm. They may also play off one group against another for their own benefit. If management prioritizes the requirements, then trade-offs can be made by dropping conflicting lower priority items in favor of higher priority requirements.

Unambiguous. Requirements are expressed in human language. Unfortunately, that means that the vagaries of language come into play. In one hospital, a nonfunctional requirement existed for "24-hour service" of a CCU computer used to monitor patients. The vendor assumed the customary computer industry standard meaning (". . . a repair technician will arrive on site within 24 hours after the call is placed"), while the hospital meant that a repair technician would arrive, even if in the middle of the night, within an hour or so of being called by a CCU nurse who is caring for an unstable patient connected to the computerized monitor.

Concise and understandable. Good requirements are written using good grammar and simple structure. If multiple complex or compound sentences are used, it is probable that communication with the developer will suffer.

Implementation free. A good requirement specifies a need, not a solution. While the end users may have preferred solutions (even preferred brands), the requirements document is not the place for them. A good test of this attribute is that *a good requirement can be satisfied by more than one potential solution.* Guard against the tendency to write requirements that are so narrowly focused that they lead inexorably to a single solution or brand. One hospital found itself drawn into an expensive all-digital patient monitoring system based on a wireless LAN concept, when a simple hard-wired system would have satisfied the real requirement. Members of the committee kept adding features without proper rationale, until only one manufacturer's product (the most expensive) would be responsive to the published RFP.

Proper. A requirement is a demand on the next lower or more detailed level of planning or design. Your requirements document "flows down" to become binding guidance on the developers. The developers may, in turn, flow subrequirements down to their own suppliers. A "proper" requirement is one that is placed on the correct level, i.e., it states what is needed, not how the need should be met.

Traceable. Each level of document specifies a "what is needed" to lower level documents. The

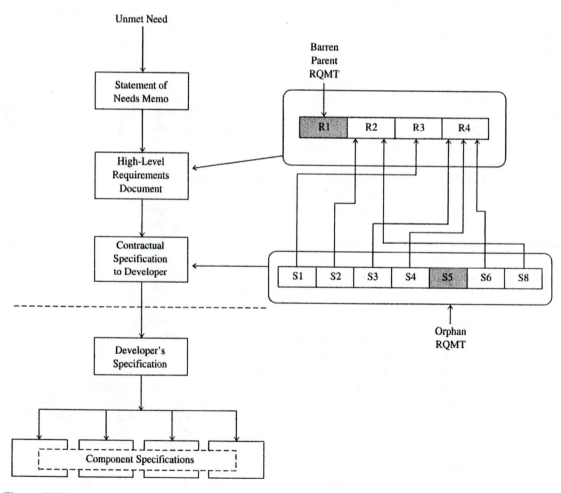

Figure 27-3

relationship between higher and lower levels is referred to as "parent" and "child." The child document becomes the "how" to its higher level parent's "what." Every item in the parent document should have at least one counterpart in the child document Figure 27-3). A requirement that does not flow down is called a "barren parent," while one that does not trace to a parent is called an "orphan." Both orphan and barren parent requirements indicate a flaw in the requirements process that should be investigated and resolved.

27-17 How are good requirements written?

The REAM process has three main activities: *definition, verification,* and *management. Requirements definition* is the eliciting and validating of requirements from the various interested parties ("stakeholders"). Elicitation is done by some combination of interviews with users and managers, focus groups, and experts; questionnaires; and surveys. There is no fixed approach, but all of these methods can be used. When recording the raw requirements, you should record: 1) the requirement statement, 2) who provided the requirement, 3) their function in the organization, and 4) their rationale or justification (no more than a single paragraph).

Part of the definition phase of requirements elicitation is validating the raw requirements and turning them into formal statements of need. This is the process of ensuring that all of the proposed requirements possess the characteristics previously described.

Once the requirements are validated, then the process of *conflicts must be eliminated.* This is necessary because the raw requirements might contain elements that are inconsistent, i.e., you can have one but not the other. In some cases, negotiation between the submitting parties under the guidance of a disinterested facilitator may remove the problem, which is why you recorded that information. In other cases, management may have to in-tervene by prioritizing the requirements, so that a rational and firm decision can be made.

Verification is the activity that determines whether or not the delivered system is what was ordered. The verification techniques used can be inspection, demonstration, test, or analysis. The goal of verification is to show that the delivered system meets the contract requirements and is the basis for a decision to pay the vendor. If the system does not meet requirements, then either the system should be rejected or a lower price negotiated in consideration of delivering less than what was ordered.

Management of the requirements is extremely important to containing costs. It is quite common for a vendor to "buy in" to a contract at an unrealistically low price, knowing they cannot profitably deliver what was promised at the contract price, and then depend on the seemingly inevitable changes to requirements to "get well." If you keep the requirements constant or defer desired changes to a preplanned future upgrade, you can control cost growth and schedule slip.

During the elicitation and validation period some form of spreadsheet or database matrix is usually created to provide requirements traceability and management insight. For larger projects or in cases where a number of projects are anticipated, there are software tools (e.g., Vital-Links) available to assist in capturing and managing requirements. There are also software decision tools, such as Expert Choice, that will help sort out conflicting requirements and other issues.

27-18 Requirements do not reflect actual needs of the user

Both users and engineers find it easier to think in concrete, rather than abstract, terms. As a result, they will often state a design solution as part of their requirements document. The requirement statement should address a need, not an implementation solution.

For example, a specification for an optical laboratory, in which a laser and sensitive photosensors were to be used, called for the interior to be painted a certain, highly specific shade of dull black. That requirement was difficult to test because it depended on matching a color patch in a published standard with the finished paint job, even though color perception varies markedly from one person to another.

The skilled systems engineer would ask: "Why do you need this particular shade of black?" The answer was ". . . to prevent light reflections from polluting the data collected by entering the sensors." The real need was to prevent any light source, either interior or exterior to the room, from reflecting from interior surfaces of the laboratory and entering the sensor aperture.

27-19 Inconsistent requirements

In a long or complex requirements documents it sometimes happens that a specific requirement will be stated in different and inconsistent ways in different parts of the document. This situation may arise because different people wrote the different sections, and they naturally come to the task with different viewpoints and writing styles. Inconsistency may, however, also indicate that the concept behind the requirement is not developed well enough to state it explicitly. Some work needs to be done to reconcile the inconsistencies.

27-20 Incomplete requirements

Although human beings are generally pretty good at pattern recognition, that ability often does not extend to finding missing elements in a pattern (Gause, 1989). When examining a collection of requirements, any one individual is likely to overlook many requirements through unfamiliarity. The use of a diverse group of reviewers, modeling and simulation (M & S), and scenario playing can help ferret out missing requirements.

The issue of missing requirements can become terribly important if something that is important to the user is left out of the requirements documents. The contractor usually deems it unimportant if it is

not explicitly stated. An example might be a computerized imaging system in which the normal default mode is not specified. The contractors may assume that some other mode is a reasonable default and incorrectly state it as such in their own internal design specifications. If an M&S effort is used, customer personnel who would normally operate the system may discover the defect when they are invited to "fly" the contractor's computer model.

27-21 Conflicting requirements

During a normal requirements elicitation effort, it is likely that inputs will be received from numerous sources. Each stakeholder community will likely offer requirements to the team. Unfortunately, not all requirements are compatible with each other. Meeting one requirement may preclude or at least impede meeting the other. For example, one might demand that an electronics box be painted white, while another will demand that it be painted blue. A box cannot be painted both white and blue at the same time.

One of the tasks of the systems engineer is to analyze the requirements set for conflicts, and then conduct negotiations amongst the stakeholders to eliminate or harmonize the problems. This is the point where trade-offs are made. But to conduct a proper trade-off, one must first prioritize the requirements according to which is more valuable and which is less valuable to the overall system.

27-22 Misunderstood or misinterpreted requirements

Requirements are expressed in human language. Unfortunately, that's where the problems start. Words can be ambiguous or vague. For example, a requirement that demands an item be "lightweight" means different things to different people. If you install the device on an ambulance, the meaning of "lightweight" is different from the meaning if that device has to be hand-carried up several flights of stairs. Sometimes, misinterpretations occur because different stakeholder communities use different jargon or different definitions for the same words.

27-23 Ambiguous requirements

One of the ways that requirements are misunderstood is that words can be ambiguous, i.e., a word can have more than one correct meaning. For example, instead of "lightweight" the requirement statement is that the desired product be "light." This can mean lightweight (whatever that means), that it is painted a light color such as white, or that it have some source of illumination. If it is a food product, then "light" can mean fewer calories than the "normal" product that it replaces or a lighter, less intense flavor than the "normal" product.

27-24 Vague requirements

A vague requirement is one that is unclear or fuzzy, rather than crisp. If the statement of the requirement fails to elicit an image or understanding of what is desired in the reader, then perhaps it is too vague to be correctly interpreted.

27-25 Introduced requirements

This type of requirement is derived from a decision made about other requirements. If some interface or environmental requirement is expected to drive the design, then issues pertaining to those factors will become requirements. For example, a requirement that the desired device must operate outdoors in arctic regions may imply that it operate, or at least safely start, at temperatures down to $-60°F$.

27-26 Spurious requirements

These "requirements" are statements that are either erroneous or fall into the category of preferences of some, but not most, stakeholders. It includes "nice to have" features that do not add any real value to the system in the eyes of most stakeholders.

27-27 Unintended consequences

All decisions have consequences. If you elect to spend your money on one thing, you cannot spend the same money on something else. Economists call this "opportunity cost." Whatever decision is made, a de facto situation is created that admits some things and eliminates certain other things. Some thought must be given to what must be given up for each alternative solution to be selected.

27-28 Approaches to requirements: stakeholder viewpoint

Good requirements elicitation requires good input from the stakeholders. As the computer folks say: GIGO (garbage in, garbage out). Below are several strategies used by some stakeholders that can result in less than ideal requirements documents.

I can't explain it, but I'll know it when I see it. The lazy way out is to push all of the responsibility for eliciting requirements onto the systems engineer or the supplier's marketer. The problem is that the systems engineer may design the wrong product if there is no consensus with the stakeholders on exactly what is to be produced. This approach may work for art, but not for engineering.

Kitchen sink. This approach is to include virtually every feature that every possible stakeholder could possibly want, plus a few more. Unfortunately, many of those requirements will be in conflict with each other. And even if there are not conflicts, the cost of the system will soar astronomically if a lot of low-valued added features are provided.

Same thing as before. The stakeholder will pass the buck by telling you to "provide what we had before, only better." That is hardly useful. If what they had before only needs to be better, then perhaps an incremental upgrade to the old system is a better business approach than an entirely new design. This approach to requirements elicitation is often a symptom of either a reluctance to change or a lack of vision of a better way of doing things in the future.

Smoke gets in your eyes. Systems requirement documents, like budgets, are often padded with unwanted, but costly things that can be "horse-traded" away. A clever stakeholder might add things to the "wish list" that are known to be beyond the scope of the new system, beyond current technology, too expensive for the current budget, or simply unneeded. Their idea is to appear reasonable at requirements negotiation time by backing off on those requirements they didn't really want in the first place.

If you can't dazzle them with your brilliance, then baffle them. Some people cannot seem to help using multitudinous, polysyllabic technical words to describe the system they want. Sometimes it is mere ego, i.e., they want to appear really, really smart. Other times, however, it is a ploy to cover up the fact that they really haven't thought through their requirements and want to put the monkey on your back.

All of these strategies may be encountered at one time or another. The job of a skilled systems engineer is to elicit the real requirements from these people by clever probing and gentle guidance.

27-29 Elements of a good requirements document

Requirements documents are designed to be read by people, so they should be laid out in a highly readable manner. All of the necessary information should be provided in the document, even if only by reference. The elements below are generic, but should exist to one degree or another in all specifications and other requirements documents at each level in the process hierarchy.

Overview. The overview should tell the reader what the system is supposed to do in high-level terms. It should spell out the benefits of developing the system and the consequences of not developing the system. It should answer the question, "Why is this system required?" In other words, the overview should make a good business case for the new system. If the business case is weak, then the system probably won't be developed.

Glossary. This glossary is a dictionary of all special terms, professional or domain-specific jargon, acronyms, or ordinary terms with either special or limited meaning used in the document. Although some developers do not hold the glossary in high esteem, it is actually a critical element for establishing a basis for communication among the participants.

Define services and functions. All of the services provided and functions performed by the system should be discussed. The attributes and properties should also be stated. Don't overlook the nonfunctional requirements: they can be as important as the functional requirements.

Constraints Every system faces constraints on its design. Some constraints may be budgetary or time-oriented. A solution that cannot come in on time at the agreed cost is not acceptable. Other constraints might be environmental. There may be mechanical, electrical, or other interfaces that must be met. If a constraint is not enumerated in the specification, the designer is justified in assuming that it does not exist.

Define the environment and likely changes. The physical, mechanical, electrical, and electromagnetic environments may all have a profound effect on the design solutions that are acceptable. This information must be provided to the designer in sufficient detail to permit a successful design effort.

Environmental details may include physical factors, such as the space in which it is installed and the pathways to that space. If an item is designed for use aboard an ambulance, for example, physical factors that would be acceptable in a hospital, home, factor, or warehouse might render the system unacceptable. Can it be mounted in the space allotted to it and still be operated by the EMT? Can the EMT carry it along with all the other gear?

27-30 Wordsmithing

There are certain words and phrases to avoid when writing requirements. Anything that is either unverifiable or ambiguous will lead to problems. Avoid indefinite words such as: minimum, maximum, flexible, adaptable, fast, rapid, user-friendly, nominal, may, can, precisely, real-time, approximately, various, multiple, many, few and limited.

All wording must pass the test of verifiability: How do you verify a requirement such as "all on-screen menus shall be accessible using a *minimum* number of keystrokes?" Adjectives and adverbs should be considered carefully to determine whether or not a reasonable and prudent person would misconstrue their modifying effects on the statement. Indefinite forms of the verb "to be" can be particularly troublesome.

Avoid concatenated slash-bar words, such as "and/or." If you require the vendor to supply "A and/or B" then the contract is fully met by the vendor if either A, B, *or* both A and B are supplied. Slash-bar concatenations are generally taken to indicate a series of *interchangeable* items. If you state "the vendor shall provide installation/training/initial consumables" then the contract may be deemed as fully met if *any* of these items are supplied.

Use the term "shall" to indicate a requirement. "Will" indicates a statement of future fact: "the hospital will make the operating room available to the vendor's installation team between 1800 hours and 0500 hours daily for a period of 2 weeks." "Should" indicates goals or objectives that are not true requirements (e.g., the "nice-to-have" items) but which might be used to differentiate between two otherwise equivalent proposals.

27-31 How do you manage requirements?

The traditional approach to managing requirements is to determine all of the requirements early, set them in concrete, and threaten the mortal destruction of anyone who proposes a change. Unfortunately, in the practical world, that approach does not work. It is rare that all of the requirements are both known and well-defined early in the process, so it is necessary to tolerate some

vagueness, incompleteness, and inconsistency until the process matures. An additional problem is that the various people who submit requirements may speak different professional languages and therefore do not communicate well with each other. In either case, it often takes several iterations of the process to finally arrive at a workable set of requirements.

Once a requirements document is prepared, it should be placed under a strict *configuration management* regime. This means that no one is permitted to make changes without formal approval. In practical terms, it means appointing one person to be the official keeper of the document and guardian of its integrity. Proposed changes should be made in writing to either this official or a small control board. Before any changes are made to the document, they must be examined by all people concerned to ferret out any conflicts with other requirements or plans being made in response to requirements.

27-32 Summary

1. Managing high technology is difficult. In one study of 8,380 information systems development projects, only 9% came in on time, under budget, and fully functional.

2. The major cause of problems is requirements engineering and management.

3. A requirement is a formal written statement of the needs and expectations of the customer, including the entire set of capabilities, functions, behaviors, characteristics, attributes, and constraints on a proposed system.

4. Requirements engineers and management (REAM) is the application of a disciplined, scientific approach to eliciting, validating, specifying, and verifying requirements.

5. Requirements are important because they formally describe what is needed or desired and because they are contractually binding on the developer or vendor.

27-33 Recapitulation

Now return to the objectives and self-evaluation questions at the beginning of the chapter and see how well you can answer them. If you cannot answer certain questions, place a check mark next to each and review appropriate parts of the text. Next, try to answer the following questions using the same procedure.

Questions

1. _____ is the major cause of problems in project design.
2. Define requirements in your own words.
3. Define REAM in your own words.
4. Why are requirements important?
5. List three types of requirements.
6. List examples of constraints on a bedside monitor.
7. List symptoms of bad requirements.
8. List examples of nonfunctional requirements on a bedside monitor.
9. A _____ _____ is an activity required to produce some product or service.
10. List eight attributes of good requirements.

Suggested readings

Andriole, Stephen J. (1996). *Managing Systems Requirements: Methods, Tools and Cases.* New York: McGraw-Hill.

Feather, M.S. (1991) "Requirements Engineering: Getting Right from Wrong," *ESEC'91,* pp. 485-488.

Forsberg, Kevin and Harold Mooz (1996). *System Engineering Overview.* Cupertino, CA: Center for Systems Management. Monograph reprinted in Thayer and Dorfman (1997).

GAO-U.S. General Accounting Office (1992). *Mission Critical Systems: Defense Attempting to Address Major Software Challenges.* GAO/IMTEC-93-13, December 1992.

Gause, Donald C. and Gerald M. Weinberg (1989). *Exploring Requirements: Quality Before Design.* New York: Dorset House.

Harwell, Richard, Erik Aslaksen, Ivy Hooks, Roy Mengot, and Ken Ptack. (1993). "What is a Requirement?" *Proceedings of the 3rd Annual International Symposium, National Council Systems Engineering.*

Jorgensen, Raymond (1999). "Requirements Management for True System Reusability." Proceedings of the 9th Annual Symposium INCOSE (CD-ROM Edition), Brighton, England, June 6-10.

Leveson, Nancy G. and Clark S. Turner, "An Investigation of the Therac-25 Accidents," *IEEE Computer,* Vol. 26(7), July 1993, pp. 18-41.

Macaulay, Linda A. (1996). *Requirements Engineering.* London: Springer-Verlag Applied Computing Series.

Rawlinson, J.A. (1987). "Report on the Therac-25," *OCTRF/OCI Physicists Meeting,* Kingston, Ont., Canada, 7 May 1987. Cited in Leveson and Turner.

Reason, James (1990). *Human Error.* Cambridge Univ Press. Cambridge (UK).

Rechtin, Eberhardt and Mark W. Maier (1997). *The Art of Systems Architecting.* Boca Raton, FL: CRC Press.

Sage, Andrew P. (1992). *Systems Engineering.* New York: John Wiley & Sons.

Scharer, Laura (1981). "Pinpointing Requirements". *Datamation.* April 1981, pp. 139-151.

Sommerville, Ian and Pete Sawyer (1997). *Requirements Engineering: A Good Practices Guide.* Chichester (UK): John Wiley & Sons.

Stone, Donald R. and Waldmann, *"Recent Developments in the U.S. Medical Device Regulatory System."* (FDA policy changes in regulating development and use of medical devices coincident with the explosion of medical technology and innovative new techniques, including breakthrough in therapies and new disciplines, such as interventional neurology and biotechnology, 1990, 1997, 1998), (Medical Device Manufacturing and Technology Business Briefing Report and CD-ROM, Aspen Market Services, World Markets Research Center, Academic House, 24-28 Oval Road, London, NWI 7DP, June, 1999, Phone: +44-171-526-2400, Internet: www.wmrc.com)

APPENDIX A
Some Math Notes

This textbook was originally designed for use by students who may not have studied calculus. But as work progressed, it became apparent that we could not adequately explain matters such as *cardiac output* and *mean arterial pressure* without using the *notation* used in calculus mathematics. Keep in mind that you need not know how to *work* calculus problems (after all, the electronic instruments *do* the calculus), but you should understand what is meant when the *symbols* used in calculus are encountered in the text.

There are two fundamental operations in calculus: *integration* and *differentiation.* In electronic instruments, circuits are used to perform these functions.

In brief, integration is the mathematical process of finding the total *area* under a curve on a graph. Differentiation, on the other hand, is the process of finding the *instantaneous rate of change* of a curve.

The curves in electronic circuits are the graph of *voltage-versus-time* in most cases. We would say, then, a *graph of the voltage as a function of time.*

A-1 Differentiation

Differentiation is the process of finding the instantaneous rate of change of the curve. Rate of change is given by the *slope* of the curve. If the curve is a straight line (Figure A-1*a*), then finding the rate of change (slope) is very easy. In that simple case, the *change* in E is divided by the *change* in T:

$$\text{Slope} = \frac{E_2 - E_1}{T_2 - T_1} \tag{A-1}$$

We use a special notation to indicate the quantities $(E_2 - E_1)$ and $(T_2 - T_1)$. These quantities are *changes,* so we can use the Greek letter delta (Δ) to replace the expressions:

$$\Delta E = E_2 - E_1 \tag{A-2}$$
$$\Delta T = T_2 - T_1 \tag{A-3}$$

It is standard mathematical practice to use Δ whenever we wish to denote a *small change* in some quantity. If we use the delta notation in Equation A-1, then, we would write:

$$\text{Slope} = \frac{\Delta E}{\Delta T} \tag{A-4}$$

The preceding equations work very well if the curve is a straight line. But what if the curve is not a straight line (Figure A-1*b*)? What do we do if we need to know the instantaneous rate of change at

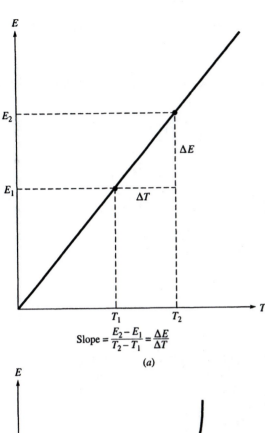

$$\text{Slope} = \frac{E_2 - E_1}{T_2 - T_1} = \frac{\Delta E}{\Delta T}$$

(a)

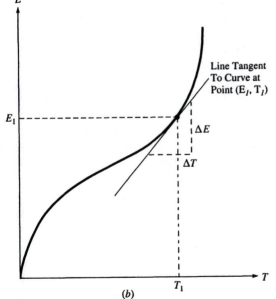

(b)

Figure A-1
Finding the instantaneous rate of change of a curve.
(a) The curve is a straight line. *(b)* The curve is not a
straight line.

some specific point on that curve? Although the
answer to that question goes right to the heart of
calculus mathematics, we can sum it up adequately for our purposes very simply. The instantaneous rate of change, also known as the *derivative,* can be found by taking the slope of a line
tangent to the curve at the point of interest. Any
calculus book will be able to prove to you that this
is true.

When speaking of derivatives, we still use the
concept of Equation A-1, but we change the notation from $\Delta E/\Delta R$ to:

$$\text{Derivative} = \frac{dE}{dT} \qquad \text{(A-5)}$$

When you see *dE/dT,* then, you should recognize that we are asking for the instantaneous rate
of change of *E* with respect to *T.* This may sometimes be written in the form *E* but is merely shorthand for *dE/dT:*

$$E = \frac{dE}{dT} \qquad \text{(A-6)}$$

An operational amplifier circuit that will differentiate signals is discussed in Section 4-8-3.

A-2 Integration

Integration is the process of finding the *area* under
a curve. This is shown in Figure A-2, where we see
two *voltage-versus-time* curves (E_1 and E_2). Assume that we want to measure the areas under
these curves over the time interval T_1 to T_2. For E_1,
the problem is very easy because the region of interest forms a rectangle. The area is:

$$A = (E_1 - 0)(T_2 - T_1) \qquad \text{(A-7)}$$
$$A = (E_1)(T_2 - T_1) \qquad \text{(A-8)}$$
$$A = E_1 \times \Delta T \qquad \text{(A-9)}$$

But what do we do when confronted with a
curve such as the signal labeled E_2 in Figure A-2?
This curve is not so well behaved, so we must revert to calculus.

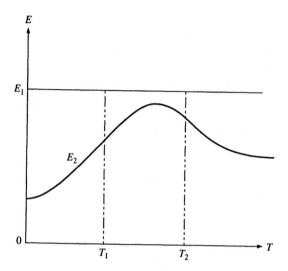

Figure A-2
Signal with an irregular curve.

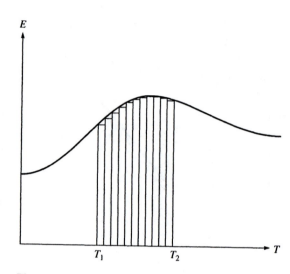

Figure A-3
Breaking the area of interest into rectangles to determine the approximate area.

The mathematical techniques of integration tell us that the solution is to break up the area of interest into rectangles (Figure A-3). We can easily calculate the area of each rectangle as $(E_1 \times \Delta T)$. By summing up the areas of all of the rectangles, we gain an approximation of the area under the curve.

If the rectangles are large, then the approximation is poor. But as the width of the rectangles becomes smaller, the approximation becomes better. Finally, when ΔT becomes very, very small (as $\Delta T \to 0$), the approximation is exact.

The symbol used for integration is shown in Equation A-10:

$$\text{Area} = \int_{T_1}^{T_2} E_2 dT \qquad (A\text{-}10)$$

The S-shaped symbol is the integral symbol. T_1 and T_2 denote the boundaries, or limits, over which integration is desired. The dT tells us that we are integrating with respect to time (T). Equation A-10 is read: "integral of E_2 with respect to T, over the interval T_1 to T_2."

When dealing with electronic signals, integration is also called *time averaging;* hence the use of integrators to calculate quantities such as mean arterial blood pressure from the arterial waveform.

Electronic integration is performed by accumulating a charge in a capacitor. An example of an electronic integrator, using an operational amplifier, is discussed in chapter 4.

APPENDIX B
Medical Terminology

Some medical terminology sounds like jargon to the layperson but is a reasonable, concise method of communication. Medical terms are made of combinations of roots, suffixes, and prefixes with highly specific meaning. For example, *hepatitis,* meaning an inflammation of the liver, is made of a root *hepar* (meaning liver), and a suffix *it is* (inflammation). Many of the long, polysyllabic words used in medical environments become quite simple in their meaning when broken down into roots, prefixes, and suffixes. Some of the more commonly encountered terms are listed here.

Roots	Meaning
aden	gland
arteria	artery
arthros	joint
auris	ear
brachion	arm
cardium	heart
cephalo	brain
cholecyst	gall bladder
colon	intestine
costa	rib
cranium	skull, head
derma	skin

Roots	Meaning
enteron	intestine
epithelium	skin
esophagus	gullet
gaster	stomach
hema, hemo	blood
hepar	liver
hydro	water
hystera	womb
kypsis	bladder
larynx	throat
myelos	marrow
nasus	nose
nephros	kidney
neuron	nerve cell
odons	tooth
odynia	pain
opsikas	eye
os	bone
osteon	bone
ostrium	mouth
otis	ear
pes	foot
pharynx	throat
phlebos	vein
pleura	chest

Roots	Meaning
pneumones	lungs
psyche	mind
pulmones	lungs
pyelos	kidney
pyretos	fever
ren	kidney
rhin	nose
rhythmos	rhythm
spondylos	vertebra
stoma	mouth
thorax	chest
trachea	windpipe
trophe	nutrition
vene	vein
vesica	bladder

Prefixes	Meaning
a-	absence, not
ab-	away from, off
ad-	toward
amphi-	on both sides, bilateral
an-	absence of
ante-	before, in front of
antero-	in front
anti-	against
ap-	separation
apo-	separation
bi-	two
bio-	pertaining to life
brady-	slow
cardio-	pertaining to the heart
cephalo-	head
chiro-	hand
chole-	bile
co-	together
con-	with
costo-	rib
cysto-	sac, bladder
dactylo-	digit (finger, toe)
derma-	skin
dermato-	skin
di-	twice
dia-	apart, through
dys-	difficult, painful

Prefixes	Meaning
ec-	out of
ecto-	outside
ex-	out of
en-	within
endo-	within
ento-	within
entero-	intestines
epi-	upon
ex-	away from
exo-	outside of
extro-	outside
eu-	well, good
gastro-	stomach
hema-, hemo-	blood
hemato-	blood
hetero-	different
homo-	the same, or the same sort
hydro-	water
hypno-	sleep
hypo-	beneath, deficient, lower than
hystero-	uterus
ileo-	ileum
in-, il-, ir-	within, not, inside
infra-	beneath
inter-	between
intra-	within
iso-	equal, same
kilo-	1000
leuko-	white, clear
litho-	stone
macro-	abnormally large, large
mal-	bad
media-	middle
mega-	great size; 1,000,000
melano-	black
meso-	middle
meta-	more than, change, after, next
micro-	small; 0.000001 (i.e., 1/1,000,000)
mono-	one
morpho-	form
multi-	many
myelo-	bone marrow; pertaining to the spinal cord

Prefixes	Meaning
myo-	muscle
neo-	new
nephro-	kidney
neuro-	nerves
ob-	in front of
odonto-	tooth
ophthalmo-	eye
ortho-	straight, normal
osteo-	bone
oto-	ear
pan-	all
para-	beside
patho-	pertaining to disease
peri-	around
pneumo-	lungs, respiration
pod-	foot
poly-	many
pre-	before
pro-	before
procto-	rectum
pseudo-	false
pyo-	pus
pyr-	fire, heat
quadra-	four
retro-	located behind, backwards
rhino-	nose
semi-	half
sphygmo-	pulsel
sub-	near, moderately, under
super-	excessive, above
supra-	above
sym-	union
syn-	union
tachy-	fast, extremely fast
trans-	across
tri-	three

Prefixes	Meaning
ultra-	beyond
uni-	single

Suffixes	Meaning
agogue	inducing agent
-agra	sudden acute pain
-algia	painful
-cele	tumor, swelling
-centesis	puncture into
-clasia	remedy
-ectomy	surgical excision of
-ecstasis	dilation
-edema	swelling
-emia	blood
-graph	graphic record
-ia	diseased condition
-iasis	process or procedure
-itis	inflammation
-logy	study, or science, of
-mania	abnormally excessive preoccupation
-meter	resembling
-oid	resembling
-oma	tumor
-opia	vision
-osis	fullness, excess
-pathy	morbid disease
-phobia	dread, fear
-plasty	plastic surgery repair
-rrhea	discharge or flow
-sclerosis	hardening
-scope	instrument for examining
-scopy	visual examination of
-stomy	artificial opening
-tomy	incision

APPENDIX C
Glossary

accretion growth or enlargement

accuracy expression of how precise each step of the analog signal can be represented in an ADC, for example. Contrasted with resolution, which is the smallest signal increment that can be detected by a measurement system. Both expressed in bits, LSBs, or percent of full scale. Accuracy is measuring how much a signal changed to some defined error, but resolution: just noting some change.

A/D analog-to-digital converter, which converts analog (continuous) signals to digital (ones and zeros); sometimes referred to as ADC.

ALU arithmetic logic unit, which performs mathematical operations

alveolus air sac or cell in lungs

amnion thin membrane around fetus

amniotic pertaining to the amnion

angstrom unit of length (1 angstrom = 10^{-10} meters)

ANSI American National Standards Institute (ANSI standard is consensus standard, not law)

anterior situated in front of

aorta great artery carrying blood from the left side of heart

aortic pertaining to the aorta

arborization form resembling a tree

arrhythmia alteration in rhythm

arteriole one of the smallest arteries that becomes a capillary

artifacts error in a test result, graph, or written record

ASIC application-specific integrated circuit (performs dedicated functions)

asynchronous property of a function: hardware (arbitrary time with synchronization to a reference clock) or software (begins an operation and returns before completion of operation)

ATE automatic test equipment (typically computer based)

atria (pl.) see atrium

atrioventricular located between the upper and lower chambers of the heart

atrium upper chamber of the heart

auricle see atrium

autonomic action independent of free volition

axon long, thin portion of a nerve cell that carries the impulse away from the neuron

bandwidth a range of frequencies over which a circuit or device operates

baud rate serial communication data transmission rate expressed in bits per second

bioelectricity electrical activity pertaining to a living cell

biophysics branch of science that applied the concepts of physical science to biology and medicine

bipolar a signal range that includes both positive and negative values

block-mode a high-speed data transfer in which a data address is sent followed by a number of data words

bit one binary digit, either 0 (zero) or 1 (one)

brachial related to, or pertaining to, the arm

bradycardia slow heart rate

break-before-make a switching contact that completely disengages from one connection before it connects to another

bronchi (pl.) see bronchus

bronchus tube leading from trachea to either left or right lung

bus group of conductors that interconnect individual circuitry in a computer, such as AT bus, NuBus, Micro Channel, EISA bus, Microwire by National Semiconductor (used in COP800 series microcontrollers)

byte eight (8) related bits of data, such as 11111111 or 00000000

cache high-speed processor memory that buffers instructions or data to increase processing throughput or the time it takes to complete a process operation

capillaries smallest vessels in the body

cardiac pertaining to the heart

cardiology study of the heart and its diseases

cardiovascular relating to the circulatory system

catheter small tube that is inserted into the body to permit injection of fluids, introduction of medication, withdrawal of fluids, or keep a vessel open

CD-ROM computer disk, read only memory

cell smallest body capable of life

cephalic pertaining to the skull or head

cerebellum large dorsal brain structure

cerebrum anterior portion of the brain

compiler software that converts a source program within a high-level programming language (such as BASIC, C-Language, or PASCAL) into an object or compiled programming in machine language

computer electronic device that performs basic calculations, such as add/sub/mul/div/logic, and operates higher-level software, such as word processors, spreadsheets, graphic programs, and instrumentation

conversion time time required for a system to acquire data after initiated to do so

cornea transparent covering of the center portion of the eye

cortex outer layer of tissue on an organ

cortical pertaining to the cortex

cranium portion of the skull covering the brain

cross talk an undesired signal on one channel due to a signal on another channel

curare drug that produces muscle relaxation

cytoplasm the matter inside of a cell, except the nucleus

D/A digital-to-analog converter, which converts digital (ones and zeros) to analog signals (continuous); sometimes referred to as DAC

DAQ data acquisition (collecting, measuring, and/or digitizing electrical signals from sensors, transducers, and other sources)

DAS data acquisition system (includes all hardware and software for data acquisition)

data flow model for programming that uses instruction or operators to execute inputs

dB decibel (a logarithmic measure of the ratio of one signal to another, usually a reference); dB $= 20\ LOG_{10}$(Vsignal/Vreference in volts per volt) or dB $= 10\ LOG_{10}$(Psignal/Preference in watts per watt)

DCS distributed control system (large-scale process control system with distributed network of process and input/output subsystems; performs control, interfacing, data collection, and system management

DDE dynamic data exchange (standard software protocol in Microsoft Windows)

defibrillator electrical machine used to stop fibrillation of the heart by application of an electrical shock

delta-sigma (sometimes called *sigma-delta*) modulating ADC (high-accuracy, high-resolution digitizer of 16 to 24 bits that samples at a high rate, then decimates to remove in-band noise)

dendrite portion of the nerve cell that conducts impulses toward the cell

depolarized state of being partially or totally depolarized

dialysis process of removing substances from the body

diastole expansion of the chambers of the heart so that they may fill with blood

diastolic pertaining to diastole

dicrotic double humped waveform

dicrotic notch feature of arterial pressure waveform

differential input analog input made up of two terminals, a plus and a minus connection, in which the signal is measured between one input referenced to ground and another signal also referenced to ground; contrasted with unipolar, which describes an analog signal measured with respect to a ground

DIO digital input/output

DLL dynamic link library (software module in Microsoft Windows with executable code and data that can be called or used by Windows applications)

DNL differential nonlinearity: measure of the worstcase variation in ADC or DAC code widths, usually expressed in LSBs (least significant bits); essentially shows how uneven the digital steps are inside the converter (e.g., a DNL of 1/2 LSB in a 12-bit converter means the steps are uneven by 0.012 percent or 1/2 step in 2^{12} or 4096 codes)

DMA direct memory access (fastest method by which data can be transferred to and from computer memory)

dorsal situated near or toward the back

drivers software that controls a hardware device; can also be a circuit that delivers a signal to an electrical line, such as a differential line driver

dynamic range ratio of the maximum signal level in a circuit to the smallest it can handle (at the noise floor); expressed in volts per volt, watts per watt, or dB

ECG electrocardiograph

ectopic located in other than normal position

EEG electroencephalograph

EEPROM electrically erasable programmable read only memory (ROM) (memory that can be erased with an electrical signal and reprogrammed)

EKG German abbreviation for ECG

electrocardiogram tracing of the electrical signals produced by the heart

electrode conductor used to make electrical contact between a wire and a conductive surface

electrodermograph recorder for measuring galvanic skin resistance

electroencephalogram recording of brain biopotentials

electroencephalograph machine for making electroencephalograms

electrogastrogram recording of the simultaneous electrical and physical activity of the stomach

electrolyte solution in which electrical current is due to ion mobility

electromyogram recording of the biopotentials produced by skeletal muscles

electromyograph machine for making electromyograms

embolus abnormal solid or gaseous particle in bloodstream

embryo undeveloped stage of fetus

EMG electromyograph, electromyogram

Emulator software program that is the equal of another for the purpose of allowing an operator to program in one language while performing operations in another

encoder device that converts linear or rotary displacement into digital or pulse signals

EPROM erasable programmable read only memory, usually erasable by intense ultraviolet light

extracellular outside the cells

extracorporeal outside the body

fibula smaller of the two bones in the leg, between the ankle and knee

fieldbus all-digital communication network for connecting process control instrumentation to control systems; medical information bus connects medical instrumentation to other equipment and medical control systems

FIFO first-in-first-out memory buffer

fixed-point format for storing or processing digital integers in which the decimal point for example is fixed (e.g., 1,500.50)

floating point format for storing or processing digital numbers in scientific exponential notation (multiples of a power of 10) in which the decimal point, for example, floats or moves left or right to accommodate the power of 10 (e.g., 1.50050×10^3)

gain factor or multiplier by which a signal is amplified, expressed in volts per volt, watts per watt, or dB

galvanic that which produces a direct current

GPIB General Purpose Interface Bus (named by Hewlett-Packard Company as HP-IB); a standard used for controlling electronic instruments via a computer; based on the IEEE 488 bus (Institute of Electrical and Electronic Engineers)

GUI graphical user interface (intuitive, easy-to-use, graphical display technique for transferring information to and from computer programs; GIUs resemble front panels of instruments or other objects)

hardware physical components of a computer system

hemisphere half of a spherical object

hemodialysis machine removes salts, water, and toxins, artifically from the body via circulating blood through external tubes.

hierarchical method of organizing computer programs in levels or a tree structure

high-flux dialysis fast removal of salts, water, and toxins from the body

homogeneity all of the same sort, state of

homogeneous of the same sort

IAC interapplication communication (protocol by which computer applications pass messages, information, or commands)

IMD intermodulation distortion: ratio, in dB, of the total rms signal level, in voltage or power, of the harmonics, to the overall rms signal level (often two sinewaves); standards: SMPTE (60-Hz and 7-kHz sinewaves added in 4:1 amplitude ratio), DIN (250 Hz and 8 kHz added in 4:1 amplitude ratio), CCIF (14 and 15 kHz added in 1:1 amplitude ratio); RMS is the root-mean-square or steady-state dc level that would transfer the same amount of heat energy (e.g., into a resistor) as the full ac waveform

infarct area of necrotic tissue due to loss of blood perfusion

inhomogeneity not homogeneous

INL integral nonlinearity: measure of the worst-case variation in ADC or DAC of the ideal minimum to code, usually expressed in LSBs or least significant bits; essentially shows how far off the digital steps are inside the converter (e.g., a DNL of 1/2 LSB in a 12-bit converter means the steps are uneven by 0.012 percent or 1/2 in 2^{12} or 4096 codes)

interpreter software utility that executes source code from a high-level language, such as BASIC, C-Language, or PASCAL

intracellular inside the cell

I/O input/output (data is transferred to and from a computer system)

ion atom or molecule that carries an electrical charge

iris colored portion of the eye behind the cornea

isoelectric having the same electrical charge (i.e., a state of zero potential difference)

isolation voltage voltage that one circuit can normally withstand with respect to another circuit; digital hardware lines are sometimes isolated from one another with opto-couplers or capacitive-couplers

isothermal having the same temperature in all portions

isotropic having the same properties in all directions

kidney organ that removes salts, water, and toxins from the blood

latency apparent inactivity

linearity measure of how well a device's transfer function adheres to an ideal straight line, such as how closely an ADC's output codes double in response to the doubling of its input analog signal

listener device on the GPIB or HP-IB that receives information from a talker on the bus

lobe rounded portion of an organ

LSB least significant bit (smallest step an ADC or DAC takes)

laptop portable, battery-powered, notebook-size computer that fits on your lap and today often has as much power as a desktop computer

lumen hollow portion of a tubular organ

manometer gas pressure meter

membrane thin layer of tissue

metabolism total of all life processes

MIB Medical Information Bus (standard for hardware configuration and software communication protocol by which electronic medical instruments communicate with each other and with a central processing system)

micron unit of length, 1/1,000,000 meters

microcomputer small fully contained computer

MIPS million of instructions per second (unit for the speed of code instructions in a processor)

microprocessor computing portion of a micro computer

mitochondria small granules or rods

mitral stenosis narrowing of the orifice between left atrium and left ventricle

MMI man-machine interface, also called human-machine interface (means by which an operator interacts with an electronic measurement and control system)

multitasking property of an operating system describing that several processes are run simultaneously

mux multiplexer (switching device containing multiple inputs that can be connected to an output by selection; exists in hardware and software)

MXIbus Multisystem eXtension Interface bus (multidrop, 32-bit parallel bus architecture for more than 20 megabytes per second, high-speed

data rate communications between devices; acts like a backplane computer bus but connects physically separate devices together

myocardium a muscle layer of the heart

myograph instrument for measuring muscle contraction

necrosis death of cells or tissue

neuron nerve cell

noise undesirable electrical signal arising from external direct and radiated sources (e.g., ac power lines) and internal sources (e.g., semiconductors, resistors, and capacitors)

nucleus central structure (in cells, atoms, etc.)

Nyquist sampling theorem law of sampling or digitizing stating that an original signal can be recovered without distortion error if that continuous bandwidth-limited signal contains no frequencies components higher than half the frequency at which it is sampled. Stated another way, you must sample at least twice the frequency bandwidth of a bandwidth-limited signal to digitize it without distortion. This can apply to any waveshape, but with a sinewave it is easy to see that if two points in one cycle are taken, the frequency and amplitude can be determined. Since the sinewave is an exact known function, the particular sinewave can be drawn perfectly. Anything less than this results in an uncertainty about the sinewave.

occipital related to or pertaining to the rear portion of the head

operating system fundamental-level software that controls a computer, runs programs, and interacts with users and peripheral devices

organ group of specialized cells that perform a special function

orthogonal at right angles to, normal to

overhead amount of computer processing resources in time, memory, or tasks

parallel bus many conductors or lines that act together to communicate or transfer data

parietal pertaining to the upper rear portion of head

PCI peripheral component interconnect (high-performing [theoretical 132 megabytes per second] expansion bus architecture that was originally developed by Intel to replace ISA [International Standards Association])

PCMCIA Personal Computer Memory Card International Association (expansion bus architecture for notebook-size computers or laptops, originally intended for add-on memory cards but now includes entire modules, such as those used in data acquisition)

PDA personal digital assistant, or palmtop computer

permeable allows material to pass through pores

peroneal pertaining to the outer side of lower leg

PID control control mechanism encompassing three terms: proportional (ratio), integral (summation), and derivative (slope) actions

piezoelectric electrical activity due to deformation of a crystalline structure

pipeline high-performance processor approach in which an instruction is sped up by breaking it into several elements that can be processed simultaneously from different instructions

peripheral device device located outside a main unit

PLC programmable logic controller (performs logic functions)

plethysmography recording volume changes due to blood flow

plug and play ISA International Standard Association specification of Microsoft, Intel, and other personal computer companies describing plug-in boards that can be fully configured by software without the need of jumpers; refers to software reconfigurable and programmable

pneumatic pertaining to or operated by gases

pneumograph measuring instrument for recording respiration

pneumotachygraph instrument for measuring respiration rate

port communication connection on a computer or remote terminal or controller

posterior pertaining to the rear

propagation delay time it takes for a signal to pass through a circuit or system (sometimes referred to as latency)

protocol exact sequence of bits, characters, and control codes used to transfer data; at least three types exist: IP (internet protocol, low-level service such as paging), TCP (transmission control protocol for high-reliability transmissions), UDP (user datagram protocol for low overhead transmissions)

protoplasm material making up portions of the cell

psychogalvanic electrical activity produced by mental or emotional stress

pulmonary pertaining to the lungs

pupil variable diameter aperture of the eye

quantization error inherent uncertainty in digitizing analog signal level due to the finite resolution of the conversion process (e.g., in an ADC or DAC)

radical group of atoms that can be replaced by a single atom

radioisotope artificially produced radioactive element

real time property of a system in which data is processed as it is acquired instead of being accumulated and processed later

relative accuracy measure usually in LSBs of how well an ADC digitizes an analog signal that includes nonlinearity, quantization, and noise errors but not offset or gain errors

resolution smallest signal increment that can be detected by a measurement system; contrasted with accuracy, i.e., how precise each step of the analog signal can be represented in an ADC, for example; both can be expressed in bits, LSBs, or percent of full scale; resolution is just noting some change, but accuracy is measuring how much it changed to some defined error

retina light-sensitive membrane in the eye

rheobase smallest electrical current that will produce stimulation

sagittal pertaining to or parallel to the midline of the body

SCADA supervisory control and data acquisition (common personal computer function used in process control applications)

scalp skin of the head covered by hair

SCPI standard commands for programmable instruments (extension of the IEEE 488.2 standard)

semipermeable permeable only to certain substances

single-ended describes an analog signal measured with respect to a common, usually ground; contrasted with differential, in which the signal is measured between one signal referenced to ground and another signal also referenced to ground

self-calibrating property of a data acquisition board or system that measures its own analog circuits and ADC or DAC accuracy with an extremely stable reference

sensor device that responds to a physical stimulus such as heat, light, sound, pressure, motion, flow, or ions from body electrodes; same as a transducer, which converts one form of energy into another

S/H amplifier sample-and-hold amplifier (acquires and stores an analog voltage on a capacitor for a brief time to allow an ADC to digitize it)

sinoatrial (SA) node collection of heart cells that automatically discharge to function as a natural pacemaker

sinus irregular cavity

SNR signal-to-noise ratio (ratio of the overall rms signal level to rms noise level, expressed in percent volts per volt, percent watts per watt, or dB)

software computer programs and accompanying commands that control a computer

SPC statistical process control (statistical analysis methodology for characterizing a process; used to evaluate, track, and improve the performance of a process)

simultaneous sampling property of a system that captures a number of channels at the same time

sphygmomanometer apparatus for measuring blood pressure

spirometer instrument for measuring respiratory volumes

stereotaxic precision positioning

successive-approximation ADC analog-to-digital converter that sequentially compares a series of binary-weighted values with an analog input voltage or current level to produce an output digital word with some number of steps

synapse junction where impulse transmits from one nerve cell to another

synchronous property of a function: hardware (specific time with synchronization to a reference clock) or software (begins an operation and returns upon completion of operation)

syntax set of rules to which statements must conform in a specific programming language

systemic pertaining to the entire body

systole period during which heart contracts

tachycardia excessively fast heart rate

THD total harmonic distortion (total rms signal level from harmonics to overall rms signal level; can be expressed in percent volts per volt, percent watts per watt, or dB)

THD+N total harmonic distortion plus noise (sometimes called SINAD or signal-noise-ratio and distortion): total rms signal level from harmonics plus noise to overall rms signal level; can be expressed in percent volts per volt, percent watts per watt, or dB

thermistor electrical component that exhibits changes in electrical resistance with changes in temperature

thermocouple device that uses a bimetallic strip to produce voltage proportional to temperature

thoracic pertaining to the thorax

thorax section of the body between the abdomen and neck

thrombus clot of blood remaining at its site of origin

throughput rate data time rate, in bytes per second, for a given continuous operation that includes software overhead; hardware delays and processing times are included in software overhead; throughput rate = transfer rate − software overhead factor

tibia larger of the two bones in the leg, between the ankle and knee

tissue collection of similar cells that perform a specific function or have a similar form

torso trunk of the human body

trachea main tube passing air from the atmosphere into the lungs

transducer device that converts energy from one form to another for purposes of measurement or control

transfer rate time rate, in bytes per second, at which data is moved from source to destination after the software has initialized and operations have been set up; maximum rate at which the hardware can operate

UART universal asynchronous receiver transmitter (integrated circuit that converts parallel data to serial data and serial data to parallel data; commonly used as a computer bus interface for serial communication)

ulnar pertaining to the larger of the two bones in the forearm

unipolar signal range that is always positive or always negative

utero Latin dative for uterus

uterus organ in the female body for protection and nourishment of the fetus

vasoconstrictors agents that narrow blood vessels

vasodilators agents that widen blood vessels

vasomotor agent affecting the size of a blood vessel

ventricle lower chamber of the heart

venule small vein connected to capillaries

viable capable of living

VXI open instrumentation standard developed by a consortium of instrument companies in 1987 to accomplish the *instrument on a card,* in which any company's printed circuit card can be plugged in to a card cage or mainframe; with VXI plug and play systems alliance, multivendor integration is possible

word standard number of bits that a processor or memory can handle at one time; usually 8, 16, or 32 bits

windows applications software that displays separate computer screens at the same time; usually uses pull-down menus for commands

APPENDIX D
Electrical Safety
in the Medical Environment

D-1 Objectives

1. Be able to define electrical safety as applied to medical institutions.
2. Be able to describe the scope (electrical equipment and specific environmental areas) of electrical safety in medical institutions.
3. Be able to list major publications and organizations concerned with electrical safety.
4. Be able to identify degree of involvement and nature of responsibilities of various hospital personnel for electrical safety.
5. Be able to describe how preventive maintenance (equipment inspection and documentation) can reduce electrical hazards.
6. Be able to list legal and insurance requirements relating to electrical safety in medical institutions.
7. Be able to list the major areas of concern in setting up a hospital electrical safety program.
8. Know how to describe the physiological effects of electricity on humans (the theory of *macroshock* and *microshock*).
9. Be able to list macroshock (arm to arm) and microshock (through the heart) 60-Hz shock current levels that produce adverse effects.
10. Be able to define leakage current.
11. Be able to describe the subtle hazards and cautions of microshock in hospitals.
12. Be able to describe monitoring instrument design considerations for reducing electrical shock hazards.
13. Be able to describe a power isolation transformer system and line isolation monitor and their use in reducing electrical shock hazards.
14. Be able to describe an equipotential grounding system and its use in reducing electrical shock hazards.
15. Be able to describe a ground fault interrupter.
16. Be able to draw a diagram for a proper power wiring, distribution, and ground system for providing a safe patient environment.
17. Be able to list specialized electrical safety test equipment and its use in electrical safety testing programs.

D-2 Self-evaluation questions

These questions test your knowledge of the material in this chapter. Look for the answers as you read the text. After you have finished studying the chapter, try answering these questions and those at the end of the chapter.

1. What is the definition of *electrical safety* as applied to medical institutions?

2. What specific medical equipment causes electrical hazards?

3. List the major publications and organizations concerned with electrical safety.

4. Who is responsible for electrical safety in medical institutions?

5. State specific legal and insurance problems that can arise from electrically hazardous environments.

6. Define the terms *macroshock* and *microshock*.

7. Explain why leakage current is potentially dangerous.

8. What is a line isolation transformer and monitor?

9. Explain what is meant by an equipotential ground system.

10. How does a ground fault interrupter operate?

11. How is a proper power wiring, distribution, and ground system used to provide a safe patient environment?

12. What special test equipment is used in hospital electrical safety testing programs?

D-3 Definition of electrical safety

Electrical safety is the *containment* or *limitation* of hazardous electrical shock, explosion, fire, or damage to equipment and buildings.

Electrical shock refers to both *macroshock* (high-value arm-to-arm current ultimately passing through the heart) and *microshock* (low-value current passing directly through the heart). A difference of potential must be present (two points of contact in either case). Shock may occur to patients, employees, and visitors to a hospital or healthcare facility. Shock results from improperly wired or maintained electrical equipment or power systems.

Explosion may result from electrical contact sparks that ignite a variety of explosive gases, such as ether or cyclopropane anesthetic.

Fire may result from heat produced by overloaded, incorrectly wired, or improperly maintained equipment or power systems.

Damage to equipment and buildings may result from explosion, fire, or electrical overload.

Safety may be defined as the condition of being safe from pain, injury, or loss. Actually, safety is often referred to as a situation that is harmless. However, in reality, no situation can be rendered *completely* safe. As such, electrical safety in the medical environment refers only to the limitation of hazardous situations.

In the practical daily routine of hospital life, it is important to remember that electrical safety is not so much a static state as it is a dynamic, continuous course of action involving hazard *detection* and *correction*.

D-4 Scope of electrical safety in medical institutions

A multitude of articles appearing in health care-oriented publications in the early 1970s represented an attempt to define the vague hazard of electrical microshock. *Microshock*, now called *cardiac shock*, is defined as a low-value (10-μA) current passing *directly* through the heart of a *catheterized* patient, causing *ventricular fibrillation* and possible death. The 10-μA limit is believed to be too conservative, and higher limits are now in effect.

D-5 Major organizations that produce electrical safety publications

Electrical safety in medical institutions is now entangled in a vase array of codes and standards. Some of these involve *national law,* such as the Occupational Safety and Health Administration *(OSHA),* Health, Education and Welfare *(HEW),* Public Health Service *(PHS),* and Food and Drug Administration *(FDA).* Others involve *voluntary consensus standards* (nationally agreed-on specifications), such as the National Fire Protection Association *(NFPA),* National Electrical Code *(NEC),* American National Standards Institute *(ANSI),* Underwriters Laboratories *(UL)* Association for the Advancement of Medical Instrumentation *(AAMI),* and Joint Commission on Accreditation of Healthcare Organizations *(JCAHO).* Furthermore, local codes and standards are also influential in defining electrical safety specifications.

D-6 Responsibilities of hospital personnel

The responsibility for electrical safety in medical institutions rests with *every* employee and patient. However, the scope of responsibilities differs. The *patient* should report any suspected electrical hazard to the attending physician or nurse, who in turn should report this to the safety officer/technician, if the condition is questionable. Even though the patient should be alert, he or she will probably be unaware of most of the potential electrical hazards. Therefore, the *bulk* of responsibility rests with the following hospital personnel:

1. *Medical staff*—includes physicians, nurses, and medical technicians who should constantly inspect all electrical equipment connected to the patient and report any suspicious electrical hazards.

2. *Support staff*—includes biomedical engineers (BMEs), biomedical equipment technicians

(BMETs), safety officer/technicians, plant operations personnel, and medical technicians, who must be able to recognize, test for, and correct all electrical hazards and educate other hospital personnel.

3. *Administration staff*—includes administrators, managers, and supervisors, who must hire competent employees and sponsor electrical safety educational programs.

D-7 Preventive maintenance to reduce electrical hazards

One description of *preventive maintenance* is "the performance of nonfunctional repairs, component replacements, cleaning, and general service in order to prevent improper and/or inadequate operation, thus extending the period between possible malfunctions and also extending the service life of the instrument by months and years." *Calibration* is "the assessment and correlation of instrument performance against standards traceable to the National Institutes of Standards and Technology." *Repairs* are "effected either during the scheduled preventive maintenance interval or on an unscheduled immediate-need basis."

Preventive maintenance (PM) differs from *corrective maintenance (CM)* in that PM involves *routine* inspection and testing, while CM involves *total* calibration or replacement of defective parts. Electrical safety test measurements made during PM can reduce electrical hazards by uncovering early signs of degradation. Faults can then be corrected during CM. By replacing broken plugs, faulty power receptacles, and poor ground connections, the medical environment can be made safer for the patient.

PM involves *testing* to specific *standards.* These standards or specifications are stated in the publications listed in section 19-5. For example, AAMI publishes *Safety Standards for Electromedical Apparatus, Safe Current Limits.* Its objectives are to provide techniques for measuring risk currents and to provide the user-authority with basic guidelines for proper use and care of equipment. This standard sets risk current limits for *all categories of electrical apparatus* used on or in the vicinity of any patient.

Following the functional and electrical safety testing of any biomedical instrument, a *sticker* should be affixed to the equipment. This denotes the date on which the equipment was tested. Another sticker gives the location of the *manufacturer's operation and service manual.* This manual typically describes general equipment setup procedures, installation, operational conditions and procedures, underlying theory of operation, preventive maintenance and test procedures, and spare parts. For specific details on particular biomedical instrumentation, consult the AAMI manual.

Special electrical safety test equipment is required to perform the specific tests.

All testing must ultimately be *documented,* and data recording schemes are numerous. Although the JCAHO inspection team reviews individual documentation techniques, they neither recommend nor designate a specific documentation structure. However, they do require a fixed logical documentation system and proof that the hospital is following it. They point to the AAMI standards and the procedures in the operation and service manuals. In addition, they may wish to review data recorded on a standard form. This record is part of a testing system that ensures patient safety.

D-8 Legal and insurance requirements for electrical safety

Legal requirements for electrical safety programs are varied and confusing. Dr. Martin Lloyd Norton, associate professor of anesthesiology and adjunct professor of law at Wayne State University, gave some clarification regarding negligence. He stated that failure of a hospital to have a PM program and/or use of adequately trained personnel could be considered *negligence* under "reasonable man" standards. Since electrical safety refers to limitation and not elimination of hazards, personnel car-

rying out PM programs must perform and document tests that are consistent with current acceptable practices (reasonable). In the case of Butler v. Northwestern Hospital of Minnesota, the court opinion was that "general rule is that equipment furnished by a hospital for a patient's use should be reasonably fit for the uses and purposes intended under the circumstances, and injury suffered because of failure of this duty leads to liability based on negligence." Believed to have suffered a wrongdoing any person may initiate a lawsuit. Cases of negligence involve *standard of conduct, damages,* and *appropriate relationship.* If hospital personnel are adequately trained, take reasonable care to test equipment, and document the test results, negligence and malpractice lawsuits can be reduced.

Insurance of the hospital is obviously a functional requirement. *Malpractice insurance* is costly and often nebulous. The escalated cost of malpractice insurance premiums for anesthesiologists are well documented in current hospital-oriented periodicals. Even the BMET may be sued under modern guidelines. Therefore, blanket policies taken by hospitals cover support as well as medical personnel.

In any event, *the patient comes first,* and that legal liability can be reduced by proper performance of and adequate documentation from a PM program.

D-9 Setting up an electrical safety program in the hospital

Every BME and BMET should be familiar with procedures for setting up or running an electrical safety program in the hospital. BMETs may be called on to give electrical safety *instruction* to nurses, physicians, and other medical care personnel. A video presentation should not exceed 20 min. Lecture and group discussions should not exceed 45 min per session. The instruction program is, briefly, as follows:

1. Introduction—purpose and objectives of safety instruction.

2. Basic concepts of electricity.

3. Physiological nature of electrical shock.

4. Macroshock (arm to arm shock) and microshock (cardiac shock) hazardous situations.

5. Identifying electrically hazardous equipment and situations.

6. Reporting all suspicious conditions.

7. Avoiding electrically hazardous situations.

8. Establishing responsibility.

9. Relating to pertinent publications.

10. Making a friend of the BME/BMET, safety officer/technician.

11. Demonstration.

12. Conclusion, discussion.

BMETs in the hospital usually give such presentations periodically, but they may also be involved in setting up an entire electrical safety program. This is coordinated with the *hospital safety committee* and consists of the following:

1. Purposes and objectives—patient safety at a cost.

2. Scope—hospital size/type, personnel available, safety committee.

3. Pertinent publications—law, codes, standards.

4. Test procedures—in-house, nationally published.

5. Inspections—specific operations, time schedule, preventive maintenance.

6. Documentation—in-house, commercially available.

7. Education—medical staff, users.

8. Assessment of effectiveness—feedback.

9. Cost of operation—dollars versus benefit.

D-10 Physiological effects of electricity on humans (macroshock and microshock)

Electrical current passing through the human body has *three primary effects:* injury to tissues, uncontrollable muscle contraction or unconsciousness, and fibrillation of the heart. Appreciation of these effects rests with knowledge of cellular action potentials. *Muscle and nerve cells* in the body act as tiny batteries or *polarized units.* Polarized, depolarized, or reversed-polarized cellular potentials arise from sodium, potassium, and chlorine ion concentration differences across semipermeable cell membranes. At rest, cells polarized at resting potentials of -70 mV can be stimulated to depolarization by any of the following means: mechanical, chemical, thermal, optical, and electrical. It is the electrical stimulation of muscle and nerve cells that is of primary interest in electrical safety.

Electrical shock involves electrical stimulation of tissue, and its effects range from a *tingling sensation* to the violent reactions of *muscle tetanus* to ventricular fibrillation. Thus, electrical shock is measured in terms of current *intensity* at specific *frequencies. Macroshock* is defined as a *high-value current* level (mA), which passes arm to arm through the body by (skin) contact with a voltage source. There must be two points of body contact. The resulting current eventually passes through the heart and may cause ventricular fibrillation or death.

Microshock or *cardiac shock* is defined as a *low-value current* (μA), which passes *directly through the heart* via a needle or catheter in an artery or a vein. The catheter may touch the interior surface of the heart, where blood pressure is measured or cardiac pacing is effected.

Larger currents are required to cause death from macroshock because the skin is a relatively good insulator. Table 19-1 shows the effect of 60-Hz arm-to-arm electric current shock. These currents range from *1 mA* threshold of sensation) to *10 mA*

TABLE 19-1   EFFECTS OF 60-HZ ELECTRIC SHOCK ON HUMAN BODY

Current intensity (1-s contact)	Effect
1 mA	Threshold of perception.
5 mA	Accepted as maximum harmless current intensity.
10–20 mA	"Let-go" current before sustained muscular contraction.
50 mA	Pain. Possible fainting, exhaustion, mechanical injury; heart and respiratory functions continue.
100–300 mA	Ventribular fibrillation will start, but respiratory center remains intact.
6 A	Sustained myocardial contraction followed by normal heart rhythm. Temporary respiratory paralysis. Burns if current density in high.

(can't let go) to *100 mA* (respiratory failure and ventricular fibrillation—death) to *1 A* and larger (tissue damage—burns). In contrast, microshock currents of *10* to *100 µA* can cause ventricular fibrillation and death.

The *frequency of the current* is also important when considering the shock phenomenon. For example, an arm-to-arm shock at 50 to 60 Hz is particularly potent compared to higher or lower frequencies. A 1-mA, 60-Hz current establishes the threshold of perception for most people, and a 60-Hz, 100-mA current may cause respiratory difficulty, ventricular fibrillation, and/or death. However if the frequency is raised above 1 kHz, these current levels no longer produce such sensations or *life-threatening phenomena*. High frequencies in the megahertz region, for example, rarely cause shock, but do cause serious burns. This relates to the function of the *electrosurgical* unit described in chapter 18. This unit cuts, burns, and cauterizes tissue but does not induce electrical shock.

Most danger from macroshock or microshock is *ventricular fibrillation*. This is defined as a condition of the heart in which the myocardium quivers instead of pumping rhythmically. The result is an ineffective heart pump. Heart tissue is one of the most sensitive tissues in the body. Normal internal electrical stimulation of the heart, beginning with the sinoatrial node in the right atrium, initiates *synchronous* cardiac activity. This electrical activity of the heart gives rise to the electrocardiogram (ECG).

Ventricular fibrillation may result when the heart is *externally* stimulated. A few heart cells become deranged and can trigger off a chain reaction of chaotic activity. The *ectopic foci* of electrical impulses spread and cause *asynchronous* cardiac function. Death follows in minutes if the patient is not treated by *cardiopulmonary resuscitation* (CPR) or defibrillation with a *defibrillator unit.* Defibrillation requires large instantaneous currents of 6 A or more passing through the chest to "reset the heart."

Since 10 mA or less is the let-go shock level, a safe 5-mA leakage current has become the standard. In fact, for a manufacturer to receive a *UL listing* (approval), the equipment must have a 60-Hz leakage current from power line to equipment metal case of less than 5 mA.

D-11 Leakage current

Leakage current is defined as the low-value electrical current (µA) that inherently flows (leaks) from the energized electrical portions of an appliance or instrument to the metal chassis. All electrically operated equipment has some leakage current. This current is not a result of a fault but is a natural consequence of electrical wiring and components.

Leakage current has two major parts: capacitive and resistive. *Capacitive leakage current* results from distributive capacitance between two wires or between a wire and a metal chassis/component case. For example, the "hot" cooper wire (black

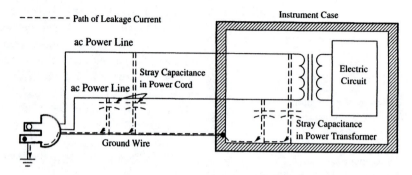

Figure D-1
Origins of leakage current (stray capacitance). (Reprinted courtesy of Hewlett-Packard)

for power systems) forms one plate, the wire insulation forms the dielectric, and the metal chassis (ground) forms the other plate of a capacitor. This capacitor is actually distributed over the entire length of the power cord, and the longer the cord, the greater the capacitance. A capacitance of 2500 pF at 60 Hz on a 120-V power system gives approximately 1 MΩ of capacitive reactance and 120 μA of leakage current. Components that cause capacitive leakage current are radio frequency (RF) filters, power transformers, power wires, and any device that has stray capacitance.

Resistive leakage current arises from the resistance of the insulation surrounding the power wires and transformer primary windings. Modern thermoplastic dielectrics or power lines and cords are of such high resistance that the resultant leakage current is negligible compared to capacitive leakage. Figure D-1 shows the *origins,* of leakage current and Figure D-2 the increased leakage with use of RF filters.

The *classical remedy* for excessive leakage current is the third or safety ground wire. Understanding of electrical power *wiring distribution* and *grounding* is a prerequisite to understanding the leakage current phenomena. The *hot-wire* in U.S. systems is *black* and is the *ungrounded* wire. The *neutral ground wire* is *white* and is the return wire that is connected to earth ground in the main power/fuse panel. The *safety ground wire* (which

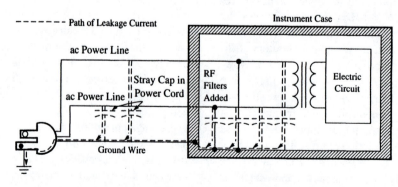

Figure D-2
The RF filters increase leakage current. (Reprinted courtesy of Hewlett-Packard)

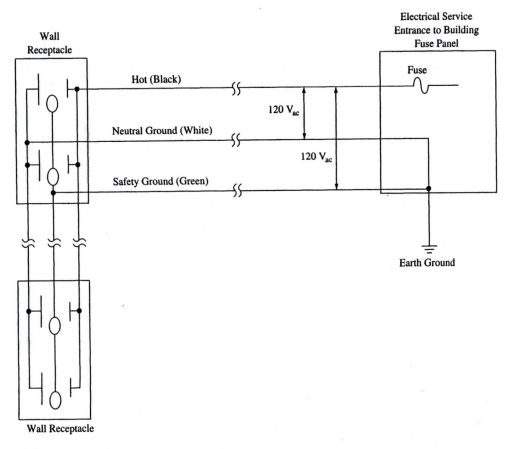

Figure D-3
Receptacles connected to fuse panel.

normally carries no current) is *green* and is the ground current return only under leakage and fault conditions. Actually, two purposes of safety grounding are to drain off leakage current and blow the fuse in the hot line in case of catastrophic fault (such as hot-wire shorts to grounded metal case or over-load). The NEC clearly specifies wiring distribution and grounding techniques. Figure D-3 shows two electrical receptacle outlets connected to a power/fuse panel.

As an example of the effect of safety ground, consider an electrical instrument connected to a power system in which the leakage current through a 1-Ω ground resistance is assumed to be 100 μA (no patient connection). If a patient of 500-Ω resistance touches the instrument metal case, 0.2 μA of leakage current flows through the patient, and 99.8 μA flows through the safety ground. Clearly, the safety ground is a much lower resistance connected in parallel with the patient. Hence, most of the leakage current flows through safety ground. Figure D-4 shows the normal ground system. If the safety ground connection should become broken or defeated by using a 3 to 2 adapter or two-wire extension cord, *all* leakage current flows through the patient. Figure D-5 shows a broken ground system that is potentially hazardous to the patient.

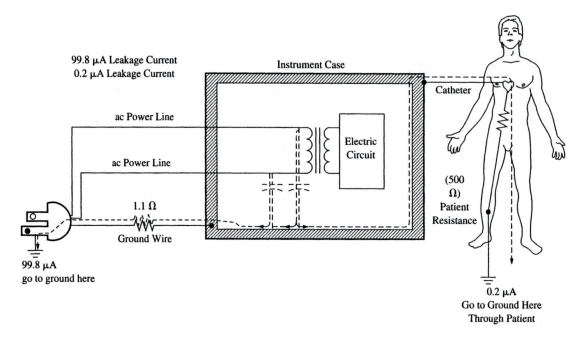

Figure D-4
Normal path for leakage current. (Reprinted courtesy of Hewlett-Packard)

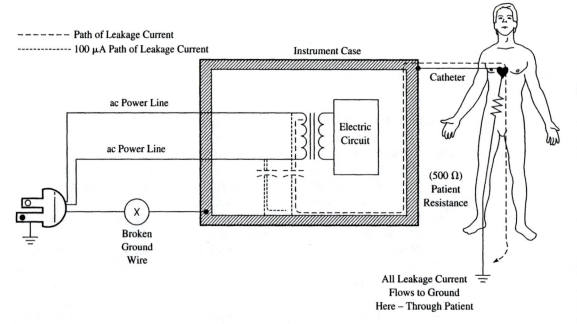

Figure D-5
Path of leakage current with defective ground wire. (Reprinted courtesy of Hewlett-Packard)

In the case of the three-wire (safety ground) failure, the following measures could prevent patient shock or electrocution:

1. Reduce internal equipment leakage current to below standard level.

2. Continuously monitor ground-wire continuity.

3. Add an additional ground wire in parallel with the power cord safety ground.

4. Periodically inspect ground-connection integrity.

5. Use a power-isolated system that isolates the equipment, and hence the patient, from neutral ground.

D-11-1 Current Definitions

In medical device maintenance it is necessary to distinguish between several types of current: *fault current, risk current,* and *source current.* The fault current flows when a fault occurs in the device; that is, when a defect occurs or something breaks, the fault current is the maximum current that will flow.

The risk current, of which there are several types, refers to currents likely to flow when the device is operating normally. It specifically excludes fault currents. The *general risk current (GRC)* flows when the device is operating normally but is ungrounded and is not working in conjunction with other devices. The last of these three requirements is implied and is not in the standard. The implication is reasonable because of the *apparatus interconnection risk current (AIRC).*

The AIRC is the risk current that flows when the device is connected to other devices, modules, or accessories attached to the device in the manner, quantities, and combinations specified by the manufacturer.

The *sterilization risk current (SRC)* is the risk current that flows after the device has been exposed to the sterilization process or disinfectant agents, as specified by the manufacturer.

The *environmental conditions risk current (ECRC)* is expected to flow when the device is subjected to the worst-case and nonoperational environmental conditions specified by the manufacturer.

The source currents are divided into two categories: *chassis source current (CSC)* and *patient source current (PSC).* The CSC flows between the power line service ground (an earth connection) and the chassis of the device, or any of its exposed conductive (e.g., metallic) hardware, or any grounding conductor. The PSC flows between any patient connection and the earth ground, or any exposed conductive hardware or the chassis. In both cases, the source current also includes the current flowing through a 200-cm^2 metal foil in direct contact with the insulating enclosure of the device. Also, the currents must be specified for any combination of conditions shown below.

ac Power source	Polarity normal	Polarity reversed
Power switch:	On	Off
Ground:	Intact	Open

The root-mean-square *(rms)* current levels permitted by standard are:

CSC (ac cord connected), portable

Ground open:	300 μA
Ground intact:	100 μA

GSC (ac cord connected), permanent connection

Ground open:	5000 μA
Ground intact:	100 μA

Lead-to-ground current

Isolated patient connection

Ground open:	50 μA
Ground intact:	10 μA

Non-isolated patient connection

Ground open:	100 μA
Ground intact:	50 μA

D-12 Line isolation systems

Power isolation transformers produce isolated systems by breaking direct electrical connection to neutral ground. (*Note: Auto-transformers* will *not* produce isolated systems.) The power used inside the electrical equipment is not effectively referenced to ground. This amounts to *reducing if not eliminating low-voltage hazards* since contact with either side of

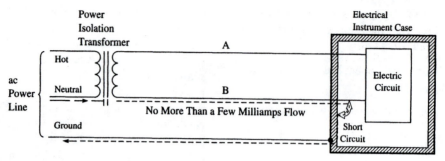

Figure D-6
Short circuit with power isolation transformer. (Reprinted courtesy of Hewlett-Packard)

the isolation transformer secondary and ground produces no shock. Patient isolation through a driven (RL) amplifier amounts to *reducing possible current paths through the patient.* While these approaches are different, they both aim at preventing excessive electric currents from flowing through the myocardium via an indwelling catheter.

Power isolation transformer design is geared toward reducing differential voltages to 5 mV between the catheter and equipment chassis or earth ground. These devices are used in the operating room. If the standard patient resistance of 500 Ω is used, no more than 10 μA will flow. This design

goal is not easy to achieve, and such transformers can add $1000 to $3000 to the cost of each bed for the monitoring installation. Furthermore, if the isolated hot-wire should short to the grounded metal case, the fuse or circuit breaker will not blow since this isolated power is not ground referenced. In this case, excessive leakage current will flow and be detected only by the line isolation monitor buzzer. Figure D-6 shows a short circuit with a power isolation transformer.

In terms of historical perspective, the original isolation transformer systems were designed to *prevent heating and sparking* due to the hot-wire

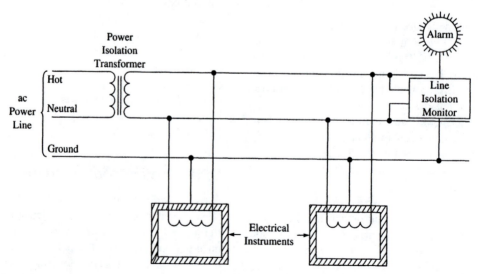

Figure D-7
Power line isolation transformer with fault detector. (Reprinted courtesy of Hewlett-Packard)

shorting to the metal case. This caused explosion of flammable anesthetic gases, such as ether. To understand this phenomenon, consider a *ground-referenced (non-isolated) system* and an ECG monitor. If the *hot-wire shorts to the metal case* in a *two-wire system,* the floating case (not grounded) becomes 120 V with respect to ground. The fuse does not blow, and this is a very serious macroshock and microshock hazard. For this reason, *two-wire systems are never used in the hospital.* If the *hot-wire shorts to the metal case* in a *three-wire system,* the grounded case passes a large current (15-30 A) until the fuse blows. This disconnects the power from the equipment and removes the shock hazard. However, this large current causes heating and may jump small gaps to cause sparking. At levels near the floor, where anesthetic gases collect, this can cause explosion. *In a non-grounded (isolated) system,* if the *hot-wire (either isolation transformer secondary wire) shorts to the grounded metal case,* no large currents flow through the case. Only leakage current flows (a few milliamperes) and *sparking is nonexistent.* This system protects against explosion, and corrective action is taken when the line isolation monitor sounds (loud buzzer) or the monitor leakage meter reads in the red (2-3 mA).

The *line isolation monitor (LIM)* is a device that continuously monitors the impedance of either isolated power line to ground. The modern *dynamic LIM* monitors this impedance several times per second. The effect is to monitor leakage current. This device is used with power isolation transformer systems. Figure D-7 shows a power LIM system with fault detector.

Essentially, there are several ways in which one could be shocked: by touching one power line and ground, one metal chassis and ground, and two metal chassis. For example, if the patient touches two metal chassis (devices A and B), both of which are grounded, and the *insulation on device B breaks down,* the *patient can be protected by the LIM system* (Figure D-8). Only 2 μA will flow through the 500-Ω patient and 998 μA through the ground wire as a result of the LIM (alarm) limit of 1 mA total fault current.

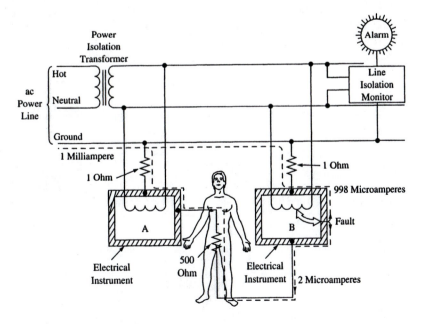

Figure D-8
Single insulation failure. (Reprinted courtesy of Hewlett-Packard)

One class of *faults is not eliminated* by the LIM system: the *open ground*. The fuse does not blow and the LIM alarm does not sound. This is a relatively difficult hazard to solve, and the leakage currents depend on relative leakage capacitance values that generate a total leakage current. A separate ground-wire, equipotential ground system provides added security in which all equipment chassis are connected through a separate wire to the same ground terminal.

D-13 Equipotential grounding in reducing electrical shock

An *equipotential ground system* simply consists of separate connections from each equipment chassis to a common ground terminal. This is achieved by adding another grounding wire from each chassis to a central point that is parallel with the third wire in the power cord. These ground wires have nearly the same length, and, as such, each metal chassis is at or near the same potential with respect to the other. Also, all metal surfaces are connected to the common terminal. If the maximum differential potential between any two metal surfaces is held to under 5 mV, then no more than 10 μA will flow

through a 500-Ω patient. These systems can be recognized by the large bulky ground wires (AWG 8) drooping from the equipment. Such systems are used in the OR, ICU, an CCU.

D-14 Ground fault interrupters in reducing electrical shock

A *ground fault interrupter (GFI)* is an *automatic switch* that disconnects power if excessive leakage current is present. These devices utilize a toroidal coil on which several turns of the hot and neutral conductors are wrapped. Figure D-9 shows a block diagram of a GFI. When the current in the hot and neutral wires is equal, no net magnetic flux is present, which indicates no leakage current. The relay remains closed. When these currents are unequal, a net magnetic flux is present, which indicates the presence of leakage current. The sensing coil presents a signal to the relay coil via the sensing amplifier, and the relay contacts open, removing power from the wall receptacle. The sensitivity can be set to detect up to 6 mA of leakage current. The GFI is usually used in *wet areas of the hospital,* such as the hemodialysis ward. However, it would be hazardous to see it in the operating room on all

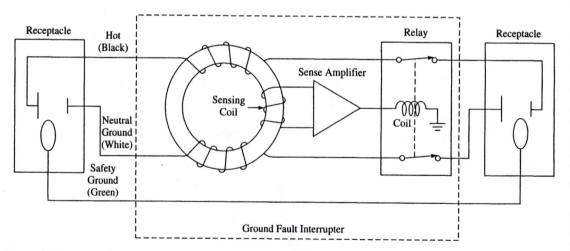

Figure D-9
Ground fault interrupter.

biomedical equipment because electrical power interruption could remove life-support equipment function from the critically ill patient.

D-15 Proper wiring, distribution, and ground in reducing shock hazards

Electrical power wiring, distribution, and grounding are as important in electrical safety as the electrically operated equipment. Four diagrams illustrate proper wire distribution and grounding. The general guidelines are to distribute power from a central junction box connection and to keep wires to all outlets approximately equal length, especially ground wires. Ground wires between outlets should be less than 15 ft long. The NEC specifies wiring

standards. Figures D-10 and D-11 show isolated input systems with a reference ground near the bed to reduce voltages between equipment chassis. Figure D-12 shows a single bed system with isolation transformer wired in the common-ground point configuration. Figure D-13 shows an isolated wiring system for multiple beds in which differential voltages are reduced by short grounding wires.

D-16 Specialized electrical safety test equipment

To conclude our discussion on electrical safety, it will be instructive to reread section D-7. To be knowledgeable in electrical safety, a BMET should know the material presented in this chapter. However, to be functional in the hospital, a BMET

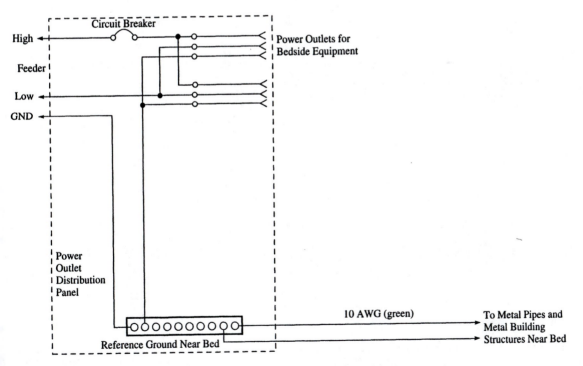

Figure D-10
Wiring installation for grounded line outlet cluster near bed. (Reprinted courtesy of Hewlett-Packard)

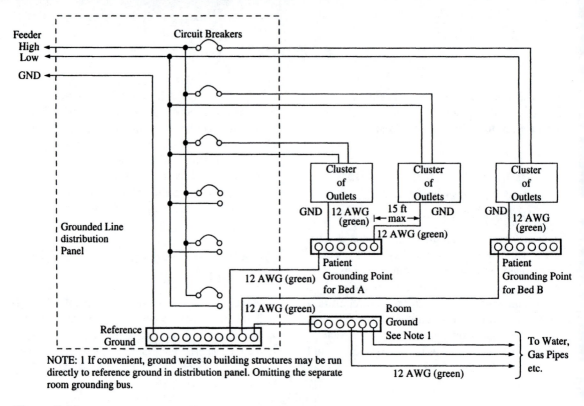

Figure D-11
Wiring installation for grounded line (beds remote from distribution panel). (Reprinted courtesy of Hewlett-Packard)

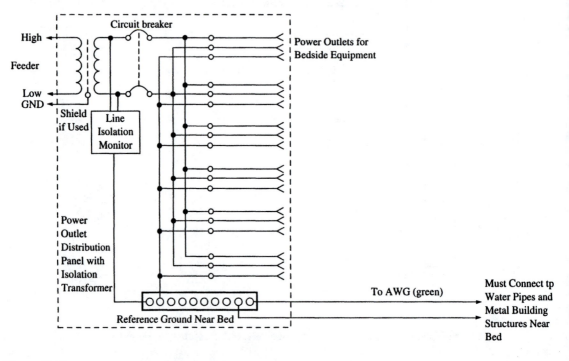

Figure D-12
Isolated line system near patient's bed. (Reprinted courtesy of Hewlett-Packard)

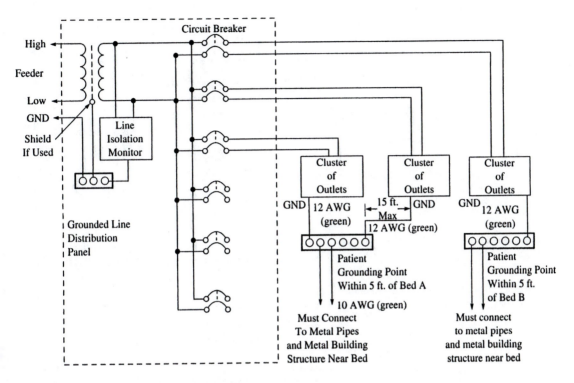

Figure D-13
Isolated line system remote. (Reprinted courtesy of Hewlett-Packard)

should be able to perform equipment/system PM and document the results of the electrical safety inspection and tests. These tests are intended to uncover hazards such as those shown in Figure D-14. The following special test equipment is required to ensure proper measurement and tests:

1. *Tension tester* to test the spring tension on the hot, neutral, and ground lugs of the wall receptacle. Tension should be at least 8 ounces of pull to ensure good physical contact of the plug in the receptacle.

2. *Ground wire loop resistance tester* for resistance measurement between safety (green) and neutral (white) wires from the power system.

3. *Receptacle polarity tester* for correct wiring. This can be accomplished with a separate tester.

4. *Resistance* between *third wire prong* on the plug to equipment metal *chassis* tester.

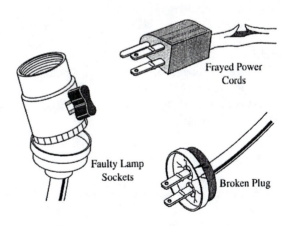

Figure D-14
Common lethal electrical hazards. (Reprinted courtesy of Hewlett-Packard)

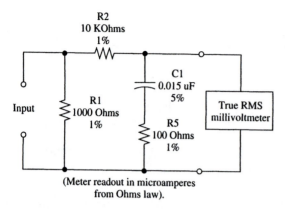

(Meter readout in microamperes
from Ohms law).

Figure D-15
Millivoltmeter.

5. *Resistance* from *hot* (black) wire to *chassis* and
   neutral (white) wire to chassis insulation
   resistance tester.

6. *Leakage current tester* for chassis to ground
   and separate ECG leads to ground.

D-16-1 Weighted risk current measurement

The *weighted risk current,* in microamperes, can
be read using a millivoltmeter calibrated to read
true rms value voltage if the AAMI standard test
load (Figure D-15) is connected between the test
terminals and the voltmeter. This load must be
manufactured using precision metal film resistors
with a rated tolerance of 1% or better. The 0.015-
µF capacitor must be either mica dielectric or
plastic dielectric of the extended foil design and
must have a tolerance of 5% or better.

D-17 Summary

1. *Electrical safety* in medical institutions is
   defined as the containment or limitation of
   hazards: (a) electrical shock to patients,
   employees, and visitors (macroshock and
   microshock); (b) explosions; (c) fire; and
   (d) damage to equipment and buildings.
   Hazards can be minimized but not eliminated.

2. The *scope* of electrical safety in medical
   institutions includes any electrically operated
   equipment used in (a) public, (b) general care,
   and (c) critical care areas of the hospital.

3. The following organizations produce
   pertinent documents for hospital electrical
   safety: (a) OSHA, (b) FDA, (c) NFPA, (d)
   NEC (e) ANSI, (f) UL, (g) AAMI, and (h)
   JCAHO.

4. *Responsibility* for electrical safety in the
   medical institutions rests with all personnel
   and, more specifically, with the *medical staff*
   (physicians, nurses), *support staff* (BMETs,
   safety technicians, plant operation personnel),
   and *administrative staff* (administrators,
   managers, supervisors).

5. *Preventive maintenance* involving frequent
   equipment inspections and safety checks
   can reduce electrical hazards by uncovering
   early signs of degradation and allowing for
   correction of faults, such as broken plugs
   and poor electrical ground contacts.

6. *Legal and insurance requirements* of
   electrical safety involve possible negligence
   under the "reasonable man" standards.
   BMETs in the hospital could be sued.
   Insurance requirements revolve around the
   cost of claims to insurance companies, but
   proper PM and documentation can reduce
   premiums through reduced hazards. *The
   patient should come first.*

7. Electrical safety *instruction sessions* may
   be delivered by BMETs to nurses and other
   medical staff and should include such topics
   as purposes and objectives, basic electricity,
   nature of shock, identification and avoidance
   of shock hazard, reporting of hazardous
   situations, responsibilities, pertinent

publications, demonstration, conclusion, and discussion.

8. Hospital electrical safety programs should cover objectives, scope, pertinent publications, PM, test procedures, inspections, documentation, education, assessment of effectiveness, and cost versus benefit analysis.

9. The *physiological effects* of electricity on the human body involve injury to tissues, uncontrollable muscle contractions, and fibrillation of the heart.

10. *Macroshock* or *cardiac shock,* is a large-value electrical current (mA) that passes arm to arm and eventually through the heart. It may be lethal. Accepted values are (a) 1 mA, sensation (b) 10 mA, can't let go, (c) 100 mA, respiratory failure/fibrillation of the heart, and (d) 1 A and above, burns.

11. *Microshock* is a small-value electrical current (μA) that passes directly through the heart. It may be lethal.

12. *Leakage current* is a naturally occurring current that results primarily from distributed capacitance within equipment or power cords and leaks from the hot side (black wire) to equipment metal chassis to safety ground (green wire).

13. The *subtle hazards of cardiac shock* have caused the primary interest in hospital electrical safety. On a case-by-case basis, the description of parameters and technical analysis pave the way for recommendations of hazard limitation. Hazards include faulty ac power cord ground connections, use of two-wire cord on appliances, and long ground-wire connections between ac power outlets. Hazard containment is accomplished through personnel education and PM programs.

14. The *LIM* is a device that monitors the impedance of either isolated power line to ground. In effect, the modern dynamic LIM continuously monitors leakage current in an isolated power system. It is used with power isolation transformer systems.

15. An *equipotential ground system* consists of separate additional ground-wire connections from each equipment chassis and metal surface to a central ground terminal. This reduces differential potentials between metal surfaces to near zero. Consequently, leakage current hazards are greatly reduced. Such systems are used in the OR, ICU, and CCU.

16. The *GFI* is an automatic switch that disconnects power if excessive leakage current is present. It is used in wet areas of the hospital, such as the hemodialysis ward.

17. Proper *power wiring, distribution, and grounding* is as important in electrical safety as electrically operated equipment. Correct polarity and ground-wire integrity are the underlying safety features of the medical equipment system. The NEC specifies wiring standards.

18. *Special electrical safety test equipment* must be included in the hospital electrical safety inspection, testing, and PM program. This includes an electrical output tension tester, outlet and line cord ground-wire resistance tester, outlet polarity tester, and leakage current tester.

D-18 Recapitulation

Now return to the objectives and self-evaluation questions at the beginning of the chapter and see how well you can answer them. If you cannot answer certain questions, place a check mark next to each and review appropriate parts of the text. Next, try to answer the following questions using the same procedure.

Questions

1. Electrical safety in medical institutions involves the limitation of _____, _____, and _____ to _____ as well as electrical shock hazards.

2. Electrical shock hazards exist in _____, _____ _____, and _____ hospital areas.

3. Eight major organizations producing pertinent publications related to electrical safety in medical institutions are _____, _____, _____, _____, _____, _____, _____, and _____.

4. The medical, administrative, and _____ staff are responsible for hospital electrical safety.

5. Electrical safety test measurements made during _____ _____ can reduce electrical hazards by uncovering early signs of _____.

6. Faults are corrected during _____ _____.

7. AAMI publishes safety standards for _____ _____ _____ _____ _____.

8. All electrical safety tests must ultimately be _____.

9. Typically, the manufacturer's operation and service manual has six sections describing _____ _____, _____, _____ _____, _____ of _____, _____ _____, and _____ _____.

10. Electrical safety test equipment measures outlet polarity, ground-wire resistance, and _____ _____.

11. The JCAHO inspection team reviews hospital _____ techniques.

12. Legal requirements for hospital electrical safety PM programs relate to "_____ _____" standards.

13. Lawsuits may be avoided if hospital personnel are _____ trained.

14. Poor electrical safety PM programs may result in _____ insurance premiums.

15. One ultimate goal of an electrical safety PM program is to protect the *patient/hospital.*

16. BMETs are often required to give electrical safety presentations to _____ and _____.

17. A hospital electrical safety program should include objectives, scope, pertinent _____, test _____, inspection, practices, documentation, education, assessment of _____, and cost of _____.

18. The effect of electrical current passing through the body includes injury to tissues, _____ muscle contractions, and _____ of the heart.

19. Fibrillation refers to (a) asynchronous skeletal contractions, (b) synchronous heart waves, or (c) asynchronous heart contractions.

20. Macroshock results from *high/low* current passing arm to arm.

21. Microshock results from *high/low* current passing directly through the heart.

22. Leakage current results primarily from *inductive/capacitive* effects of ac power cords and electrical transformers.

23. Leakage current can be reduced by adding a _____ wire from equipment metal chassis to a common _____ terminal.

24. In power systems, the black wire is _____, the white wire is _____, and the green wire is _____ _____.

25. The third wire in power systems serves to blow the _____ _____ if the hot-wire shorts to equipment metal case, and to drain off _____ _____ _____ to earth ground.

26. Subtle hazards exist in biomedical equipment systems as a result of *open/shorted* ground connections and the use of two/three-wire extension cords.

27. In the ECG "ground-referenced differential amplifier," the patient's _____ leg is connected to safety ground.

28. The UL standard for leakage current is _____ milliamps.

29. The driven right-leg ECG amplifier system *increases/decreases* ECG recording noise.

30. A signal isolation transformer (ECG am modulation scheme) isolates the patient from *neutral/safety* ground and reduces _____ _____.

31. A power isolation transformer breaks direct electrical connection from *neutral/safety* ground and reduces _____ _____.

32. The modern equivalent patient resistance is _____ Ω.

33. The maximum differential voltage standard in critical care areas is _____ mV.

34. The LIM monitors _____ current and is used with the *signal/power* isolation transformer.

35. The maximum differential voltage between any two _____ surfaces in an equipotential ground system is _____ mV.

36. A GFI disconnects _____ power if excessive _____ current exists.

37. GFI devices are usually used in the (a) operating room, (b) EEG laboratory, or (c) hemodialysis ward.

38. Electrical power wiring, distribution, and grounding is detailed in the _____ _____ Code.

39. Specialized hospital electrical safety test equipment measures _____ _____ resistance, _____ polarity, _____ spring tension, and _____ current.

References

1. *Patient Safety—Electrical Safety,* Hewlett-Packard applications note AN718 (Waltham, Mass., 1971).

2. *Using Electrically Operated Equipment Safely with the Monitored Cardiac Patient,* Hewlett-Packard applications note AN735 (Waltham, Mass., 1970).

3. *AAMI Safety Standards for Electromedical Apparatus, Safe Current Limits,* Association for the Advancement of Medical Instrumentation (Arlington, Va., 1977).

4. National Fire Protection Association, *National Electrical Code* (Boston, Mass., 1977).

5. *Joint Commission on the Accreditation of Hospitals* Manual (Chicago, Ill., 1978).

6. Walter, Carl W., "Green Wire Spells Electrical Safety in Hospitals," *Hospital Topics, 50* (2): 25-29 (February 1972).

7. Friendlander, G. D., "Electricity in Hospitals—Elimination of Lethal Hazards," *IEEE Spectrum* (September 1971).

8. Butler *v.* Northwestern Hospital of Minneapolis, 202 MINN. 282 278 N.W. 37, legal case.

9. Norton, M. L., "Biomedical Instrumentation and Liabilities," *J. AAMI Mag* (June 1971).

10. *Operating and Service Manual,* Safety Analyzer for Model 431A/431F, Neurodyne-Dempsey, Inc. (Napa, Calif., 1975).

11. *Operating and Service Manual,* Microspector, Model 449, Neurodyne-Dempsey, Inc. (Napa, Calif., 1975).

12. *Operating and Service Manual,* Cordometer, Model 447, Neurodyne-Dempsey, Inc. (Napa, Calif., 1974).

13. Strong, Peter, *Biophysical Measurements,* Measurement Concepts Series, Tektronix, Inc. (Beavertown, Ore., 1970).

14. Leeming, Michael N. and Eric Perron, *Electrical Safety Program Guide,* Biotek Instruments, Inc. (Shelburne, Vt., 1975).

15. Roth, Herbert H., Erwin S. Teltscher, and Irwin M. Kane, *Electrical Safety in Health Care Facilities,* Academic Press (New York, 1975).

16. *National Safety News*—Periodical, October 1976, Data Sheet, "Electrical Safety in Health Care Facilities."

17. Hoenig, Stuart A. and Scott H. Daphne, *Medical Instrumentation and Electrical Safety—The View from the Nursing Station,* Wiley (New York, 1977).

18. Simmons, David A., *Medical and Hospital Control Systems, The Critical Difference,* Little, Brown Co. (Boston, 1972).

19. Spooner, Robert B., *Hospital Instrumentation Care and Servicing for Critical Care Units,* Instrument Society of America (Pittsburgh, Pa., 1977).

20. Caceres, Cesar A. and Albert Zara, *The Practice of Clinical Engineering,* Academic Press (New York, 1977).

INDEX